INFECTIOUS DISEASES OF THE EYE

Infectious Diseases of the Eye

EDITORS

ALEXANDER A. BIALASIEWICZ

KLAUS P. SCHAAL

BUTTERWORTH HEINEMANN

BOSTON LONDON OXFORD SINGAPORE

SYDNEY TORONTO WELLINGTON

Notice

...The authors and editors of this book have been careful to ensure that dosage recommendations are precise and in agreement with standards officially accepted at the time of publication.

It does happen, however, that dosage schedules are changed from time to time in the light of accumulating clinical experience and continuing laboratory studies. This is most likely to occur in the case of recently introduced products.

It is essential that you check the manufacturer's warnings and recommendations for dosage, especially if the drug to be administered or prescribed is one that you use only infrequently or have not used for some time.

THE PUBLISHER

ISBN 9070 43005 3

Europe, Africa, Asia, Australia, Oceania, South and Central America

Æolus Press Science Publishers, P.O. Box 740, 4116 ZJ Buren, The Netherlands

ISBN 7506-9586-2

USA, Canada, Mexico

Butterworth-Heineman US, 80 Montvale Avenue, Stoneham, MA 02180 USA

EDITORIAL

One hundred years of genuine cooperation between medical microbiology, virology, immunology, dermato-venerology, internal medicine, pediatrics and tropical medicine have resulted in substantial progress in the

- etiopathogenetic characterization,
- prevention and prophylaxis,
- clinical and laboratory diagnosis and
- medical and surgical management

of infectious eye disease. With the advent of effective antibiotics interest in infectious eye diseases was temporarily lost. The surging interest over the last two decades has primarily been due to the

- detection of new pathogens,
- introduction of modern laboratory diagnostic techniques, and the
- advent of AIDS with its manifold infectious complications.

In this book a survey of the state of the art in basic sciences achievements fertilising clinical ophthalmology as well as controversial opinions in clinical diagnosis and therapy on an international scale has been attempted. The contributions have been conceived to help interested readers define their own specific research problems, get new ideas and recognize the work done by others. A selection of pertinent clinical and scientific topics has been made, since a complete textbook covering every facet of ocular infections is beyond the scope of this work. The various contributions herein shall bring about a lively and contemporary discussion of ocular infections.

Table of Contents

- Bacterial: Lyme Borreliosis

- Other Bacterial

- Viral

- Parasitic: Toxoplasmosis

I. BASIC CONSIDERATIONS

Theodor Axenfeld and the History of Microbiology in Ophthalmology

Hans Schadewaldt

The German historian Heinrich von Treitschke (1834-1896) once said, "History is made by men".

Nowadays this is not strictly true, but it is nonetheless accurate to say that the introduction of findings from the young science of bacteriology and the newly developing field of immunology by Theodor Axenfeld (1867-1930) (Fig.1) led to major new insights into the etiology, pathogenesis, diagnosis and therapy of numerous eye diseases.

Axenfeld was born in Smyrna (Izmir) and died in Freiburg im Breisgau at the age of 63. His greatest contribution to medical science was his now classic work "Bacteriology in Ophthalmology", published in Jena by Gustav Fischer-Verlag 1907 (3). It is perhaps not inappropriate to compare the impact of Axenfeld's work with the effect of Helmholtz's ophthalmoscope which was put into practical use by Albrecht von Graefe (1828-1870). It was Graefe's work on the fundus of the eye, which revealed the many causes of blindness and made the global term "amaurosis" redundant. In the same way, Axenfeld's work led to a considerable differentiation of the diagnosis "conjunctivitis".

In the history of medicine, infectious diseases of the eye are innately linked to the work of Theodor Axenfeld and the influence of immunology on Ophthalmology, a topic which will be further outlined by Arthur Silverstein in this book (22). The only living ophthalmologic relative is Theo Waubke, professor and director of the Department of Ophthalmology in Essen/Germany (born in 1928), whose great-uncle was Theodor Axenfeld.

Axenfeld's obituaries were just one indication of the high regard in which his contemporaries held him (1,11,23,24). The most impressive obituary was written by the famous pathologist Ludwig Aschoff (1866-1942) (1), one of Axenfeld's colleagues in the Medical Faculty at Freiburg. Axenfeld's international renown is probably best illustrated by the enthusiasm with which his Japanese colleagues greeted the lectures, which he gave at the Eighth All-Japan Ophthalmology Congress in Osaka shortly before his death. His son, Helmut Axenfeld, put together an exceptionally interesting description of this Congress in 1932, drawing on the correspondence and diaries of his father (2). Even today, the name of Axenfeld is spoken with the same reverence in Japan as the names of the men who laid the foundations of modern Japanese medicine in the 1870s at the start of the Meiji period (21). Memorials were erected in honor of the first two military medics appointed to this task, Major Leopold Müller (1824-1893) and Naval Lieutenant Commander Theodor Eduard Hoffmann (1837-1894), and their important successors, the surgeon Julius Scriba (1848-1905) and the internist Erwin

Baelz (1849-1913). These memorials still exist, and Axenfeld laid a wreath there during his visit to Japan (Fig.2).

Captain Emil Behring (1854-1917) worked very successfully with his Japanese assistant Shibasaburo Kitasato (1856-1931) at the Berlin Institute of Hygiene under Robert Koch (1843-1919) and they jointly published their now famous treatise "On the Development of Diphtheria Immunity and Tetanus Immunity in Animals" in the "Deutsche Medicinische Wochenschrift" on December 4, 1890. In 1906 Axenfeld's Freiburg colleague Aschoff and his Japanese student Sunao Tawara (1873-1952) described the node in the conduction system of the heart which was subsequently named after them. In the same way, Axenfeld worked with a number of Japanese colleagues (Fig.3) who later became professors of Ophthalmology in their native country and always remembered their German training with gratitude. This gratitude lasted well beyond the First World War.

In order to understand the full significance of Axenfeld's achievements in ophthalmic microbiology, we must take a brief look at the ideas, which predominated before the concept of bacteriology was introduced into the study of inflammations of the eye. I would like to mention the publication by my Zurich colleague Huldrych Koelbing entitled "Early Modern Concepts of Ocular Inflammation" (15). In particular, Koelbing contrasted the views held in antiquity with inflammations being due to humoral imbalances and the concept of inflammations having local causes, a theory which did not become widespread until the 19th century. The inflammatory process was described by a non-medic, Aulus Cornelius Celsus (25 b.c.-50 a.d.) in terms of its signs calor, rubor, dolor and tumor, a description which is still used today. Inflammation was thought to be due to "materia peccans", or offending substances, which were either formed in the body or passed into the body. The four humors, whose balanced proportions in the body were supposed to bring about "eucrasia", were thought to be weakened by the effect of "materia peccans" (Fig.4). Equally, the offending substances were thought to cause increased secretion of one of the humors. This "dyscrasia" was to be fought with all the means available, either by procedures designed to evacuate the superfluous humor from the body such as bloodletting, enemas, sweating therapies, induced vomiting or diarrhea, or by certain drugs which were thought either to stimulate or to moderate the effects of the humors. It was also thought that substances were excreted at certain sites in the organisms; these excretions were termed apostasis or metastasis and were treated with topical agents. It was quite common to apply leaches or cupping glasses, a practice which has been used widely since antiquity. These thoughts were also applied to the eye and targeted at radical therapeutic measures such as enucleation, first described in 1583 by the famous oculist Georg Bartisch (1535-1606) in his "Ophthalmodouleia, der Augendienst". Usually, however, radical surgery was generally confined to true tumors of the eye. Felix Platter (1536-1614), a physician in Basle, classified ocular inflammations as three groups in his "Praxis Medicinae", which appeared in 1602. He described "Ophthalmia Vera", "Ophthalmia non Vera aut Pseudo-ophthalmia" and the "Aigilops" syndrome, or goateye, which in modern terms was probably dacryocystitis, often associated with a "Fistula Lacrimalis". Platter identified the standard signs of inflammation, as described by Celsus, and chemosis, an extreme swelling of the conjunctiva which probably equivalent to Celsus' tumor. The main cause of this ophthalmia was thought to be a constitutional weakness of the organism. The only other causes of disease that were admitted at the time were secondary external noxae such as extreme coldness or heat or too dry atmosphere.

The quality of the blood evacuated from the body played a very important role in humoral pathology, but it was also believed that, apart from blood, mucosal substances could pass into the eye. The medics of the era thought that a mucosal gland in the brain excreted substances which caused coryza in the nose, asthma in the lungs and ophthalmia in the eyes. Accordingly, some fairly radical therapeutic measures were developed, such as cauterization of the "fontanelles", the areas thought to be most affected. One especially popular therapy was to attach a seton to the back of the neck; this thread was signed to draw pus out of the wound and was often covered with dirt from the street to enhance its effect. A wide range of ointments were also in use at the time; these collyria were mainly based on metal compounds such as white lead, lead acetate and zinc oxide. The most commonly used eye remedies, however, contained extracts of belladonna. They were without a doubt effective in the treatment of infectious processes of the iris as they induced mydriasis and also had a local analgetic effect. From about 1805, John Cunningham Saunders (1773-1810), the founder of London's first eye hospital, made extensive use of these important properties of belladonna preparations.

Almost nothing was known about the causes of these diseases until Robert Koch carried out his epoch-making research. A wide variety of theories came into existence; in Germany the concept of vitalism was wide-spread, the British tended more towards the neuropathological approach. In 1843 even the young Rudolf Virchow (1821-1902) described "Famus Illud Acre Rheumaticum" in his Latin dissertation on "corneal rheumatism", as it was then called. Virchow later went on to found the science of cellular pathology, but at the time he was unable to furnish a scientifically satisfactory definition for many infectious eye diseases.

The breakthrough in Ophthalmology came as a result of Robert Koch's fundamental work on wound Infections in 1878. This work led to the introduction of asepsis in Germany (8); the first establishment to adopt this practice was the private clinic run by Gustav Adolf Neuber (1850-1932) in Kiel. Joseph Lister (1827-1912) had, of course, established surgical antisepsis with carbolic acid in 1867 already, but its impact on Ophthalmology was limited because, understandably, it is not possible to use carbolic acid in the eye. Robert Koch's work led to a second important discovery; he found that a specific organism was the causative agent in tuberculosis (20). This finally put an end to the controversies that had been raging for almost a century. The contagionists believed that diseases were transmitted by miasma, and found this belief supported by the work of Louis Pasteur (1822-1895) and Robert Koch. The non-contagionists did not believe that epidemic diseases could be transmitted and continued to insist that diseases were generated spontaneously. Koch's work ultimately decided the argument in favor of the contagionists.

It was during this phase that Axenfeld came onto the scene. He passed the "Matura" in Bonn at the age of 17 and completed medical school at 22. He then studied Physiology under the renowned pathologist Jakob Felix Marchand (1846-1928), who was particularly interested in the problems of inflammation, and under the hygienist Max Ruber (1854-1932), who coauthored the first comprehensive handbook on hygiene with Max Ruber (1853-1927) and Martin Ficker (born 1868) from 1911 through 1913.

In 1894 Axenfeld then moved on to Ophthalmology in Marburg and gained his doctorate one year later under Wilhelm Uhthoff (1853-1927). In 1896, Uhthoff and Axenfeld moved to Dresden. Axenfeld's doctoral thesis on purulent metastatic ophthalmia was a particularly well-thought piece of bacteriological work and was awarded the von Graefe prize by the Heidelberg Ophthalmological Society. One year later in 1897, Axenfeld was appointed to a Chair at the University of Rostock at the age of 30, and in 1901 became Director of the University Eye Hospital in Freiburg, his alma mater, where he stayed until his death (6,8,9,10, 11).

By then it was generally accepted throughout the medical society that very specific pathogenic organisms were the causes of infectious diseases and thoughts that every wound infection had been caused by a single pathogen (as even the great surgeon Theodor Billroth (1829-1894) had believed for some time) were abandoned. In 1894, Axenfeld wrote about the classic features of metastatic endophthalmitis dealing with the various septic foci in puerperal fever, surgical sepsis, cryptogenic pyemia and other infectious diseases. After this publication, one discovery after another was made. Axenfeld identified the pneumococcus as the pathogen in ulcus serpens corneae. In 1896, he and Victor Morax (1866-1935), an ophthalmologist and scientist at the Institute Pasteur in Paris, independently discovered the diplobacilli responsible for chronic contagious conjunctivitits. The diplobacilli were later named after both scientists. Axenfeld also succeeded in identifying Löffler's Pseudo-Corynebacterium diphtheriae as the causative agent of xerosis. In 1893, Koch travelled to the Near East and isolated a pathogenic agent of a certain conjunctivitis not identical with trachoma, but which was very common in Egypt at that time. The thin, inflexible organisms had already been identified by John Elmer Weeks (1852-1949) in New York in 1887 and was subsequently named after both scientists.

Axenfeld was particularly concerned with the identification of the various forms of tuberculosis of the eye. This field was of particular interest because his predecessor in Freiburg, Wilhelm Manz (1833-1911), had observed tubercles in the choroid as a manifestation of generalized miliary tuberculosis in 1858 - shortly after the introduction of ophthalmoscopy. When other forms of scrophulosa of the eye were examined, these lesions turned out of be often observed phenomena. Axenfeld and his French friend Morax had recommended that in unexplained cases of iritis the aqueous humor should be extracted and injected into the anterior chamber of a rabbit eye. This method provided far better evidence of tuberculosis than was obtainable with the staining techniques of the era. Tuberculin was discovered before its importance was fully realized and there was a mess about its apparent therapeutic failure. Thereafter, however, tuberculin became an increasingly important diagnostic aid, and Axenfeld immediately turned his attention to a detailed investigation of the method.

It must be remembered that Axenfeld was editor-in-chief of the "Klinische Monatsblätter für Augenheilkunde" from 1900 until his death, the "Klinische Monatsblätter für Augenheilkunde" being a citable journal enjoying an international reputation (17). In 1926, on the 25th anniversary of his accepting this position he expressed a wish, which is still being enacted up to date: "...to promote thought and practical work in ophthalmology and to encourage a lively scientific exchange."

A comment made by Axenfeld, which nowadays may be even more relevant should end this review:

In 1877, Koch published a widely acclaimed article on the techniques for the photography of bacteria and produced some outstanding photographic material. Axenfeld published a lengthy article in the 1903 "Handbook of Pathogenic Microorganisms" coauthered by August von Wassermann (1866-1925) and Wilhelm Kolle (1868-1935) and followed by his own textbook on Bacteriology in Ophthalmology (3). In the foreword to this book Axenfeld emphasized the importance of the illustrations, which had been done by a specially trained artist:

"I believe that colorful illustrations are far better than micro photographs for learning diagnoses. While the latter are undoubtedly important, even the best technique may sometimes fail to reproduce the finest details in such a way that every student can clearly appreciate the situation".

Today, greater emphasis is again given to illustrations in both Pathology and Bacteriology, as they in some instances provide better teaching material. The "Netter atlas" drawn by the American physician Frank Henry Netter (born in 1906) is an outstandingly fine example of this "new" feeling. It is fair to put Axenfeld's Bacteriology in Ophthalmology into the same category of impressive educational books, which remain unsurpassed.

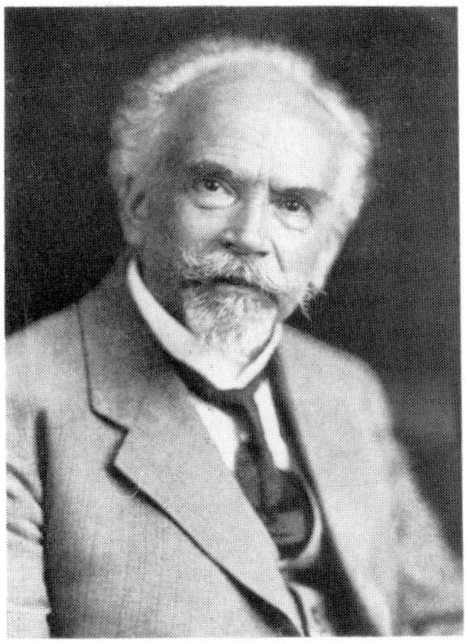

Fig.1

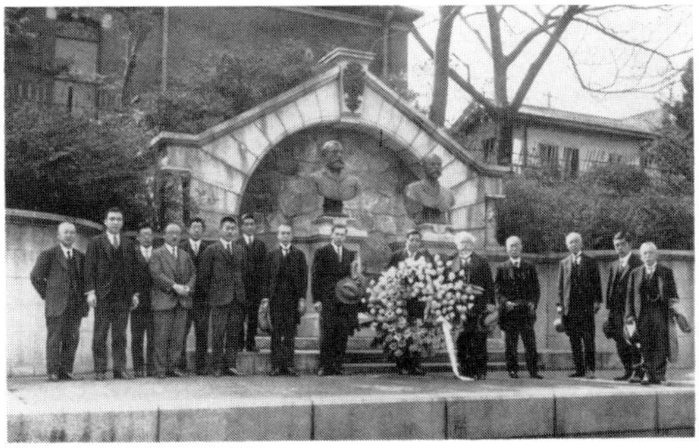

Fig. 2

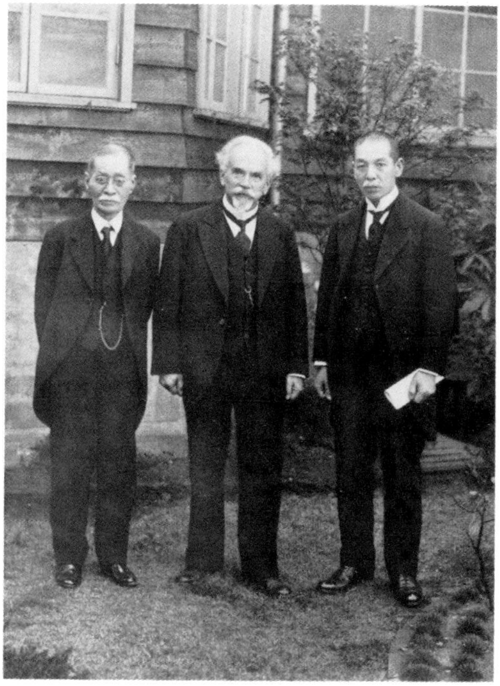

Fig. 3

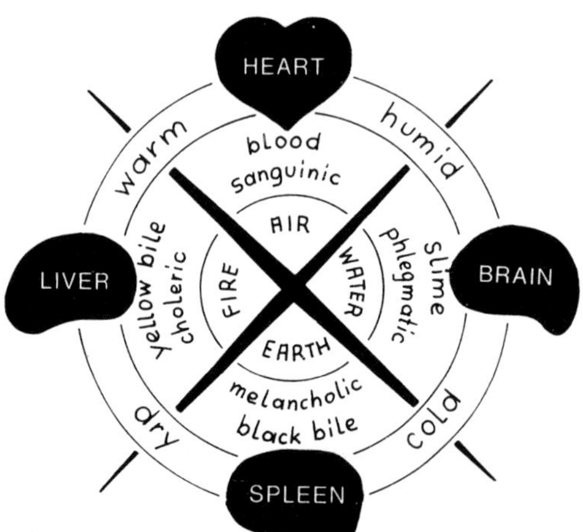

Fig. 4 Galen's scheme of the elements, temperatures, cardinal fluids, primary qualities, and main organs

References

1. Aschoff L (1969) In memoriam Theodor Axenfeld.(Aus der Grabrede) Klin Mbl Augenheilk 192:47-49
2. Axenfeld T (1932) Theodor Axenfelds Briefe und Tagebuchblätter. Enke Stuttgart
3. Axenfeld T (1907) Die Bakteriologie in der Augenheilkunde. Gustav Fischer, Jena
4. Axenfeld T (1909) Lehrbuch und Atlas der Augenheilkunde. Gustav Fischer, Jena
5. Axenfeld T (1928) Zum Gedächtnis am Albrecht von Graefe. Enke, Stuttgart
6. Bader A (1933) Entwicklung der Augenheilkunde im 18. und 19. Jahrhundert. Schwabe, Basel, p.73
7. Chance EB (1962) Ophthalmology. Hafner, New York,pp.94-95
8. Diepgen P (1965) Geschichte der Medizin. Bd.II,2,2.Aufl.,Gruyter, Berlin p.115 ff and p.248
9. Esser A (1957) Geschichte der Deutschen Ophthalmologischen Gesellschaft. Bergmann, München p.19
10. Fischer I (1962) Biographisches Lexikon der hervorragenden Ärzte der letzten fünfzig Jahre. Bd 1, 2. und 3.Auflage, Urban & Schwarzenberg, München-Berlin p.52
11. Franz R (1968) Lotsen durch 125 Jahre ophthalmologischer Wissenschaft und Praxis. Theodor Axenfeld (1867-1930). Klin Mbl Augenheilk 192:47-49
12. Gorin G (1982) History of Ophthalmology. Publish or Perish, Wilmington, Delaware p.162
13. Heinsius E (1971) Die Entwicklung der medikamentösen Therapie am Auge in den letzten 100 Jahren. Med Mschr 25:443-447
14. Hirschberg J (1918) Geschichte der Augenheilkunde.In: Graefe, Saemisch (eds) Handbuch der gesamten Augenheilkunde Bd.5 II, 2.Auflage, Engelmann, Leipzig-Berlin, p.263
15. Koelbing HM (1966) Early Modern Concepts of Ocular Inflammation. In: Fowler

PD, Birdwood GFB (eds) The Importance and Treatment of Inflammation in Ophthalmology. Manchester, p.1,6
16. Küchle HJ (1974) 75 Jahre Geschichte des Vereins Rheinisch-Westfälischer Augenärzte. Lautemann, Düsseldorf, p.41
17. Münchow W (1969) Karl Wilhelm von Zehender zum 150. Geburtstag (1819-1916). Klin Mbl Augenheilk 154:858-863
18. Münchow W (1984) Geschichte der Augenheilkunde. Enke, Stuttgart 2.Auflage (Erstauflage in "Der Augenarzt" Bd.9) pp.682-683
19. Rohrschneider W (1966) Die Einflüsse der allgemeinen Medizin auf Fortschritte der Augenheilkunde in den letzten 60 Jahren. Document Ophthal (Den Haag) 21:285-300
20. Schadewaldt H (1983) Die Entdeckung des Tuberkuloseerregers. Krankenhausarzt 56:157-166
21. Schadewaldt H (1984) 100 Jahre deutsch-japanische medizinische Zusammenarbeit. Berichtsband Deutsch-Japanischer Kongress der Angiologischen Gesellschaften Deutschlands und Japans in Heidelberg, pp.1-8
22. Silverstein A (1989) A History of Immunology. Academic Press, San Diego
23. Szily A von (1930) Theodor Axenfeld. Klin Mbl Augenheilk 85:1-16
24. Velhagen K (1938) Theodor Axenfeld und A.v.Szily. Erinnerungen. Klin Mbl Augenheilk 101:316-320

History of Ocular Immunology

Arthur M. Silverstein

Abstract. Early immunology was concerned with protective vaccination and serotherapy of infectious diseases, and ophthalmologists paid little attention.
But when Metchnikoff suggested that the immune response could be directed against the body's tissue, and when anaphylaxis, serum sickness, and the Arthus reaction were shown to be mediated by antibodies, it became clear that immunological disease was possible. Ophthalmologists immediately attributed the pathogenesis of sympathetic ophthalmia and diseases of the lens to an (auto-)immune response, and initiated a collaboration with basic experimental immunology that has continued to the present day.
Even when immunology turned away from biomedical interests to immunochemistry, ophthalmology maintained this interest, and contributed to the modern revival of activity in immunobiology and immunopathological processes.

Introduction

The development of subdisciplines in medicine is an interesting study. In some cases, the intellectual content of the subspecialty area derives from developments within the parent discipline itself (retina, uveitis etc.);

in others, it is borrowed fully formed from the cognitive content of some other rapidly moving and highly popular discipline. This latter mechanism was responsible for the growth of ocular immunology, which adapted from the vibrant young field of immunology early in this century the directions for its development.

Ophthalmologists seized upon the concepts and techniques of the early immunologists, and slowly ocular immunology developed as a subdiscipline within the larger field of ophthalmology. Of equal interest is the fact that while many other clinical fields of medicine attempted to integrate the turn-of-century immunological excitement into their clinical and research programs, ophthalmology is perhaps unique in having maintained that interest from that time up to the present day. This was true even during the half-century or so when mainstream immunology abandoned its biomedical concerns in favor of more parochial immunochemical approaches (67). Throughout this history, ophthalmology continued to adapt newer advances in immunology to its own purposes, and occasionally immunologists utilized the special characteristics of the eye to design experiments to answer non-ophthalmic questions. The interaction of these two disciplines accelerated when the immunobiological revolution got fully under way in the early 1960s.

The Research Program of Early Immunology

The demonstration by Louis Pasteur in 1880 of the ability to attenuate pathogens and utilize them for preventive vaccination in the case of chicken cholera (50), anthrax, rabies, and other diseases excited the interest of the world, and assured that many prominent scientists would interest themselves in this field. These successes were reinforced by the discovery by von Behring and Kitasato in 1890 that circulating antibodies can neutralize the toxins of diphtheria (4). No wonder that by the end of the 19th century, the doctrines of this-not-yet organized or even named discipline were proving so popular and attracting the attention of the academic community in all of the medical specialties.

Three components of the research program of the young field of immunology were applied by ophthalmologists to the explanation of their own clinical disease problems. The first of these was the "doctrine" of cytotoxic antibodies. The immune response had been viewed initially as an evolutionary development for the protection of the individual from harmful disease agents. This view seemed appropriate at a time when the immune response appeared to be limited to mechanisms aimed at the destruction of pathogenic organisms and the neutralization of their deadly toxins. But antibody formation was found to be a more general phenomenon in the late 1890s, and antibodies against such bland proteins as albumins were observed. Then Jules Bordet showed in 1899 (6) that antibodies could even be formed against erythrocytes, which they hemolyse with the help of the nonspecifically-acting serum factor complement. Investigators everywhere asked why other tissues and organs might not also stimulate an immune response that might account for the tissue destruction seen in so many diseases of unknown etiology and pathogenesis. In the following years, suspensions or extracts of almost every available tissue and organ were injected into animals to search for specific antibodies and for cytotoxicity, and theories were advanced to link the pathogenesis of one or another disease to this mechanism.

The concept of autoimmunity was the second relevant component of the immunological research program that interested ophthalmology. When Jules Bordet reported the finding of anti-erythrocyte antibodies able to hemolyze red blood cells, Ehrlich and Julius Morgenroth wasted no time in testing whether an animal could form antibodies against its own erythrocytes (15). This they never observed, and Ehrlich advanced the dictum of Horror Autotoxicus(16), which held that even if autoantibodies could be demonstrated, internal regulatory mechanisms would operate to prevent self-destructive consequences. Ehrlich's prestige was so great that his concept was accepted as law, and even the demonstration by Donath and Landsteiner that autoantibodies may cause paroxysmal cold hemoglobinuria (13) failed to shake this belief. As a result, progress in autoimmune disease research was retarded for over 50 years (68). Only the ophthalmologists worked consistently on this problem during this period.

The third important component of the immunological research program that influenced ophthalmology was that of anaphylaxis. In 1902, Paul Portier and Charles Richet reported that animals could be sensitized by a first exposure to antigen, such that a second challenge with the same antigen would lead to shock-like symptoms and even death (52). Anaphylaxis the word and the concept became so popular that it penetrated into all branches of medicine, and not least into ophthalmological concepts of disease. We shall now see how these three concepts affected ideas of pathogenesis in a number of clinically important ophthalmic diseases.

Autoimmune Diseases of the Eye

Sympathetic Ophthalmia

In 1906, Santucci drew attention to the possibility that sympathetic ophthalmia might be caused by the formation of cytotoxic antibodies, following resorption of damaged ocular tissue in the first eye. These antibodies would then attack the hitherto normal contralateral eye (68). Golowin pointed out that he had advanced this idea in 1904, in a Russian journal apparently unread in the West (23,56). Golowin claimed that the seat of attack in the sympathizing eye was the iris and ciliary body, and so named these antibodies "cyclotoxins".

The famous Prague ophthalmologist Elschnig quickly became the leading advocate of an autoimmune pathogenesis of sympathetic ophthalmia (17), suggesting that the resorption of antigen in the damaged eye leads to a "hypersensitivity" that also involves the second eye. Elschnig identified uveal pigment as the offending antigen. The foremost supporter of this thesis was ophthalmologist Alan Woods, who published extensively on this subject starting as early as 1916 (90). Woods employed uveal pigment as antigen in an intracutaneous test for sensitization in patients with sympathetic ophthalmia, and his colleague Jonas Friedenwald demonstrated that the histopathology of the uveal pigment skin test was "consistent with an allergic reaction" (19), thus reinforcing the concept.

The absence of a satisfactory animal model of the disease was one of the chief obstacles to progress in understanding the etiology and pathogenesis of sympathetic ophthalmia. Finally, in two landmark papers (10), Collins reported on the production of uveo-retinitis in guinea pigs induced by uveal extracts injected in adjuvant. These observations (along with others) helped to ensure the modern revival of interest in autoimmune diseases. Then Wacker and Lipton showed that retinal extracts are much more efficient in producing autoimmune disease than uveal extracts, and this initiated the search for the organ-specific antigens involved. Three such antigens were found initially, localized by immunofluorescent analysis to the outer segments of the retina (84). Then, simultaneously, two different laboratories isolated and identified a soluble retinal antigen (S-antigen) able to induce autoimmune disease in animals (14,85). Since then, a number of other organ-specific antigens have been implicated, including an interphotoreceptor retinoid-binding protein (IRBP) and even the visual pigment itself, rhodopsin. By varying the dosage and sensitizing regimen, it has been possible to alter the previously observed chronic inflammatory picture to that of a granolomatous form more typical of human sympathetic ophthalmia (54).

Phacoanaphylaxis

A new chapter in the history of immunology was opened by Paul Uhlenhut when he reported in 1903 that the antigens of the lens of the eye are organ-specific (80). This was the first intimation that unique antigens might exist within a single organ and might be shared among widely divergent species. Other workers showed (3,36) that these lens antigens could mediate both active and passive anaphylaxis in test animals. A guinea pig could even be rendered sensitive to its own lens protein and sent into anaphylactic shock with the protein from any other lens (81). When Krusius demonstrated that rupture of the lens capsule in a normal guinea pig would both sensitize the animal and serve as the disease-producing challenge (37), the true implications of this system for ocular disease became apparent.

The clinical condition was named endophthalmitis phacoanaphylactica by Verhoeff and Lemoine in 1922, and these investigators reported positive skin test responses in patients with this disease (83). Perhaps the most significant contributions to our understanding of this autoimmune process were made by Marak and coworkers (39,40), who produced a disease in rats histopathologically similar to that seen in the human, and were able to transfer the disease adoptively using immune serum. There is little evidence that T cell mechanisms contribute significantly to the pathogenesis of "phacoantigenic uveitis".

The story of lens immunology would not be complete without mention of its application to the problem of evolution. This approach was elegantly pursued by Halbert and Manski (25,26), using lens antigens from many species and a battery of antilens antisera. Given the evolutionary conservation of these structures, cross-reactions were detectable across the entire vertebrate spectrum.

Sjögren's Syndrome

Sjögren's syndrome was first described clinically in 1933 (70), but autoantibodies were only reported in 1958 (31). It is a disease characterized by an autoimmune attack on the lacrimal and salivary glands, involving a chronic inflammatory destruction of acinar cells and ductular epithelium (78). Recent experiments appear to confirm the existence of lacrimal and Harderian gland-specific antigens, able to induce organ-specific, T cell-mediated autoimmune dacryoadenitis in the rat (38).

Immunogenic Keratitis

Corneal Arthus Reactions

Wessely first reported that the injection of antigen intrastromally in the central cornea of a sensitized rabbit would produce an opaque ring of interstitial keratitis (87), and von Szily devoted an entire book to the study of this phenomenon (77). Germuth, Maumenee, and coworkers, employing modern techniques such as immunohistochemical staining, proved that the Wessely ring was in fact a true intracorneal Arthus reaction, i.e., an immune complex deposit with local fixation of complement and the release of pharmacologic agents that attract polymorphonuclear leukocytes to the site (21).

Tuberculosis

The tuberculin test and developments in the field of delayed hypersensitivity led to another approach to the problem of immunogenic interstitial keratitis. During the early period, Calmette proposed his "ophthalmoreaction" (8), in which tuberculin dropped on the eye of a sensitized individual resulted in a more-or-less severe conjunctivitis. While too dangerous, this test did stimulate experiments using other ocular tissues. Intracorneal injection of tuberculin into sensitized guinea pigs produced keratitis, whereas intracorneal injection of antigen into an anaphylactically sensitive animal did not lead to corneal inflammation. A different mechanism seemed to be involved, one that depended on the normal avascularity of the cornea. This difference was long used as one of the principal criteria to differentiate these two phenomena.

The hypersensitivity that accompanies tuberculosis may also be expressed by the spontaneous development of phlyctenular keratoconjunctivitis. This is seen most frequently at the corneal limbus, and presents as an inflammatory infiltrate or nodule composed of epithelioid cells surrounded by lymphocytes, resembling a small tubercle. Descriptions of such nodules appear in the 2nd century in the writings of Paul of Aegina and of Ali ben Isa, and more recently in the 18th century treatise on ocular diseases by St. Yves (75). The condition was produced experimentally by Weekers and Riehm in the tuberculin-sensitive rabbit (57,86).

Herpesvirus Keratitis

While herpesvirus destruction of the corneal epithelium (and of the retina in intraocular infections) appears to be the result of direct viral cytopathogenicity, the corneal stromal pathology associated with this virus seems to be based upon hypersensitivity mechanisms (46). Most investigators have favored a Tcell-mediated pathogenesis (47,55,64).

Corneal Transplantation

The history of attempts to transplant cornea is a long one, but only around the turn of this century did technical improvements in trephines and sutures permit the ophthalmic surgeon to begin to attain consistent success in this venture. When, as frequently happened, a graft would fail, it was usually attributed to some unknown physiological factor. Although the immunologic "laws of transplantation" were well worked out by tumor transplanters early in this century (68), the information appears to have been unknown outside that field. Peter Medawar finally clarified the immunologic basis of allograft rejection in his elegant series of studies in the 1940s (45), and these immediately caught the attention of transplant surgeons everywhere. Maumenee was chiefly responsible for bringing these findings to the attention of ophthalmologists, and for bringing to the attention of the transplanters the special characteristics of the cornea that allows keratoplasty to succeed, while most other tissue and organ grafts fail (41). The important mechanism responsible for the occasional graft rejection was shown to be the cellular immune response mediated by effector T lymphocytes, and the high success rate of allokeratoplasty was shown to reside in an immunological privilege of the cornea, involving both the afferent and efferent limbs of the immune response. This is due to the avascularity and lack of lymphatic drainage in the cornea (5,35).

Immunogenic Uveitis

The fact that the eye shares in the general hypersensitivity of the immunized or infected host, and that such sensitization can be induced also by intraocular administration of antigen was well known. But it remained for Sattler (59) to show in 1909 that bland antigen introduced into the vitreous of the rabbit eye would cause in addition a local ocular hypersensitivity, an observation extended by the elegant studies of the Seegals (63). Such a sensitized eye will respond for many months thereafter with an acute anterior uveitis when specific antigen is introduced intravenously or even by feeding. Here was a possible animal model of human recurrent nongranulomatous anterior uveitis that stimulated later workers to investigate its pathogenesis. Similar studies found that the tissues of the eye can support the local formation of antibody, much like a regional lymph node. This emerged initially from work with equine periodic ophthalmia, a leptospiral infection (22,88). It was later postulated that the inflammatory response accompanying intraocular antibody formation might be the primary pathogenetic contributor to recurrent anterior uveitis, due to the persistence of specific memory cells within the uveal tract of the sensitized eye (65).

Intraocular Infections and the Focal Reaction

It was widely speculated that the hypersensitivity that often accompanies infection might contribute to the pathogenesis of such granulomatous diseases of the eye as tuberculosis, syphilis, toxoplasmosis, and others. This idea received support from the old observation that quiescent tubercles in the eye (and elsewhere) may be reactivated during attempts to desensitize tuberculosis patients with tuberculin, the so-called focal reaction. For many years, ophthalmologists searched for the trigger of attacks of uveitis (i.e., a source of inciting antigen) at distant sites of infection, including the teeth and appendix. The possible role of hypersensitivity in these infectious uveoretinopathies was first advanced by the foremost exponent of this thesis, Alan Woods (92).

Anterior Chamber Privilege

The studies of H.S.N. Greene on the transplantation of tumors and endocrine tissues into the anterior chamber of the eye (24) implied that this site might enjoy a degree of immunological privilege. This phenomenon has been examined in detail in the laboratories of Streilein and his collaboraters, who suggest that an anterior chamber-associated immune deviation (ACAID) results from the induction of suppressor T cells when antigens are presented to the immune system by this route (74).

Ocular Immunopathology and Systemic Disease

Recent developments in immunogenetics have led to increasing collaboration between ophthalmologists and other specialists. A significant group of systemic diseases known or suspected to involve immunopathogenetic mechanisms have been shown to manifest ocular complications, most usually uveitis or uveoretinitis. The clinical and pathogenetic factors involved in the ocular components of these HLA-associated systemic diseases are reviewed in detail by Faure and colleagues (18).

Allergic Conjunctivitis

As indicated above, the conjunctiva may become inflamed by instillation of tuberculin in the sensitized individual. When hayfever and asthma were shown to be immunologic reactions also, it became apparent that immunogenic conjunctivitis was a more general phenomenon, and ophthalmic clinicians became more interested in its pathogenesis and treatment (1,38). This stimulated research on the possible immunopathogenesis of such diseases as vernal catarrh, a seasonal papillary conjunctivitis most often associated with pollen allergy (2,49).

Among the most interesting development along these lines was the suggestion that a chronic immune response to the antigens of Chlamydia trachomatis might account for the primary lesions seen in trachoma (12) and in other follicular conjunctivitides. The exuberant development of germinal centers beneath the conjunctival epithelium in trachoma led Barrie Jones to liken the conjunctival sac to a lymph node cut open, where antigenic stimuli enter through an overlying epithelium (32,66).

Contact Allergy

The widespread use of ophthalmic medications and especially of cosmetics has made contact allergy an increasingly important problem in industrialized societies. While the conjunctiva may be involved in the process, it is more often as a secondary complication of an allergic reaction of the skin of the eyelids. The mechanisms involved, and the many agents that may elicit this disease, are reviewed in detail by Theodore and Schlossmann (79).

Institutionalization of the Discipline

The assignment of an exact date to the establishment of a scientific discipline is always difficult. In the case of ocular immunology, a specific research program (involving sympathetic ophthalmia, lens-induced disease, "anaphylactic" keratitis and conjunctivitis, etc.) had already been identified by 1912, and an interacting community of clinical and laboratory researchers had formed. The first monograph devoted to ocular immunopathology, by von Szily, appeared in 1914, and many other texts and monographs in general immunology (9,11,20,60,71,91) and in immunopathology (7,18,53) followed. Departments of ophthalmology throughout the world added immunological research laboratories to their facilities. These ocular immunology units soon began to hire basic science faculty members, a trend that accelerated after the Second World War with the expansion of interest in all biomedical specialties. The establishment of the National Eye Institute at the U.S. National Institutes of Health in 1968 testifies to the growing scientific and political strength of ophthalmic and vision research, from the fruits of which research in ocular immunology has benefited immeasurably.

One of the hallmarks of the institutionalization of a discipline is the development of first informal and then formal net-works of individuals with common scientific interests. In the mid-1940s, Phillips Thygeson, James Allen, and Fred Theodore oganized an informal group to discuss epidemic keratitis and other problems in ocular microbiology. Immunological discussions quickly entered, and in 1966 Thygeson formalized the meeting at the Proctor Foundation in San Francisco as the Ocular Immunology and Microbiology Group. This Group served as the model for the Section on Ocular Immunology and Microbiology, when the Association for Research in Vision and Ophthalmology (ARVO) was reorganized into disciplinary sections in 1968 (28). Both the Group and the ARVO Section continue to meet annually, and the latter has grown from a few dozen persons at the start to a current membership of over 400. The earliest investigators were almost all clinicians with a bent for research; more than 50% of current ARVO members are basic scientists with formal training in such fields as immunology, molecular biology, bacteriology, and virology.

Another prerequisite for the formation of a new discipline is the definition of its scope. A significant step in this direction was the organization in the late 1950s of a series of

Macy Foundation meetings by Alan Woods and A.E. Maumenee. Prominent basic immunologists were invited to interact with clinicians in highly productive exchanges (42-44). A similar set of meetings was assembled in a series of workshops sponsored by the National Eye Institute (27,72,74). Immunology had been identified by the Eye Institute as one of the principal research areas for further exploitation, and these meetings were designed to define the current status of the field and to identify new and fruitful approaches.

Perhaps the most significant organizational development in this field was the founding in 1974 of a series of quadrennial International Symposia on the Immunology and Immunopathology of the Eye by W. Böke of Germany, R. Campinchi and E.Bloch-Michel of France, and M. Luntz of South Africa. Five such symposia have been held, whose sessions and resulting publications (48,61,67, 73,82) have consolidated this specialized community of scientists, recorded the progress in the field, and stimulated new interest and activity by promoting the exchange of information with other scientific disciplines.

References

1. Allansmith MR (1982) The Eye and Immunology. Mosby, St. Louis
2. Allansmith MR, Frick OL J.Allergy 34:535
3. Andrejew P, Uhlenhuth P (1908) Arb Kaiserl Gesundheitsamt 30:450
4. vBehring E, Kitasato S (1890) Dt Med Wchschr 16:1113
5. Billingham RE, Boswell T (1953) Proc Roy Soc London (Biol) 141:392
6. Bordet J (1899) Ann Inst Pasteur 12:688
7. Böke W (1968) Immunpathologie des Auges. Karger, Basel
8. Calmette LCA (1907) C R Acad Sci 144;1324
9. Campinchi R, Faure JP, Bloch-Michel E et al (1970) L'uvéite, phénomènes immunologiques et allergiques. Masson, Paris
10. Collins RC (1949) (1953) Am J Ophthalmol 32:1687; 36:150
11. D'Ermo F (ed) (1983) Allergia ed immunologia oculare. Masson,Milano
12. Dhermy P, Coscas G, Nataf R et al (1968) Rev Int Trachom 44:295
13. Donath J, Landsteiner K (1904) Münch Med Wchschr 51:1590
14. Dorey C, Faure JP (1977) Ann Immunol (Inst.Pasteur) 128:229
15. Ehrlich P, Morgenroth J (1901) Berl Klin Wchschr 28:251
16. Ehrlich P (1901) Verhandlung 73 Ges.Dtsch.Naturforsch.Ärzte
17. Elschnig A (1910-1911) Graefes Arch Ophthalmol 75:459; 76:509; 78:549; 9:428
18. Faure JP, Bloch-Michel E, Le Hoang P et al (1988) Immunopathologie de l'oeil. Masson, Paris
19. Friedenwald JS (1934) Am J Ophthalmol 17:1008
20. Friedlander MH (1979) Allergy and Immunology of the Eye. Harper & Row, New York
21. Germuth FG, Maumenee AE, Senterfit L et al (1962) J Exp Med 115:919
22. Goldmann H, Witmer RH (1953) Ophthalmologica 127:323
23. Golowin S (1909) Klin Mbl Augenheilk 47:150;
24. Greene HSN (1942) (1947) Cancer Res 2:669; 7:491.
25. Halbert SP, Manski W (1963) Prog Allergy 7:107
26. Halbert SP, Manski W, Auerbach T (1961) In: Smelser GK (ed) The Structure of the Eye. Acad Press, New York

27. Helmsen RJ, Suran A, Gery I et al (eds) (1981) Autoimmune phenomena and ocular disorders. Information Retrieval, Washington (II)
28. Henkind P (1978) History of the Association for Research in Vision and Ophthalmology. Invest Ophthalmol Vis Sci 17 (Suppl):2
29. Immunology: A History of Immunology Note 68, pp 275-295
30. Jabs DA, Prendergast RA (1988) Invest Ophthalmol Vis Sci 29:1437
31. Jones BR (1958) Lancet II:773
32. Jones,BR (1965) In:Duke-Elder S (ed) System of ophthalmology Kimpton, London, Vol.8, pp 4-5;
33. Kalsow CM, Wacker WB (1973) (1975) Int Arch Allergy Appl Immunol 44:11; 48:287
34. Kaplan HJ, Streilein JW (1978) J Immunol 118:809; 120:689;
35. Khodadoust AA, Silverstein AM (1972) Invest Ophthalmol 11:137
36. Kraus R, Doerr R, Sohma M (1908) Wien Klin Wchschr 21:1084
37. Krusius FF (1910) Arch Augenheilk 67:6
38. Lagrange H, Delthil S (1932) Les conjunctivites de nature anaphylactique. Doin, Paris
39. Liu SH, Prendergast RA, Silverstein AM (1987) Invest Ophthalmol Vis Sci 28:270; 28:276
40. Marak GE, Font RL, Czawlytko LN et al (1974) Exp Eye Res 19:311
41. Marak GE, Font RL, Alepa FP (1976) (1977) Mod Probl Ophthalmol 16:75; Ophthalm Res 9:162
42. Maumenee AE (1955) Ann NY Acad Sci 59:453
43. Maumenee AE (ed) (1959) Uveitis. Survey Ophthalmol 4 (part 2):212
44. Maumenee AE (ed) (1962) Toxoplasmosis. Williams & Wilkins, Baltimore
45. Maumenee AE, Silverstein AM (eds) (1964) Immunopathology of Uveitis. Williams & Wilkins, Baltimore
46. Medawar PB (1956) Harvey Lect 52:144
47. Metcalf JF, Kaufman HE (1976) Am J Ophthalmol 82:827
48. Metcalf JF, Hamilton DF, Reichert DW (1979) Infect Immunity 26:1164
49. O'Connor GR, Chandler JW (eds) (1985) Advances in Immunology and Immunopathology of the Eye. Masson, New York
50. Oguchi M (1954) Acta Soc Ophthalmol Japan 58:735
51. Pasteur L (1880) C R Acad Sci 90:239, 952.
52. Porter R, Knight J (eds) (1973) Corneal Graft Failure. Elsevier Amsterdam
53. Portier P, Richet C (1902) C R Soc Biol 54:170
54. Rahi AHS, Garner A (1976) Immunopathology of the Eye. Blackwell, Oxford
55. Rao NA, Wacker WB, Marak GE (1979) Arch Ophthalmol 97:1954
56. Russel RG, Nasisse MP, Larsen HS et al (1984) Invest Ophthalmol Vis Sci 25:938
57. Russky Vratch (1904)22; May 29.
58. Riehm W (1931) Arch Augenheilk 105:55
59. Santucci S (1906) Riv Ital Ottal Roma 2:213
60. Sattler CH (1909) Arch Augenheilk 64:390
61. Secchi AG (ed) (1984) Immunologia ed immunopathologia oculare. Masson, Milano
62. Secchi AG, Fregona IA (eds) (1989) Modern Trends in Immunology and Immunopathology of the Eye. Masson, New York
63. See EG, Leigh AG (1966) Corneal Transplantation. Blackwell, Oxford pp 1-5
64. Seegal D, Seegal BH (1930) (1931) Proc Soc Exp Biol Med 27:390;J.Exp.Med. 54:265
65. Sery TW, Nagy RM, Nazario H (1972) Ophthalmic Res 4:137.
66. Silverstein AM (1964) In: Maumenee AE, Silverstein AM (eds) Immunopathology of Uveitis. Williams & Wilkens, Baltimore pp 83-110

67. Silverstein AM, Prendergast RA (1971) In: Lindahl-Kiessling K et al (eds) Morphological and Functional Aspects of Immunity. Plenum, New York p. 583
67. Silverstein AM, O'Connor GR (eds) (1979) (1982) Immunology and Immunopathology of the Eye. Masson, New York; Seattle
68. Silverstein AM (1989) A history of Immunology. Acad Press,New York pp 160-189
69. Silverstein AM (1991) The Dynamics of Conceptual Change in Twentieth Century Immunology. Cell Immunol 132:515
70. Sjögren H (1933) Acta Ophthalmol 2 (Suppl):1
71. Smolin G, O'Connor GR (1986) Ocular Immunology 2nd edn. Little Brown, Boston
72. Steinberg GM, Gery I, Nussenblatt RB (eds) (1980) Immunogenetics and Transplantation Immunity. Information Retrieval, Washington
73. Strassbourg (1974) Böke W, Luntz MA (eds) (1976) (1978) Ocular Immune Responses. Karger, Basel; San Francisco
74. Streilein JW, Niederkorn JY (1984) J Immunol 134:603
75. St. Yves C (1922) Nouveau traité des maladies des yeux. Le Mercier, Paris
76. Suran A, Gery I, Nussenblatt RB (eds) (1981) Immunological aspects of ocular diseases. Information Retrieval, Washington
77. v.Szily A (1914) Die Anaphylaxie in der Augenheilkunde. Ferdinand Enke, Stuttgart
78. Talal N (1985) In: Rose NR, Mackay IR (eds) The Autoimmune Diseases. Academic Press, New York pp 145-159
79. Theodore FH, Schlossman A (1958) Ocular Allergy. Williams & Wilkins, Baltimore pp.281-298
80. Uhlenhuth P (1903) Festschrift zum 60. Geburtstag von Robert Koch. Fischer-Verlag, Jena pp 49-74
81. Uhlenhuth P, Haendel W (1910) Z Immunitätsforschg 4:761
82. Usui M, Ohno S, Aoki K (eds) (1990) Ocular Immunology Today. Excerpta Medica, Milano, Tokyo, Amsterdam
83. Verhoeff F, Lemoine AN (1922) Am J Ophthalmol 5:737
84. Wacker WB, Lipton MM (1965) (1968) Nature 206:253; J.Immunol. 101:151
85. Wacker WB, Donoso LA, Kalsow CM et al (1977) J Immunol 119:1949
86. Weekers L (1909) Arch Ophthalmol 23:577
87. Wessely K (1911) Münch Med Wchschr 58:1713
88. Witmer RH (1953) (1955) Am J Ophthalmol 37:243; Arch Ophthalmol 53:811
89. Woodruff MFA (1960) The Transplantation of Tissues and Organs. Chas C Thomas, Springfield Illinois
90. Woods AC (1916-1918) Arch Ophthalmol 45:557; 46:8, 503; 47:161
91. Woods AC (1933) Allergy and Immunity in Ophthalmology. Johns Hopkins Press, Baltimore
92. Woods AC (1961) Endogenous Inflammations of the Uveal Tract. Williams & Wilkins, Baltimore

Morphology of the Eye as it Relates to Infection Pathogenesis

W. Richard Green

Abstract. Classification of ocular infectious inflammatory diseases based on pathologic features, location and origin are reviewed.
While many microbes may involve most ocular structures, there are numerous infectious agents that are highly selective in the ocular structures that they involve. The reasons for this selectivity are reviewed, but such reasons are not always evident.
The most common causes of microbial conjunctivitis, keratitis, endophthalmitis and periocular infections are reviewed with special emphasis on the morphological aspects when pertinent.

Introduction

We may review some basic features of inflammation:

Inflammation is the local reaction of living tissue to injury and may be classified on the basis of clinical and histopathologic features. Acute and chronic inflammation are distinguished by duration and the type of inflammatory response. Suppurative inflammation is an acute inflammation characterized by numerous polymorphs and tissue destruction.

Classification of chronic inflammation into granulomatous and nongranulomatous is determined by the presence of foci of macrophages in the former and absence in the latter.

Classification of inflammation by site has value for certain infectious agents that are selective in the areas of involvement. Endophthalmitis involves the vitreous and inner coats of the eye and in panophthalmitis all coats of the eye are involved and extension to the orbit may occur.

With more localized inflammation, identification by the structure and the suffix "-itis" is utilized. Examples include blepharitis, conjunctivitis, keratitis, iritis, cyclitis, vitritis, retinitis and choroiditis.

It is also helpful to identify inflammation by the source as in exogenous endophthalmitis associated with keratitis and after accidental and surgical trauma and endogenous endophthalmitis from hematogenous spread.

In practice, various combinations of these classifications are commonly used. Examples include exogenous suppurative endophthalmitis, endogenous multifocal granulomatous choroiditis, chronic vitritis, etc.

Morphologic aspects of the eye and ocular adnexa may influence the clinical features of some infections. In most instances, however, it is not clear why certain structures are involved by specific infectious agents.

Clinicopathologic Correlations
Canaliculitis

One condition that is influenced by the relative anaerobic site is lacrimal canaliculitis due to Arachnia propionica (Fig.1).

Conjunctivitis

A relatively lower temperature of the surface of the eye favors infection with Mycobacterium leprae (Fig.2).

Some generalization are recognized in regards to the appearance and inflammatory response of the many causes of conjunctivitis. An injected and edematous conjunctiva with a purulent discharge is characteristic of acute bacterial conjunctivitis. An injected and edematous conjunctiva with a watery discharge is characteristic of viral conjunctivitis. Conjunctival hemorrhage may be seen in any severe conjunctivitis, but is characteristically seen in conjunctivitis due to Streptococcus pneumonia, Hemophilus aegypticus and some adenoviruses.

A pale and milky edematous appearance is characteristic of allergic conjunctivitis.

The presence of papillae often means vernal conjunctivitis and the presence of follicles is characteristic of viral and chlamydial conjunctivitis.

The conjunctival inflammatory response as seen in smears is helpful in categorizing the possible causes of conjunctivitis. Neutrophils are seen with bacterial infections, eosinophils with an allergic and vernal disease, lymphocytes with viral conjunctivitis and lymphocytes and polymorphs with chlamydial conjunctivitis. The hyperacute conjunctivitis due to Neisseria (Fig.3) and the mixed polymorphs and lymphocytic response with a follicular reaction to Chlamydia trachomatis (Fig.4) are examples.

Pseudomembranes may be seen with any severe conjunctivitis but they are characteristically seen with several agents such as some adenoviruses, Herpes simplex, C.diphtheriae and Streptococcus species and in bullous conditions. Pseudomembranes consist of fibrinous material and are indicative of damage to the epithelium and blood and lymphatic vessels.

Some agents that cause conjunctivitis typically have regional adenopathy (Parinaud's Oculoglandular Fever). These include infectious mononucleosis, cat-scratch disease, syphilis, tuberculosis, sarcoidosis, and others.

Keratitis

The lamellar structure of the corneal stroma influences the features of keratitis due to some organisms of low pathogenesis. The bacteria extend between collagen lamellae and give a crystalline-like pattern (Fig.5).

Acanthamoeba keratitis is commonly associated with the use of contact lenses and has two principal characteristic features - pain and a ring infiltrate (Fig.6).

Intraocular Sequestration

Sequestration of organisms within the capsular bag after extracapsular cataract extraction may lead to a recalcitrant lowgrade inflammatory process. Propionibacterium acnes (9) (Fig.7), Staphylococcus epidermidis, Corynebacterium species and Torulopsis candida have been associated with this special form of postsurgical ocular inflammatory disease.

Systemic Infections

Invasion of the retina and vitreous by macrophages with bacillary forms in varying stages of degradation is characteristicin Whipple's disease (10) (Fig.8).

There are a variety of infectious agents that localise in the retina. These include Toxoplasma gondii, Candida species, Cytomegalovirus, Cryptococcus neoformans, Herpes simplex, and Varicella zoster. Most of these will be discussed in detail elsewhere in this book.

A number of infectious agents are known to produce multifocal choroiditis and these include Mycobacterium tuberculosis (miliary tuberculosis), Histoplasma capsulatum (Fig.9), Blastomyces dermatitidis, Coccidioides immitis, and more recently, Pneumocystis carinii (Fig.10) and Mycobacterium intracellulare (Fig.11).

Endogenous Bacterial Endophthalmitis

Endogenous bacterial endophthalmitis may occur in association with foci infection in many areas of the body such as meningitis, abdominal infections, endocarditis, renal infections, pneumonia, otitis media, breast abscesses, paronychia, pharyngitis and lymphangitis. The ocular sites of involvement are seemingly random with early retinal, choroid, ciliary body and iris involvement. In many instances the presentation is endophthalmitis as in a patient with meningococcemia (Fig.12). Prompt diagnosis and treatment of this patient resulted in clearing of the endophthalmitis with only the sequelae of high intraocular pressure - the post-congestive triad including iris necrosis, pigment dispersion and Glaukomflecken (Fig.12B).

In Fig.13, an example of retinitis and endophthalmitis due to Staphylococcus is provided in a 15 year old boy with chronic glomerulonephritis and peritonitis.

In early ocular involvement multifocal lesions may be observed in the retina and choroid (Fig.14). Those in the retina may have the appearance of a hemorrhage with a white center (Roth spot).

One patient with bacterial endocarditis was found to have septic choroiditis post mortem (Fig.15).

One patient with bacterial meningitis had multiple septic foci in the choroid (Fig.16A) and one in the ciliary body (Fig.16B) and optic nerve.

A septic focus in retina (Fig.17) was observed in a patient with hepatic encephalopathy and sepsis. Here is an example of endogenous retinitis/endophthalmitis due to Streptococcus in a patient with bronchopneumonia (Fig.18).

A retinal focus of Gram-negative rods in a patient with acute leukemia is shown (Fig.19).

One patient developed endogenous endophthalmitis (Fig.20) associated with a Klebsiella perinephritic abscess.

Endogenous Listeriosis has a predilection for location in the iris where it leads to high pressure glaucoma, iris necrosis and a pigmented hypopyon (2).

Endogenous Fungal Endophthalmitis

Candida is the most common cause of endogenous fungal endophthalmitis. There are numerous underlying illnesses and factors that predispose to Candida sepsis and endogenous endophthalmitis and these include antibiotics, corticosteroid therapy, chemotherapy, radiotherapy, malignancy, hyperalimentation, organ transplantation and gastrointestinal surgery.

In an autopsy study of 133 patients with fungemia or invasive fungal infection, the eyes were the fifth most commonly involved organ (6). It seems reasonable that screening ophthalmologic examinations be performed on patients with fungemia and on patients at high risk for development of fungal infection.

Endogenous spread to the eye occurs at random sites including the choriocapillaris (Fig.21A), retina (Fig.21B), choroid (Fig. 22A) and ciliary body (Fig.22B). Here is an example (Fig.23) where there was extension from the choroid into the retina and vitreous.

Indeed, the extension into the vitreous has become quite characteristic (Fig.24). Here the principal location of the fungus is in the vitreous. Such cases had been successfully treated with antifungal agents in the past but were often accompanied by fibrosis and traction retinal detachment (Fig.25).

With the evolution of vitreous surgery, diagnosis can be more readily accomplished and fibrosis can be avoided by surgical excision of the infected vitreous (7) (Fig.26).

Indeed the combined use of surgical excision and antimicrobial therapy has become the standard treatment for endophthalmitis due to fungi and some bacteria.

Parasites

Parasites are an important cause of ocular inflammatory disease. Fly larvae characteristically burrow under the retina and leave a tract of hypo- and sometimes hyperpigmentation. This case reported by Gass (3), illustrates how the organism burrowed out to the periphery and turned around and returned to the posterior pole (Fig.27).

The larvae are light sensitive and may gain access to the vitreous cavity and anterior chamber.

A 12 year old girl with suspected ocular myiasis interna was operated upon with removal of the cloudy vitreous, which contained a granulomatous inflammation, eosinophils (Fig.28), and the organism - an instare stage of a Hypoderma species (8) (Fig.29).

The second stage larvae of Toxocara canis may produce an epibulbar nodule (Fig.30A), a condition that Ashton termed allergic granulomatous conjunctivitis (1). He noted remnants or intact parasites in a few cases along with eosinophils, granulomatous inflammation and deposits of eosinophilic material (Fig.30B) - the Hoeppli-Splendore phenomenon.

Toxocara larvae may localise under the retina posteriorly (Fig. 31) and in the vitreous cavity and lead to traction retinal detachment (Fig.32).

Maguire and coworkers (5) reported the case of a 27 year old man who developed ocular inflammatory disease three months after acquiring a puppy. He developed an epiretinal membrane with traction for which he was operated. The vitreous specimen contained a dense granulomatous inflammation with rare eosinophils and, to our surprise, the secondary stage larva of Toxocara canis (Fig.33) with rounded cephalic and tapered caudal ends.

Comment

The foregoing are but a few examples of specific and non-specific localisations of infectious ocular diseases and how morphology may contribute to the clinical features.

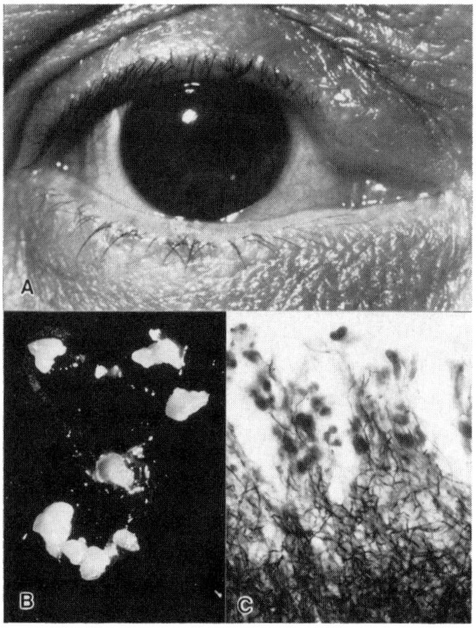

Fig. 1. Lacrimal canaliculitis. A.: The right upper lid is swollen in the area of the lacrimal canaliculitis. B: Concretions removed from the canaliculus. C: Gram-positive appearance of branching filamentous organism of Arachnia proprionica (x1300).

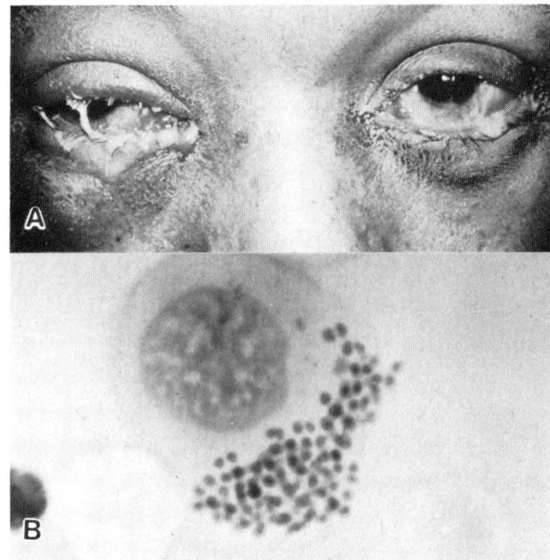

Fig. 3. Gonococcal conjunctivitis. A: Hyperacute conjunctivitis with extensive purulent exudate. B: Gram-negative intracellular diplococci in conjunctival scarring (x1300).

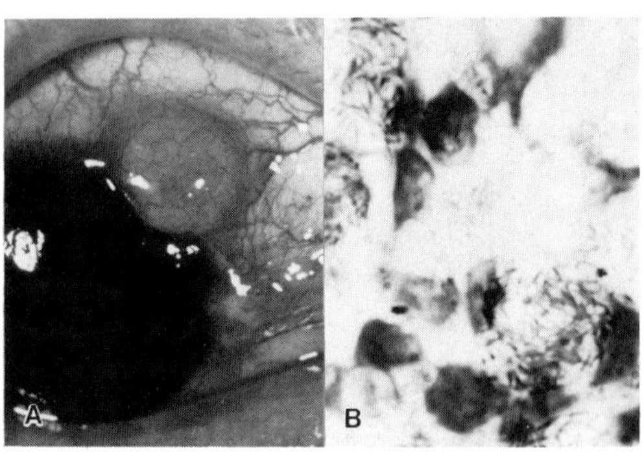

Fig. 2. Leprosy. A: (AFIP 220937) Elevated epibulbar nodule. B: Large macrophages distended by acid-fast bacilli (Ziehl Neelsen 1300).

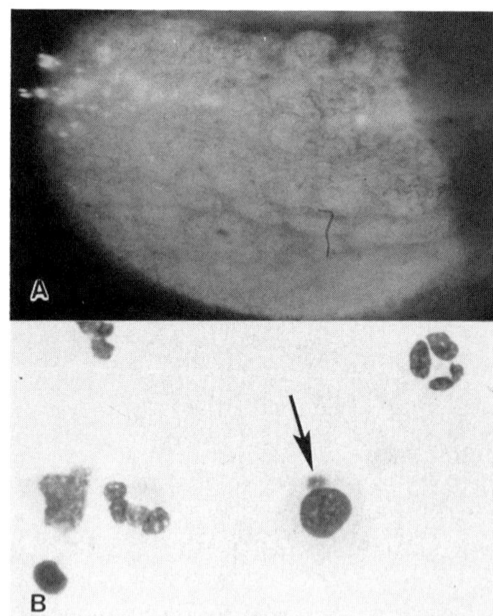

Fig. 4. Chlamydial conjunctivitis. A: Follicular conjunctivitis. B: Scraping of conjunctiva with mixture of neurophils and lymphocytes and epithelial cells with cytoplasmic perinuclear inclusion (arrow) (Giemsa x525).

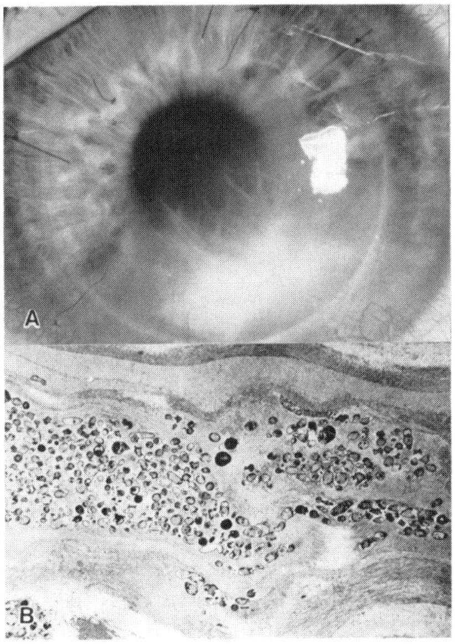

Fig. 5. Bacterial crystalline keratopathy. A: Branching fern-like configuration of extension of bacteria into the cornea. B: Ultrastructural appearance of bacteria located between the collagen lamellae of cornea (x 3800).

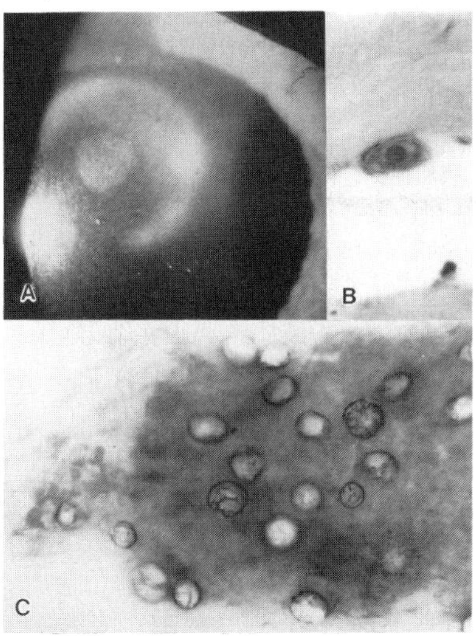

Fig. 6. Acanthamoeba keratitis. A: Ring infiltrate. B: Large trophozoite of Acanthamoeba polyphaga in corneal button (Hematoxylin/Eosin x1300). C: Corneal scraping with numerous acanthamoeba cysts (Hematoxylin/Eosin x1300).

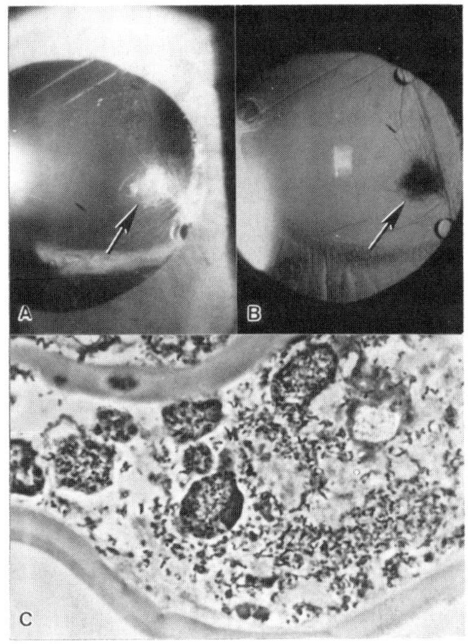

Fig. 7. Chronic postoperative inflammation due to Propionibacterium acnes. Direct (A) and retroillumination (B) slit lamp views of a 1.2mm whitish plaque (arrow) between the intraocular lens optic and posterior capsule near margin of the anterior capsulotomy. (C) Phase contrast microscopy of the capsulectomy specimen with bacilli both free and in macrophages contained within a fold of lens capsule (PPDA x 1200). (From Sawusch MR et al (1989) Ophthalmic Surgery 20:90-92).

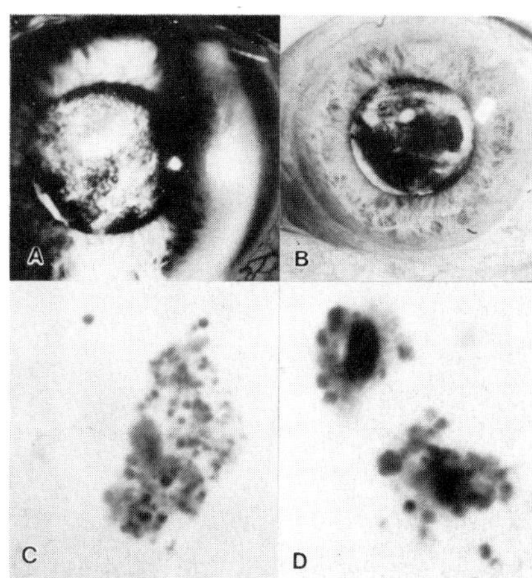

Fig. 8. Whipple's Disease. A: Initial appearance of vitreous opacities. B: Partial clearing of opacities after seven days of tetracycline therapy. C and D: Macrophages distended by periodic Acid-Schiff material in cytoplasm (membrane filter and Periodic acid-Schiff: C.x390; D.x640). (From Selsky EJ et al (1984) Retina 4:103-106.

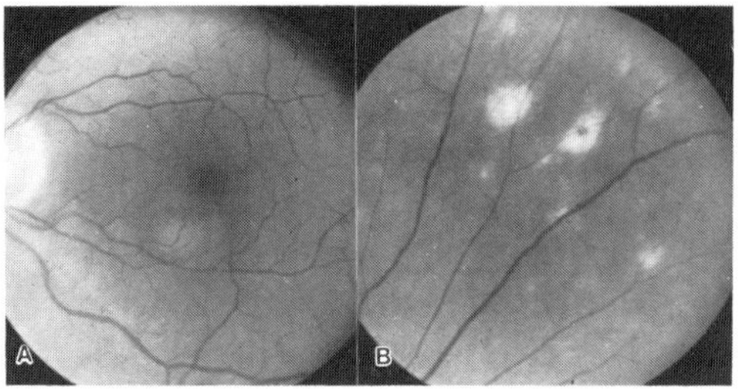

Fig. 9. Ocular histoplasmosis. Multifocal healed scars in the macular and peripapillary areas (A) and in midperiphery (B).

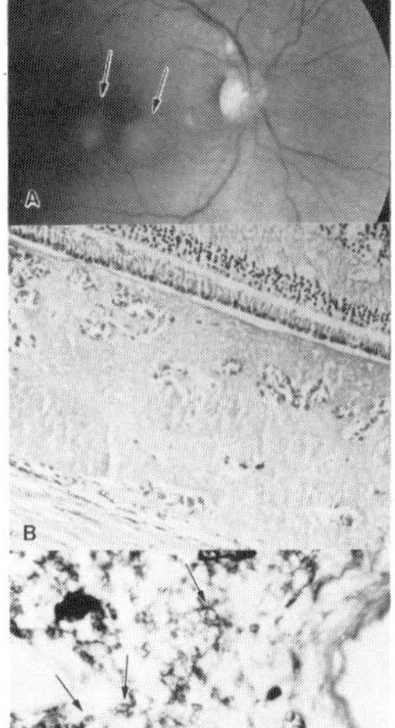

Fig. 10. Pneumocystis carinii choroidopathy. A: Ophthalmoscopic appearance of two choroidal lesions (arrows) in patient with acquired immune deficiency. B: Area of one of the lesions discloses the choroid to be thickened by a coagulum (Hematoxylin/Eosin x137). C: Cysts of Pneumocystis carnii (arrows) (Grocott-Gomori-Methenamine-Silver x525).

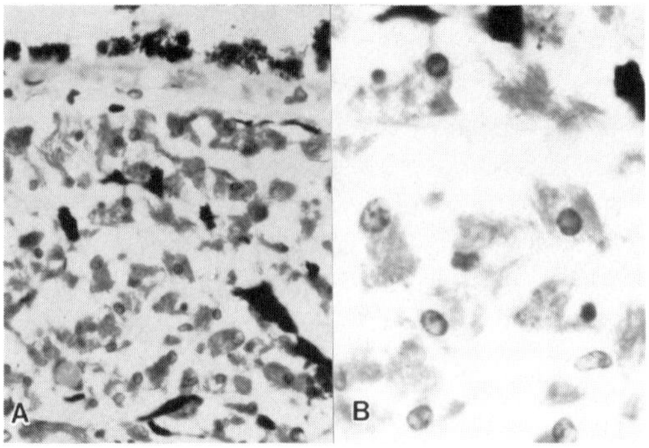

Fig. 11. Atypical Mycobacterium choroidal lesions. A and B: Area of choroid with numerous macrophages that are distended by acid-fast bacilli (Ziehl-Neelsen A.x325; B.x525).

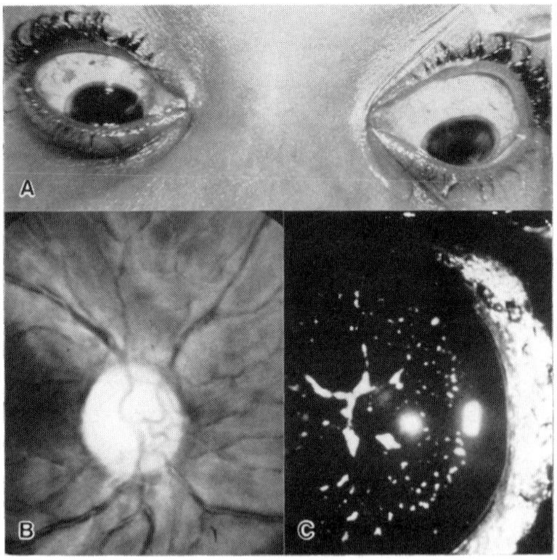

Fig. 12. Bilateral endogenous meningococcal endophthalmitis. A: Early appearance revealed moderate conjunctival injection with petechial hemorrhages, diffuse corneal haze and no view of the fundus of both eyes. B: Clear view of optic nerve head after antibiotic therapy. C: Three weeks after acute infection, pupils were widely dilated with patches of iris atrophy. Lenses had small, irregular patches of white subcapsular opacities (glaukomflecken) (From Jensen AD and Naidoff MA (1973) Arch Ophthalmol 90:396-398.

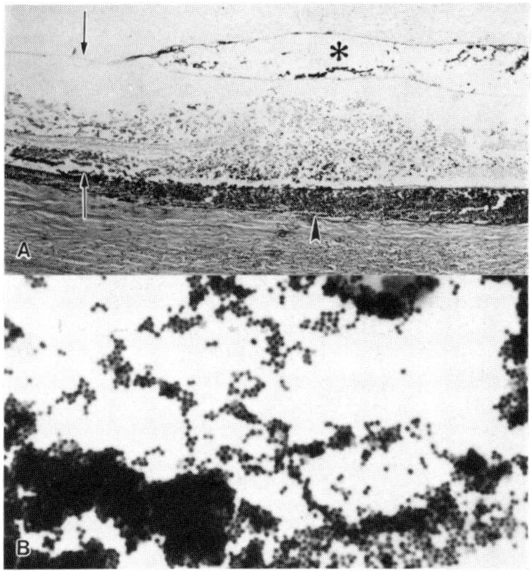

Fig 13. Endogenous bacterial retinitis. A: Area with retinal necrosis (between arrows), much bacteria (asterisk), and an intense inflammatory cell infiltrate in the choroid (arrowhead) (Brown and Hopps x37). B: High power view of Gram- positive cocci in retina (Brown and Hopps x1300).

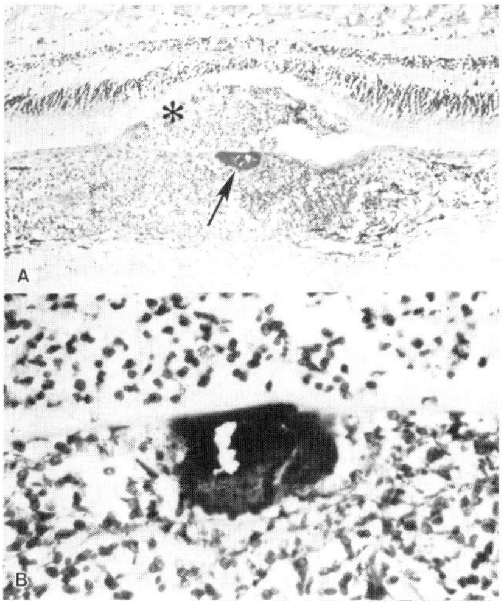

Fig. 15. Endogenous bacterial choroiditis. A: Septic focus in choroid with a large colony of Gram-positive cocci (arrow) and an intense infiltration of polymorphonuclear leucocytes in the choroid and subretinal space (asterisk) (Hematoxylin/Eosin x137). B: Higher power view of large colony of bacteria in choroid (Hematoxylin/Eosin x525).

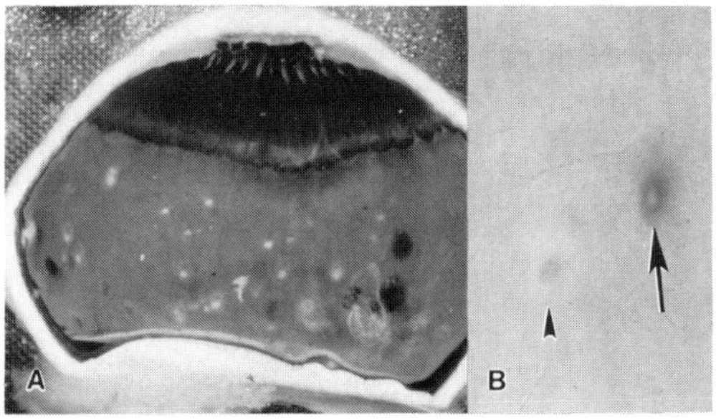

Fig. 14. A: Endogenous bacterial lesions involving retina and choroid. B: Area discloses septic foci in choroid (arrowhead) and retina (arrow) with a white-centered hemorrhage.

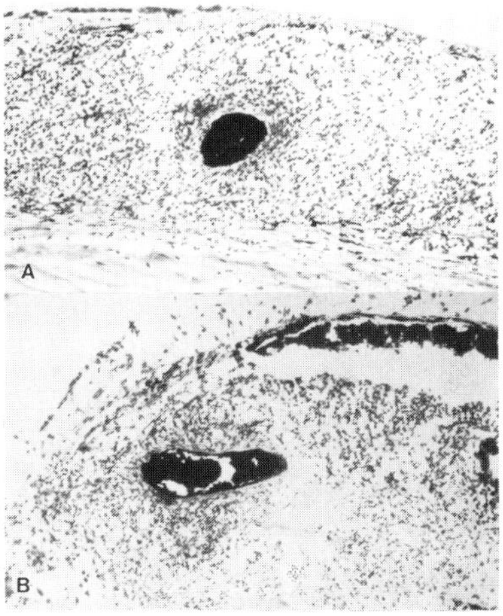

Fig. 16. Endogenous bacterial choroiditis and cyclitis. Focus of Gram-positive cocci surrounded by an intense neutrophilic infiltrate in the choroid (A) and ciliary body (B) (Brown and Hopps; A&B. x137).

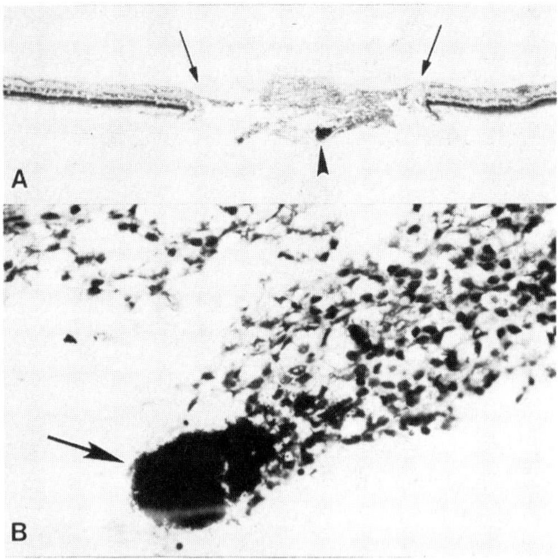

Fig. 17. Endogenous bacterial retinitis. A: Area of acute retinal necrosis (between arrows) with a focus of bacteria (Hematoxylin/Eosin x37). B: Higher power view of focus of Gram-positive cocci (arrow) (Brown and Hopps x525).

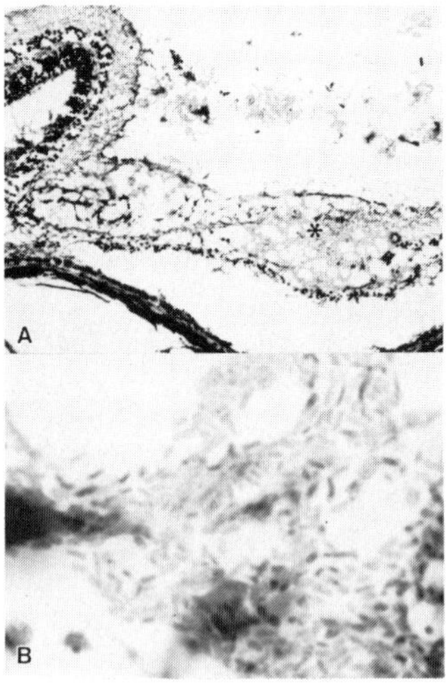

Fig. 19. Endogenous bacterial retinitis. A: Area of retinal necrosis (asterisk) with Gram-negative rods (Brown and Hopps x135). B: Higher power view of Gram-negative rods in the retina (Brown and Hopps x2000).

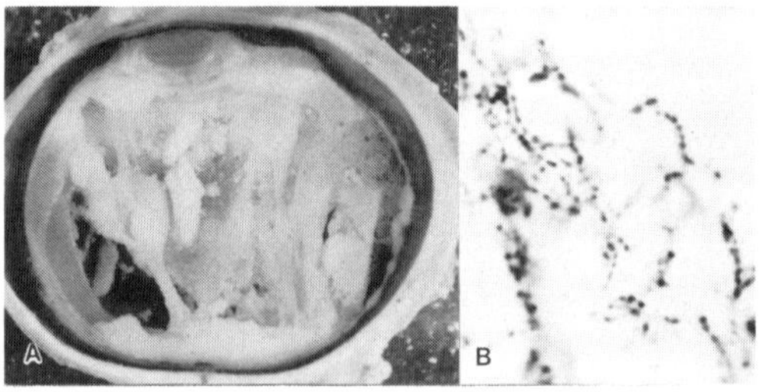

Fig. 18. Endogenous bacterial endophthalmitis, Gross appearance (A) with Gram-positive cocci , in chains (B). (B.Brown and Hopps x1300).

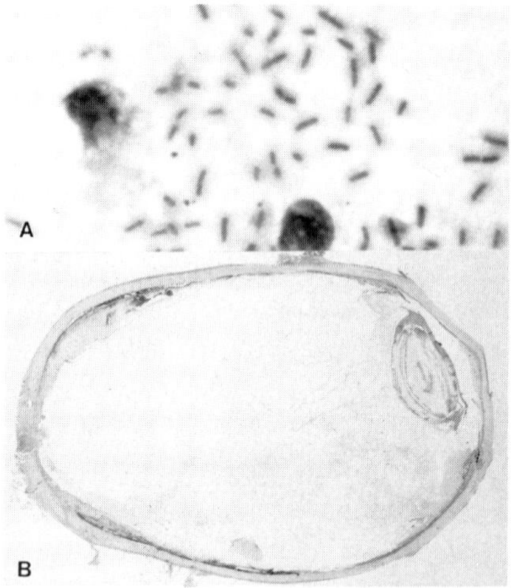

Fig. 20. Endogenous endophthalmitis from a Klebsiella perinephric abscess. A: Smear of vitreous reveals large Gram-negative rods (Brown and Hopps x2000). B: Low power view of surgically enucleated eye with near total necrosis of retina (Hematoxylin/Eosin x2.7).

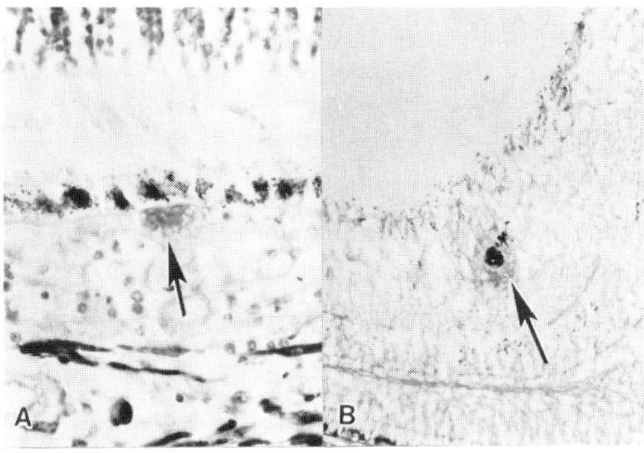

Fig. 21. Candida sepsis with early small foci involving the choriocapillaris (A) and retina (B) (arrows) (Periodic Acid-Schiff: A. x137; B. x328).

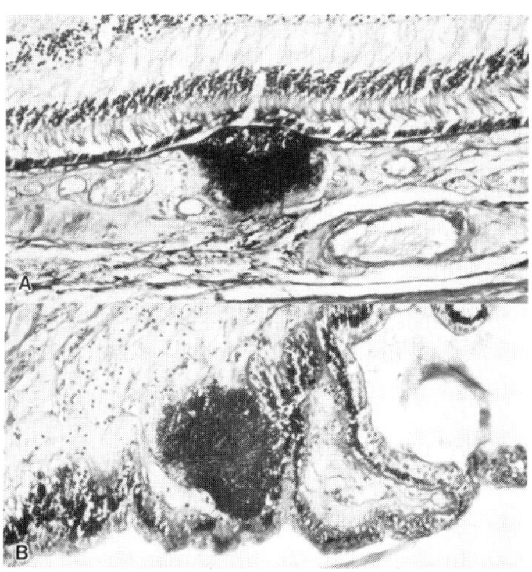

Fig. 22. Candida sepsis with large focus in choroid (A) and ciliary body (B) (arrows) (Periodic Acid-Schiff: A. and B. x137).

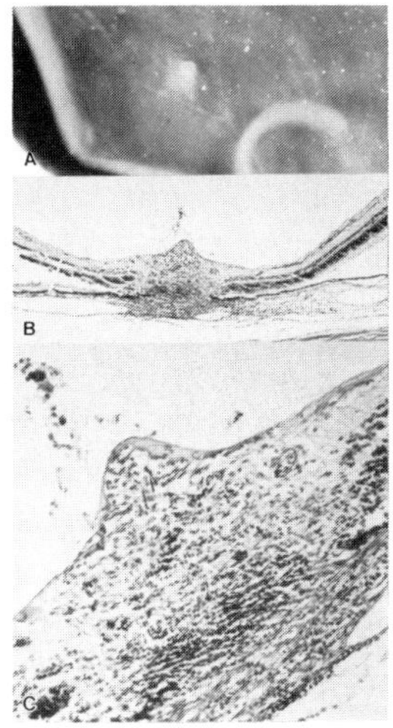

Fig. 23. Gross (A) and microscopic (B and C) appearance of endogenous Candida lesion that apparently started in the choroid and extended into the retina and vitreous (Periodic Acid-Schiff: B. x137; C. x328).

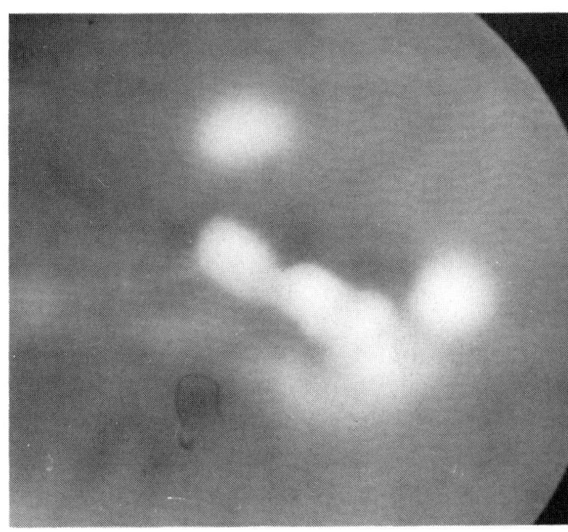

Fig. 24. Typical appearance of endogenous Candida endophthalmitis with whitish vitreous lesions with ill-defined margins.

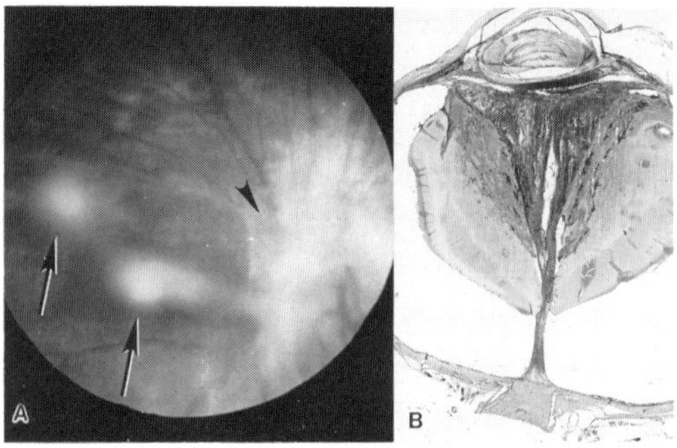

Fig. 25. Endogenous Candida endophthalmitis in 25 year-old-woman with inflammatory bowel disease. A: Appearance of vitreous fungal lesions (arrows) and area of vitreous fibrosis (arrowhead). B: Low power view of surgically enucleated eye with vitreous fibroinflammatory lesion and traction retinal detachment (Hematoxylin/Eosin x2).

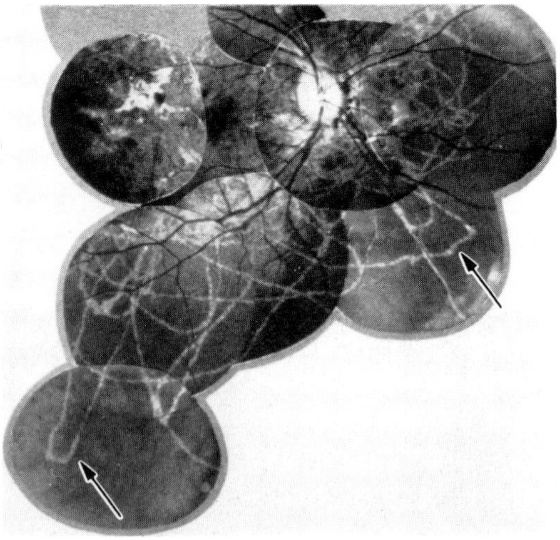

Fig. 27. Ophthalmomyiasis interna posterior. Composite photo illustrates subretinal tracks. In two areas (arrows), the parasite makes a U-turn and heads back to the posterior pole. (From: Gass JDM and Lewis RA (1976) Arch Ophthalmol 94:1500-1505

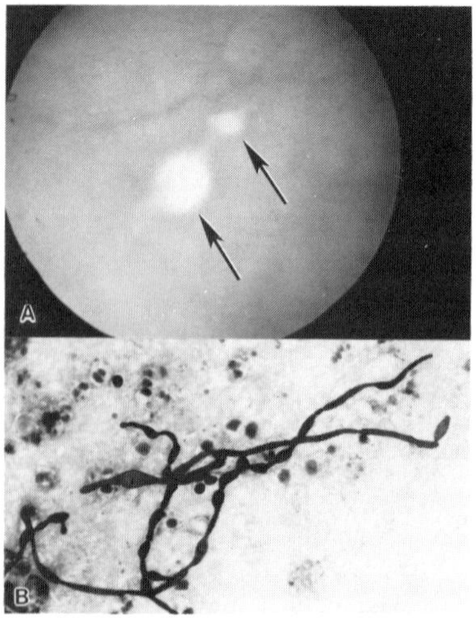

Fig. 26. Endogenous Candida endophthalmitis. A: Two white fluff balls (arrows) in posterior aspect of vitreous taper toward the retina. B: Fungus removed the vitreous cavity demonstrate pseudohyphae and budding blastospores characteristic of Candida species (Periodic Acid-Schiff x900). (From Snip RC and Michels RG (1976) Am J Ophthalmol 82:699-704).

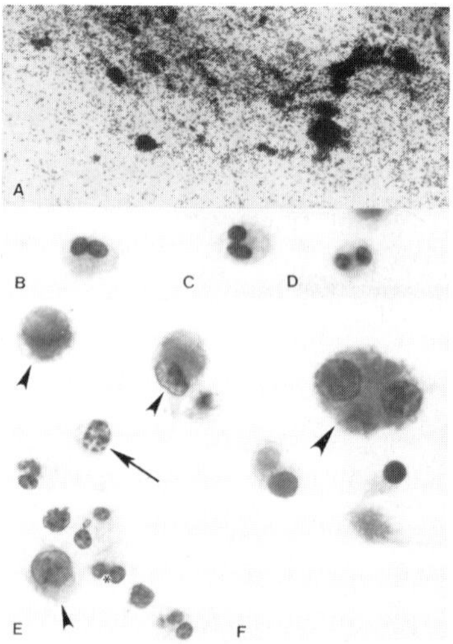

Fig. 28. Ophthalmomyiasis interna posterior. A: Millipore filter concentration of vitreous specimen stained by a modified Papanicolaou technique shows intense chronic inflammatory infiltrate (x55). B-D: Higher power views of eosinophils with typical bilobed nuclei (x1450). E: Area with large epithelioid cells (arrowheads), plasma cell (arrow), and eosinophil (asterisk) (x1450). F: Multinucleated giant cell (arrowhead) (x1450).

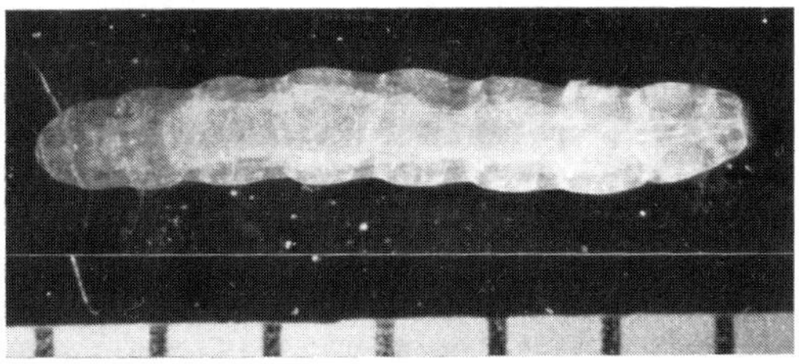

Fig. 29. Gross appearance of early instar larva of Hypoderma species with eight segments and a central tubular structure. (From: Rapoza PA et al (1986) Retina 6:99-104

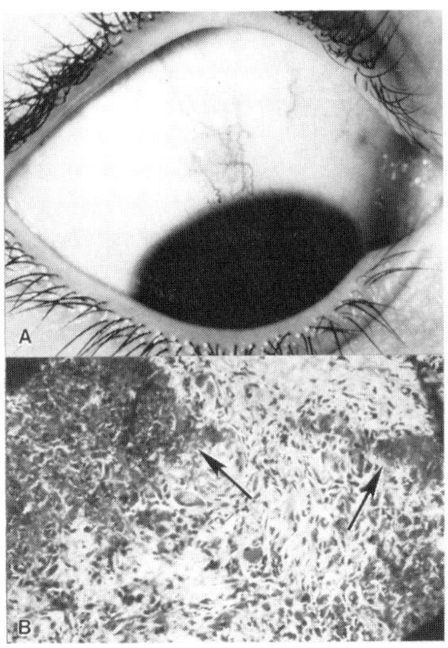

Fig. 30. Allergic granulomatous conjunctivitis. A: Epibulbar nodule in six-year-old girl. B: Lesion contains eosinophils, epithelioid and giant cells and deposits of eosinophilic material (arrows) (Hematoxylin/Eosin x525).

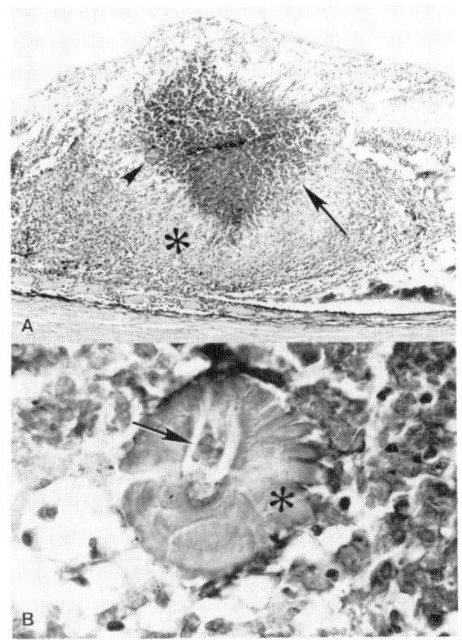

Fig. 31. Ocular Toxocariasis. A: Lesion is located posteriorly under the retina where an eosinophilic material (arrow) with eosinophils, the partially degenerated parasite, and a partially surrounding area of fibroinflammatory tissue (asterisk) is present (Hematoxylin/Eosin x60). B: Higher power view of degenerated nematode larva (arrow) surrounded by a dense eosinophilic material (Hematoxylin/Eosinx800).

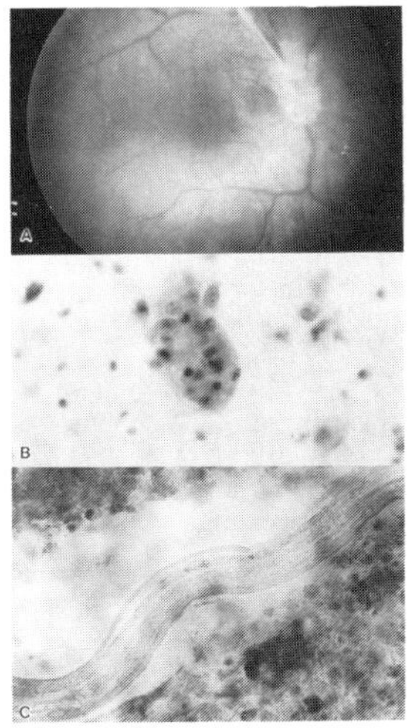

Fig. 32. Ocular Toxocariasis. A: Diffuse type with fibroinflammatory lesion in the peripheral vitreous with traction retinal detachment. B: Area of fibroinflammatory lesion in vitreous with partially degenerated nematode larva (arrow) (Hematoxylin/Eosin x228).

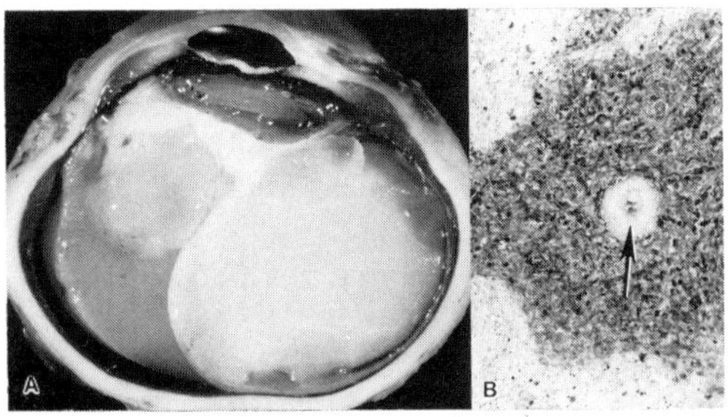

Fig. 33. Toxocariasis. A: Ophthalmoscopic appearance of a vitreopapillary traction band from an equatorial inflammatory lesion located in the 11 o'clock meridian of right eye of an 18-year-old man who had acquired a puppy 5 months before the onset of ocular symptoms. B: Vitreous aspirate by pars plana vitrectomy contained an intense inflammatory cell infiltrate with neutrophils, epithelioid cells, multinucleated giant cells and the second-stage larva of Toxocara canis (C) (Millipore filter, modified B Papanicolaou stain A and D x525; C. x340).(From Maguire et al. Ophthalmology (1990)97:675-680.

References

1. Ashton N (1979) Allergic Granulomatous Nodules of the Eyelid and Conjunctiva. Am J Ophthalmol 87:1-28
2. Eliott D, O'Brien TP, Green WR et al (to be published) Ophthalmology
3. Gass JDM, Lewis RA (1976) Subretinal Tracks in Ophthalmomyiasis. Arch Ophthalmol 94:1500-1505
4. Jensen AD, Naidoff MA (1973) Bilateral Meningococcal Endophthalmitis. Arch Ophthalmol 90:396-398
5. Maguire AM, Green WR, Michels RG et al (1990) Recovery of Intraocular Toxocara canis by Pars Plana Vitrectomy. Ophthalmology 97:675-680
6. McDonnell PJ, McDonnell JM, Brown RH et al (1985) Ocular Involvement in Patients with Fungal Infections. Ophthalmology 92:706-709
7. Rapoza PA, Michels RG, Semeraro RJ et al (1986) Vitrectomy for Excision of Intraocular Larva (hypoderma species). Retina 6:99-104
8. Sawusch MR, Michels RG, Stark WJ et al (1989) Endophthalmitis Due to Proprionibacterium acnes Sequestered Between IOL Haptic and Posterior Capsule. Ophthalmic Surg 20:90-92
9. Selsky EJ, Knox DL, Maumenee AE et al (1984) Ocular Involvement in Whipple's Disease. Retina 4:103-106
10. Snip RC, Michels RG (1976) Pars Plana Vitrectomy in the Management of Endogenous Candida Endophthalmitis. Am J Ophthalmol 82:699-704

Mucosal Immunity and the Eye

Brian J. Underdown

Abstract. The immune system includes a number of cell types and antibody molecules specially adapted to function at mucosal surfaces of the body, including the conjunctiva and lacrimal gland. Initiation of the immune response is facilitated by specialized M cells overlying lymphoid aggregates within the epithelium, through which antigen is delivered to antigen presenting cells, as well as lymphocytes of the T and B lineage. Lymphocytes at mucosal sites form a recirculating pool which offer the potential to use oral immunisation to protect distal mucosal sites from infectious agents. Some T cells within the gut have the capacity to promote systemic unresponsiveness to mucosally presented antigen while others promote the synthesis of IgA antibodies which are transported across the mucosal epithelium via a receptor specific for polymeric immunoglobulins. Secreted IgA antibodies prevent infection by restricting attachment to and entry of microorganisms into the epithelium. The ability of T cells to promote different functions is related to their ability to secrete different cytokine molecules.

Mucosal tissue contains mast cells and large granular lymphocytes, which appear specially adapted to function in mucosal tissue. The nervous and immune systems may regulate each other through the direct innervation of mast cells and the ability of cytokines and neuropeptides to promote communication between the two systems.

Introduction

The eye has a close anatomical and functional relationship with two mucosal structures, namely the lacrimal gland and the conjunctival epithelium. The lacrimal gland supplies on a continuous basis the surface of the eye with tear fluid containing antibody. The major antibody isotype in tears is IgA, which is characteristic of most mucosal secretions (4,19,22,28). Thus, the common mucosal immune system (10,12,42) provides the surface of the eye with protection against infectious agents with which it comes into contact frequently. In contrast to the lacrimal gland, the conjunctival epithelium does not appear to be capable of transporting IgA antibodies to its mucosal surface and does not appear to provide immune protection to the eye, except perhaps in the rabbit (14).

In this review, I will attempt to summarize the general features of the mucosal immune system, as well as to distinguish those features which may be relevant to ocular tissue from those which are not. Much of the information available on the mucosal immune system comes from studies of the respiratory and gastrointestinal tracts, where many of the general features of the mucosal immune system have been studied in greatest detail.

Induction of Immune Responses at Mucosal Surfaces

A central paradigm of mucosal immunology is that immunocytes stimulated at one mucosal site may travel through the lymphatic and blood circulation to distant mucosal sites. This process is aided by specific receptors on high endothelial venules within mucosal tissue, which are capable of selecting lymphocytes of mucosal origin from the recirculating pool and transferring them to the mucosal tissue (35,41,46). Thus, immune cells stimulated initially within the gastrointestinal tract circulate through the intestinal lymphatics, thoracic duct lymph and blood circulation and are distributed to other mucosal sites such as the lacrimal gland (32,39,41,but see ref.29).

Within the gastrointestinal tract, the Peyer's patches are thought to be prime sites where IgA-specific T helper cells are located and where IgA antibody synthesis commences (8,24). The ability of the host to take in antigen is enhanced by M cells which form the lumenal face of the Peyer's patch (3,36). M cells are thought to be active in taking up particulate and/or replicating antigens from the lumen and delivering them to the antigen-presenting cells and associated lymphocytes within the Peyer's patch.

Immune responses can also be generated directly at mucosal sites other than the gastrointestinal tract. Evidence exists that Peyer's patch-like lymphoid aggregates exist in the bronchial tree and immunization at this site results in the appearance of antibody in the respiratory secretion, but not in other mucosal sites (49). Thus, it is possible that the gastrointestinal tract may be the only mucosal site with the capacity to generate immune responses sufficient to seed other mucosal sites (50).

There is little doubt that immune responses appear within the lacrimal gland and IgA antibody is secreted there following topical administration of antigen or infection on the ocular surface (15,26). It is not clear to what extent these immune responses can be generated directly in the lacrimal gland, particularly since the mucosal tissue associated with the eye does not contain germinal centers, a characteristic feature of tissues where immune responses develop. Nor does the lacrimal gland or conjunctival epithelium contain specialized M cells, which are commonly associated with uptake of antigen for presentation to the mucosal immune system (3). It seems possible that the initiation of the response following introduction of antigen at the ocular surface may depend on antigen reaching the gut, which in turn would generate an immune response which migrates to the eye. Evidence exists to support this hypothesis. Sullivan and coworkers reported that topical radiolabelled antigen applied to the ocular surface was found primarily in the stomach, presumably having travelled there via the nasolacrimal duct (45). In support of the possibility that immune responses may be stimulated locally in the eye are the findings by one group that the extent of the local response was greater following topical immunization compared to immunization via the gastrointestinal route (37). Once immune cells arrive in the lacrimal gland, it is likely that they may be amplified locally by antigen present in the ocular tissue, but it is not clear whether memory remains within the lacrimal gland sufficient to respond briskly to subsequent infection.

The Enrichment of Mucosal Tissue with IgA-Producing Cells

The generation of IgA antibody is the best characterized of mucosal immune responses. The production of IgA-secreting cells appears to be substantially influenced by a subset of T-lymphocytes known as T_H2 cells (33). These cells secrete a number of soluble cytokines, which may act synergistically on B cells to produce a variety of effects. For example, some of the cytokines such as Interleukin-5 and Transforming Growth Factor-ß have been shown to promote the differentiation of relatively immature B cells bearing IgM on their surface into B cells, which express IgA on their surface. IgA-bearing B cells are the direct precursors of IgA-secreting cells. Other cytokines, e.g. Interleukin-4, Interleukin-5, Interleukin-6 and Transforming Growth Factor-ß act as differentiation and growth factors driving the B--Cell pool to secrete IgA (30,31). An additional mechanism, which promotes IgA synthesis is the occurrence of T cells, which have receptors for IgA on their surface. Such T cells (T_{alpha} cells) have the capacity to interact closely with B--Cells expressing IgA on their surface, which is thought to increase the local concentration of cytokines such as Interleukin-5 and enhance the production of cells committed to IgA synthesis (30). Indeed, clones of T_H2 cells have been described recently, which display Fc_{alpha}-receptors on their surface (40).

Transcytosis of IgA and the Poly Ig Receptor

Following secretion from plasma cells, dimers and higher polymers of IgA are selectively transported from the interstitial fluid bathing the basal surface of the epithelium to the mucosal lumen (4). This is accomplished by a specific receptor, which is expressed at the basal surface of most mucosal epithelial cells (but not conjunctival epithelia). This receptor, known as the poly Ig receptor, has a high affinity for dimers and higher polymers of IgA, but not monomeric IgA (1,2,4). The poly Ig receptor is a 100kD protein, which in humans has five extracellular domains, a transmembrane region, and a cytoplasmic tail (34). The five extracellular domains of the poly Ig receptor were discovered first in its soluble form and correspond to the secretory component. The transport of IgA across mucosal epithelia is known as transcytosis, and depends on high affinity binding between poly IgA antibodies and the poly Ig receptor, which ensures that the poly IgA ligand remains with its receptor throughout the transport process. This includes its transition through the multivesicular compartment for uncoupling ligands and receptors (CURL (17)). The poly IgA.poly Ig receptor complex migrates to the apical face of the epithelial cell where it is cleaved by proteolysis resulting in the release of secretory IgA (48). Secretory IgA consists of the dimer or higher polymers of IgA complexed to the five extracellular domains of the poly Ig receptor known as secretory component.

The cell biology of IgA transcytosis has been studied in some detail and is summarized in several reviews (47,48). The cytoplasmic tail of the poly Ig receptor appears to be crucial for the transcytotic process to occur, since specific alterations in the amino acid sequence of this region of the molecule affect transport. In addition, phosphorylation of a serine within the cytoplasmic tail occurs just prior to the appearance of the receptor at the basal surface of the epithelial cell and appears crucial for effective function of the receptor (6).

The vast majority (>95%) of polymeric IgA antibody taken up by the epithelium is synthesized at the site of transport. Polymeric IgA antibody synthesized at one mucosal site is not redistributed to other mucosal sites. This is because IgA, which diffuses via the lymphatics to the blood circulation remains primarily intravascular due to its size and is eventually catabolized by the liver (11).

It should be noted that in some species including humans the poly Ig receptors also bind IgM with high affinity. However, the amount of IgM found normally in human mucosal secretions including tears is relatively small, except in IgA-deficient individuals where often compensatory increases of IgM are observed (25).

Hormonal Control of Poly Ig Receptor Expression

Sullivan and colleagues have described an interesting regulatory effect of androgens on the expression of the poly Ig receptor and secretory IgA. Thus, male rats have higher levels of IgA in tears and this was shown to be associated with increased levels of secretory component (the soluble form of the poly Ig receptor) in tears. Administration of testosterone in orchiectomized male rats mimicked this effect (42,43).

Expression of the poly Ig receptor is also increased by cytokines, which presumably act in synergy with other inflammatory processes designed to maximize the immune elimination of foreign microorganisms (47).

Cellular Elements of the Secretory Immune System

In addition to IgA, a number of other immune elements appear to be specialized to function in mucosal tissue. Of particular interest are the intraepithelial lymphocytes, a heterogeneous population of cells, which have several characteristics of T cells, but may represent in part a lineage distinct from the T cell pool within peripheral lymphoid tissue (9,21). For example, some intraepithelial lymphocytes do not express CD3, CD4 and CD8 structures on their surface, but do express T cell receptors for antigen-Major Histocompatibility Complex class II complexes displayed by antigen-presenting cells. Moreover, the T cell receptors on intraepithelial lymphocytes are enriched for the gamma-delta phenotype, compared to peripheral T cells, which express primarily the alpha-beta phenotype. In humans, the enrichment of the gamma-delta phenotype was not reported in normal subjects, but individuals with inflammatory bowel disease had substantially greater numbers of gamma-delta cells than normal individuals. The gamma-delta phenotype of the T cell receptors may be enriched for recognizing antigens common to bacterial flora found normally in the intestine.

Intraepithelial lymphocytes have cytotoxic function, which may be detected as a constitutive property (i.e., they may behave as "natural killer" cells). Intraepithelial lymphocytes have also been reported to function as cytotoxic lymphocytes with specificity for alloantigens and virus-infected cells (5). It has also been suggested that intraepithelial lymphocytes may play an immunoregulatory function normally associated with contrasuppressor cells and in so doing, may be one of the mucosal elements responsible for so-called orally-induced systemic unresponsiveness (i.e. oral tolerance). Intraepithelial lymphocytes have been implicated in inflammatory bowel disease as well as intestinal infections.

In addition to intraepithelial lymphocytes, mucosal mast cells have properties, which are different from tissue mast cells in a number of important ways including the content of their granules, the affinity of their receptors for IgE and their response to pharmacologic agents. Moreover, recent evidence suggests that mast cells secrete cytokines (18). The importance of mucosal mast cells in inflammatory processes at the mucosa is well documented (38).

Approximately 50% of B cells in the intestine appear to arise from a lineage, which appears distinct from the peripheral B cell pool and express the CD5 cell surface phenotype. $CD5^+$ B cells appear to be enriched for synthesis of IgM and IgG_2 (IgG_3 in mice) antibodies directed to glycolipid and carbohydrate antigenic determinants, which are common on many microbial surfaces (20). Thus, several cell types (intraepithelial lymphocytes, mucosal mast cells and $CD5^+$ B cells) in addition to IgA antibody appear to be specially adapted to function within mucosal tissue.

Finally, inflammatory cells such as neutrophils, macrophages and eosinophils, which are distributed throughout the body, have been reported to express Fc_{alpha}-receptors, which in the presence of IgA antibody might enhance their ability to eliminate foreign microbes at the mucosal surface (7).

Interaction of the Mucosal Immune System with the Nervous System

Recently, a number of investigators including Perdue, Bienenstock and coworkers have pointed out that mucosal tissue is highly innervated. Many mucosal cells have receptors for neuropeptides and some immune cells such as macrophages can secrete neuropeptides (e.g., substance P). In addition, neuropeptides have been demonstrated to affect the function of immune-related cells or responses (13,23).

To explore the potential for interaction between the nervous and mucosal immune systems, several groups have set up conditioning paradigms in which allergic responses in the intestine and respiratory tracts have been generated by a conditioning stimulus (presented first, together with the primary sensitizing allergen) to a degree, which was as great as that produced by challenge with the sensitizing antigen (16,27).

However, Sullivan and coworkers carried out transsection of the nerves that innervate ocular tissue without observable changes in the local immune responses (44). Clearly, this area of investigation will receive considerable attention in the next few years.

Vaccine Development

Many of the infectious diseases of the eye pose problems for vaccine development. If the generation of the responses in the lacrimal gland depends on the antigen reaching the intestinal mucosae, a key issue is whether memory can be maintained within the eye tissue itself or whether secondary responses too may need to be re-stimulated in the gut with subsequent redistribution to the eye. This would seem inefficient and confer on the infectious agent a "head start", so to speak. A number of groups have reported attempts to stimulate protective immunity to Chlamydia trachomatis. While antibody and cell-mediated responses to whole cell bodies and purified components have been elicited, none of these responses have provided adequate protection to experimental challenge of monkeys with infectious chlamydia (see Whittum-Hudson in this volume). This may be related to the inability of the vaccine regimen to induce appropriate protective immunity, but could underlie a more fundamental problem, which relates to the possibility that following vaccination memory resides not in the lacrimal gland, but in the gut.

Comment

The mucosal immune system appears to function best as a first line of defence, as has been emphasized by many investigators. The provision of the surface of the eye with a continuous supply of IgA antibody reduces the probability of entry to many of the infectious agents found commonly in the environment. Agents which are common in the environment likely stimulate specific IgA antibody responses frequently and thus, provide tear fluid with an immune barrier to common enemies of the host.

On the other hand, the effectiveness of this barrier is probably seriously compromised in cases where trauma breaches the outer surface of the eye and permits easier internal access of foreign microbes, or when the invading organism can establish itself within the epithelium and thus escape the action of IgA antibody.

References

1. Ahnen DJ, Brown WR, Kloppel TM (1985) Secretory Component: The Polymeric Immunoglobulin Receptor. Gastroenterology 89:667-682
2. Allansmith MR, Gillette TE (1980) Secretory Component in Human Ocular Tissue. Am J Ophthalmol 89:353-361
3. Bockman DE, Cooper MD (1973) Pinocytosis by Epithelium Associated with Lymphoid Follicles in the Bursa of Fabricius, Appendix and Peyer's Patches. An Electron Microscopic Study. Am J Anat 136:455-478
4. Brandtzaeg P (1981) Transport Models for Secretory IgA and Secretory IgM. Clin Exp Immunol 44:221-232
5. Carman PS, Ernst PB, Rosenthal KL et al (1986) Intraepithelial Leukocytes Contain a Unique Subpopulation of NK-Like Cytotoxic Cells Active in the Defence of Gut Epithelium to Enteric Murine Coronavirus. J Immunol 136(5):1548-1553
6. Casanova JE, Apodaca G, Mostov KE (1991) An Autonomous Signal for Basolateral Sorting in the Cytoplasmic Domain of the Polymeric Immunoglobulin Receptor. Cell 66:65-75
7. Childers NK, Bruce MG, McGhee JR (1989) Molecular Mechanisms of Immunoglobulin A Defense. Ann Rev Microbiol 43:503-536
8. Craig SW, Cebra JJ (1971) Peyer's Patches: An Enriched Source of Precursors for IgA-Producing Immunocytes in the Rabbit. J Exp Med 134:188-196
9. Croitoru K, Ernst PB (to be published) Leukocytes in the Intestinal Epithelium: An Unusual Immunological Compartment Revisited. Regional Immunology.
10. Czerkinsky C, Prince SJ, Michalek SM et al (1987) IgA Antibody Producing Cells in Peripheral Blood After Antigen Ingestion: Evidence for a Common Mucosal Immune System in Humans. Proc Natl Acad Aci USA 84:2449-2453
11. Dahlgren U, Ahlstedt S, Hedmkan L et al (1981) Dimeric IgA in the Rat is Transferred from Serum into Bile but not into Milk. Scand J Immunol 14:95-98
12. Franklin RM (1989) The Ocular Secretory Immune System: A Review. Curr Eye Res 8:599-606
13. Franklin RM, Malaty R, Amirpanahi F et al (1988) Neuroregulation of the Lacrimal

Gland Function. Invest Ophthalmol Vis Sci (Suppl):66
14. Franklin RM, Remus LE (1984) Conjunctival-Associated Lymphoid Tissue: Evidence for a Role in the Secretory Immune System. Invest Ophthalmol Vis Sci 25:181-187
15. Friedman MG (1990) Antibodies in Human Tears During and After Infection. Survey of Ophthalmology 35:151-157
16. Gauci M, Husband AJ, King MG (to be published) Conditioned Allergic Rhinitis: A Model for Central Nervous System and Immune System Interaction in IgE-Mediated Allergic Reactions. In: Husband AJ (ed) Behaviour & Immunity. CRC Press, Boca Raton
17. Geuze HJ, Slot JW, Strous GJ et al (1984) Intracellular Receptor Sorting During Endocytosis: Comparative Immunoelectron Microscopy of Multiple Receptors in Rat Liver. Cell 37:195-204
18. Gordon JR, Burd PR, Galli SJ (1990) Mast Cells as a Source of Multifunctional Cytokines. Immunology Today 11(12):458-464
19. Gudmuudsson OG, Sullivan DA, Bloch KJ et al (1985) The Ocular Secretory Immune System of the Rat. Exp Eye Res 40:231-238
20. Herzenberg LA, Herzenberg LA (1989) Toward a Layered Immune System. Cell 59:953-954
21. Janeway CA, Jones B, Hayday A (1988) Specificity and Function of T-Cells Bearing gamma-delta Receptors. Immunol Today 9:73-76
22. Josephson AS, Lockwood DE (1964) Immunoelectrophoretic Studies of the Protein Composition of Normal Tears. J Immunol 93:532-539
23. Kelleher RS, Hann LE, Edwards JA et al (1991) Endocrine, Neural and Immune Control of Secretory Component Output by Lacrimal Gland Acinar Cells. J Immunol 146:3405-3412
24. Kiyono H, Cooper MD, Kearney JF et al (1984) Isotype Specificity of Helper T-Cell Clones. Peyer's Patch T-Cells Preferentially Collaborate with Mature IgA B Cells for IgA Responses. J Exp Med 159:798-811
25. Kuizenga A, Stolwijk TR, van Agtmaal EJ et al (1990) Detection of Secretory IgM in Tears of IgA Deficient Individuals. Curr Eye Res 9:997-1005
26. MacDonald AB, McComb D, Howard L (1984) Immune Response of Owl Monkeys to Topical Vaccination with Irradiated Chlamydia Trachomatis. J Infect. Dis.149:439-442
27. MacQueen G, Marshall J, Perdue M et al (1989) Pavlovian Conditioning of Rat Mucosal Cells to Secrete Rat Mast Cell Protease II. Science 243:83
28. McClellan BH, Whitney CR, Lawrence P et al (1973) Immunoglobulins in Tears. Am J Ophthalmol 76:89-101
29. McGhee D, Franklin RM (1984) Lymphocyte Migration Into the Lacrimal Gland is Random. Cell Immunol 86:75-82
30. McGhee JR, Mestecky J, Elson CO et al (1989) Regulation of IgA Synthesis and Immune Response by T Cells and Interleukins. J Clin Immunol 9(3):175-199
31. Mestecky J, McGhee JR (1987) Immunoglobulin A (IgA): Molecular and Cellular Interactions Involved in IgA Biosystesis and Immune Response. Adv Immunol 40:153-245
32. Mestecky J, McGhee JR, Arnold RR et al (1978) Selective Induction of an Immune Response in Human External Secretions by Ingestion of Bacterial Antigen. J Clin Invest 6:731-737
33. Mossman TR, Coffman RL (1989) TH1 and TH2 Cells: Different Patterns of Lymphokine Secretion Lead to Different Functional Properties. Ann Rev Immunol 7:145-174
34. Mostov KE, Friedlander M, Blobel G (1984) The Receptor for Transepithelial

Transport of IgA and IgM Contains Multiple Immunoglobulin-Like Domains. Nature (London) 308:37-43
35. Nakache M, Lakey Berg E, Streeter PR et al (1989) The Mucosal Vascular Addressin is a Tissue-Specific Endothelial Cell Adhesion Molecule for Circulating Lymphocytes. Nature 337:179-181
36. Owen RL (1977) Sequential Uptake of Horseradish Peroxidase by Lymphoid Follicle Epithelium of Peyer's Patches in the Normal Unobstructed Mouse Intestine: An Ultrastructural Study. Gasteroenterolog. 72:440-451
37. Peppard JV, Randolph VM, Montgomery PC (1988) Antibody Production in Rats Following Ocular-Topical or Gastro-intestinal Immunization: Kinetics of Local and Systemic Antibody Production. Curr Eye Res 7:471-481
38. Perdue MH, Bienenstock J (1991) Immunophysiology of the Gut. Curr Opinion in Gastroenterol.7:421-431
39. Rudzik O, Clancy RL, Perey DYE et al (1975) Differential IgA Repopulation After Transfer of Autologous and Allogeneic Rabbit Peyer's Patch Cells. J Immunol 114(1):40-44
40. Sandor M, Gajewski T, Thorson J et al: CD4+ Murine T Cell Clones that Express High Levels of Immunoglobulin Binding Belong to the IL-4 Producing T_H2 Subset.
41. Schmitz M, Nunez D, Butcher EC (1988) Selective Recognition of Mucosal Lymphoid High Endothelium by Gut Intraepithelial Leukocytes. Gastroenterology 94:576-581
42. Sullivan DA: Hormonal Influence on the Secretory Immune System of the Eye. In: Freier,S (ed) The Neuroendocrine-Immune Network in CRC Reviews Chap.15
43. Sullivan DA, Allansmith MR (1987) Hormonal Influence on the Secretory Immune System of the Eye: Endocrine Interactions in the Control of IgA and Secretory Component Production by the Rat Exorbital Gland. Immunol 60(3):337-343
44. Sullivan DA, Hann LE, Soo C et al (1990) Neural Influence on the Secretory Immune System of the Lacrimal Gland. Invest Ophthalmol Vis Sci (Suppl)31:45
45. Sullivan DA, Yee L, Conners AS et al (1990) Influence of Ocular Surface Antigen on the Postnatal Accumulation of Immunoglobulin-Containing Cells in the Rat Lacrimal Gland. Immunology 71:573-580
46. Tseng J. Than A, Rosado A (1990) In Vivo Adherence of Lymphocytes to High Endothelial Venules of Peyer's Patches and Peripheral Lymph Nodes. In: MacDonald TT et al (eds) Advances in Mucosal Immunology. Kluwer Academic Publishers, London pp 227-229
47. Underdown BJ: Transcytosis by the Receptor for Polymeric Immunoglobulin. In: Metzger H (ed) Fc Receptors and the Action of Antibodies.pp 74-92
48. Underdown GJ, Schiff JM (1986) Immunoglobulin A: Strategic Defense Initiative at the Mucosal Surface. Ann Rev Immunol 4:389-417
49. van der Brugge-Gamelkoorn GJ, Claassen E, Siminia T (1986) Anti-TNP-Forming Cells in Bronchus-Associated Lymphoid Tissue (BALT) and Paratracheal Lymph Node (PTLN) of the Rat After Intratracheal Priming and Boosting with TNP-KLH. Immunology 57:405-409
50. Yednock TA, Rosen SD (1989) Lymphocyte Homing. Adv Immunol 44:313-378

Immunopathologic Consequences of Ocular Immune Privilege

J.Wayne Streilein

Abstract. The eye requires immune protection against pathogens as do other organs and tissues of the body. Recent experimental evidence indicates that the patterns of immunity evoked by antigens and pathogens in the eye are unusual and distinctive. The internal compartments of the eye - anterior chamber and vitreous cavity - represent immunologically unique and privileged sites. Antigenic materials placed in the anterior chamber and vitreous cavity reach the systemic immune apparatus primarily by blood vascular, rather than lymphatic pathways, and as a consequence a distinctive systemic immune response is elicited.
This response, termed Anterior Chamber Associated Immune Deviation, is characterized by a selective antigen-specific deficiency of T-cells that mediate delayed hypersensitivity, and of B-cells that secrete complement-fixing antibodies. Induction of Anterior Chamber Associated Immune Deviation depends upon the presence of antigen-containing eye, and an anatomically intact spleen. When these conditions are met, a unique Anterior Chamber Associated Immune Deviation-inducing signal arises from within the eye itself. This signal is carried by eye-derived dendritic cells, which migrate via the blood to the spleen. In this organ, the deviant immunity of Anterior Chamber Associated Immune Deviation is generated among T and B lymphocytes. Anterior Chamber Associated Immune Deviation and immune privilege are important in the pathogenesis of experimental models of ocular inflammatory and malignant diseases, such as progressively growing intraocular tumors, stromal herpes keratitis during the course of corneal infection with Herpes simplex virus type 1, and experimental autoimmune uveitis induced by soluble autoantigens of the retina. The existence of immune privilege in the eye represents a physiologic adaptation of the immune response to ocular antigens so that the visual axis is preserved. This is accomplished by the induction of immune effectors that mediate antigen elimination without inducing nonspecific inflammation. However, this selective immune deficiency renders the eye and the host susceptible to pathogens for which delayed hypersensitivity and complement-fixing antibodies are essential.

Introduction

Immune reponses that occur on the surface of the eye and within the internal compartments of the eye have been studied extensively over the past 20 years. The ocular surface - cornea and conjunctiva - is served by a specialization of the systemic immune apparatus that is appropriate to and protective of mucosal surfaces - the Mucosa Associated Lymphoid Tissues. Responses at the ocular surface are virtually identical to immune responses to antigens and pathogens on the mucous membranes of the oropharynx, the epithelial surfaces of the gastro-intestinal, the respiratory and the urogenital tracts of the eye, such as the anterior chamber and

(4). By contrast, the internal compartmentsvitreous cavity are not provided with conventional systemic immunity. The long-known phenomenon of immunologic privilege at these ocular sites is an expression of the fact that immune reponses to antigens and pathogens within the eye are distinctive and unusual.

Evidence that ocular immunity is unusual: Experimental studies of the immune responses directed at antigens and pathogens in the eye have provided evidence that either impaired, or excessive immune responses are possible. Moreover, the consequences of both types of responses correlate with clinical disease. Among the data that indicate that ocular immunity is impaired are the following: (a) Corneal allografts in experimental animals and in man are extraordinarily successful when compared to all other types of solid tissue allografts;
(b) Opportunistic infections occur frequently in immunocompromised patients; among the tissues particularly at risk for these infections is the eye, especially the retina;
(c) The eye is particularly prone to infections by conventional pathogens that infrequently cause infections at other tissue sites in immunocompetent individuals; and
(d) Foreign and incompatible tissue grafts can usually be placed in the anterior chamber or vitreous cavity of the eye without eliciting a destructive systemic immune response and such grafts can persist indefinitely - an expression of immunologic privilege.

Despite this evidence of impaired immunity within the eye, there is another body of experimental and clinical evidence that indicates that ocular immune responses can be excessive and damaging to the eye. Several examples can be cited:
(a) Sympathetic ophthalmia and phakoanaphylaxis are rare, but devastating complications of trauma to the eye; after injury of one eye, blindness can result from an immune response directed at unique tissue-restricted antigens of the retina and lens;
(b) Infection of the anterior surface of the eye with the Herpes simplex virus type 1 sometimes results in stromal keratitis, a serious inflammatory disorder of the stroma that is an important cause of blindness in man; experimental evidence strongly suggests that an inappropriate, vigorous immune attack upon Herpes simplex virus type 1 infected cells produces the pathology; and
(c) Acute Retinal Necrosis, a rare Herpes virus infection of the eye, occurs in immunocompetent individuals; and experimental analysis implicates a pathogenic role for Herpes-specific T effector cells.

It is the thesis of this review that in order to preserve vision, immune privilege is established in the eye by regulatory cells, which down-regulate and impair immunity to ocular antigens and pathogens. Although this altered immunity is essential for maintaining vision, in certain circumstances it renders the eye susceptible to disease. Moreover, the down-regulation of immune responses within the eye is selective, so that a few pathogens can induce an excessive immune response resulting in immunopathologic destruction of normal ocular tissue.

Anterior Chamber Associated Immune Deviation

More than 15 years ago, Kaplan and Streilein (6) discovered that alloantigenic cells placed in the anterior chamber of rat eyes elicited a deviant form of systemic immunity in which circulating antibodies were present, but the animals' ability to display cell-mediated immunity was grossly impaired. Since then, considerable experimental data have been assembled to confirm that antigens placed in the anterior chamber induce a deviant form of systemic immunity termed Anterior Chamber Associated Immune Deviation (13,16). The characteristics of Anterior Chamber Associated Immune Deviation include impaired delayed hypersensitivity resulting from an inability to activate T-cells that mediate delayed hypersensitivity (T_{DH}), and absence of antigen-specific cmomplement-fixing antibodies. At the same time, the sera of animals with Anterior Chamber Associated Immune Deviation contain antigen-specific antibodies that do not fix complement (22), and their secondary lymphoid organs contain primed antigen-specific cytotoxic T-cell precursors (pTc). The antigen-specific, selective immune deficiencies of Anterior Chamber Associated Immune Deviation are mediated in part by multiple populations of suppressor T-cells that down-regulate the induction and expression of T_{DH}-cells and B-cells that secrete complement-fixing antibodies (21). As a consequence of these deficiencies, animals with Anterior Chamber Associated Immune Deviation are unable to reject orthotopic skin allografts bearing transplantation antigens identical to antigens placed originally in the eye. In addition, they are unable to eliminate soluble antigen from the blood, since elimination is accomplished by complement fixation through opsonization of antigen-antibody complexes.

Induction of Anterior Chamber Associated Immune Deviation occurs during the initial 4-5 days following injection of antigen (or pathogen) in the anterior chamber, and during this time both an anatomically intact eye and a spleen are essential (23). Enucleation of the antigen-containing eye during this interval, or extirpation of the spleen, aborts Anterior Chamber Associated Immune Deviation induction; such animals develop conventional immune responses to the anterior chamber injected antigen.

These results have given rise to the concept of a camerosplenic axis in which immunologic information in the form of an Anterior Chamber Associated Immune Deviation-inducing signal is transmitted from the antigen-containing eye to the spleen via the blood. In the spleen, the Anterior Chamber Associated Immune Deviation inducing signal is recognized by T and B lymphocytes in a distinctive manner, giving rise to the unique spectrum of effectors associated with Anterior Chamber Associated Immune Deviation.

Features of the Anterior Chamber Pertinent to Its Privileged Status

Microanatomical and molecular features of the anterior chamber are known to be important in conferring immune privilege upon this site. Among the important features are the following:

(a) Blood-Ocular Barrier:

The blood vessels that supply the internal compartments of the eye possess (directly or indirectly) a barrier, which dictates the type and amount of leukocytes and macromolecules that can enter the eye from the blood. Lymphocytes, monocytes and granulocytes normally enter the anterior chamber under controlled conditions, presumably mediated by cell-adhesion molecules rather than by simple diapedesis. Tight junctions uniting the endothelial cells of iris capillaries, and similar unions among ciliary epithelial cells, stringently control the entry of molecules from the blood into the eye.

(b) Lymphatic Drainage Pathway:

Under normal circumstances the internal compartment of the eye virtually lacks a demonstrable lymphatic drainage system. Thus, antigens within the eye are denied access to the lymphatics and draining regional lymph nodes which is a primary pathway for antigens in the periphery to mobilize conventional immune responses. Instead, the aqueous humor of the anterior chamber drains via the trabecular meshwork directly into the blood vasculature. In general, antigens injected directly into the blood stream are first recognized immunologically in the spleen, rather than lymph nodes and therefore antigens from the anterior chamber would also be expected to impact the systemic immune apparatus first within the spleen.

(c) Eye as an Antigen Depot:

Soluble antigens (and other molecules) injected into the anterior chamber rapidly exit via the trabecular meshwork and can be easily detected in the blood. However, a significant portion of the injected material is also retained in the eye, only to be released into the blood very slowly over the next several days to weeks (20). The capacity of the eye to function as a depot, which is not a significant feature of subcutaneous injection sites, allows for antigen to be present in the blood for protracted intervals of time. It is known that this pattern of antigen availability strongly influences the character of systemic immune responses.

(d) Intraocular Antigen Presenting Cells:

During conventional immune responses, professional antigen presenting cells that express class II major histocompatibility complex (MHC) molecules on their surface play a central and critical role in preparing antigens for presentation to T and B lymphocytes. Most tissues of the body are replete with these types of bone marrow-derived (dendritic) cells. However, the tissues that surround the anterior chamber - cornea, iris, ciliary body - contain far fewer class II MHC^{+}cells than do other tissues (24). In the stroma of the iris and ciliary body there are numerous bone marrow-derived dendritic appearing cells that express class I but not class II MHC molecules. These cells have been shown to be capable of capturing antigens in the anterior chamber and delivering an Anterior Chamber Associated Immune Deviation-inducing signal via the blood to the spleen (19).

(e) Immunosuppressive Intraocular Microenvironment:

The aqueous humor has been demonstrated to be profoundly immunosuppressive by virtue of its content of cytokines, such as Transforming Growth Factor-beta and alpha-Melanocyte Stimulating Hormone (17). These, and perhaps other cytokines and mediators are constitutively present in normal aqueous humor due to their continuous synthesis and release by parenchymal cells of the iris and ciliary body (presumably the epithelial cells). Aqueous humor and TGF-ß possess the capacity to inhibit antigen-processing and presentation by professional antigen-presenting cells, and to impair the activation of primed T-cells exposed to antigen-bearing antigen presenting cells. An expression of the immunosuppressive nature of the anterior chamber, at least in mouse eyes, is the inability of this site to display delayed hypersensitivity responses and graft-versus-host reactions (3).

In the aggregate, these features of the anterior chamber, as well as features yet to be described, account for the facts that induction and expression of immune response to ocular antigens is unusual and deviant.

Anterior Chamber Associated Immune Deviation and Ocular Immunopathology

Study of the Anterior Chamber Associated Immune Deviation phenomenon in mice and rats has included an exploration of several experimental diseases with important clinical counterparts: Intraocular tumors, stromal keratitis and autoimmune uveoretinitis. The role of Anterior Chamber Associated Immune Deviation in the immunopathogenesis of each of these experimental models will be related and discussed in this section.

Immune Privilege and the Threat of Intraocular Tumors: Although immunogenic tumor cells are rejected promptly when implanted at subcutaneous or other conventional body sites, these tumors are frequently not rejected when injected into the anterior chamber of the eye. Niederkorn and Streilein and their many collaborators (7,8,9,14,15) have studied extensively the nature of immune responses to immunogenic intraocular tumors in order to determine why these tumors are not rejected, and in an effort to develop immunotherapeutic strategies that could be used to eliminate intraocular tumors. One model system has been used extensively and utilizes the mast cell tumor, P815, which was originally derived from DBA/2 mice. Inoculation of P815 cells into the anterior chamber of BALB/e mice (in which tumor cells express multiple minor transplantation antigens) results in a progressively growing intracameral tumor that will eventually spread throughout the globe, penetrate through the scleral capsule, and kill the host by direct extension into the cranial vault. Mice bearing P815 tumors in the anterior chamber display Anterior Chamber Associated Immune Deviation: They are unable to reject DBA/2 skin grafts, and they cannot mount delayed hypersensitivity to DBA/2 antigens. However, their secondary lymphoid organs contain large numbers of DBA/2-specific pTc, which eventually infiltrate and accumulate within the tumor-containing eye. However, this infiltration does not lead to tumor rejection. Ksander and coworkers (1,10) have found that the central defect in mice with P815-induced Anterior Chamber Associated Immune Deviation is the absence of T-cells that mediate delayed hypersensitivity and secrete lymphokines (such as IL-4, gamma-interferon). These lymphokines are required for the terminal differentiation of pTc into fully functional cytotoxic T-cells.

When P815 cells are injected subconjunctivally, a conventional immune site, a measurable tumor never develops, and complete rejection of the tumor cells occurs within 8-12 days. Elimination of tumor cells is correlated early with infiltration of the subconjunctival site with pTc, followed by infiltration of T_{DH} cells (11). Shortly thereafter, cytotoxic T-cells emerge, and these cells then proceed to destroy the tumor cells. Based on these results, it has been proposed that the failure of pTc that infiltrate anterior chamber P815-tumors to cause tumor rejection is due to the inability of the host immune system to deliver lymphokine-secreting T_{DH}-cells to the tumor site. In addition, since the aqueous humor is profoundly immunosuppressive, and since its suppressive influence is particularly effective against T_{DH}, even if T_{DH} were generated by mice with Anterior Chamber Associated Immune Deviation it is unlikely that they could respond to P815 antigens and release lymphokines in this hostile intraocular environment.

The failure of the immune system to restrain P815 tumors in the eyes of BALB/e mice results from the induction of the deviant systemic immune response that is deficient in those types of immune effectors (T_{DH}) that are required for rejection. This failure is compounded by the resistance of the anterior chamber to expression of cell-mediated immunity which further reduces the likelihood that an effective anti-tumor immune response could be mounted (3). We suspect that similar immune factors operate in human intraocular tumors, and it is hoped that experimental analysis of murine intraocular tumors will guide us to develop immunotherapies that could be directed at human tumors.

Immunopathogenesis of Herpes Simplex Virus Type 1-Induced Stromal Keratitis: Stromal keratitis occurs as recurrent disease in a subset of human beings with corneal Herpes Simplex Virus Type 1 infections. In experimental animals, strong circumstantial evidence links the pathogenesis of acute stromal keratitis to an immune attack directed at Herpes Simplex Virus-infected corneal cells. According to this concept, stromal keratitis is not the direct consequence of virus-induced cellular pathology, but rather represents damage to virus-infected cells attacked by virus-specific T lymphocytes. Sundmacher (18) has proposed that stromal keratitis as well as other forms of deep ocular disease associated with Herpes Simplex Virus Type 1 infection, is due to excessive, Herpes Simplex Virus specific delayed hypersensitivity. We became interested in this hypothesis when it was discovered that stromal keratitis developed in eyes of Herpes Simplex Virus Type 1 infected mice that previously contained corneal degeneration (25). In uninfected eyes with corneal degeneration, the overlying epithelium of the cornea is infiltrated with Langerhans cells. Under normal circumstances, the corneal epithelium, except at the limbus, is virtually devoid of Langerhans cells; however, Langerhans cells can be induced to migrate into the corneal epithelium by light cauterization of the central corneal surface. The reason why this is important is that Anterior Chamber Associated Immune Deviation cannot be induced in eyes in which the cornea already contains Langerhans cells in the central epithelium.

Thus, it was speculated, that there may be a relationship between the presence of corneal Langerhans cells, the induction of delayed hypersensitivity to Herpes Simplex Virus Type 1 antigens during corneal infection with this virus, and the development of stromal keratitis. To test this possibility, an experimental model system was devised in which BALB/e mice received a snout infection with a strain of Herpes Simplex Virus Type 1 (SC16) that spreads in zosteriform fashion to infect the ipsilateral anterior ocular segment within 3-4 days. In the vast majority of mice only a mild (or no) inflammation develops in these eyes, and the virus is cleared within 6-8 days.

In the experiment, the corneal surfaces of eyes of mice to be infected in this manner were cauterized in order to deploy Langerhans cells within the central epithelium at the same time as virus was expected to reach the anterior segment. The mice were then evaluated for (a) the incidence and severity of stromal keratitis and (b) the time of onset of Herpes Simplex Virus-specific delayed hypersensitivity.

It was found (12) that mice with Langerhans cell-containing corneas developed a high incidence of stromal keratitis, and the intensity of keratitis was quite severe. By contrast, mice with normal corneas at the time of Herpes Simplex Virus Type 1 infection developed a very low incidence of keratitis, and in these mice only mild disease was observed. In concert with these findings, mice with Langerhans cell-containing corneas displayed virus-specific delayed hypersensitivity as early as four days after snout infection, whereas mice with normal corneas did not give systemic evidence of virus-specific delayed hypersensitivity until 6 days after snout infection. It was concluded that stromal keratitis occurs in Herpes Simplex Virus Type 1 infected corneas only when host mice had already acquired the capacity to respond to virus-infected cells with delayed hypersensitivity. If systemic delayed hypersensitivity reactivity was delayed in onset until after virus had been cleared from the cornea, stromal disease did not develop.

Although the factors that appear to govern stromal keratitis in this system are multiple, and their interactions are undoubtedly complicated, we feel that the following scenario presents a reasonable explanation of the pathogenic process. Stromal keratitis results from a vigorous delayed hypersensitivity attack upon corneas simultaneously infected with Herpes Simplex Virus Type 1. Under normal circumstances, zosteriform spread of virus from a mucocutaneous infection site to the anterior segment of the eye is rapid, and viral antigens present in the eye induce a transient state of Herpes Simplex Virus-specific Anterior Chamber Associated Immune Deviation. The result is that systemic emergence of virus-specific delayed hypersensitivity is delayed until virus has been largely eliminated from the corneal tissue, presumably by non-specific host defense mechanisms. However, if Langerhans cells are already present in the corneal epithelium at the time virus first arrives in the anterior segment of the eye, then delayed hypersensitivity, rather than Anterior Chamber Associated Immune Deviation, is induced. Since viral antigens are still present within the cornea, T_{DH} cells infiltrate and generate a local delayed hypersensitivity response that is manifest as stromal keratitis.

In this scenario, the normal state, in which Langerhans cells are absent from the cornea, promotes Anterior Chamber Associated Immune Deviation induction which turns out to protect the eye from a blinding immunopathogenic process. Thus, under these circumstances, the impaired immune response of Anterior Chamber Associated Immune Deviation acts to the host's advantage rather than its detriment.

Anterior Chamber Associated Immune Deviation in the Pathogenesis of Autoimmune Uveitis: The retina of the eye contains numerous soluble molecules which can be used as antigens to induce experimental uveoretinitis. Retinal S-antigen and Interphotoreceptor-Retinol-Binding-Protein are two examples. The latter molecules, when combined with adjuvant and injected subcutaneously along with pertussis toxin in to B10.A mice, produce within 12-16 days bilateral uveoretinitis that persists for at least 14 days (2). In this disease, intraocular inflammation is initiated and mediated by immune effectors specific for the Interphotoreceptor-Retinol-Binding-Protein molecule as an autoantigen. Since anterior chamber injection of soluble antigens has been demonstrated to induce Anterior Chamber Associated Immune Deviation, and since Anterior Chamber Associated Immune Deviation lacks immune effectors that cause intense inflammation, we wondered whether Anterior Chamber Associated Immune Deviation could be induced by Interphotoreceptor-Retinol-Binding-Protein, and if so, whether Anterior Chamber Associated Immune Deviation would correlate with a reduced incidence and severity of uveoretinitis. To examine this question, B10.A mice received an anterior chamber injection of Interphotoreceptor-Retinol-Binding-Protein; 7 days later, the animals received a uveitogenic regimen comprised of adjuvant and pertussis toxin (5). Mice that first received Interphotoreceptor-Retinol-Binding-Protein via the anterior chamber failed to develop Interphotoreceptor-Retinol-Binding-Protein-specific delayed hypersensitivity, whereas mice that received Interphotoreceptor-Retinol- Binding- Protein first via the subconjunctival space displayed vigorous delayed hypersensitivity. More importantly, none of the mice that encountered Interphotoreceptor-Retinol- Binding- Protein via the anterior chamber developed posterior retinitis, whereas virtually all positive controls developed bilateral ocular disease. In subsequent experiments, spleen cells were harvested from mice with Interphotoreceptor-Retinol-Binding-Protein-induced Anterior Chamber Associated Immune Deviation, and used as possible suppressors of Interphotoreceptor-Retinol-Binding-Protein-induced experimental allergic uveoretinitis in normal mice. It was found that Anterior Chamber Associated Immune Deviation-spleen cells were able to suppress experimental allergic uveoretinitis if the cells were injected prior to immunization, or prior to onset of ocular inflammation. More impressive, Anterior Chamber Associated Immune Deviation-spleen cells were even able to suppress already established intraocular inflammation; inflammation disappeared clinically from eyes of mice with experimental allergic uveoretinitis within 24-48 hours of systemic injection of Anterior Chamber Associated Immune Deviation suppressor cells. These results not only indicate that Anterior Chamber Associated Immune Deviation can be used to prevent experimental allergic uveoretinitis, but that the suppressor cells of Anterior Chamber Associated Immune Deviation can be used as specific immunotherapeutic entities to eliminate ongoing intraocular disease.

It is known that soluble molecules of retinal origin, such as S-antigen and Interphotoreceptor-Retinol-Binding-Protein, are released albeit in small quantities, from the normal retina and can be found in the aqueous humor and even in the blood. Similarly, resting unprimed S-antigen specific T lymphocytes have been detected within the peripheral blood of normal human beings. Thus, it would appear that the potential to respond to retinal antigens exists in normal individuals, and that exposure to these antigens is a daily occurrence. We suspect that continuous release of retinal antigens from the eye via the trabecular meshwork may represent a "natural" Anterior Chamber Associated Immune Deviation experiment, in which soluble intraocular antigens induce protracted antigen-specific suppression of the immune system. The fact that only some genetically defined strains of animals can develop experimental allergic uveitis implies that host genes govern the expression of this autoimmune disease. We suspect that polymorphic host genes may dictate the effectiveness with which Anterior Chamber Associated Immune Deviation can be induced and/or maintained and therefore, abrogation of Anterior Chamber Associated Immune Deviation may be an important component of experimental allergic uveoretinitis susceptibility.

Discussion

The need for immune protection against pathogens is universal for all tissues including the eye. Therefore, immune privilege can not be ascribed to an inability of the immune system to become aware of antigens and pathogens in the eye. The explanation and importance of immune privilege stems from the realization that antigens placed in, or arising from the eye make a significant impact on the host's immune apparatus resulting in a highly regulated, stereotypic, antigen-specific systemic immune response.

In carrying out its responsibilities of protecting the body against an enormous array of potential pathogens, the immune system has acquired a wide range of effector modalities, each of which addresses particular types of pathogens in particular types of situations. No single immune effector is able to eliminate all pathogens, and no single immune effector is appropriate within each and every unique tissue microenvironment. Although in the aggregate the diverse immune effectors, acting in concert, can provide complete protection against the universe of pathogens, the specific array of effectors that is appropriate for eye tissue and organ other varies considerably.

Delayed hypersensitivity and complement-fixing antibodies are unique among immune effectors to the extent to which recruitment of non-specific host inflammatory defenses is required in order to accomplish elimination of the offending pathogen. Unfortunately, the inflammation that accompanies delayed hypersensitivity and complement-fixing antibody-induced responses is usually intense and because the inflammation is inherently nonspecific, "innocent bystander" cells in the vicinity of the response are often harmed.

Maintenance of the precise microanatomy of the visual axis is essential to the preservation of vision. Distortions of tissue architecture that would have trivial consequences at many other tissue sites can profoundly disturb the visual axis and significantly alter the fidelity with which retinal images are formed; blindness is an inevitable consequence. In this setting, the amplified inflammation that typically accompanies delayed hypersensitivity and complement-fixing antibody-mediated immunity represents a serious threat to vision, and therefore life. Based on these considerations, we believe that immune privilege and its cellular mechanism, Anterior Chamber Associated Immune Deviation, is a physiologic adaptation that provides the eye with a limited array of immune effector modalities to ward off pathogens, and the expression of these effector modalities is appropriate within the eye, since maintenance of the visual axis is assured.

However, this adaptation represents a compromise between the eye and the immune system. As in all compromises, each participant realizes gains and losses. In the case of the eye, preservation of vision is achieved while rendering the eye susceptible to those pathogens for which delayed hypersensitivity and complement-fixing antibodies are essential for eradication. Examples for pathogens of this type include intraocular tumors, infections with Herpes Simplex Virus Type 1, and Onchocerciasis. It is likely that the success of immunogenic intraocular tumors, persistent infections with Herpes Simplex Virus Type 1, and ocular onchocerciasis may be circumstances that reveal the price the eye pays for the compromise that creates immune privilege. In the case of the immune system, Anterior Chamber Associated Immune Deviation induced by ocular antigens represents a systemic pattern of immune reactivity, not merely a unique immune response limited to the eye. Therefore, the ocular vulnerabilities to pathogens first encountered through the eye extend to all other tissues of the body, where impaired cell-mediated immunity may prove life-threatening.

It is now well appreciated that immune privilege in the eye is not absolute. That is, not all foreign tissue grafts placed in the anterior chamber survive indefinitely. Moreover, while Anterior Chamber Associated Immune Deviation induced by antigens first introduced into the eye, is a universal response, Anterior Chamber Associated Immune Deviation may be transient as is the case with alloantigens encoded by the Major Histocompatibility Complex. The factors that determine whether immune privilege and Anterior Chamber Associated Immune Deviation are permanent have yet to be described completely.

However, it is clear that under certain circumstances the systemic immune response to ocular antigens avoids, or overcomes Anterior Chamber Associated Immune Deviation, and is characterized by the entire array of immune effectors including delayed hypersensitivity and complement-fixing antibodies. It is presumed that these circumstances will be found to concern life-threatening infections with pathogens. In these instances, host survival becomes the paramount concern, and destruction of the visual apparatus, and blindness, are the unfortunate result.

Reaching an understanding of the cellular and molecular factors that determine whether Anterior Chamber Associated Immune Deviation or conventional immunity will be elicited by antigens and pathogens within the eye will eventually prove to be important to developing immunotherapeutic strategies for many chronic and blinding ocular inflammatory and malignant diseases.

Acknowledgement. Part of this work was supported by USPHS grant EY-05678.

References

1. Bando Y, Ksander BR, Streilein JW (1991) Characterization of Specific T-Helper Cell Activity in Mice Bearing Alloantigenic Tumors in the Anterior Chamber of the Eye. Eur J Immunol 21:1923-1932
2. Caspi RR, Roberge FG, Chan CC et al (1988) A New Model of Autoimmune Disease: Experimental Autoimmune Uveoretinitis Induced in Mice with Two Different Retinal Antigens. J Immunol 140:1490-1502
3. Cousins SW, Trattler WB, Streilein JW (1991) Immune Privilege and Suppression of Immungenic Inflammation in the Anterior Chamber of the Eye. Curr Eye Res 10:287-297
4. Franklin RM, Remus LE (1984) Conjunctiva-Associated Lymphoid Tissue: Evidence for a Role in the Secretory Immune System. Invest Ophthalmol Vis Sci 25:181-187
5. Hara Y, Caspi RR, Wiggert B et al (1991) Effect of Anterior Chamber Associated Immune Deviation Induction on Expression of IRBP-Specific Delayed Hypersensitivity and EAU in Mice. Invest Ophthalmol Vis Sci 32:791
6. Kaplan HJ, Streilein JW (1977) Immune Response to Immunization Via the Anterior Chamber of the Eye. I. F_1 Lymphocyte Induced Immune Deviation. J Immunol 118:809-814
7. Knisely TL, Luckenbach MW, Fischer BJ et al (1987) Destructive and Non-Destructive Patterns of Immune Rejection of Syngeneic Intraocular Tumors. J Immunol 138:4515-4523
8. Ksander BR, Mammolenti M, Streilein JW (1991) Immune Privilege in the Anterior Chamber of the Eye Terminates When Tumor Infiltrating Lymphocytes Acquire Cytolytic Function. Transplantation 52: 128-132
9. Ksander BR, Streilein JW (1989) Analysis of Cytotoxic T-Cell Responses to Intracameral Allogeneic Tumors. I. Quantitative and Qualitative Analysis of Cytotoxic Precursor and Effector Cells. Invest Ophthalmol Vis Sci 30:323-329
10. Ksander BR, Streilein JW (1989) Immune Privilege to MHC Disparate Tumor Grafts in the Anterior Chamber of the Eye. I. Quantitavite Analysis of Intraocular Tumor Growth and the Corresponding Delayed Hypersensitivity Response. Transplantation 47:661-667
11. Ksander BR, Streilein JW (1989) Recovery of Activated Cytotoxic T-Cells from Minor H Incompatible Tumor Graft Rejection Sites. J Immunol 143:426-431
12. McLeish W, Rubsamen P, Atherton SS et al (1989) Immunobiology of Langerhans Cells on the Ocular Surface. II.Role of Central Corneal Langerhans Cells in Stromal Keratitis Following Experimental HSV-1 Infection in Mice. Regional Immunol 2:236-243
13. Niederkorn JY (1990) Immune Privilege and Immune Regulation in the Eye. Adv Immunol 48:191-226
14. Niederkorn JY, Streilein JW, Shadduck JA (1980) Deviant Immune Responses to Allogeneic Tumors Injected Intracamerally and Subcutaneously in Mice. Invest Ophthalmol Vis Sci 20:355-363
15. Streilein JW, Niederkorn JY (1985) Characterization of the Suppressor Cell(s) Responsible for Anterior-Chamber Associated Immune Deviation (Anterior Chamber Associated Immune Deviation) Induced in BALB/e Mice by P815 Cells. J Immunol 134:1381-1387
16. Streilein JW (1987) Immune Regulation and the Eye: A Dangerous Compromise. The FASEB J. 1:199-208
17. Streilein JW, Cousins SW (1990) Aqueous Humor Factors and Their Effect on the Immune Response in te Anterior Chamber. Curr Eye Res 144:175-182

18. Sundmacher R (1987) Clinical Aspects of Herpetic Eye Diseases. Curr Eye Res 6:183-188

19. Wilbanks GA, Mamolenti M, Streilein JW (1991) Studies on the Induction of the Anterior Chamber Associated Immune Deviation (Anterior Chamber Associated Immune Deviation). II.Eye-Derived Cells Participate in Generating Blood Borne Signals that Induce Anterior Chamber Associated Immune Deviation. J Immunol 146:3018-3024

20. Wilbanks GA, Streilein JW (1989) The Differing Patterns of Antigen Release and Local Retention Following Anterior Chamber and Intravenous Inoculation of Soluble Antigen. Evidence that the Eye Acts as an Antigen Depot. Regional Immunol 2:390-398

21. Wilbanks GA, Streilein JW (1990) Characterization of Suppressor Cells in Anterior Chamber Associated Immune Deviation (Anterior Chamber Associated Immune Deviation) Induced by Soluble Antigen.Evidence of Two Functionally and Phenotypically Distinct T-Suppressor Cell Populations. Immunology 71:383-389

22. Wilbanks GA, Streilein JW (1990) Distinctive Humoral Responses Following Anterior Chamber and Intravenous Administration of Soluble Antigen. Evidence for Active Suppression of IgG_{2a}-Secreting B-Cells. Immunology 71:566-572

23. Wilbanks GA, Streilein JW (1991) Studies on the Induction of the Anterior Chamber Associated Immune Deviation (Anterior Chamber Associated Immune Deviation). I. Evidence that an Antigen-Specific, Anterior Chamber Associated Immune Deviation-Inducing Cell-Associated Signal Exists in the Peripheral Blood. J Immunol. 146:2610-2617

24. Williamson JSP, Bradley D, Streilein JW (1989) Immunoregulatory Properties of Bone Marrow Derived-Cells in the Iris and Ciliary Body. Immunology 67:96-102

25. Williamson JSP, DiMarco S, Streilein JW (1987) Immunobiology of Langerhans Cells on the Ocular Surface. I. Langerhans Cells Within the Central Cornea Interfere with Induction of Anterior Chamber Associated Immune Deviation. Invest Oph thalmol Vis Sci 28: 1527-1532

II. THE OUTER EYE

Staphylococci and the Outer Eye: Relationship of Colonisation and Immunity to Disease

Peter Wright, Linda Ficker and David Seal

Abstract. Animal studies have shown that cell-mediated immunity to S.aureus is an absolute necessity for the production of ulcerative blepharitis, phlyctenules and marginal infiltrates. In patients with blepharitis of mixed etiology, only 40% showed enhanced cell-mediated immunity to S.aureus. It was associated with folliculitis and marginal keratitis requiring topical steroid therapy. It was not associated with meibomianitis.
High counts of S.aureus were found on the lids of all atopes and patients with acute folliculitis. S.aureus was present on lids of 9% of patients with chronic blepharitis, both those with and without enhanced cell-mediated immunity. Coagulase Negative Staphylococci colonised all lids. Normal controls and patients with blepharitis showed similar quantitative cultures and biotypes. All isolates of S.aureus produced alpha lysin whilst 73% of coagulase negative Staphylococci isolates produced epsilon toxin. No evidence was found of toxin-producing strains specific for blepharitis. The frequency of marginal keratitis was not different in patients with and without enhanced cell-mediated immunity to S.aureus protein A.
The enhanced group showed an increased need for corticosteroid therapy compared to those without enhanced cell-mediated immunity. No relationship could be shown between atopy and enhanced cell-mediated immunity to S.aureus.

Introduction

The expression of acute infection by S.aureus can include purulent conjunctivitis, ulcerative folliculitis and microbial keratitis but these conditions are uncommon and easily managed compared to chronic blepharitis. The acute infection responds well to anti-staphylococcal antibiotics such as Fucidin and Gentamicin but recurrences occur. Secondary effects of blepharitis include involvement of the cornea with a phlyctenular response or marginal ulceration.

The etiology of chronic blepharitis and recurrent marginal keratitis is more complex. Both S.aureus and coagulase-negative Staphylococci can intermittently be isolated from the lid margins. Many theories have been proposed for their role in disease including toxins (18), lipases (4) (splitting meibomian triglycerides to toxic fatty acids) and delayed-type hypersensitivity (12). A clinical classification has been suggested to separate patients with "staphylococcal" blepharitis and its complications from those with seborrhoea, meibomianitis and other types of inflammatory lid disease (16). Unfortunately, most of these theories have not been supported by later clinical and laboratory studies.

We have explored the area of interaction between colonisation and immunity as a mechanism for causing disease in 116 patients with blepharitis. One hundred and eleven suffered from chronic disease, five had recurrent acute infections (folliculitis) and thirty-seven suffered from marginal keratitis.

Role of Lid Colonisation by Staphylococci

The expected number of S.aureus and coagulase-negative Staphylococci organisms on the normal lid margin has been assessed in 100 volunteers using soluble alginate swabs (1) when values were expressed as colony forming units (cfu) per ml swab. S.aureus was isolated from 6% of the volunteers at a count of 1-10 cfu/ml swab. A count of >15 cfu/ml swab represented an expected distinction between colonisation and infection ($p=0.01$). For coagulase-negative Staphylococci, counts were expressed for each Baird-Parker Scheme biotype.

There was an overall isolation rate from lids of 88%, with 74%, 11% and 3% of these isolates belonging to biotypes II/III, IV/V and VI. Counts of type II/III did not occur at >1000 cfu/ml swab and IV-VI at not >100 cfu/ml swab.

In a study of 116 patients with chronic blepharitis (5), S.aureus counts occurred in 5 patients with recurrent acute folliculitis at 194, 206, 400, 178 and 46 cfu/ml swab indicating active infection (>15 cfu/ml swab).

We isolated S.aureus from 8 (7.2%) patients with chronic blepharitis at counts <15 cfu/ml swab. We compared isolation rates between patients without and with enhanced delayed-type hypersensitivity to S.aureus protein A (refer to next section), and between the traditional lid "scrub" and soluble swab techniques (5). Results for the lid "scrub" technique were 22% for patients without and 26% with enhancement and for the soluble swab technique were 8.6% and 10.6% respectively. There was no significant difference in lid colonisation rates for blepharitic patients with and without enhanced delayed-type hypersensitivity to S.aureus. In addition, in an earlier study using the lid "scrub" technique, only 5% of blepharitic patients had increased numbers of S.aureus (21).

Numbers and biotypes of coagulase negative Staphylococci present on the lid margin have been compared between normals (found in 88% of volunteers) and 116 patients with chronic blepharitis (19,21).

We have shown in two studies, using both swab techniques, that there is no difference between normal volunteers and patients in quantitative counts of coagulase negative Staphylococci lid isolates for each Baird-Parker Scheme biotype. Overall isolation rates of coagulase negative Staphylococci from lids of the blepharitic patients were not significantly different at 74% (21) (lid "scrub") and 63% (19) (soluble swab). Coagulase negative Staphylococci exist on blepharitic lids in normally-expected numbers.

Role of Staphylococcal Immunity

Monteil and coworkers described how the response to S.aureus infection may be affected by selective immunodeficiency (14). They investigated patients, mostly children, with failure of opsonisation and polymorphonuclear leucocyte killing of S.aureus and found they could be treated successfully with normal plasma or IgG. Some of their patients with recurrent staphylococcal infection, however, had normal staphylococcal inhibition titers. Disease that occurred was thought due to defective chemotaxis secondary to failure of C5a generation (Leiner's disease) (14) or the lazy phagocyte syndrome (6). Such children can present with recurrent carbuncles, styes, blepharitis or marginal keratitis. We suggest that patients with defective phagocytosis or intracellular polymorphonuclear leucocyte killing of S.aureus have recurrent severe inflammatory lesions due partly to the development of enhanced cell-mediated immunity to staphylococcal antigens (20).

It was Panton and coworker who first demonstrated that repeated dermal injection of the rabbit with S.aureus at different concentrations, induced delayed-type hypersensitivity due to the development of cell-mediated immunity (17). After repeated challenge, the inflammatory effect of a large inoculum of S.aureus was considerably reduced, but inocula diluted 100fold and 1000fold gave rise to inflammatory lesions where no such effect had occurred prior to challenge. Animals challenged seven times gave similar skin reactions but also developed agglutinating antibodies. These antibodies gave partial immunity to intravenous doses of S.aureus, which were fatal to control rabbits.

Johanovsky also created a rabbit model of delayed-type hypersensitivity to S.aureus. His original work demonstrating cell mediated immunity used an inoculum of homogenised spleen cells to transfer staphylococcal delayed-type hypersensitivity to normal rabbits with negative skin tests (8). Boe in 1949 had previously failed to transfer such delayed-type hypersensitivity using serum (2). Johanovsky also showed with controlled experiments that animals with delayed-type hypersensitivity to S.aureus had an increased susceptibility to, and mortality, from intravenous challenge with $2x10^6$ live cells.

Johnson and coworkers in 1961 further investigated delayed-type hypersensitivity to S.aureus in the rabbit. They injected the knee joint and the anterior chamber of the eye (9) in addition to giving intradermal injections. They induced delayed-type hypersensitivity in the skin with injections of 10^9 killed cells and elicited more severe infections in knee joints injected with 10^4 cells than occurred in controls. Susceptibility to infection in the anterior chamber, injected with $6x10^2$ S.aureus cells (this being the Infective Dose 50) was, however, similar for rabbits with and without delayed-type hypersensitivity. This demonstrated that local delayed-type hypersensitivity to S.aureus was not induced within the anterior chamber by dermal immunisation.

Boe in 1949 found that large doses of coagulase negative Staphylococci produced abscesses when injected subcutaneously as whole cells into rabbits previously given delayed-type hypersensitivity to coagulase negative Staphylococci or S.aureus but did not occur in rabbits without such delayed-type hypersensitivity (2). Conversely he was able to produce abscesses to S.aureus in rabbits which had been immunised with killed S.aureus or coagulase negative Staphylococci but not in a control rabbit that had not been immunised. Hence, cross-over of delayed-type hypersensitivity reactivity due to a common antigen, probably teichoic acid, of S.aureus and coagulase negative Staphylococci can occur in the rabbit.

Boe pointed out the parallels between patients suffering from chronic S.aureus infections and delayed-type hypersensitive rabbits. Both give exaggerated inflammatory reactions to heat-killed whole cell S.aureus vaccines, including the formation of sterile abscesses (2). He suggested that "allergy" against Staphylococci was more important than virulence factors such as alphalysin production. Thjotta (1929) had previously found that patients with "allergic" rhinitis, yielding cultures of S.aureus, had a reduction of symptoms following immunisation with killed whole cell vaccines of the autologous S.aureus, but the author did not test for delayed-type hypersensitivity; patients with hydrorrhea, devoid of sneezing, had no benefit (23).

Boe could not desensitise his rabbits with either intradermal or subcutaneous injections. It was, however, achieved by intravenous administration of a killed whole cell vaccine (2). He also successfully desensitised the rabbits by intravenous administration of a concentrated filtrate of live S.aureus cells; their skin then proved insensitive to new infections and the filtrate did not sensitise control rabbits. Three patients with chronic S.aureus skin infection, one of whom developed sterile abscesses following subcutaneous injection of a killed whole cell vaccine, received intravenous injections of live S.aureus filtrates, which produced varying degrees of shock. Treatment was successful except in one patient who developed toxicity and relapse. This could have been due to alphalysin toxin in the filtrate.

Mudd and coworkers in 1970 investigated the use of filtered staphylococcal phage lysate (250×10^6 S.aureus cells lysed by 500×10^6 phages) for hyposensitising patients with delayed-type hypersensitivity to S.aureus (15). The first three injections produced immediate-type I reactions of a wheal and flare, as given by purified protein A, which subsided by three hours and subsequently gave a delayed-type hypersensitivity response at 24 hours; the average induration on initial testing of 52 patients was 19mm. After the sixth injection the induration was reduced to 3mm. Their experience suggested, however, that the hyposensitive state was not long-lasting and was only maintained by similar injections every 2-4 weeks. There were no reported side-effects. The crude lysate probably contained protein A, peptidoglycan and teichoic acid but this was not established.

In 1982, Mondino and Kowalski produced phlyctenulae and catarrhal corneal infiltrates in rabbits previously immunised with either staphylococcal whole cell vaccines or purified cell walls. The rabbits' eyes (lids and conjunctivae) were challenged topically with viable S.aureus (13); rabbits developed corneal vascularisation and elevated nodular infiltrates often separated from the limbus by a lucid interval. Lesions only occurred in immunised rabbits that were also challenged topically.

Mondino, Caster and Dethlefs in 1987 have since developed a rabbit model of acute ulcerative blepharitis due to S.aureus. Rabbits require immunisation to gain delayed-type hypersensitivity prior to topical challenge. They develop crusting around the lashes (collarettes) with lash loss and chronic corneal infiltrates, but the meibomian glands appear normal (12).

Marginal Keratitis and the Limbus

Thygeson isolated S.aureus from the lids of 133/156 patients with catarrhal ulcers associated with chronic catarrhal conjunctivitis (24). Hogan and coworkers noted that marginal corneal infiltrates and ulcerations occasionally occurred during the course of lid infections when lid cultures usually grew S.aureus, but cultures of the ulcers were usually sterile (7). They noted that single or multiple, rounded or crescentic lesions developed in the peripheral corneal stroma separated from the limbus by a narrow rim of normal cornea. At times the multiple lesions extended to become a confluent partial ring infiltrate, 1-2mm wide but rarely deeper than the mid-stroma. They found recurrences with ulceration to be common with vascularisation occurring from the limbus. Like Mondino (12), they obtained no pathological effect by repeated topical installations of staphylococcal antigen or toxin in non-immunised rabbits. Injection of a challenging dose of staphylococcal antigen (cell wall/toxic filtrate) or toxoid alone into the central corneal stroma of rabbits, previously immunised with staphylococcal cell wall antigen or pure toxoid, did produce corneal rings. Staphylococcal cell wall antigen was twice as likely to produce the effect as toxoid.

It is the usual finding that marginal ulcers and phlyctenulae respond to topical steroid (7). While such treatment ameliorates the condition it is not curative and patients suffer recurrent marginal ulcers over many years. It is interesting that marginal ulcers and blepharitis may be asymmetrical or even unilateral. Could it be that the corneal response is a local expression of delayed-type hypersensitivity at the limbus to the intermittent presence of S.aureus colonisation on the lids in a host who has previously developed enhanced cell-mediated immunity to the organism? Such phenomena have been tentatively documented for the respiratory mucosae in "allergic" rhinitis and asthma (15,23).

Investigation of Staphylococcal Immunity: Cell-mediated Immunity

It has previously been mentioned that patients with chronic staphylococcal infections develop sterile abscesses when injected with killed whole cell staphylococcal vaccines which contained 10^9 or more cells. It has been our experience, however, that such abscesses do not occur after injecting 0.1ml intradermally (10^7 cells) of a suspension of S. aureus (NCTC 6571) or S.epidermidis (NCTC 7292). Both preparations were heat-killed and diluted in saline to $5x10^8$ cells/ml and preserved with 0.5% phenol). Both early and late flare can be assessed as well as induration at 48 hours, which represents the delayed-type hypersensitivity response.

Taubler and coworker have investigated S.aureus cell-mediated immunity in mice and have shown a 20% inhibition of macrophage migration in the presence of homologous antigen (22). We are not aware of such tests yet used to investigate patients for staphylococcal cell-mediated immunity, but they may be useful.

The cell wall of S.aureus, but not of coagulase negative Staphylococci contains protein A. This protein has been well characterised (10); in particular it binds to the Fc (fragment crystallisable) part of the antibody molecule, forming non-specific immune complexes as well as acting as an antigen to which delayed-type hypersensitivity occurs as a cell-mediated immune response. This has been investigated in rabbits by Mondino and coworkers (13) and in humans by White and Noble (26). They gave intradermal injections and assessed erythema, rather than induration, at 48 hours. They demonstrated the response expected from normals plus a reduced response that occurred in atopes. Protein A also binds to Fc receptors of IgE bound in turn to mast cells liberating histamine and, when injected intradermally, forming a wheal at 15 minutes (type I response). Patients or volunteers can be tested for an early or late delayed-type hypersensitivity response with 2.5 nanograms of purified protein A given by intradermal injection of 0.05ml of a 50 nanograms/ml freshly prepared solution of a freeze-dried preparation (Pharmacia Fine Chemicals Ltd.).

Humoral Immunity

Traditional tests measure the circulating antibody response to extracellular staphylococcal toxins or enzymes, viz. alpha-lysin and nuclease, as markers of recent acute purulent S.aureus infection, but they do not reflect the immunological response to the staphylococcal cell wall. In their rabbit model, Mondino and co-workers found anti-teichoic acid antibodies to be raised following immunisation with staphylococcal cell walls (13), and such antibodies are variably found in the human following S.aureus infection. They can be measured by an enzyme-linked immunosorbent assay technique (5), which is sensitive enough for their assay in tears, but only limited quantities of teichoic acid are available commercially. We prepared our own antigen.

Atopic patients with hyperimmunoglobulinemia E, who also have defective polymorphonuclear leukocytes chemotaxis, can develop "cold" staphylococcal abscesses (Job's syndrome) (3). Twenty-one percent of total IgE in such patients specifically binds to the S.aureus cell wall compared with 2% in controls, but the authors were uncertain whether this was cause or effect. One of their 16 patients studied had asymmetrical polyarthritis and bilateral keratoconjunctivitis with scarred, thinned corneae attributed to an immunological reaction to S.aureus. How this syndrome relates to atopy, where lids are often colonised with large numbers of S.aureus in the absence of clinical signs is unclear as is the association between IgE specific for S.aureus and delayed-type hypersensitivity (25).

It may be that enhanced delayed-type hypersensitivity to S.aureus due to a polymorphonuclear leukocyte defect, with increased concentration of staphylococcal antigen in macrophages, is a pre-requisite in the atopic patient for the development of specific IgE to S.aureus. This may in turn result in chronic inflammation at local sites of S.aureus antigen.

Relationship of Blepharitis and Cell-Mediated Immunity, Expressed as a Delayed-Type Hypersensitivity Response to Protein A of S.aureus

We tested the response of a control group of eight normal subjects and 116 patients with chronic blepharitis to the intradermal injection of 2.5 nanograms of purified protein A (5). Values for normal subjects were a mean of 3.9mm with a standard deviation of 6.3, which are similar to those of White and Noble (26). Protein A gave a wheal and flare reaction at 15 minutes in all normal subjects and patients tested. Of 116 patients, 69 (60%) gave a normal response (0-20mms) while 28 (24%) and 19 (16%) gave enhanced and very enhanced reactions respectively at 20-60 and greater than 60mms (5).

These results showed that 40% of a randomly selected group of blepharitics attending a specialist External Diseases Clinic have enhanced cell-mediated immunity to S.aureus protein A, which is abnormal. Marginal keratitis occurred in patients with out enhancement but there was a trend in patients with enhancement for treatment with topical steroids (5).

Relationship of Blepharitis and Cell-Mediated Immunity to Killed S.aureus Cells

We tested the cell-mediated immune response of our 116 blepharitic patients to the intradermal injection of 10^7 killed cells of S.aureus (5). Patients could be divided into two groups at less than 5mm induration (n=82 mean value 2.0) and at greater than 5mm (n=34). The latter were considered to give an enhanced cell-mediated immunity effect to S.aureus, with a mean induration value of 9.5mm (standard deviation 4.1). Of these 34 patients, 21 gave an enhanced response as well to protein A. Similarly, patients with an enhanced response to protein A gave significant enhancement to killed S.aureus cells (p=0.001) but not to S.epidermidis (coagulase negative Staphylococci) cells. Patients with a normal response to protein A and normal subjects gave no significant response of induration to either S.aureus or S.epidermidis cells.

Staphylococcal phage lysate (Staphage Lysate, Delmont Laboratories Inc., Swathmoore,PA,USA) is a sterile vaccine containing components of the S.aureus cell wall, bacteriophage and culture medium. It is prepared by lysing cultures of S.aureus (serologic types I and III) with a polyvalent staphylococcus bacteriophage. Sterility is achieved by ultrafiltration. Neither heat nor preservative are used in its preparation. Mudd and coworkers showed that such a preparation of staphylococcal phage lysate could be used to desensitise the cell-mediated immunity effect shown to S.aureus (15). New patients are first tested intradermally with 0.02ml staphylococcal phage lysate. Each ml contains approximately 1.5×10^8 lysed S.aureus cells and 5.0×10^8 bacteriophage plaque units. The preparation contains protein A besides other cell wall and intra-cellular products, which gives a type I wheal and flare response 15 minutes after injection as well as a delayed-type hypersensitivity effect with induration. With repeated weekly injections of increasing dose, tolerance can be acquired ascribed to the production of IgG blocking antibodies. Monthly injections are then required to maintain tolerance. Sterile abscesses are not reported to occur as with killed whole cell staphylococcal vaccines, probably because the lysed staphylococcal cell does not act to enhance the presence of cell mediated immunity but rather leads to its suppression by stimulating production of blocking antibody. Topical use is not recommended, although the manufacturer suggests that drops of staphylococcal phage lysate may be placed in the conjunctival sac.

Relationship of Blepharitis and Cell-Mediated Immunity to Killed Coagulase-Negative Staphylococcal Cells

We could not elicit a delayed-type hypersensitivity response to killed S.epidermidis (coagulase negative Staphylococci) cells in either our eight normal subjects or our 116 blepharitic patients. This lack of response occurred despite finding a delayed-type hypersensitivity response to S.aureus in 40% of our blepharitic patients. These results contrast with those of Boe (2) and Mondino (11) and others in the past, who have been able to induce cell-mediated immunity to coagulase negative Staphylococci in the rabbit. This demonstrates the difference in expression of the immunological response to an antigen between the rabbit and the human and therefore, the danger of extrapolating results of protective or other immunity found in such animal experiments to the human situation. Mondino and coworkers could not induce acute ulcerative blepharitis in the rabbit with coagulase negative Staphylococci as they could with S.aureus, even though the rabbit developed a delayed-type hypersensitivity response to coagulase negative Staphylococci cell walls. This suggests that S.aureus protein A may be the most important cell wall component for inducing an exaggerated cell mediated immune response and contributing to the acute ulcerative blepharitic process in the rabbit.

Relationship of S.aureus and Chronic Allergic Conjunctivitis

A study has been undertaken to determine whether the expression of chronic allergic eye disease (thickening of lid margins, blepharitis, conjunctival scarring and in some patients corneal disease) in atopes could be related to lid colonisation by S.aureus (25). It was found that lids of atopes who had dermatitis, but who lacked ocular disease, were colonised with S.aureus on approximately 80% of occasions, of which 50 yielded a heavy growth. Similarly, we found eye lids of 23 adults who suffered both atopic dermatitis and chronic allergic conjunctivitis to be heavily colonised with S.aureus (25). We investigated these S.aureus isolates from both groups of patients but found no difference in protein A or toxin production between them. We also found no difference between the two groups in their serum IgG or IgE antibodies to S.aureus ribitol teichoic acid (25). A delayed-type hypersensitivity response to S.aureus was not given on intradermal testing of seven patients with chronic allergic keratoconjunctivitis. These results have suggested that the humoral (IgG/IgE) or cell-mediated immunity (delayed-type hypersensitivity) response to S.aureus does not play a role in the expression of disease in chronic allergic conjunctivitis.

Relationship of Blepharitis, Atopy and Cell-Mediated Immunity to S.aureus

We have found that 28% of our 116 patients with chronic blepharitis suffered from atopy. This compares with an expected prevalence rate in the normal population of 30%. We also found that atopy was not related to the presence of cell-mediated immunity to S.aureus protein A as 27%, 27% and 29% of patients in the non-enhanced, enhanced and very enhanced groups respectively were atopic.

Although White and coworker showed that atopes can react less strongly than normals in their delayed-type hypersensitivity response to protein A (26), this effect did not occur with our blepharitic patients. We did find total suppression of delayed-type hypersensitivity to protein A in seven patients with atopic keratoconjunctivitis (25). A conundrum clearly exists.

Conclusion

Colonisation of lids with S.aureus occurs intermittently in the normal host but is excessive in the atopic patient. No direct relationship has been found between the presence of cell-mediated immunity to S.aureus and lid colonisation except in recurrent acute folliculitis. We have found that 40% of 116 patients with chronic blepharitis had enhanced cell-mediated immunity to S.aureus not found in the normal population. In addition, patients with marginal keratitis requiring treatment with steroids were more likely to have enhancement. The possibility that recurrent ulceration is due to the expression of a cell-mediated immune response at the limbus to S.aureus on the lids in patients with systemic enhancement has been discussed including the possible role for selective desensitisation. The development and requirement of cell-mediated immunity to S.aureus in animal model experiments has been reviewed and contrasted with the human situation. Coagulase negative Staphylococci were found to exist on blepharitic lids in normally-expected numbers and biotype distribution.

References

1. Badiani D, Bron A, Elkington A et al (1988) Use of a Novel Transport Method for the Quantification of the Normal Flora of the External Eye. Microb Ecol Health Dis 1:57-59
2. Boe J (1949) Investigation on the Importance of Bacterial Allergy for the Development of Cutaneous Infections due to Staphylococci. Acta Dermatol Venereol 26:111-136
3. Donabedian H, Gallin J (1983) The Hyperimmunoglobulin E Recurrent Infection (Job's Syndrome). Medicine 62:195-208
4. Dougherty JM, McCulley JP (1986) Bacterial Lipases and Chronic Blepharitis. Invest Ophthalmol Vis Sci 27:486-491
5. Ficker L, Ramakrishnan M, Seal DV et al (1991) Role of Cell-Mediated Immunity to Staphylococci in Blepharitis. Am J Ophthalmol 111:473-479
6. Foroozanfar N, Grohmann PH, Hobbs JR (1984) Abnormal Fluorescent Actin Pattern of Lazy Phagocyte Syndromes. Diag Immunol 2:25-29
7. Hogan MJ, Diaz-Bonnet V, Okumoto M et al (1962) Experimental Staphylococcal Keratitis. Invest Ophthalmol Vis Sci 1:267-272

8. Johanovsky J (1958) Role of Hypersensitivity in Experimental Staphylococcal Infection. Nature 182:1454
9. Johnson JE, Cluff LE, Goshi K (1960) Studies on the Pathogenesis of Staphylococcal Infection. J Exp Med 113:235-247
10. Langone JJ (1983) Protein A of Staphylococcus aureus and Related Immunoglobulin Receptors Produced by Streptococci and Pneumococci. In: Easmon CSF, Adlam C (eds): Staphylococci and Staphylococcal Infections. Academic Press, London 157-252
11. Mondino BJ, Adam S (1988) Ocular Immune Response to Staphylococcus Epidermidis. In: Dwight Cavanagh H (ed) The Cornea. Transactions of the World Congress on the Cornea III. Raven Press, New York 431-433
12. Mondino BJ, Caster AI, Dethlefs B (1987) A Rabbit Model of Staphylococcal Blepharitis. Arch Ophthalmol 105:409-412
13. Mondino BJ, Kowalski RP (1982) Phlyctenulae and Catarrhal Infiltrates - Occurrence in Rabbits Immunized with Staphylococcal Cell Walls. Arch Ophthalmol 100:1968-1971
14. Monteil M, Hobbs J, Citron K (1987) Selective Immunodeficiency Affecting Staphylococcal Response. Lancet ii:880-883
15. Mudd S, Taubler J, Baker AG (1970) Delayed-Type Hypersensitivity to S.aureus in Human Subjects. J Reticuloendothel Soc 8:493-498
16. McCulley JP, Dougherty JM, Deneau DG (1982) Classification of Chronic Blepharitis. Ophthalmology 89:1173-1179
17. Panton PN, Valentine FCO (1929) Staphylococcal Infection and Reinfection. Brit J Exp Pathol 10:257-262
18. Seal DV, Ficker L, Ramakrishnan M et al (1990) Role of Staphylococcal Toxin Production in Blepharitis. Ophthalmology 97:1684-1688
19. Seal DV, Ficker L, Wright P (1992) The Role of Coagulase-Negative Staphylococci in Chronic Blepharitis. Microb Ecol Health Dis. 5: 69-75
20. Seal DV, Lightman S (1987) Immunodeficiency, Immunity and Staphylococcal Infection. Lancet ii:1522
21. Seal DV, McGill JI, Jacobs P et al (1985) Microbial and Immunological Investigations of Chronic Non-Ulcerative Blepharitis and Meibomianitis. Brit J Ophthalmol 69:604-611
22. Taubler JH, Mudd S (1968) Staphylococcal Delayed Hypersensitivity in Mice. J Immunol 101:550-555
23. Thjotta TH (1929) Treatment of Rhinitis Vasomotorica with Vaccines; Preliminary Report. Acta Otolaryngol 13:329-334
24. Thygeson P (1946) Marginal Corneal Infiltrates and Ulcers. Tr Am Acad Ophthalmol 51:198-209
25. Tuft SJ, Ramakrishnan M, Seal DV et al (1992) The role of Staphylococcus aureus in Chronic Allergic Conjunctivitis. Ophthalomology 99: 180 - 184
26. White MI, Noble WC (1985) The Cutaneous Reaction to Staphylococcal Protein A in Normal Subjects and Patients with Atopic Dermatitis or Psoriasis. Br J Dermatol 113:179-183

Diagnosis and Management of Chronic Blepharitis

James P.McCulley, Ward Shine, R. Wayne Bowman

Abstract. Chronic blepharitis is a commonly encountered disease process in ophthalmologists' offices world-wide.
In order to understand better the disease process and formulate appropriate therapeutic plans, a classification system has been developed. The vast majority of chronic blepharitis can be categorized into one of six diagnostic groups as follows: staphylococcal, seborrheic alone, seborrheic with mixed staphylococcal component, seborrheic with meibomian seborrhea, seborrheic with secondary meibomianitis, and meibomian keratoconjunctivitis.
In dealing with patients, the first and most important step is to convince the patient that he/she has a chronic disease for which we have no cure, but one that can be initially treated and brought under control. Once the disease is brought under control, maintenance therapy must be established and continued indefinitely.
The mainstay of therapy includes mechanical and hygienic maneuvers. Topical antibiotics play a significant role and should be selected based on the susceptibility patterns of the bacteria that are typically encountered. Systemic tetracyclines or tetracycline analog antibiotics are useful in the therapy of meibomian keratoconjunctivitis but have no proven role in the therapy of the anterior blepharitis.

Introduction

Chronic blepharitis is a frequently encountered disease in an ophthalmologist's office. It represents a very frustrating problem, not only for the afflicted patients, but for the treating ophthalmologist as well. Very little attention has been paid to chronic blepharitis by the ophthalmic clinical scientist since the 1930's and 40's. Therefore, many of the dogma were based on data from the pre-antibiotic pre-corticosteroid era. The different expressions of the disease in recent times as well as the ability to apply current laboratory techniques to understanding the disease led to my interest in evaluating the pathophysiology and therapy of chronic blepharitis. My interest began in 1974 and has continued to the present. The long-term laboratory work has been supported by the National Institutes of Health as well as Research to Prevent Blindness.

We previously were taught that chronic blepharitis fell into one of three diagnostic groups: staphylococcal, seborrheic, or a mixture of the two. We also were taught that meibomianitis, when present, was the result of staphylococcal infection of meibomian glands. Additionally, the teaching was that corneal epithelial disease was by and large the result of the deleterious effect of Staphylococcos aureus. My impression was that the presentation of disease as it was being seen could not be placed comfortably simply into the above three diagnostic categories, that meibomianitis was not the result of direct meibomian gland infection, and that the surface disease associated with chronic blepharitis could not be adequately, or even appropriately, explained by the action of exotoxin.

A classification system was, therefore, developed that more appropriately reflected chronic blepharitis as it was being seen (17,18). The classification system includes six major diagnostic groups that are as follows:

- staphylococcal,
- seborrheic alone,
- seborrheic with associated staphylococcal superinfection,
- seborrheic with meibomian seborrhea, or with
- secondary meibomianitis; or
- primary meibomianitis (meibomian keratoconjunctivitis).

This classification system evolved over time and resulted in the vast majority of patients with chronic blepharitis being classifiable into one of these six categories (12,2).

There are other uncommon forms of chronic blepharitis that will not be addressed in this manuscript that include atopy, psoriasis, fungal infections, etc.

Only chronic blepharitis will be dealt with, and there will be no attempt to address the many issues related to the various forms of acute blepharitis.

Dermatological Association

All patients with chronic blepharitis were examined by a masked dermatologist who was unaware of whether the person being evaluated was a normal control or a patient with chronic blepharitis. Normal controls were found to have no dermatological abnormality. Similarly, patients with chronic staphylococcal blepharitis were found to have no dermatological abnormality.

Patients with the four different types of seborrheic blepharitis were found 95% of the time to have an associated seborrheic dermatitis. Typically, the dermatitis was not severe, and was accepted by the patient as a minor irritant with which they had to live. Patients with meibomian keratoconjunctivitis were found to have associated seborrheic dermatitis 36% of the time and acne rosacea 63% of the time (19,20). In other words, patients with chronic blepharitis, with the exception of those with staphylococcal blepharitis, were found to have a frequent association with dermatitis centered around the sebaceous glands as manifest by the presence of seborrheic dermatitis or acne rosacea (15). It may, therefore, be assumed that these patients have a tendency to develop abnormalities diffusely of sebaceous-like glands, not only of the skin, but those of the lids, including the glands of Zeis and the meibomian glands.

Clinical Manifestations

Staphylococcal Blepharitis

Patients with staphylococcal blepharitis had involvement principally of the anterior portion of the lid. Lids were relatively inflamed compared to the various types of seborrheic blepharitis. There frequently was loss of lashes, i.e. madarosis. The debris deposited on the lashes characteristically had collarettes as a prominent feature. Fluctuating bacterial activity most likely accounts for the waxing and waning of these patients' signs and symptoms. The most typical patient in this disease category was a relatively young female; however, both males and females of all age groups were encountered.

There was a frequent associated keratoconjunctivitis sicca in that 50% of patients with chronic staphylococcal blepharitis had associated keratoconjunctivitis sicca. As previously stated, these patients were normal from a general dermatological standpoint.

Seborrheic Blepharitis (alone)

These patients principally had the disease process located on the anterior portion of the lid. There was minimal to moderate inflammation in contrast to the marked inflammation in patient with staphylococcal blepharitis. The debris on the lids and lashes was of an oily, greasy nature and has been characterized as scurf.

These patients fell into two groups from a symptomatic standpoint. There were those who had chronic, persistent symptoms and who most likely had no periods of staphylococcal overgrowth.

Another segment of these patients gave a past history of exacerbations and marked increase in inflammation which most likely represent previous episodes of staphylococcal overgrowth and tipping over into a mixed seborrheic staphylococcal picture. Surprisingly, there was also a relatively high frequently associated keratoconjunctivitis sicca in these patients, as it was found in 33%.

Seborrheic with Staphylococcal Superinfection

A segment of seborrheic blepharitis give a history of exacerbations associated with a marked increase in inflammation representing episodes of staphylococcal overgrowth, resulting in a mixed sebor-rheic/staphylococcal picture. These patients were found to be relatively inflamed to a similar degree as those patients with staphylococcal alone, with the inflammation being centered along the anterior portion of the lids. The debris on the lids and lashes, however, had characteristics of both those of seborrheic and staphylococcal disease, i.e. collarettes as well as scurf.

These patients gave a history of a chronic disease process with periodic exacerbations similar to the level of symptoms with which they were presenting. Keratoconjunctivitis sicca was found to be concomitantly present in 35% of these patients.

Seborrheic Blepharitis with Meibomian Seborrhea

These patients had an appearance of chronic seborrheic blepharitis involving the anterior portion of the lids. The differentiating characteristic in these patients was that they had the appearance of excessive meibomian secretions that could be seen through the tarsal plate. The meibomian glands appeared to be dilated and expanded by meibomian secretions. These secretions were easily expressed, and there was no evidence of secretion inspissation near the orifice, i.e. plugging. The tears in these patients appeared to have more foam than any of the other disease groups. There was very minimal bulbar conjunctival injection and no tarsal conjunctival abnormality.

There was a 40% incidence of associated keratoconjunctivitis sicca. These patients typically had complaints of severe ocular burning far out of proportion to the observed signs. Most likely, patients with this disease entity go undiagnosed and are thought to have psychosomatic disease, as they frequently complain markedly of burning. On examination often there will be only minimal seborrheic changes of the anterior lids, along with foamy tears, and possibly minimal bulbar injection.

The key to recognizing this disease entity is the observation of excessive meibomian secretions that are easily expressed from the glands onto the ocular surface.

Seborrheic Blepharitis with Spotty or Secondary Meibomianitis

These patients have a typical anterior seborrheic blepharitis with the inflammatory process having spread posteriorly to involve scattered patches of meibomian glands. The meibomian glands that are involved typically are less severely involved and demonstrate less intense meibomianitis than that which is seen in meibomian keratoconjunctivitis.

Historically, these patients often give a history of periodic exacerbations that most likely represent a chronic seborrheic blepharitis spilling posteriorly to involve glands with resultant meibomianitis. As with the other forms of anterior blepharitis, there was a 25% diagnosis of concomitant keratoconjunctivitis sicca.

Primary Meibomianitis, Meibomian Keratoconjunctivitis

Patients with meibomian keratoconjunctivitis in contrast to all of the above described forms of blepharitis, have the inflammatory process centered not in the anterior portion of the lid, but in the posterior portion of the lid, with the meibomian glands apparently being the focus of inflammation.

Meibomianitis is characterized by inflammation around the meibomian glands with pouting of the meibomian gland orifices above the lid margin (13). It is possible to see through the tarsal conjunctiva a build-up of secretions within the glands; however, in contrast to meibomian seborrhea, there is marked inspissation of the meibomian secretions near the gland orifice, resulting in plugging. When one attempts to express the secretions, one may find either that they are nonexpressable or that one must express an inspissated plug or tube of secretion before fluid meibomian secretions are encountered. There may be minimal to moderate inflammation of the anterior portion of the lid. The inflammation also extends posteriorly, in that there typically is tarsal papillary conjunctival hypertrophy as well as bulbar conjunctival injection.

The preocular tear film is found to be unstable and there is an associated interpalpebral fissure rose bengal staining characteristic of an unstable tear film. Often, the surface disease will be sufficiently severe that one can observe a punctate corneal epithelial erosions even without stain. It was possible to stabilize the tear film by expressing from deep within the meibomian gland fresh meibomian lipids, suggesting that an abnormal lipid layer of the tear film was responsible for the instability.

Once the meibomianitis was effectively treated, it was possible to identify a 33% association with concomitant keratocon-junctivitis sicca (1).

Laboratory Evaluation

Bacteriology

Extensive aerobic and anaerobic cultures were taken from the lid margin, conjunctival culde-sac, and meibomian secretions of all patients and controls. The detailed results of these studies has been previously published (2).

S.aureus was recovered in statistically significantly higher frequency only from patients with clinical staphylococcal blepharitis and clinical mixed seborrheic/staphylococcal blepharitis at the rate 46% and 83%, respectively. It was recovered in 13% of normals, which compared to the recovery rate from all of the other diagnostic categories.

Coagulase-negative Staphylococci were recovered from 94% of normals, as well as on average 94% from each of the patient groups.

Propionibacterium acnes and Corynebacterium species were also frequently recovered from normals and patients with there being no statistically significant difference between groups.

It would, therefore, appear that there is evidence only for a primary role of a single bacterial species, i.e. S. aureus, in the production of the clinical disease entities of staphylococcal blepharitis and mixed seborrheic/staphylococcal blepharitis (14). There may well be roles for other bacteria in the production of disease; however, no single bacterial species appears to be an identifiable agent. However, there may be common pathways shared by multiple bacteria that might contribute to the production of disease as will be addressed below.

Bacterial Antimicrobial Susceptibility

The susceptibility patterns of S.aureus and coagulase negative Staphylococci were very similar and almost identical, whether recovered from normals or those with disease. There was a high susceptibility rate to

- Tetracyclinet,
- Erythromycin,
- Bacitracin, the
- aminoglycosides, and
- Chloramphenicol.

Remarkably, the most frequently used antimicrobial for this disease in the United States, the sulfanilamides, were found to be ineffective against the majority of the isolates. It would, therefore, seem prudent to select as a topical antimicrobial one of the antibiotics found to be effective in vitro. My personal choice is that of Bacitracin over Erythromycin, because of its bactericidal rather than bacteriostatic function. Also, because Bacitracin is not used systemically, there is a lower likelihood of patients being allergic to it, and even if they do develop an allergy, we do not lose the ability to use an important oral agent. I hold in reserve the aminoglycosides for more difficult patients and do not use as a first-line of choice Chloramphenicol because of the medicolegal climate relative to the Chloramphenicols in the USA. Chloramphenicol is also bacteriostatic.

Meibomian Lipids (Meibum)

The possible role of alterations in meibum have been extensively evaluated by our laboratory.

As is known, normal meibum is clear in its fluid state, but becomes turbid as it either solidifies or when abnormal. Many of the components of meibum have a relatively high melting point and therefore have a great propensity to solidify and lead to inspissation and plugging.

We have carefully evaluated the meibomian secretions and have found that expressible meibum from the lids of normals or patients weighs approximately 0.6mg, with a protein content of between 6.6 and 7.9%. We have confirmed that the majority of the lipid composition of meibum is accounted for by wax esters (32%), sterol esters (27%), polar lipids (15%), hydrocarbons (7%), triglycerides (4%), free sterols (2%), and free fatty acids (2%) (16).

It is theorized that meibum can be involved in the production of disease in several different ways, including stagnation and plugging of the secretions as the result of generation of lipids with higher melting points, destabilizing the tear film by the production of excessive polar lipids or free fatty acids, direct toxicity to the ocular surface by noxious lipids, e.g. free fatty acids, and the encouragement of bacterial overgrowth by a shift to lipids that are more favorable to bacterial growth. An alternate explanation for the tendency to develop "plugging" is keratinization of the cells near the orifice of the meibomian gland. Whether this is a primary abnormality or a secondary phenomenon caused by chronic irritation from either noxious lipids or inflammation is not clear.

To date, we have looked very carefully at the free fatty acid, wax ester, and sterol ester component of meibum. We did find an alteration in the free fatty acids of patients with all forms of seborrheic blepharitis and those with meibomian keratoconjunctivitis (4). The free fatty acid component was normal in patients with staphylococcal blepharitis. The importance of these differences is not clear; however, free fatty acids are recognized to be potent molecules and minor changes might have great biological significance.

In evaluating the wax esters and sterol esters, we found a shift toward individual esters with higher melting points in patients with meibomian keratoconjunctivitis as compared to normals (21). This has the obvious potential clinical relevance of a shift toward lipids in patients with meibomian keratoconjunctivitis that are more apt to solidify, stagnate, and cause congestion within the meibomian glands (21).

We also have found in the wax and sterol esters an increase in mono unsaturated fatty acids in all of the disease groups as compared to normals (10). Also, the fatty acid methyl esters derived from the fatty acid component of the wax and sterol esters showed variability among normals as well as in the disease groups (22). In fact, it was possible to predict with a high degree of accuracy into which group the individual patient fell simply by looking at this fraction.

These changes in the wax and sterol fatty acids cannot be explained by random chemical alterations, but represent highly specific biological changes regulated either by the meibomian gland or postproduction meibum changes, e.g. bacterial lipases.

In looking at the cholesterol ester component in the normal controls, we found two populations, those with and those without a cholesterol ester component. It was found that patients with cholesterol esters tended to have an unsaturated fatty acid component; whereas, it tended to be saturated in normals without cholesterol esters.

In looking at the fatty acid chain in the cholesterol ester containing disease groups, there was a correlation with disease of the presence of long chains (C-20-28) and a correlation with unsaturated C-18 in patients with meibomian keratoconjunctivitis. We also have preliminary data to suggest that cholesterol esters may have a stimulating role in bacterial growth and therefore may represent another method by which cholesterol esters might contribute to the production of disease (23).

The demonstrated differences in meibum in the patient groups compared to normals may be genetic, developmental, or degenerative, e.g. related to bacterial production of lipolytic exoenzymes.

Bacterial Lipolytic Exoenzymatic Activity

Dermatologists have noted for years that Propionibacterium acnes produces a triglyceride lipase that has been theorized as being contributory to the development of acne vulgaris. We, therefore, evaluated S.aureus, P.acnes, and coagulase-negative Staphylococci for the production of cholesterol esterase, fatty wax esterase, and triglyceride lipase (6).

We found that S.aureus uniformly produced all three lipolytic exoenzymes, whether the organism was recovered from normal controls or disease groups.

P.acnes was found not to produce a cholesterol esterase but 90% of the isolates produced a fatty wax esterase and 99% of the isolates produced a triglyceride lipase. There were no significant differences among any of the patient groups.

Among the coagulase-negative Staphylococci, 40% of the isolates produced a cholesterol esterase, 82% a fatty wax esterase, and 83% a triglyceride lipase. There was a statistically significant difference comparing isolates from patients with meibomian gland disease to controls for the production of one or more of the lipolytic exoenzymes.

It therefore appears that the three most frequently isolated bacteria from patients with blepharitis, i.e. S.aureus, P.acnes, and coagulase-negative Staphylococci may share a common characteristic that contributes to the production of disease, i.e. the production of lipolytic exoenzymes that in turn alter the meibomian secretions.

Other Laboratory Evaluations

Lid margin and conjunctival cytology was performed on all groups, including controls, and no significant differences were observed.

The presence of Demodex on cilia similarly was found to be similar among groups; however, there was a tendency toward there being more organisms in patients with seborrheic blepharitis with meibomian seborrhea.

This is not unsurprising considering the affinity of Demodex for lipid secretions.

The possibility that local defense mechanisms might be altered was considered as a possible contributory factor to the production of disease.

As an indicator of this, tear lysozyme was evaluated in controls, as well as all patient groups (7,8). We found the tear lysozyme concentration in tears in normals to be 3760±320μg/ml, in patients with blepharitis without keratoconjunctivitis sicca, 4070±3080, and in patients with blepharitis with concomitant keratoconjunctivitis sicca 2503±320. The difference, therefore, between normals and patients blepharitis without keratoconjunctivitis sicca was similar; however, patients with blepharitis with keratoconjunctivitis sicca had a statistically significant decrease in tear lysozyme at the $p<0.01$. The sensitivity of the test was 71%, and specificity 77% in our study, and the test was reproducible within 4% (±160μg/ml). We could find no significant correlation with age or with sex. Therefore, tear lysozyme correlated with the predictability of approximately 75% with keratoconjunctivitis sicca and had no correlation with blepharitis per se.

We, therefore, found no evidence for decreased local defense mechanisms as measured by tear lysozyme concentrations in patients with blepharitis.

Therapy

The most important point for the treating physician and the patient to understand relative to therapy is that we are dealing with a chronic disease for which we have no cure, and that therapy will be directed initially at bringing the disease under control with intensive therapy, and then establishing the minimal amount of chronic long-term therapy that will maintain control of the disease process.

In other words, there are two phases to therapy, an acute intensive phase followed by a tapering of intensity and number of therapeutic modalities, to the minimum amount of chronic therapy that will maintain control. It is important to keep in mind that patients with all forms of seborrheic blepharitis as well as meibomian keratoconjunctivitis have associated dermatological disease that must be treated with a similar philosophy, often with the assistance of a dermatologist (3,11).

All forms of blepharitis require topical therapy. The mainstay of topical therapy are mechanical and hygienic maneuvers. Topical antibiotics most likely also have a place in the therapy of all forms of chronic blepharitis. Systemic therapy is indicated only in patients with meibomian keratoconjunctivitis and rare patients with severe seborrheic blepharitis with secondary meibomianitis who are not controelable with topical therapy alone.

Patients are directed to apply warm compresses to closed lids by using a face cloth placed first under the hot water faucet and then to the lids. They are instructed to maintain the warm compresss as hot as is tolerated and to maintain the heat for 5-10 minutes. This necessitates the repeated soaking of the face cloth or sterile towel in the running hot water, and then reapplying to the closed lids. Patients with any type of meibomian gland involvement are then instructed to massage effectively both upper and lower lids. They are instructed to take the tip of a clean index finger and to press the lid against the globe with the finger being placed just beyond the lash line and to press until secretions flow from the glands. It is possible for the treating ophthalmologist to determine how firmly to press by observing the expression of secretions from the meibomian gland at the slit lamp. The firmness of massage should then be demonstrated to the patient.

Following the massage, in those with meibomian gland involvement, and after the application of warm compresses in those not massaging, patients are instructed apply to a moist face cloth a non-irritating, "no-tears" baby shampoo and to scrub the brows, lids, and lashes with a left to right motion. They are informed that the maneuver is directed at the removal of debris from the base of the eyelashes and they therefore are not to squeeze the lids tightly together; otherwise the lashes will be buried and inaccessible. A face cloth is preferred over a cotton swab for practical reasons. Additionally, the face cloth provides somewhat of an abrasive surface and is more effectively and safely used.

Bacitracin/Erythromycin

Following the mechanical and hygienic maneuvers, the patient is instructed to rub into the lid and lash margin an antibiotic ointment of choice. These maneuvers are typically prescribed to be done on arising in the morning and in early evening. Additionally, patients are instructed to instill the antibiotic ointment into the inferior cul-de-sac at bedtime. As indicated above, my antibiotic of choice is Bacitracin over Erythromycin, while holding the aminoglycosides in reserve. Also, as indicated, in the United States, it is our feeling that it is medicolegally unwise to use chloramphenicol. We do select one of the aminoglycosides as our antibiotic of choice if it is felt that an antibiotic needs to be in the preocular tear film during the awake hours. In that case, an aminoglycoside ointment will be utilized as described above and an aminoglycoside drop will be instilled onto the ocular surface 3-4 times a day. This approach is taken because of the poor acceptance by patients of ointment in the preocular tear film and the impracticality of trying to force this upon them when dealing with a chronic disease. Acute therapy is maintained until the disease process is under control.

An attempt then is made to define the minimum amount of chronic therapy that will maintain control. This typically represents mechanical and hygienic maneuvers once or twice a day, with the most important treatment time being on arising in the morning. Rarely, patients will require long-term chronic antibiotics, in which case we alternate on a weekly basis two different antibiotics, e.g. Bacitracin one week, alternating with Erythromycin the next week.

Systemic antibiotic therapy is indicated only in patients with meibomian keratoconjunctivitis and very rare patients with seborrheic blepharitis with severe secondary meibomianitis. There is no evidence to support the efficacy or usefulness of such oral therapy in any of the forms of anterior blepharitis.

Tetracyclines

On the other hand, oral tetracyclines or one of its analogs has been shown to be effective in the treatment of patients with meibomianitis. The exact mechanism of action of the tetracyclines is not clear; however, the mechanism does not appear to be through the drug's antimicrobial abilities. Tetracyclines are known to have many effects, including that of a chelator, an antichemotactic, as well as to have an ability to decrease serum cholesterol. As already stated, its antimicrobial abilities do not appear to account for its efficacy in the treatment of meibomianitis.

We have evaluated the ability of tetracyclines to inhibit lipolytic enzymes. Since the production of triglyceride lipase by P.acnes has a potential role in the therapy of Acne vulgaris, we evaluated the ability of tetracyclines to inhibit production of triglyceride lipase, cholesterol esterase and fatty wax esterase produced by the ocular flora.

We found that the cholesterol esterase and fatty wax esterase produced by coagulase negative Staphylococci was inhibited by tetracyclines prior to any effect being noted on the bacteria itself or its growth patterns (9).

We were unable to separate out the effect of tetracyclines on the cholesterol esterase and fatty wax esterase produced by S.aureus apart from a concomitant effect on bacterial growth. It may, therefore, be that the therapeutic effect of tetracycline and its analogs in the treatment of meibomianitis is through its inhibitory effect on the production of the lipolytic enzymes produced by the ocular flora (9).

Sulfanilamides

Specifically, it is our recommendation not to use topical sulfanilamides as the antimicrobial of choice as there is poor in vitro susceptibility by the bacteria in question to this drug. It may be that the sulfanilamides have some other mechanism of action other than an antimicrobial one that may bestow upon its therapeutic efficacy; however, this has not yet been demonstrated. Until there is evidence to support the use of sulfanilamides, given the poor in vitro susceptibility of the bacteria in question, it would seem prudent to use available antimicrobials with good in vitro effectiveness against the bacteria in question.

Corticosteroids

Finally, the avoidance of topical corticosteroids in the management of chronic blepharitis cannot be overemphasized. Since this is a chronic disease, it is recommended that topical corticosteroids not be used. Although corticosteroids will decrease lid and ocular inflammation, it is better to treat effectively the cause of the inflammation rather than suppressing it. Unfortunately, the suppression of inflammation by corticosteroids may provide the patient with greater comfort than direct therapy will. The patient's comparison, then, of their symptoms while on corticosteroids to their state when being treated effectively and directly for their disease may stimulate them to want to be on topical corticosteroids chronically. This clearly is inappropriate in a chronic disease given the many potential side-effects of the topical corticosteroids.

Both from a patient management and an art of medicine standpoint it is unwise to expose these patients to topical corticosteroids, especially since, by following the treatment guidelines outlined above all forms of chronic blepharitis can be safely and effectively managed.

References

1. Bowman RW, Dougherty JM, McCulley JP (1987) Chronic Blepharitis and Dry Eyes. Internat Ophthalmol Clin 27:27-35
2. Bowman RW, Miller K, McCulley JP (1989) Diagnosis and Treatment of Chronic Blepharitis. In:Focal Points: Clinical Modules for Ophthalmologists. Am Academy of Ophthalmol Vol 7, Mod 10
3. Brown DD, McCulley,JP (1990) Staphylococcal and Mixed Staphylococcal/ Seborrheic Blepharoconjunctivitis. In: Fraunfelder FT, Roy FH (eds), Current Ocular Therapy III, W.B. Saunders, Philadelphia pp 525-527
4. Dougherty JM, McCulley JP (1986) Analysis of Free Fatty Acid Component of Meibomian Secretions in Chronic Blepharitis. Invest Ophthalmol Vis Sci 27:52-56
5. Dougherty JM, McCulley JP (1984) Comparative Bacteriology of Chronic Blepharitis. Br J Ophthalmol 68:524-528
6. Dougherty JM, McCulley JP (1986) Bacterial Lipases and Chronic Blepharitis. Invest Ophthalmol Vis Sci 27:486-491
7. Dougherty JM, McCulley JP (1985) Tear Lysozyme Measurements in Chronic Blepharitis. Ann Ophthalmol 17:53-57
8. Dougherty JM, McCulley JP, Meyer DR (1986) Keratoconjunctivitis Sicca and Tear Lysozyme in Chronic Blepharitis. In: Holly FJ (ed) The Preocular Tear Film. Dry Eye Institute, Lubbock pp 176-181
9. Dougherty JM, McCulley JP, Silvany RE et al (1991) The Role of Tetracycline in Chronic Blepharitis: Inhibition of Lipase Production in Staphylococci. Invest Ophthalmol Vis Sci 32:2970-2975
10. Dougherty JM, Osgood JK, McCulley JP (1991) The Role of Wax and Sterol Esters Fatty Acids in Chronic Blepharitis. Invest Ophthalmol Vis Sci 32:1932-1937
11. Halsted M, McCulley JP (1990) Seborrheic Blepharitis. In:Fraunfelder FT, Roy FR (eds). Current Ocular Therapy III. W.B. Saunders, Philadelphia pp 522-524
12. McCulley JP (1984) Blepharoconjunctivitis. Int Ophthalmol Clin 24:65-77
13. McCulleyJP (1988) Meibomitis. In: Kaufman HE, Waltman S, McDonald M et al (eds): The Cornea. Churchill Livingston, New York pp 125-138
14. McCulley JP, Dougherty JM (1986) Bacterial Aspects of Chronic Blepharitis. Trans Ophthalmol Soc UK 105:314-318
15. McCulley JP, Dougherty JM (1985) Blepharitis Associated with Acne Rosacea and Seborrheic Dermatitis. Int Ophthalmol Clin 25:159-172
16. McCulley JP, Dougherty JM (1986) Meibomian Lipids in Chronic Blepharitis. In: Holly FJ (ed) Preocular Tearfilm: In Health, Disease, and Contact Lens Wear. Holland Ophthalmic Publishing Center, Amsterdam pp 626-631
17. McCulley JP, Dougherty JM, Deneau DG (1981) Chronic Blepharitis: Classification and Mechanisms. In: Suran A, Gery I, Nussenblatt RB (eds): Proceedings of "Immunology of the Eye; Workshop III", Sp.Supp.Immunology Abstracts pp 55-72
18. McCulley JP, Dougherty JM, Deneau DG (1982) Classification of Chronic Blepharitis. Ophthalmology 89:1173-1180
19. McCulley JP, Sciallis GF (1977) Meibomian Keratoconjunctivitis. Am J Ophthalmol 84:788-793

20. McCulley JP, Sciallis GF (1983) Meibomian Keratoconjunctivitis: Oculodermal Correlates. CLAO J 9:130-132
21. Osgood JK, Dougherty JM, McCulley JP (1989) The Role of Wax and Sterol Esters in Meibomian Keratoconjunctivitis. Invest Ophthalmol Vis Sci 30:1958-1961
22. Shine WE, McCulley JP (1991) The Role of Cholesterol in Chronic Blepharitis. Invest Ophthalmol Vis Sci 32:2272-2280
23. Shine W, Silvany RE, McCulley JP (1193) Relation of Cholesterol-Stimulated Staphylococcus aureaus Growth to Chronic Blepharitis. Invest. Ophthalmol Vis Sci 34: 2291-2296

Blepharitis - A Report on 450 Consecutive Cases

Veronika Huber-Spitzy, Kornelia Böhler-Sommeregger, Günther Grabner

Abstract. Recently, the incidence of patients with chronic bilateral blepharitis has markedly increased.
From January 1985 through 1990, 450 patients with this diagnosis underwent complete ophthalmological and dermatological work-ups at the out-patient clinic for infectious eye diseases of the 2nd Department of Ophthalmology of the University of Vienne. When the spectrum of organisms reportedly isolated from the affected sites by several authors was compared to our own data, it seemed that during recent years the range of microorganisms associated with this chronic localized inflammation had shifted. The prevalence of S.aureus apparent in the pre-antibiotic era had markedly decreased, although there still seems to be a distinct entity of staphylococcal blepharitis alone or in combination with seborrheic blepharitis (63.5%).

Introduction

In any of its various forms, blepharitis is one of the most commonly encountered diseases in Ophthalmology. In spite of that, the condition still remains a diagnostic and therapeutic challenge. Few details are known about the underlying etiology, and management is both time-consuming and often ineffective with frequent recurrences in the course of the disease. The merely descriptive term "blepharitis" comprises a number of conditions with inflammatory changes of varying degrees with secondary changes of the conjunctiva.

Nearly all of the blepharitis patients have abnormal sebaceous gland functions ranging from seborrhea sicca to seborrheic dermatitis or acne rosacea, suggesting a generalized sebaceous gland dysfunction including the Meibomian glands (13,27,28).

This report describes the clinical, microbiological and dermatological findings in a large consecutive series of patients who presented to the out-patient clinic for infectious eye diseases of the 2nd Department of Ophthalmology of the University of Vienna with the signs of chronic inflammatory changes of the lids from 1985 through 1990.

Material and Methods

Dermatologic and ophthalmologic examinations were performed on all of 450 patients (246 male, 204 female) with the primary diagnosis of "chronic blepharitis". Their ages ranged from 13 to 85 years (mean of 38.7 - 12.4 years). Each patient was seen by the same dermatologist (K.B.-S.) and particular attention was directed to the function of the sebaceous glands.

Aerobic as well as anaerobic cultures were collected from the eyelash roots of each patient by an eyelid scrub technique. To optimize recovery of microorganisms, a broth-soaked sterile calcium alginate swab was passed along the anterior lid margin and a second one over the conjunctiva of the inferior fornix. For aerobic cultures, different media (trypticase soy broth with 5% sheep erythrocytes, chocolate agar, mannitol-salt agar, endo agar) were used and subsequently incubated in a 5% CO_2 atmosphere for a minimum of 12 to 24 hours (if any growth was observed) up to a maximum of 72 hours for the detection of anaerobic microorganisms. For the cultures of anaerobic agents, Schaedler's broth gassed with 97% CO_2 and 3% hydrogen was used. They were placed into GasPak^R Jars (BBL).

A group of 60 normal controls (30 men, 30 women, aged 20 to 80 years, mean 43.2 - 18.3 years) were sampled in an identical way.

Sensitivity patterns to usually applied ophthalmic antibiotics and sulphonamides for all rapidly growing aerobic isolates were determined by the Barry agar overlay method (3), using commercially available antimicrobial discs and Mueller Hinton Agar (BBL). We used the broth disc method of Wilkins and Thiel (30) for culture of P.acnes.

In this study, isolation of Pityrosporon ovale or Demodex folliculorum was attempted in the last fifty patients, because these yeasts may play an important role in the pathogenesis of folliculitis.

A lash from each eyelid was selected, epilated, and placed in a drop of peanut oil on a microscope slide that was covered with a cover slip. The presence or absence of Demodex was determined by light microscopy. Huismans has reported a new topical therapy (3% isoptocarbachol) of chronic eczematous blepharitis due to Demodex folliculorum (12).

Pityrosporum yeasts can hydrolyse triglycerides into free fatty acids, and it has been postulated that an overgrowth of the yeast in a follicle produces folliculitis by a combination of fatty acid production and blockage of the follicular ostium by scale (26).

Results

Ophthalmologic findings: The clinical classification according to McCulley divides "blepharitis" into the following categories:

- staphylococcal blepharitis,
- seborrhoeic blepharitis,
- mixed forms,
- seborrhoeic blepharitis with Meibomian seborrhea,
- seborrhoeic with secondary Meibomitis and
- primary Meibomitis and keratoconjunctivitis (17).

The last condition is characterized by an inflammation centering around all of the Meibomian glands with concomitant plugging of the ducts and a keratoconjunctivitis (16). In this series patients were evaluated for signs of keratoconjunctivitis sicca additionally by observation of the tear meniscus, Schirmer's tests and break-up time. Schirmer's tests were reduced (less than 15mm of wetting according to our standard series) in 21.7%. The incidence of keratoconjuntivitis sicca in conjunction with blepharitis was 15.8% of the patient population also suffering from acne rosacea.

According to Lemp and coworkers (15) the incidence and coexistence of asymptomatic acne rosacea and asymptomatic keratoconjunctivitis sicca is quite high in the general population, particularly in the older age group (fourth to sixth decades).

Forty-six of those patients presented with a significantly reduced Schirmer's test and in 25 only the break-up time had been abnormal.

It has been postulated by Seal and coworkers in 1985 that the effects on the tear film must be due to disturbance of the tear film components themselves (23), perhaps due to the excessive secretions from the lid margins. Whatever the underlying pathomechanism, therapeutic regimens are similar to those used in keratoconjunctivitis sicca without involvement of the lids. It is a fact, however, that keratoconjunctivitis sicca does not show any improvement without additional therapy, even if the signs of blepharitis respond well to the treatment.

According to the clinical picture of 450 cases, we have made up a classification using the following three categories only:

1. Blepharitis Sicca is defined as a superficial, non-destructive inflammation of the lid margins with dry scaling being the prominent clinical feature in this group. We have diagnosed this condition in 188 patients (=41.7%). This form of lid affection represents an anterior blepharitis and it can be considered to represent a local eczematous dermatologic disease, so-called seborrhea sicca.

2. Blepharitis Seborrhoica (squamosa) is characterized by excessive sebaceous gland secretion with marked inflammation of the posterior lid margins (without ulceration) and large yellow or greyish, "greasy" scales that are loosely attached to the eye lashes. Secondary Meibomitis associated with seborrheic blepharitis (with or without Meibomian seborrhea) tended to have a spotty distribution involving scattered clusters of Meibomian glands. Most of these patients (212 patients = 47.1%) additionally complained of itching and a "burning sensation". They regularly complained about a constant cosmetically disturbing "redness of the eyes". This group also includes patients with the diagnosis of primary Meibomitis, which is charaterized by diffuse inflammation surrounding the Meibomian gland orifices. Solidification of the lipid secretions is prominent, with resultant "plugging" of the gland orifices and build-up of secretions within the gland ducts (56 patients =12.44%).

3. Blepharitis Ulcerosa has only been diagnosed, if the follicles of the lashes had been involved, always covered by thickmatted, hardened crusts. When trying to remove these scales with a pair of forceps, frequently small, bleeding ulcerations in the area of the hair follicles appear. This most severe form of blepharitis was observed in 50 patients (=11.1%).

Frequent findings in the latter two types of blepharitis are dilated blood vessels on the lid margins (83%), poliosis (32%),madarosis

(54%), trichiasis (43%) and "collarettes" (82%). Collarettes are thin, small, fibrinous scales that surround the eyelash like a small piece of paper impaled on a stick (22).

The role of staphylococci in the pathogenesis of all of the three forms of blepharitis is not clear - in each of the three groups we have been able to isolate these bacteria (sicca and seborrhoica up to 50%). It would be possible to construct a "pure" staphylococcal group and a mixed staphylococcal/seborrheic group, but in our opinion this would make the diagnosis more complicated. As the percentage of staphylococci has nearly been the same in our control group, it is thus quite likely that many reported isolates of staphylococci in association with blepharitis may represent commensals/non-pathogenic flora.

Dermatological Findings (Tab.1)

316 (=70.2%) of our patients with blepharitis presented with evidence of an associated dermatologic disease.

Seborrheic dermatitis was diagnosed in 143/450 (=31.7%) cases and most commonly involved the scalp and the "cool" areas of the face, such as the glabella, the brows and lids. In this group the young male patients in the second and third decade of life were mostly affected, "blepharitis sicca" was diagnosed in 11.7%, blepharitis seborrhoica in 21.8%.

Acne rosacea was found in 121/450 (=26.8%) individuals, the dermatological findings classically characterized by erythema, teleangiectasia, papules, pustules, and hypertrophy of the sebaceous glands. It was apparently a disease of the older age groups (fifties and sixties) and women were affected twice as often as men (4,5). The clinical pictures of blepharitis seen in these patients was predominantly of the seborrhoeic type (24.4%).

From our own series it appears that patients with acne rosacea have an increased predisposition to staphylococcal infections; in this group, marginal corneal infiltrates were occasionally observed. In all of these patients S.aureus could be isolated, which supports the concept that delayed type hypersensitivity to ribitol teichoic acid, the major antigenic determinant of S.aureus may play some role in the development of marginal corneal infiltrates (19,20).

Atopic dermatitis was diagnosed in 50/450 patients (=11.1%). Nearly all of them (44/450 =9.7%) presented with a severe ulcerative type of inflammation of the lid margins. Their ages ranged from 12 to 29 years.

Microbiological Findings (Tab.2)

The results of aerobic and anaerobic cultures from both the lids and conjunctivae of patients and controls are listed in Tab. 2. 427 (94.88%) of the samples taken from the affected lids showed some growth of microorganisms, and 408 (=90.6%) cultures were established from the conjunctival fornix.

In the control group, 56 (93.33%) samples from the lids showed growth of bacteria, 57 conjunctival cultures grew organisms.

In almost all of the cases, the right and left conjunctivas showed the same flora. In case of infectious blepharitis the predominant microorganisms were the same as found in the conjunctival sac, variations being only the different amounts cultured.

Within the bacterial genus, Staphylococci (S.aureus, S.epidermidis and S.saprophyticus) were the most frequently isolated organisms (273 cultures =63.5% of culture-positive samples). In the control group a very similar figure (57.14%) was obtained.

The second most frequent isolates of the lids were Corynebacteria and Propionibacteria, which constitute normal inhabitants of the skin and were isolated in both groups (18).

It was quite interesting that a significant number of gramnegative rods could be isolated. When cultures were obtained from lids with severe inflammation and marked scarring, Pseudomonas sp. was most frequently growing on special media (51 cases =11.9%). In the control group, Citrobacter could be isolated only once.

A total of 34.5% of the Staphylococci isolates was found to be resistent to gentamicin, most probably as a consequence of the widespread use of this antibiotic by general practitioners and clinics. We suggest - as previous authors have done - that antibiotics should be only prescribed after results of the sensitivity tests have been gathered (6,14).

Cultures for Candida sp. were positive in 48 samples (=11.24%), the predominantly affected group being atopic patients with ulcerative blepharitis. We were never able, however, to isolate fungi from the conjunctival sac or from patients of the control group.

To the best of our knowledge this is the first report of a very high incidence (94%) of Candida sp. in patients suffering from ulcerative blepharitis. Only one patient with this isolate was found to have a different type of lid inflammation (seborrhoeic blepharitis). Most of the affected individuals showed the signs of atopic skin disease. Since atopic patients have been reported to exhibit a defect in their cell-mediated immunity and, possibly, also a defective local IgA antibody response we propose that this might constitute the major contributing factor for the development of fungal infections. On the other hand, all of these patients had had a long history of lid disease and they had all been treated with a broad range of antibiotics over prolonged periods of time; two thirds of these patients had received topical steroids in addition; both factors are known to contribute to fungal superinfection.

It is, therefore, advisable to perform repeated scrapings and cultures in every case of recalcitrant blepharitis. This is the only reliable way to rule out a coinfection with fungi.

Treatment

Topical antibiotic treatment - in the majority of cases for a duration of thre weeks - was initiated according to the results of the microbiological cultures and the respective sensitivity tests in 323 of the patients. In most cases of a clinically manifest infectious component either gentamicin or bacitracin-neomycin were prescribed in accordance with the antibiotics sensitivity results. In Austria, only five antibiotic ointments are available. The topical use of chloramphenicol seems to be dangerous, because bone marrow aplasia may occur, as has been reported by Abrams and Fraunfelder (1,11). Because of the high resistance rate of bacteria towards sulfonamides and tetracyclines, only two antibiotics remain as alternative, although we are well aware of the fact that neomycin is a highly allergenic substance.

Each patient with a confirmed fungal infection received systemic therapy with two single doses of 100mg Ketoconazole per day and Miconazol ointment or Fluconazol solution topically for a duration of 6 weeks. In all of these cases, control cultures after this period were negative.

Only when corneal involvement (like marginal catarrhal infiltrates) was present, topical steroid treatment (6 drops per day, ointment for the night) was prescribed for short periods of time.

All patients were advised to start a regimen of lid hygiene (scrubbing the lids twice daily with a moist cotton-tipped applicator, soaked in mild baby shampoo, or in the severe cases with I-Scrub, which is a hypoallergenic, pH-adjusted detergent composed of both anionic and non-anionic surfactants).

Whenever the Meibomian secretions were found to be excessive, the patients were taught how to express the glands once or twice weekly with the use of a cotton swab in front of a magnifying mirror.

Whenever deemed necessary, dermatologic therapy was initiated: All patients with chronic seborrhoea received oral tetracyclines and topical ointment containing vitamin A. Acne rosacea was treated in a similar fashion, patients suffering from atopic dermatitis were placed on a diet and received specific ointments. In two cases, systemic corticosteroid treatment was found to be necessary. The symptoms of blepharitis decreased during treatment parallelling the improving skin condition.

Discussion

Patients with chronic blepharitis quite frequently represent a serious diagnostic and therapeutic challenge for the practising ophthalmologist, since both dermatologic and microbiologic factors apparently play a synergistic role in the etiology and pathogenesis of disease (7).

When comparing the spectrum of microorganisms that had reportedly been isolated from the affected sites by several other research groups with our own data, it seems apparent that over the last couple of years the spectrum of microorganisms has shifted: The prevalence of S.aureus isolated in the pre-antibiotic era (2) has markedly decreased, although there still seems to exist a distinct entity of staphylococcal blepharitis alone or in combination with seborrheic blepharitis (26,29).

Dougherty found that S.aureus and many of the coagulase-negative staphylococcal strains of patients with chronic blepharitis could hydrolyze triolein and behenyl oleate and cholesteryl oleate, which represent three different lipid classes of meibum (7). P.acnes is able to hydrolyze triolein and behenyl oleate. Therefore, it seems reasonable that bacteria present on lids and conjunctivae could alter meibum in the same fashion as the cutaneous flora alter sebum.

In the past, exotoxins from all staphylococci have been thought to play a part in producing the signs and symptoms that occur in these conditions (26), but Ficker and Seal recently showed that this may not be true. Their in vitro results (10,24) do not support a toxicogenic theory for most cases of blepharitis. Ficker has pointed out that cell-mediated immunity to S.epidermidis does not occur in either normal subjects or those with chronic blepharitis.

The importance of dermatological consultations when performing the eye examination cannot be overemphasized. It is important to know that the skin lesions that are required to confirm a specific dermatologic problem need not necessarily be severe in all cases. From our own experience it appears that the lid symptoms start to improve simultaneously with the beginning of an appropriate treatment by the dermatologist.

Meibum is a complex material. Because many different classes of lipids are represented, chemical reactions among the lipids themselves and other components of the tear film may contribute to a dazzling array of biologically significant interactions that we know little about. Comparative studies of meibum have shown significant differences of the free fatty acids (8) and the composition of the ester fraction (9,21). Shine and coworkers have found two significantly different types of normal subjects, those with and those without cholesterol esters - all the secretions from blepharitis patients containing cholesterol esters (25). Furthermore, these results suggest that lipid abnormalities are involved in the many signs and symptoms of chronic blepharitis.

A pivotal point in the management of blepharitis is the patient's ability to endure the requirement of prolonged treatment, since the disease is chronic requiring close daily attention and care.

A satisfactory - if not rapid - management of this multifaceted disease is within reach regarding the results of microbiological investigations and the dermatological considerations detailed above.

Table 1

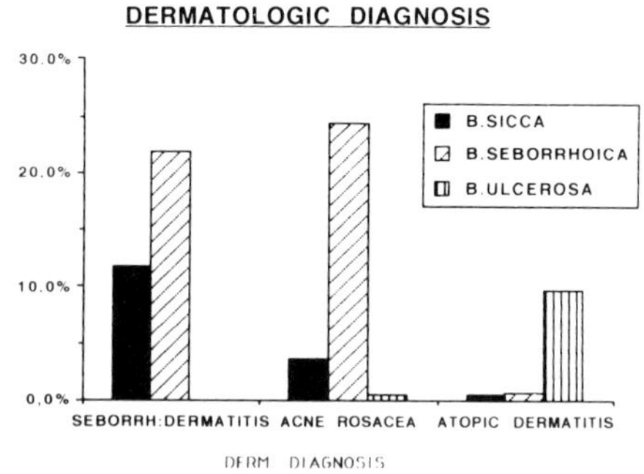

Table 2

Microbiological results

n = 427 (=94.9%) out of 450 samples taken from the lids showed a growth of microorganisms.

	Patients		B.sicca		B.seborrhoica		B.ulcerosa	
total	n= 427 (=94.9%)		n= 166 (= 88.3%)		n= 211 (=99.5%)		n=50 (100%)	
	Lid	Conj	Lid	Conj.	Lid	Conj.	Lid	Conj.
S.aureus	92	83	34	32	50	29	8	12
coag.neg.Staph	181	129	98	54	74	56	9	19
Streptococcus (A & B)	66	37	34	17	32	19	0	2
Bacillus sp.	6	6	0	0	5	4	1	2
Corynebacterium	106	91	34	37	71	41	1	13
Propionibacterium	137	82	52	38	76	49	9	5
E.coli	32	2	0	0	20	0	12	2
Pseudomonas sp.	51	12	0	0	3	0	48	12
Citrobacter	4	0	0	0	4	0	0	0
Candida species	48	0	0	0	1	0	47	0

References

1. Abrams SM, Degnan TJ, Vinciguerra V (1980) Marrow Aplasia Following Topical Application of Chloramphenicol Eye Ointment. Arch Intern Med 140:576-578
2. Allen JH (1937) Staphylococcal Conjunctivitis. Am J Ophthalmol 20:1025-1031
3. Barry AL, Garcia F, Trupp LD (1984) An Improved Single Disc Method for Testing the Antibiotic Susceptibility of Rapidly Growing Pathogens. Am J Clin Pathol 53:149-158
4. Browning DJ, Proia AD (1986) Ocular rosacea. Surv Ophthalmol 31:145-157
5. Browning DJ, Rosenwasser G, Lugo M (1986) Ocular Rosacea in Blacks. Am J Ophthalmol 101:441-444
6. Dougherty JM, McCulley JP (1984) Comparative Bacteriology of Chronic Blepharitis. Br J Ophthalmol 68:524-528
7. Dougherty JM, McCulley JP (1986) Bacterial Lipases and Chronic Blepharitis. Invest Ophthalmol Vis Sci 27:486-491
8. Dougherty JM, McCulley JP (1986) Analysis of the Free Fatty Acid Component of Meibomian Secretions in Chronic Blepharitis. Invest Ophthalmol Vis Sci 27:52-56
9. Dougherty JM, Osgood JK, McCulley JP (1991) The Role of Wax and Sterol Ester Fatty Acids in Chronic Blepharitis. Invest Ophthalmol Vis Sci 32:1932-1937
10. Ficker L, Ramakrishnan M, Seal D et al (1991) Role of Cell-Mediated Immunity to Staphylococci in Blepharitis. Am J Ophthalmol 111:473-479
11. Fraunfelder FT, Bagby GC, Kelly DJ (1982) Fatal Aplastic Anemia Following Topical Administration of Ophthalmic Chloramphenicol. Am J Ophthalmol 93:356-358
12. Huismans H (1988) Demodex folliculorum. Klin Mbl Augenheilk 193:394-406
13. Keith CG (1967) Seborrhoic Blepharo-Kerato-Conjunctivitis. Trans Ophthalmol Soc UK 87:85-103
14. Khan JA, Hoover D, Ide CH (1984) Methicillin-Resistent Staphylococcus Epidermidis Blepharitis. Am J Ophthalmol 98:562-565
15. Lemp MA, Mahmood MA, Weiler HH (1984) Association of Rosacea and Keratoconjunctivitis Sicca. Arch Ophthalmol 102:556-557
16. McCulley JP, Sciallis GF (1977) Meibomian Keratoconjunctivitis. Am J Ophthalmol 84:788-793
17. McCulley JP, Dougherty JM, Deneau DG (1982) Classification of Chronic Blepharitis. Ophthalmology 89:1173-1180
18. McGill J, Goulding NJ, Liakos G et al (1982) Pathophysiology of Bacterial Infection in the External Eye. Trans Ophthal Soc UK 102:7-10
19. Mondino BJ, Caster AL, Dethlefs LB (1987) A Rabbit Model of Staphylococcal Blepharitis. Arch Ophthalmol 105:409-412
20. Mondino BJ, Adamu SA, Pitchekian-Halabi H (1991) Antibody studies in a Rabbit Model of Corneal Phlyctenulosis and Catarrhal Infiltrates Related to Staphylococcus Aureus. Invest Ophthalmol Vis Sci 32:1854-1863
21. Osgood JK, Dougherty JM, McCulley JP (1989) The Role of Wax and Sterol Esters in Chronic Blepharitis. Invest Ophthalmol Vis Sci 30:1958-1961
22. Ostler HB (1986) Blepharitis. In: Duane TD (ed) Clinical Ophthalmology Bd 4/22 Harper & Row Publ. Philadelphia
23. Seal DV, McGill JI, Jacobs L et al (1985) Microbial and Immunological Investigati
24. Seal DV, Ficker L, Ramakrishnan M et al (1990) Role of Staphylococcal Toxin Production in Blepharitis. Ophthalmology 97:1684-1688

ons of Chronic Non-Ulcerative Blepharitis and Meibomianitis. Br J Ophthalmol 69:604-611
25. Shine WE, McCulley JP (1991) The Role of Cholesterol in Chronic Blepharitis. Invest Ophthalmol Vis Sci 32:2272-2280
26. Smolin G, Okumoto M (1977) Staphylococcal Blepharitis. Arch Ophthalmol 95:812-816
27. Thygeson P (1946) The Etiology and Treatment of Blepharitis: A Study in Military Personel. Milit Surg 98:191-203
28. Thygeson P (1946) Etiology and Treatment of Blepharitis. A Study in Military Personel. Arch Ophthalmol 36:445-457
29. Thygeson P (1969) Complications of Staphylococcal Blepharitis. Am J Ophthalmol 68:446-449
30. Wilkins TD, Thiel T (1973) Modified Broth-Disc Method for Testing the Susceptibility of Anaerobic Bacteria. Antimicrob Ag Chemother 3:350-356

Microbiological Diagnosis of Chronic Lacrimal Canaliculitis

M.F.W. Tost, C. Höhne and H.G. Struck

Abstract. It is widely known that relatively little notice has been given to chronic lacrimal canaliculitis.
In this report, avenues of establishing a sound clinical and microbiological diagnosis in 45 patients suffering from chronic canaliculitis are shown. Thus, 19 cases of Actinomyces infections could be substantiated from 54 samples. In 36 probes, further anaerobic bacteria were identified.
Sampling techniques and organising procedures, immediate identification, and evaluation of resistance patterns of aerobic and facultatively anaerobic isolates respectively, cultures of anaerobic specimens and the production of pure cultures for subcultivation have been evaluated. Special custom-made media may be useful for the identification of anaerobes and microaerophilic strains.

Introduction

Chronic canaliculitis is a rare disease: This statement can usually be found in standard textbooks of ophthalmology (5,16).

Since A.v.Graefe had reported the disease entity for the first time in detail in 1852, subsequent publications have remained case-reports or evaluations of very few cases. According to a survey by Hoffmann in 1962 (10), one hundred years of ophthalmology had only resulted in 150 publications concerning this disease. Up to date, few works have been added. From the literature it may be derived that the disease obviously presents difficulties concerning the correlation with a correct clinical and etiologic diagnosis, resulting in inadequate treatment attempts and an unfavorable prognosis.

Therefore, we have surveyed the history and microbiological work-ups of patients suffering from chronic canaliculitis in our area.

Microbiological Procedures

From 1978 through 1991, 44 patients were evalutated clinically and microbiologically.

In several patients, more than one canaliculus was involved. 54 specimens were analysed. In 34 patients, a typical clinical picture had been misdiagnosed. Duration of the disease was 26 months on average and in one case 11 years.

Clinical evaluation centered on

- the type of secretion,
- determination of the degree of ectasy of the canaliculus,
- evaluation of further abnormalities of the efferent lacrimal duct system and exclusion of post-saccus stenosis. Conjunctival swabs were taken for the evaluation of aerobic bacteria using cotton-tipped devices. When ectatic canaliculi could be verified and purulent secretion was noted and, particularly, when concrements were seen, an incision was performed using a conjunctival access parallel to and far off the lid margin. Pus and concrements were then excised with a sharp spoon and evaluated microbiologically. A 5% iodine solution was instilled and no sutures were applied. On the following days, the lacrimal duct system was rinsed with Penicillin G (200000 I.U./ml) twice or three times daily until no secretion was observed any more.

For microbiologic work-ups, prepared agar plates for aerobic and anaerobic cultivation were inoculated in the operation room, and Gram stains were performed additionally.

Aerobic cultures included 5% sheep blood, chocolate and endoagar plates as well as a nutrient broth. Cultures were evaluated after 24 and 48 hours of incubation at 35°C. Subcultivation, identification and antibiotic susceptibility testing of aerobic and facultatively anaerobic isolates was done following standard procedures.

Anaerobic cultures inoculated into two separate supplemented sheep blood agar plates (medium no.5 (7)) with one of them supplemented with Gentamicin 20μg/ml for the suppression of aerobic or facultatively aerobic bacteria. A supplemented brain-heart-infusion broth was additionally used for some specimens (7). Anaerobic conditions were achieved by the Fortner procedure, and less frequently by anaerobic jars. Both procedures were done simultaneously in some cases (7,8). Anaerobic cultures were incubated at 37°C up to 10 days or until a significant build-up of colonies or pertubation resp. had been recognized. Except from those cultures in anaerobic devices, reading of the plates was done on a daily basis.

Single colonies were taken from the agar plates containing Gentamycin for subcultivation. Each type of colony was subcultivated on supplemented sheep blood agar (3x), chocolate agar (2x) and endo agar plates. One of the subcultures on sheep blood agar plate was incubated under anaerobic conditions. Aerobic incubation was done on sheep blood and chocolate agar plates each to identify aerobic or facultatively anaerobic bacteria. For the identification of capnophilic organisms, cultivation was performed using the rest of agar plates with supplemented sheep blood and chocolate agar in an aerobic atmosphere of 10% CO_2.

For identification of obligatory anaerobic isolates and microaerophilic isolates, standard procedures according to Allen and coworkers (1), Höhne (7,9), Holdeman and coworkers (11), Moore and coworkers (13) and Sutter and coworkers (21) were performed. The Minitek-Anaerobe-II^R system (BBL, Becton-Dickinson, Cockeysville,MD,

USA mod.by Schaal) was used.

Results

Branching gram positive rods could be identified in 11 out of 54 specimens isolated from a diseased canaliculus could be observed in a direct stain already. Actinomyces could be isolated in 7 cases. Solely in culture, Actinomyces was proven in 8 cases.

With regard to all of the 54 probes, anaerobic organisms could be isolated in 56 cases. Out of these, Actinomyces was seen in 19, Peptostreptococcus in 12 and Bacteroides in 5 cases. Nineteen anaerobic bacteria belonged to rare species.

Cultivation of aerobic organisms was done in 38 cases, microaerophilic and capnophilic resp. in 6 cases (except from microaerophilic growing Actinomyces).

The main organisms found in coinfections were coagulase negative Staphylococci (11x), non-hemolysing Streptococci (8x) and S.aureus (7x). One single specimen contained up to 7 different bacterial strains (three aerobic and four anaerobic). More than four anaerobic organisms could not be verified in one single specimen.

Microaerophilic and capnophilic resp. organisms identified were S.intermedius (3x), Capnocytophaga (2x) and E.corrodens (1x).

In brief, 15 cultures out of 54 probes showed Actinomyces, and a microscopic hint for Actinomyces could be further derived from four Gram stains. In 5 patients, two different Actinomyces species were isolated from purulent canalicular samples. Differentiation of Actinomyces resulted in the detection of A.israelii (7x), A.meyeri (1x) and A.viscosus (1x); in 8 cases, Actinomyces could not be subdifferentiated. Additionally, A.propionica was found in three cases.

Discussion

Our report contradicts the standard textbook view in that chronic bacterial canaliculitis may not be as rare as has been reported. Particularly, the disease is often not recognized or has been cured by a non-directed (antibiotic) treatment in early stages without appropriate diagnostic measures. On the other hand, the infection is not severe and may obviously be tolerated by many patients for a long time. This is supported by a long history of months or years in most of our patients and the patients reported in the literature (14).

Signs and symptoms as well as the clinical diagnosis are usually pathognomonic. Epiphora combined with a slight conjunctivitis and itching of the eye lids nasally are the predominant, however, not necessarily found, symptoms.

Subsequent to this catarrhal stage, a typical chronic non-progressive purulent inflammation and secretion may follow. The efferent lacrimal ducts can usually be flushed, since even in the presence of concrements a relatively little effective mechanical stenosis occurs. Ectatic lacrimal ducts, caused by the chronic secretory stop and the replication of Actinomyces with their products (drusen and other concrements) may lead to the differential diagnosis of a neoplasm.

If even at this stage no therapeutic regimen has been instituted, the third stage of the disease may result in ulceration of the lacrimal ducts. However, even with an extremely long history of 11 years in one of our patients, we have not been able to verify this reported stage.

Typical clinical signs have been reported with elevated prominent margins of the lacrimal punctum, thickening of the lid margins nasally and a frequent purulent secretion (6,12).

The clinical differential diagnosis comprises hordeola, chalazia, tumors, post-saccus dacryostenosis just to name the most important. The difficult and extensive microbiological work-up is only justified with a sound clinical diagnosis. A smear taken from the punctum and aerobic culture is easily done. An incision of the lid margins and extraction of all concrements may be the method of choice in patients with a long history. The punctum will remain untouched, and the canaliculitis will disappear in a couple of days. We have not observed postoperative stenosis when technical guidelines were adhered to. It is important to make a broad opening for repeated daily aerosolation and flushing if necessary. If concrements, sulphur granules and drusen are found, a diagnosis of Actinomyces canaliculitis is almost certain. Even when other organisms have been found, a broad opening is indicated for expression of pus and faster healing. The microbiological diagnosis should not be waited for. Even with the best of organisation, preparation of culture media, fast transport of probes and immediate inoculation, culture of Actinomyces may only be achieved in approximately 40% of cases.

Excisional biopsies should be performed during surgical interventions, and histopathological work-ups may be done. Specific infections like tuberculosis and syphilis may thus be excluded apart from a serological diagnosis. Other infections like trachoma, zoster, varicella or vaccinia would usually not be suspected by history and other clinical signs. Mycotic infections, however, are important findings. Establishing a fungal infection requires appropriate cultivation and may be an indication for a proper histochemical evaluation (3,19,20).

Few reports of histopathological specimens of chronic canaliculitis also called "blennorrhea of the lacrimal ducts" are known. The epithelium is intact with subepithelial accumulation of lymphocytes, plasma cells, giant (epithelioid) cells and necrosis (Fig.1,2). When Actinomyces is present, granular masses and coronary shaped structures with filaments of 1μ. Drusen may have a diameter of 0.1-0.12mm. Despite the infection, most parts of the epithelial walls are conserved and naso-lacrimal ducts are therefore usually flushable (15).

It is not known why most frequently female patients and the elderly are affected and why canaliculitis is mostly one-sided and affects the lower punctum. It is hypothesized that the reduction of bactericidal activity of the tears may play some role for the colonization of Actinomyces. Dry eye syndromes, which are more frequent in elderly women may predispose for this infection. Spontaneous flux of the lacrimal duct in this condition is reduced or not at all possible even when flushing under pressure may be achieved. It may be presumed that the remaining tear secretion is sufficient to inhibit an infection in the second lacrimal duct, which has not been involved.

With regard to chronic bacterial canaliculitis due to Actinomyces, it is not known if there are regional differences. This infection may cause up to 2% of purulent naso-lacrimal duct diseases.

Chronic canaliculitis has been reported to be associated with an infection of the anterior segment of the eye, however, this event is rare (4). Coinfections may possibly be more prone to cause corneal lesions than Actinomyces organisms by themselves.

Staphylococci, Streptococci, Enterobacteriaceae, Mycobacteria, Treponemes and Chlamydia may additionally endanger the eye.

Particular risks arise from omitted cure of chronic canaliculitis prior to elective intraocular surgery (17).

The differential diagnosis has to consider a diverticle in association with an ectatic lacrimal duct (18). An embryopathy may be the cause for the development of a diverticle of the lacrimal duct involving an epithelial spread and subsequent canalisation (2). Ectasy, on the other hand, may be thought as a result of the secretory stop. If an empyema develops, this complication must be dealt with in any case.

From these observations, we may conclude:

- A high percentage of misdiagnosis may be caused by the lack of information about chronic canaliculitis.
- The diagnosis of presumed infections with Actinomyces may be more frequently established, if meticulous planning of the microbiological diagnostic techniques accompanies a smooth interdisciplinary cooperation.
- Aerobic cultures have to be inoculated additionally to evaluate for frequent coinfections.
- Actinomyces could be identified in 19/54 specimens with the standard techniques of sampling and cultivation described by us.Identification of Actinomyces species resulted in the detection of A.israelii, A.meyeri, A.viscosus; in addition, three cases of A.propionica were found. In 8 specimens, further subdifferentiation of Actinomyces was not possible.

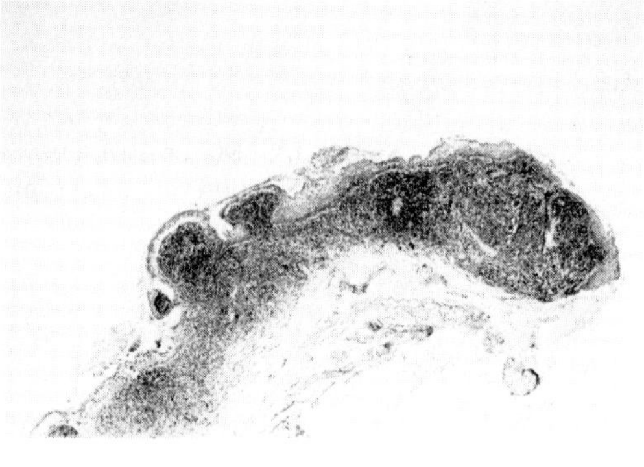

Fig.1. 51 year old male patient with a history of canaliculitis of 6 months duration. Excisional biopsy from ectatic lacrimal duct: Epithelial hyperplasia; massive subepithelial infiltration of mononuclear cells with few leukocytes and plasma cells without epithelioid giant cells. Basal papillomatosis, epithelial invaginations, scarring of connective tissue. Hematoxylin-Eosin stain, magnification 30x. Histopathologic diagnosis: Chronic nonspecific and cicatricial inflammation with a pseudoepitheliomatous and reactive lymphoid hyperplasia.

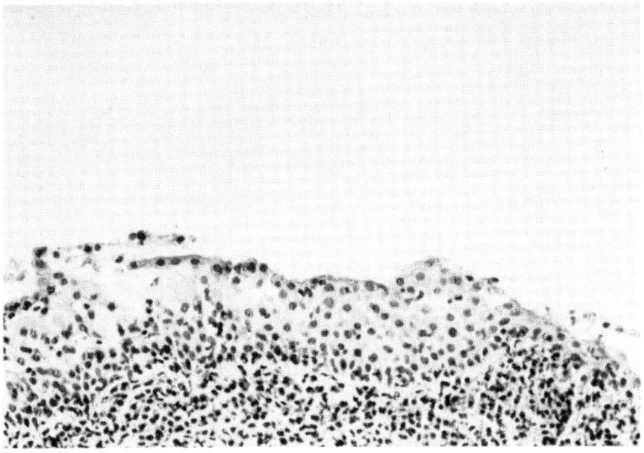

Fig.2. Mostly intact epithelium, some lymphocytes in the upper layers, massive subepithelial mononuclear infiltration. Magnification: 200x (from Fig.1).

References

1. Allen SD, Siders JA, Marer LM (1985) Isolation and Examination of Anaerobic Bacteria. In: Lenette EH, Balows A, Hausler WJ, Shadomy HJ, (eds) Manual of Clinical Microbiology, American Society for Microbiology, Washington pp.413-433
2. Badtke G, Tost M (1986) Fehler beim Aussprossen der Tränenröhrchen. In: Velhagen K (ed) Der Augenarzt, Bd.11, neu bearb. u. erweitert von Tost,M, VEB G.Thieme, Leipzig pp.779-781
3. Concini M de, Bois S, Detassis C (1985) Canalicolite lacrimale da actinomyces. Minerva oftal 27:81-83, Zbl f Augenheilk 128:628
4. Duke-Elder ST (1965) Actinomyces of the Conjunctiva. In: Duke-Elder ST (ed) System of Ophthalmology Vol. VIII, Kimpton H, London Part I:229-232
5. Duke-Elder ST (1965) Inflammations of the Lacrimal Passages: Canaliculitis. In: Duke-Elder ST, (ed) System of Ophthalmology Vol. XIII, Kimpton H, London Part II:693-699
6. Hanselmayer H, Roll P, Reich ME et al (1980) Licht- und elektronenmikroskopische Untersuchungen bei Aktinomykose des Tränenkanälchens. Klin Mbl Augenheilk 176:113-118
7. Höhne C (1985) Klinisch-mikrobiologische Untersuchungen über Kultivierung, Differenzierung, Vorkommen und Chemotherapeutikaresistenz von Bacteroides. Promotion B, Martin-Luther-Universität Halle Wittenberg, Med. Fakultät, Halle
8. Höhne C, Sandow D (1986) Effektive Modifikationen anaerober Inkubationssysteme für das klinisch-mikrobiologische Laboratorium. Z Klin Med 41:783-786
9. Höhne C (1989) Klinisch-mikrobiologische Aspekte endogener Anaerobierinfektionen. Z Klin Med 44:1125-1129
10. Hoffmann DH (1962) Ein Beitrag zur Aktinomykose der Tränenröhrchen. Klin Mbl Augenheilk 140:834-845
11. Holdeman LV, Cato EP, Moore WEC (1977) Anaerobe Laboratory Manual. 4th Edition, Virginia Polytechnic Institute and State University, Blacksburg
12. Marré M, Roder H (1978) Zur Ätiologie der chronischen Canaliculitis lacrimalis mit Konkrementbildung. Folia Ophthalmol 3:28-32
13. Moore LVH, Cato EP, Moore WEC (1987) Anaerobe Lab Manual Update. Virginia Polytechnic Institute and State University, Blacksburg
14. Müller F (1987) Erkrankungen der Tränenorgane: Canaliculitis. In: Velhagen K (ed) Der Augenarzt Bd 2,2 ergänzte u.überarbeitete Aufl. VEB G.Thieme, Leipzig pp.76-79
15. Naumann GOH (1980) Pathologie des Auges. Springer Verlag, Berlin-Heidelberg-New York

16. Radnót M (1977) Tränenableitungswege. In: Francois J, Hollwich F (eds) Augenheilkunde in der Klinik und Praxis Bd 1:7.39-7.41. Thieme Verlag, Stuttgart
17. Roussel TJ, Olsen ER, Rice T et al (1991) Chronic Postoperative Endophthalmitis Associated with Actinomyces Species. Arch Ophthalmol 1091:60-62
18. Schmidt JGH, Beyer D (1980) Zur Diagnostik und Behandlung des Tränenröhrchendivertikels. Ber Dtsch Ophthalmol Ges 77:151-154
19. Smith RE, Nobe JR (1989) Eye Infections. In: Finegold SM, George WL (eds) Anaerobic Infections in Humans. Academic Press Inc, San Diego, New York, Berkeley, Boston, London, Sydney, Toronto
20. Struck HG (1982) Zur Problematik der Pilzinfektion der ableitenden Tränenwege. Folia Ophthalmol 7:212-216
21. Sutter VL, Citron DM, Edelstein MAC et al: Wadsworth Anaerobic Bacteriology Manual. 4th Edition, Star Publishing Company, Belmont

The Treatment of Chronic Blepharoconjunctivitis: Results of Differing Approaches to Treatment

Claudia M. Vojvodic Ruzir, Horacio M. Soriano, Amalia Fernandez

Abstract. Ophthalmologists apply empirical medications in most of their patients with chronic blepharitis or blepharoconjunctivitis. The main object of this work was to determine the efficacy of those treatment regimens generally inspired by the Marketing Departments of the pharmaceutical industry.
From 1987 through 1990, 600 patients with chronic blepharoconjunctivitis were examined. A protocol was used including history, exfoliative cytology, bacteriology, culture and antibiotic sensitivity tests. 288 patients (48%) with positive cultures for bacterial chronic blepharitis and blepharoconjunctivitis were examined.
In 30% of those patients, two different bacterial strains were found. 77.3% of the isolated bacteria were Gram-positive. The most frequent were S.aureus (63.5%) and S.epidermidis (61.3%). 70% of S.epidermidis were found resistant to the antibiotics that the patients had used. All patients had been treated with corticosteroids, Chloramphenicol and aminoglycosides. All of them were sensitive to Cephalotin and 94% to Erythromicin.
We demonstrate that empirical treatment and laboratory findings differ widely. Our findings add to the explanation of known frequent therapeutic failure.

Introduction

Conjunctivitis is one of the most common affections of the eye in the Western hemisphere (9). Etiologic agents are bacteria, viruses, chlamydiae, fungi and parasites. Bacterial conjunctivitis is most frequent and may be acute or chronic.

Acute conjunctivitis may be provoked by S.aureus, S.epidermidis, pneumococci and H.influenzae, the last one being frequent in children.

S.epidermidis plays an important role in chronic bacterial conjunctivitis. Bacterial sensitivity and resistance patterns to different antibiotics in chronic conjunctivitis have not been investigated in the recent past.

In the section of ocular infections of the Jose de San Martin Hospital and Centro Optalmologico de Alta Complejidad 600 patients have been examined for chronic diseases of the lids and conjunctivae from March 1987 through February 1990. In all of these patients, systemic questionnaires were donee. Cultures and sensitivity testing of smears were performed to evaluate for bacterial infection.

In smears from 288 patients (48%), significant bacterial colony counts could be determined.

Patients and Methods

Six hundred patients with signs and symptoms of blepharoconjunctivitis were examined. A complete ophthalmologic examination including history-taking, slit-lamp examination, refraction, determination of the break-up time was complemented by a cytobacteriological study. In case of previous medication, the treatment was stopped 48 hours before the sample was taken.

Blepharitis was defined as an inflammation with lesions of the anterior and posterior lid margins, hyperemia and alterations of the eye lashes.

Conjunctivitis was defined as an inflammation with conjunctival hyperemia, chemosis and exudate. We considered conjunctivitis to be chronic when signs and symptoms prevailed for more than 15 days (with or without treatment). We defined conjunctivitis to be infectious when counted colonies in solid medium were more than 10^5 compared to saprophytic bacterial counts (7).

Bacteriological Study

Smears were taken from the conjunctivae and the free lid margins in 600 patients using a cotton-tipped swab without anesthetics under slit-lamp control.

Stewart-Ames broth was used for transportation and the following studies were done:

Bacterioscopy (Gram and MG Giemsa)

Incubation for aerobic and facultatively anaerobic bacteria was done on agar trypticase soy with 5% sheep blood, chocolate agar at 37°C and 5%-10% of CO_2. For anaerobic bacteria, smears were cultivated in Brucella agar with menadione blood and Vancomycin and Amikacin added. Incubation was done at 37°C in an anaerobic device. The plates were examined 24 hours later and, if necessary incubation was prolonged for another 48 hours. For evaluation of the cultures, the semiquantitative technique of Marcenac and coworkers to test the sensitivity of Staphylococci, Pseudomonas and Acinetobacter to different antibiotics was applied(10). In Hemophilus influenzae strains ß-lactamase activity was evaluated using the nitrocephin technique.

Out of 600 patients examined, 288 (48%) yielded positive bacterial cultures. The remaining 312 patients with chronic diseases of lids and conjunctivae but with negative cyto-bacteriologic work-up for bacterial infection were excluded. Previous ocular and systemic history of 288 patients was taken (Tab.1). All of the 288 patients with positive cultures had received previous empirical treatment with Chloramphenicol and an aminoglycoside or polypeptide antibiotic, and corticosteroids. Treatment ranged from four to 7 days (Tab.2).

Bacteriological Results

Results of the cultures are given in Tab.3. A cellular inflammatory reaction was infrequently observed. Gram-staining only rarely revealed the presence of bacteria while cultures from smears in all of the 288 patients studied were positive. One single bacterial strain could be isolated in 198 patients (68.75%), and more than one strain in 90 patients (31.25%). Gram-positive bacteria were isolated in 80.69% of the cases with 76.33% being Staphylococci and Streptococci. The most frequent Gram-negative bacteria were Pseudomonas (5.55%) followed by H.influenzae (4.77%) and A.calcoaceticus (4.23%).

Anaerobic bacteria were not found.

All of the S.aureus, S.epidermidis and other coagulase negative Staphylococci strains were sensitive to Cephalotin, Methicilin, Vancomycin and Rifampicin. More than 90% of the three different staphylococcal strains were sensitive to Erythromycin and more than 60% to Cotrimoxazole (Tab.4).

P.aeruginosa was resistent to Gentamycin and Tobramycin. 71.42% of P.aeruginosa was sensitive to Amikacin and Polymyxin B.

A.calcoaceticus was sensitive to Mezlocilin, aminoglycosides, cephalosporins, Cotrimoxazole and Polymyxin B. All were resistent to Chloramphenicol (Tab.5).

Discussion

We found that in 48% of patients with chronic blepharitis and conjunctivitis a bacterial etiology may be determined. Gram-positive bacteria had the highest incidence. The most frequently found organism were Staphylococci, particularly S.epidermidis.

Until 1960, Staphylococci were considered bacterial contaminants and had little clinical impact when cultured. Today, much attention is given to these bacteria as they may produce different types of infections.

In our study they were responsible for 66.79% of all infections determined by the comparative colony counts on solid media (7).

Before they had been referred to our Department, all of the patients had received empirical undirected topical antibiotic treatment in the course of disease. All had received Chloramphenicol and Tobramycin and 25% of them a polypeptide antibiotic or an aminoglycoside as well as topical corticosteroids, sometimes in fixed combinations with antibiotics. Duration of treatment with each antibiotic was seven days in 13.88% of patients and less than five days in 86.10% of patients. A previous history of conjunctivitis treated with these antibiotics was found in 83.68% of patients. In 54 patients with a previous hordeolum S.aureus could be isolated.

Staphylococci were resistant to Chloramphenicol and aminoglycocosides, however, 100% were sensitive to Cephalotin. The high sensitivity of P.aeruginosa and A.calcoaceticus to the antibiotics tested might be explained by the fact that the sources of contamination had not been nosocomial.

In all patients the break-up time was abnormal (under 25"), which means associated dry eye syndromes secondary to chronic infections. The break-up time was under 5" in all cases with rheumatoid arthritis. In our study, the initial undirected empirical treatment had never correlated with the sensitivity data found in cultures of the organisms, a fact, which might offer an explanation of therapeutical failures in the 288 patients evaluated.

Initial treatment with topical antibiotics should be directed toward the most frequent organisms. This means more than 90% of the Staphylococcus strains should be sensitive to the antibiotics in question and the duration of treatment should at least be ten to fifteen days.

The antibiotics which match these requirements are

- Cephalosporins of the first generation,
- Isoxazol-Penicillins, and
- Erythromycin.

In all cases of chronic conjunctivitis and blepharitis persisting for more than two weeks cyto-bacteriological and clinical evaluations with sensitivity tests are recommended. The antibiotic should be chosen according to the sensitivity testing and the type of isolated bacteria.

Conclusions

Ophthalmologists usually administer empirical antibiotics in most of the patients with chronic blepharoconjunctivitis.

In our study, the initial empirical treatment had never correlated with the eventual antibiotic sensitivity patterns found in cultures, which might offer an explanation for prior therapeutic failures.

Options for antibiotic regimens should therefore be chosen only after sensitivity testing of the cultivated organisms.

Table 1. Empirical antibiotic used in 288 patients with chronic blepharoconjunctivitis

Two antibiotics:	Chloramphenicol + Tobramicine	216 (75%)
Three antibiotics :	Chloramphenicol + Tobramicine + Gentamicine	72 (25%)
Corticosteroids :		28 (100%)
DURATION OF TREATMENT		
Days	Patients	%
4	185	64.23
5	63	21.87
7	40	13.88

Table 2. History of the treated patients

Previous Ocular History	N° Patients	%
Previous hordeolum	54	18.75
History of previously conjunctivitis	241	83.68
Contact lenses usurious	72	25.00
Ocular surgery:		
- cataract	27	9.37
- glaucoma	12	4.17
Vernal conjunctivitis	12	4.17
B U T :		
- 5"	72	25.00
- from 5 to 10"	126	43.75
- from 10 to 15"	90	31.25
Previous Systemic History	**N° Patients**	**%**
Seborrhea	54	18.75
Extraocular infections	12	4.17
Dermatological affections:		
- Plain red lichen	1	1.04
- Rosacea	12	4.17
- Allergy and asthma	72	25.00
- Rheumatoid arthritis	72	25.00
History of Systemic Medication		
- Corticosteroids	12	4.17
- Beta Block	15	5.20
- Psychopharms	24	8.34

Table 3.

Cultures	**N° Patients**	**%**
Monobacterial	198	68.75
Polibacterial	90	31.25
TOTAL	288	100,00
Bacterium	**N° Strands**	**%**
Gram (+)	610	80.69
Gram (-)	146	19.31
Gram (+) Bacterium	**N° Strands**	**%**
S.epidermidis	310	41.00
S.aureus	128	16.93
S.coagulase (-) (no S.epidermidis)	67	8.86
S.pneumoniae	36	4.77
S.viridans	36	4.77
Other Gram (+) bacterium: (corynebacterium sp., bacillus sp.)	33	4.36
Gram (-) Bacterium	**N° Strands**	**%**
P.aeruginosa	42	5.55
H.influenzae	36	4.77
A.calcoacetiens	32	4.23
Other Gram (-) bacteria (Enterobacter,S.marcescens,P.mirabilis)	36	4.77
Gram (+) Bacterium	**N° Bacterium**	**%**
Staphylococcus	505	82.80
Streptococcus	72	11.80
Other Gram (+)	33	5.40
TOTAL	610	100.00
Staphylococcus	**N° Bacterium**	**%**
epidermidis	310	61.38
aureus	128	25.34
No epi coagulase (-)	67	13.28
TOTAL	505	100.00

Table 4.

Antibiotic	concentration mg/l	S.epidermidis 310 strands		S.aureus 128 strands		S.coagulasa- (non S.epidermidis) 67 strands	
		n°strands	%	n°strands	%	n°strands	%
P	2	140	45.16	46	35.93	15	22.38
ME	5	310	100.00	128	100.00	67	100.00
CF	5	310	100.00	128	100.00	67	100.00
GM	5	137	44.19	30	23.43	21	31.34
TO	5	185	59.67	46	45.93	31	46.26
AN	5	185	59.67	46	45.93	33	49.25
ER	5	289	93.22	122	95.31	61	91.04
TMS	5	213	68.40	91	71.09	46	68.65
VA	4	310	100.00	128	100.00	67	100.00
CL	5	61	19.67	61	47.65	21	31.34
RF	5	310	100.00	128	100.00	67	100.00

P:	Peniciline	TO:	Tobramicin	VA:	Vancomycin
ME:	Methicillin	AN:	Amikacin	RF:	Rifampicin
CF:	Cephalotine	ER:	Erythromycin		
GM:	Gentamycin	TMS:	Cotrimoxazol		

Table 5.

Antibiotic concentration		P.aeruginosa		A.calcoaceticus	
	mg/l	42 strands		32 strands	
		n°	strands %	n°	strands %
MZ	80	42	100.00	32	100.00
CRO	16	42	100.00	32	100.00
CAZ	16	42	100.00	32	100.00
GM	5	--	------	32	100.00
AN	5	30	71.42	32	100.00
TO	5	--	------	32	100.00
CL	5	--	------	--	------
PO	1	30	71.42	32	100.00
NORFLO	1	42	100.00	32	100.00

MZ : Mezlocillin GM : Gentamycin CL : Chloramphenicol
CRO : Cefttriaxone AN : Amikacin PO : Polimyxin
CAZ : Ceftazidime TO : Tobramycin NORFLO : Norfloxacin

References

1. Adams LC, Cohen E et al (1983) Corneal Ulcers in Cosmetic Extended Wear Lenses. Am J Ophthalmol 96:705-711
2. Brunzini M, Sampaolesis R (1969) Importancia del Examen Clinico, Citologico y Bacteriologico Para el Diagnostico y Tratamiento de las Conjunctivitis. Arch Oftalmol Buenos Aires Vol 82-86
3. Fedukowicz HB (1978) External Infections of the Eye; Bacterial, Viral and Mycotic. Appleton Century Crafts, New York 100-101
4. Ganley J, Roberts J (1983) Eye Conditions and Related Need for Medical Care Among Persons 1-74 Years. United States 1971-1972 National Center for Health Statistics Vital and Health Statistics, Series 11 No.22B. (USPHS Publication 82-1678 Washington DC: US Government Printing Office)
5. Gigliotti F et al (1981) Etiology of Acute Conjunctivitis in Children. J Pediatr Ophthalmol Strab 98:531-538
6. Keith G (1967) Seborrheic Blepharokeratoconjunctivitis. Trans Ophthalmol Soc 87:85-101
7. Khan J, Hoover D, Ide C (1984) Methicilline Resistant Staphylococcus Epidermidis Blepharitis. Am J Ophthalmol 98:562-565
8. Lemped S, Jenkins M (1979) Chalazia and Rosacea. AO 97:1952-1953
9. Mandel G, Douglas G, Bennett J (1990) Principles and Practice of Infectious Diseases. Churchill Livingstone, New York. Section N: 975-979
10. Marcenac F, Fernandez A et al (1987) Halbquantitative Resistenzbestimmung auf Agar. Arzneiforschung (Drug Research) 28(1):582-585
11. Marcenac F, Fernandez A et al (1975) Antibiograma Semicuantitativa en Agar. Rev Asco Bio Arg 40:135-165
12. Rapoza P, Quinn et al (1990) Systemic Approach to the Diagnosis and Treatment of Chronic Conjunctivitis. 109:138-142
13. Smolin G, Okumoto N (1977) Staphylococcal Blepharitis. Arch Ophthalmol 95:812-816
14. Smolin G, Tabbara K, Whitcher J (1984) Infectious Diseases of the Eye. Wilkins, London Vol 2 Chpt.4

III ANTERIOR SEGMENT INFECTIONS

- Basics

Immune Mechanisms in Corneal Infection

Günther Grabner

Abstract. Over the last years the understanding of basic immune mechanisms of mucosal surfaces - and in particular of the ocular surface - has vastly increased. It has been shown that immunoglobulins and immunocompetent cells are localized in the conjunctiva and cornea and that both, epithelial and stromal cells can readily participate in - and possibly to a great extent modify - local immune reactions by the production and release of a variety of cytokines. Corneal infections by a large number of different organisms can lead to a wide spectrum of immune reactions that help to control and finally eradicate the pathogen.

The Role of the Tear Film as a First-Line Defense Mechanism

To function as the principal refractive part of the eye, the cornea has to maintain the high optical quality of its anterior surface, the transparency of the stromal layers and an adequate function of the endothelium.

All these requirements are easily compromised by infection and inflammation. The lack of blood vessels and lymphatics - at least in the healthy state - in addition confers to the cornea a distinct immunological privilege as witnessed by the high success rate of grafts in non-vascularized corneas.

Nevertheless the incidence of severe infections is quite low, as several non-immunological mechanisms are functioning to protect the cornea from infectious organisms and environmental noxious substances. The constant mechanical protection by the lids is crucial as it serves to moisten the corneal surface by evenly distributing the tear film. The latter contains a multitude of substances with bacteriostatic and bactericidal properties, such as lysozyme, lactoferrin, ß-lysin, secretory IgA, IgG and complement (45).

In experimental animals IgG has been shown to be the predominant isotype in serum and cornea during both primary and secondary infection, and in tears during secondary infection with P.aeruginosa. IgG and IgA have been found in similar quantities in the tears during primary infection.

Therefore both local and systemic immune responses occur and these responses may be regulated independently (39). Foster and coworkers have demonstrated a different antibody isotype response in the Igh-1 disparate congenic mice that have different susceptibilities to Herpes Simplex Virus (HSV)-induced necrotizing stromal keratitis (14). Similar studies in humans (e.g. a correlation with HLA-antigens, are lacking for obvious reasons.

In Human Immunodeficiency Virus (HIV)-positive patients a decreased tear level of lactoferrin was found to be associated with an increased bacterial colony count on the lid margins without either a history or a clinically apparent infection of the external eye (6).

This protective function can furthermore be compromised in patients with Sjögren's syndrome, where Epstein-Barr Virus DNA, a strong antigenic stimulus for T- and B- cell responses maintained latent in a very small number of normal gland cells, has been shown to be reactivated, both in the lacrimal and salivary glands during the disease and has been held responsible for the perpetuation of the autoimmune response (49). The finding of cellular receptors for Epstein-Barr virus on inner duct lacrimal gland and suprabasal epithelial cells of conjunctiva and cornea lend support to the hypothesis that these are the sites of acute and persistent infection responsible for the damage observed in the dry eye state (8).

The importance of the "conjunctiva associated lymphoid tissue" (CALT) has been previously discussed by Chandler and Gillette (5). Newer studies have shown that indeed thoracic duct B lymphocytes, but not spleen lymphocytes, preferentially interact with lacrimal gland epithelium and thereby may account for the retention of IgA-committed cells in the lacrimal gland (37). Specialized lymphocytes might then be stimulated by locally produced cytokines (e.g. Corneal Epithelial Thymocyte Activating Factor = Interleukin-1 (IL-1) to an increased IgA secretion as has been recently shown for Peyer's patch B cells (7).

Langerhans Cells

Apart from these paraimmunologic and humoral immunologic defense mechanisms it has been shown that indeed there are immunocompetent cells to be found in the conjunctiva and the peripheral cornea that are able to function as antigen-presenting cells: the Langerhans cells (52). They have been found to be markedly reduced in patients with Human Immunodeficiency Virus (HIV) infection in the presence of an increase of T-helper and T-suppressor cells (and a reduction of the CD4/CD8 ratio in the substantia propria), pointing to an early functional deficit in antigen presentation (42).

The mouse model of HSV-keratitis has shown progressive changes in corneal Langerhans cell distribution following HSV-reactivation by ultraviolet B light that closely followed the development of ocular pathology (29). It cannot be neglected, however, that both, genetically conferred susceptibility to this infectious disease, as well as HSV-strain related factors contribute to the clinical development: the disparate (Igh-1) congenic mice did not differ with regard to the resting conjunctival or corneal Langerhans cells, susceptible strains, however, showed more conjunctival Langerhans cells after inoculation and a more pronounced central corneal migration with ulcer formation that was not observed in the resistant strain (32). On the other hand, the RE-HSV-type 1 strain activates $CD4^+$ T-cells leading to a predominantly polymorphonuclear cell infiltrate in the cornea, whereas the KOS-HSV-type 1 strain activates $CD8^+$ T-cells leading to a predominantly mononuclear infiltrate (20). RE-HSV- type 1 induces a more rapid migration of Langerhans cells into the central cornea, with ultraviolet B depletion prior to infection reducing the incidence of corneal disease and stimulating a predominantly mononuclear infiltrate (50).

An additional curious finding by Williamson and coworkers has not yet been well explained: Langerhans cells within the central cornea interfere with the induction of the anterior chamber associated immune deviation, suggesting a hitherto unknown, possibly only locally acting immunoregulatory factor(s?) (53).

Class II Major Histocompatibility Complex Antigens and Adhesion Markers on Other Corneal Cells

Although many dendritic cells in the normal human conjunctiva and peripheral corneal epithelium stain positive for class II Major Histocompatibility Complex antigens they fail to be detected by conventional Langerhans cell markers, possibly pointing to functionally different cell populations (31). DR -, DP- and DQ-antigen expression was found to be significantly higher in conjunctival biopsies from patients with pemphigoid and atopic keratoconjunctivitis than in a normal control population (26).

In certain experimental conditions (addition of gamma-Interferon) corneal epithelial and endothelial cells, as well as keratocytes show an approximately 60% increase of class II antigen expression, whereas alpha-Interferon is effective to only +30%. A combination of both, on the other hand, downregulates the expression by over 50% (4). This inhibition can also be induced in vitro by the addition of 1,25-dihydroxyvitamin D3 (47). The importance of this finding lies in the fact that the human corneal epithelial cells themselves may serve as antigen presenting cells, as has been shown in vitro by Iwata and Thoft (23). This observation has been confirmed in conjunctival and corneal specimens from patients suffering from severe graft-versus-host-disease following bone-marrow transplantation (17).

Direct lysis of virus-infected class II bearing corneal cells by $CD4^{+}$ cytotoxic T lymphocytes (after depletion of $CD8^{+}$ T-cells) might be one of the mechanisms leading to stromal immunopathology in herpetic infections (9).

Although the intercellular adhesion molecule 1 (ICAM1), an inducible surface glycoprotein, which is a ligand for lymphocyte adhesion molecule 1 is not expressed on normal human corneas, organ cultures and epithelial cell cultures, it can readily be induced by gamma-Interferon and IL-1 on both, epithelial and endothelial cells.

This points to their possible participation in cell-cell interactions during inflammatory reactions in the cornea (24). Leukocyte adherence to corneal endothelium is a well-known phenomenon in keratitis, anterior ocular inflammation and corneal allograft rejection. Tumor necrosis factor alpha, in addition to Interleukin-1ß and gamma-Interferon induces a positive endothelial cell staining for ICAM1. Neutrophil-endothelial cell-binding could be blocked by monoclonal antibodies to ICAM1 and lymphocyte adhesion molecule 1 suggestive of a possible role in the above mentioned clinical conditions (38). This finding was confirmed by Howell and coworkers (22). These adhesion molecules have been demonstrated on other cells of the anterior segment as well, such as the trabecular meshwork cells and non-pigmented cells of the human ciliary body (3).

Effects of Cytokines on Immunemodulation, Chemotaxis and Tissue Degradation

The possible importance of soluble corneal factors as immune-mediators has been postulated about a decade ago (15). The corneal epithelial cell-derived thymocyte-activating factor has been found to closely resemble IL-1 in most biochemical and biological properties (16,28).

In human herpetic keratitis epithelial cells, keratocytes and stromal inflammatory cells were positive for IL-1 and IL-6, whereas control keratoconus corneas showed only a positive epithelial staining (46). These findings were confirmed for different mediators and receptors (Epidermal Growth Factor, Epidermal Growth Factor receptor, Fibroblast Growth Factor b, Tumor Growth Factor ß1, and IL-1 alpha) by in vitro studies of cultured human keratocytes and by analysis of mRNA of corneal fibroblasts and endothelial cells stimulated by a variety of methods (2,43,54).

Leukocytic infiltration of the cornea is an important process in a variety of corneal and anterior segment inflammatory diseases, allograft rejection and corneal injury models. Cytokine-stimulated cells such as vascular endothelial cells, monocytes, fibroblasts and retinal pigment epithelial cells produce a 72-amino-acid polypeptide (neutrophil chemotactic factor, Interleukin-8 (IL-8)) that elicits neutrophil chemotaxis and activation and is also a chemoattractant for lymphocytes at low concentration. IL-8 mRNA expression of human corneas and accumulation in the supernatants significantly increased following exposured to IL-1ß and Tumor Necrosis Factor-alpha (12). The release of these neutrophil chemotactic factor(s) from peroxide injured corneas can be inhibited by dexamethasone, indomethacin and inhibition of the intracellular synthesis with cycloheximide, puromycin and actinomycin (10,11). Chemotactic and chemokinetic effects on other corneal cells (fibroblasts, endothelial cells) can certainly be ascribed to other cytokines as well: IL-1, Epidermal Growth Factor, Tumor Growth Factor-ß and basic Fibroblast Growth Factor have been effective (16,19). The effect on different cell layers seems to vary, however, as Tumor Growth Factor-ß has been demonstrated to retard epithelial wound healing (34).

IL-6, previously described under a variety of different names is a key cytokine in immune regulation and has been found to be constitutively produced by human keratocytes with an increase of release into the culture medium following laser irradiation (for review see 44, and personal observation). It seems to promote corneal wound healing in a dose-dependent manner by stimulating the expression of fibronectin-receptors on the cell surface (33). The mechanisms of action seem to be different from those of epidermal growth factor and fibronectin, however (30).

Catabolic activities of cytokines, on the other hand, could be responsible for the development of corneal ulcers and scar formation: IL-1 alpha inhibits the synthesis of proteoglycans in a dose dependent manner while at the same time activating keratocytes (40). IL-1 increases the collagenolytic activity by keratocytes in a three-dimensional collagen gel, an activity reversed by anti-IL-

1 and serine protease inhibitors (36). A de novo elastase production has been shown in stromal fibroblasts of corneas with rheumatoid ulcers, but not with keratoconus and has been explained by a paracrine action of monokines (Tumor Necrosis Factor-alpha, IL-1, IL-6) released by macrophages at the limbal area (41).

Suppressive Effects of Mediators

With all the above listed stimulatory activities of a variety of cytokines produced and released in the corneal stroma and detectable in supernatants and surrounding tissue fluids inhibitory, down-regulating factors seem necessary to counterbalance the multitude of these effects.

Recent research has therefore focussed towards identifying such substances: small inhibitory factor(s?) of murine, porcine and bovine aqueous humor (Small Inhibitory Factor-A) with a molecular weight of less than 3500 D have been found to inhibit murine thymocyte costimulation and the generation of cytotoxic T-lymphocytes (18,25).

In addition, Tumor Growth Factor-ß has been found to be responsible to a significant extent for the immunosuppressive activity of normal aqueous humor that can be abolished by serum factors, such as alpha-2 macroglobulin in secondary aqueous humor (48). In experimental animals anterior chamber associated immune deviation can also be abrogated by antibodies to Interleukin-4 and Tumor Growth Factor-ß2, possibly at a non-ocular (systemic) level (13). The possible role of Tumor Growth Factor-ß has been discussed above. The identification of different proteinase inhibitors (alpha-1 antichymotrypsin, alpha-2 antiplasmin, alpha-2 macroglobulin) in the cornea is suggestive of a delicate regulatory balance to control its effects and has been postulated to be essential for the preservation of corneal clarity (51). In this regard it is also of interest that corneal endothelial cells seem to have a potent inhibitory activity on S-antigen- and Concanavalin A-stimulated T-cells that is cell-cell contact dependent (35).

Genetic Factors

It should not be overlooked, however, that these also significantly contribute to the development and outcome of infectious diseases as has been gathered mostly from animal studies.

When comparing BALB/c to C57BL/6 mice in HSV-1 keratitis using immunohistochemical methods it has been observed that strains with more severe disease have a more intense inflammatory response to HSV-antigen (1). The H-2 haplotype determines the susceptibility to recurrent herpes simplex keratitis that is induced by ultraviolet B light, the mechanism remaining unclear (27).

In an other immunohistochemical study of human HSV-keratitis, HSV-antigens were present significantly more often in avascular lesions (15/30) than in those with vascularisation (2/38). Corneal vascularisation was found to be associated with large stromal scars and a decrease of detectable HSV-antigen (21).

All of the above mentioned factors may contribute in different ways to the immunologic protection of the cornea and to an active invasion of the organ by microbial agents. Although many singular aspects require additional experimental and clinical research - in close cooperation with immunologists - in the future, their effective interaction and at the same time balance are obviously crucial for the maintainance of the corneal integrity and function.

References

1. Abgahri SZ, Zhu Z, Whitsett CF et al (1991) Immunohistochemical Study of Herpes Simplex Virus Type 1 (HSV) Keratitis in Inbred Mice. Invest Ophthalmol Vis Sci 32 (Suppl)803
2. Ansel JC, Tara D, Rosenbaum JT (1991) Synthesis of Interleukin 1 and 6 by Human Cornea. Invest Ophthalmol Vis Sci 32 (Suppl):676
3. Aoki KR, Kropp M, Bullington R et al (1991) ICAM-1 Expression by Cultured Human Ciliary Body Non-Pigmented Epithelial (NPE) and Primary Human Trabecular Meshwork Cells. Invest Ophthalmol Vis Sci 32 (Suppl):1119
4. Bergstrom LK, Holland EJ, Shapiro RS et al (1991) Interferon Interactions in the Regulation of MHC Class II Antigens in the Human Cornea. Invest Ophthalmol Vis Sci 32 (Suppl):677
5. Chandler JW, Gillette TE (1983) Immunologic Defense Mechanisms of the Ocular Surface. Ophthalmol 90:585-591
6. Comerie-Smith S, Nunez J, Hosmer M et al (1991) Tear Lactoferrin Levels and Ocular Bacterial Flora in HIV Positive Patients. Invest Ophthalmol Vis Sci 32 (Suppl):763
7. Cowdery JS, Kemp JD, Ballas ZK et al (1988) Interleukin-1 Induces T Cell Mediated Differentiation of Murine Peyer's Patch B Cells to IgA Secretion. Regional Immun 1:9-14
8. Crouse C, Pflugfelder S, Yen M et al (1991) Detection of Epstein-Barr Virus Antigens and Receptor Molecules on Ocular Surface and Lacrimal Gland Epithelia. Invest Ophthalmol Vis Sci 32(Suppl):807
9. Doymaz M, Rouse BT (1991) MHC-II Restricted, CD4+ Cytotoxic T Lymphocytes (CTL) Specific for Herpes-Simplex Virus-1: Implications for the Development of Herpetic Stromal Keratitis (HSK) in Mice. Invest Ophthalmol Vis Sci 32(Suppl):854
10. Elgebaly SA, Elkerm AF, Ehlers W (1991) Effect of Dexamethason and Indomethacin on Corneal Inflammation Induced by Factors Derived from Hydrogen Peroxide Injured Corneas. Invest Ophthalmol Vis Sci 32(Suppl):678
11. Elgebaly SA, Fishman JB, Kreutzer DL (1990) Intracellular Synthesis of Cornea-Derived Neutrophil Chemotactic Factor (NCF). 9th ICER Abstracts, Helsinki. August 2.
12. Elner VM, Strieter RM, Pavilack MA et al (1991) Interleukin-8 (IL-8) Gene Expression and Secretion by whole Human Corneas. Invest Ophthalmol Vis Sci 32(Suppl):1120
13. Ferguson TA, Mahendra S (1991) The Role of Interleukin-4 and Transforming Growth Factor-ß2 in Anterior Chamber Associated Immune Deviation (ACAID). Invest Ophthalmol Vis Sci 32(Suppl):1118
14. Foster CS, Zhao TZ, Dutt JE (1991) Investigation of the IgG-Subclass Response to Corneal Herpes Virus Infection in Mice. Invest Ophthalmol Vis Sci 32(Suppl):853
15. Grabner G, Luger TA, Smolin G et al (1982) Corneal Epithelial Cell-Derived Thymocyte Activating Factor (CETAF). Invest Ophthalmol Vis Sci 23:757-763
16. Grabner G, Luger TA, Luger BM et al (1983) Biologic Properties of the Thymocyte-Activating Factor (CETAF) Produced by a Rabbit Corneal Cell Line (SIRC). Invest Ophthalmol Vis Sci 24:589-595

17. Grabner G, Hinterberger W, Fischer M et al (1985) Ocular Manifestations of Graft-versus-Host Disease Following Bone Marrow Transplantation. Exp Hematol 13(Suppl 17):142-145
18. Granstein RD, Nazareno R, Knisely TL (1991) Inhibition of Cytotoxic Lymphocyte (CTL) Generation in Vitro by a small Factor in Aqueous Humor (A.H.) Invest Ophthalmol Vis Sci 32(Suppl):1118
19. Grant MB, Guay C, Schultz GS (1991) Effects of Epidermal Growth Factor (EGF), Basic Fibroblast Growth Factor (bFGF), and Transforming Growth Factor-Beta (TGF-ß) on Bovine Corneal Cell Chemotaxis. Invest Ophthalmol Vis Sci 32(Suppl):953
20. Hendricks RL, Tumpey TM (1991) Contribution of Virus and Immune Factors to Herpes Simplex Virus Type 1-induced Corneal Pathology. Invest Ophthalmol Vis Sci 31:1929-1939
21. Holbach LM, Seitz B, Rummelt C et al (1991) Herpes Simplex Keratitis: Biomorphometry of Disciform Corneal Scars and Immunohistochemical Identification of HSV Antigens. Invest Ophthalmol Vis Sci 32(Suppl):1076
22. Howell DN, Burchette J, Foulks GN et al (1991)
23. Antigen Expression by Human Corneal Endothelium. Invest Ophthalmol Vis Sci 32(Suppl):1178
24. Iwata M, Thoft RA (1991) HLA Class II Antigen Expression on Human Corneal Epithelial Cells: The Ability to Stimulate allo Lymphocytes as Antigen Presenting Cells. Invest Ophthalmol Vis Sci 32(Suppl):937
25. Kaminsky GM, Niederkorn JY, McCulley JP (1991) Intercellular Adhesion Molecule-1 (ICAM-1) Expression in Normal and Inflamed Human Cornea:Induction by Recombinant Interferon Gamma and Interleukin-1. Invest Ophthalmol Vis Sci 32(Suppl):677
26. Knisely TL, Nazareno R, Granstein RD (1991) Characterization of Small Molecular Weight Inhibitory Factors in Aqueous Humor. Invest Ophthalm Vis Sci 32(Suppl):936
27. Kupferman AE, Lee SJ, Rice BA et al (1991) HLA Class II Expression in Conjunctiva. Invest Ophthalmol Vis Sci 32(Suppl):937
28. Laycock KA, Miller JK, Pepose JS (1991) H-2 Haplotype Determines the Susceptibility to Recurrent Herpes Simplex Keratitis Induced by Ultraviolet-B light. Invest Ophthalmol Vis Sci 32(Suppl):804
29. Luger TA, Grabner G, Sztein MB et al (1983) A Corneal Cytokine Triggers the in Vivo Synthesis of Serum Amyloid A by Hepatocytes. Ophthalmic Res 15:121-125
30. Miller JK, Nash MM, Levy DS et al (1991) Progressive Changes in Corneal Langerhans Cell Distribution Following Herpes Simplex Virus Reactivation in a Murine Model Invest Ophthalmol Vis Sci 32(Suppl):803
31. Mishima H, Nakamura M, Murakami J et al (1991) TGF-ß Regulates Actions of EGF, Interleukin-6 and Fibronectin on the Functions of Corneal Epithelial Cells. Invest Ophthalmol Vis Sci 32(Suppl):954
32. Murchison JF, Yen MT, Pflugfelder SC et al (1991) Monoclonal Antibody Recognition of Human Ocular Surface Langerhans Cells. Invest Ophthalomol Vis Sci 32(Suppl):937
33. Neumann R, Foster CS (1991) Langerhans Cells in Cornea and Conjunctiva of Disparate (Igh-1) Congenic Mice Coincident with Differential Pathology to Herpes Simplex Virus. Invest Ophthalmol Vis Sci 32(Suppl):1077
34. Nishida T, Nakamura M, Mishima H et al (1991) Stimulation of Corneal Epithelial Wound Healing by Interleukin-6 (IL-6). Invest Ophthalmol Vis Sci 32(Suppl):1247
35. Nishida K, Taniguchi E, Ohashi Y et al (1991) Transforming Growth Factor-ß

(TGG-ß) Can Retard Epithelial Wound Healing of Organ-Cultured Corneas. Invest Ophthalmol Vis Sci 32(Suppl):1159
35. Obritsch WF, Olsen TW, Bergstrom L et al (1991) Inhibition of in Vitro T Cell Proliferative Responses by Corneal Endothelial Cells. Invest Ophthalmol Vis Sci 32(Suppl):680
36. Okamoto J, Mishima H, Nakamura M et al (1991) Interleukin 1 Induction of Collagenolytic Activity by Keratocytes Cultured in Three Dimensional Collagen Gel. Invest Ophthalmol Vis Sci 32(Suppl):1070
37. O'Sullivan NL, Montgommery PC (1991) T- and B-Cell Adhesive Interactions with Lacrimal Glands. Invest Ophthalmol Vis Sci 32(Suppl):939
38. Pavilack MA, Elner SG, Elner VM et al (1991) Intracellular Adhesion Molecule-1 in Human Corneal Endothelium: Modulation and Function. Invest Ophthalmol Vis Sci 32(Suppl):1119
39. Preston MJ, Berk RS, Hazlett LD (1991) Kinetics of Local and Systemic Immune Response to Pseudomonas Aeruginosa Corneal Infection. Invest Ophthalmol Vis Sci 32(Suppl):1167
40. Ramirez-Florez S, Watson PG, Davies ME et al (1991) Catabolic Activity of IL-1alpha in Corneal Organ Culture. Invest Ophthalmol Vis Sci 32(Suppl):1002
41. Saal JG, Fritz P, Pleyer U et al (1991) De novo Elastase Production of Corneal Fibroblasts in Rheumatoid Corneal Ulceration (RCU) Invest Ophthalmol Vis Sci 32(Suppl):1069
42. Sacks EH, Wieczorek R, Mastrobattista JD et al (1991) Immunophenotypic Analysis of Conjunctival Immunocytes in Patients with HIV Infection. Invest Ophthalmol Vis Sci 32(Suppl):764
43. Schreiner J, Grabner G, Luger TA et al (1985) Humane Hornhautfibroblasten und eine humane Bindehaut-Zellinie (Chang) produzieren einen thymozytenaktivierenden Faktor (TAF) in vitro. Klin Mbl Augenhlkd 187:403-405
44. Seghal PB, Grieninger G, Tosato G (1989)Regulation of the Acute Phase and Immune Responses: Interleukin-6. Ann NY Acad Sci Vol.557
45. Selinger DS, Selinger RS, Reed WP (1979) Resistance to Infections of the External Eye: The Role of Tears. Surv Ophthalmol 24:33-38
46. Tagawa Y, Kitagawa, Matsuda H (1991) IL-1 and IL-6 Expressed on Keratocytes in Human Herpetic Stromal Keratitis. Invest Ophthalmol Vis Sci 32(Suppl):802
47. Taniguchi E, Ohashi Y, Mano T et al (1991) 1,25-Dihydroxy-Vitamin D3 Inhibits Class II Antigen Expression in Cultured Human Corneal Epithelial Cells. Invest Ophthalmol Vis Sci 32(Suppl)937
48. Taylor AW, Streilein JW, Cousins SW (1991) Serum Neutralizes Antiproliferative Activity of Aqueous Humor. Invest Ophthalmol Vis Sci 32(Suppl):936
49. Tsubota K, Fujishima H, Toda I et al (1991) Increased Level of Epstein-Barr Virus DNA in Lacrimal and Salivary Glands of Patients with Sjögren's Syndrome. Invest Ophthalmol Vis Sci 32(Suppl):807
50. Tumpey TM, Hendricks RL (1991) Role of Langerhans Cells in HSV-1 Corneal Stromal Disease. Invest Ophthalmol Vis Sci 32(Suppl):803
51. Twining SS, Zhou X, Wilson PM (1991) Identification of Proteinase Inhibitors in the Cornea: alpha-1-Antichymotrypsin, alpha-2-Antiplasmin, alpha-2-Macroglobulin. Invest Ophthalmol Vis Sci 32(Suppl):1071
52. Vantrappen L, Geboes K, Missotten L et al (1985) Lymphocytes and Langerhans Cells in the Normal Human Cornea. Invest Ophthalmol Vis Sci 26:220-225
53. Williamson JSP, DiMarco S, Streilein JW (1987) Immunobiology of Langerhans Cells on the Ocular Surface. I.Langerhans Cells within the Central Cornea Interfere

with Induction of Anterior Chamber Associated Immune Deviation. Invest Ophthalmol Vis Sci 28:1527-1532

54. Wilson SE, Lloyd SA (1991) Growth Factor and Growth Factor Receptor Production by Cultured Human Endothelial Cells. Invest Ophthalmol Vis Sci 32(Suppl): 953

CD1-Positive Langerhans Cells in Various Inflammatory Corneal Diseases

Wolfgang Philipp, Wolfgang Göttinger

Abstract. Langerhans cells in normal human corneas lack thymocyte antigen CD1, which is a highly specific marker for non-corneal Langerhans cells. Furthermore, corneal Langerhans cells cannot be induced to express CD1 antigen when cultured with various cytokines including interleukin-1. Thus, some authors assume that corneal Langerhans cells may represent a distinct Langerhans cell subpopulation being innately inactive.

In the present study, we investigated 62 corneas from patients with various corneal diseases for the presence of CD1 and HLA-DR antigens on Langerhans cells in the central and pericentral epithelium. CD1$^+$/HLA DR$^+$ Langerhans cells at a high density similar to that observed in normal epidermis could be detected in the epithelium of five alkali-burned corneas. Furthermore, CD1$^+$/HLA-DR$^+$ Langerhans cells, albeit at lower densities could also be detected in corneas from patients with chronic herpetic stromal keratitis, zoster keratitis, with chronic allograft rejection and with bacterial corneal ulcers.

Although the functional significance of CD1$^+$ expression on corneal Langerhans cells still remains to be determined, the induction of CD1 antigen on corneal Langerhans cells may represent an important event for the antigen-presenting function of these cells in various corneal diseases.

Introduction

Langerhans cells are potent antigen-presenting dendritic cells in skin and other tissues with squamous epithelium. In the normal human cornea, Langerhans cells may only be detected at the limbus and the peripheral cornea, whereas these cells cannot be found in the central cornea. Furthermore, corneal Langerhans cells are CD1 antigen negative except for neonates and in some rare cases in very young children. The CD1 antigen can be found on 70% of cortical thymocytes and it has been shown that this antigen is a highly specific marker for Langerhans cells.

Our studies have dealt with the problem if corneal Langerhans cells express CD1 antigen in several defined disease entities. Thus, we have attempted to elucidate, if corneal Langerhans cells are specific CD1 negative phenotypes or if Langerhans cells in the normal cornea may appear as undifferentiated or non-activated cells and may only express the CD1 antigen in particular corneal diseases.

Immunologic Study

At the time of perforating keratoplasty for various degenerative and inflammatory corneal diseases, 62 human corneal buttons were investigated.
Antibodies: Two monoclonal antibodies, an anti-HLA-DR and an anti-CD1 antibody (Dakopatts,Copenhagen,Denmark) were used for identification of Langerhans cells. Several other monoclonal antibodies of Dakopatts, Copenhagen, Denmark, were used for the identification of cellular elements in mononuclear cell infiltrates:
- CD2 for the identification of developed peripheral T-cells (E-rosette receptor),
- CD4 for the identification of helper-inducer T cells,
- CD8 for the identification of cytotoxic-suppressor T cells,
- CD22 for identification of B cells and
- EBM11 for the identification of monocytes/macrophages.

Immunohistochemistry was performed using the peroxidase-antiperoxidase procedure described by Sternberg. HLA-DR or CD1 positive dendritic cells were identified as Langerhans cells.
Immunofluorescent technique: In addition to immunoperoxidase techniques, corneal buttons containing CD1 positive Langerhans cells in the epithelium or stroma were evaluated with a double immunofluorescent technique in order to prove a coexpression of HLA-DR and CD1 antigens. To achieve this, primary antibodies of various IgG subclasses, anti-HLA-DR alpha (IgG_1) and anti-CD1 (IgG_{2a}) and subclass-specific secondary antibodies coupled to Rhodamine and Fluorescein were used.

Results: Langerhans cells could be detected only very rarely in non-inflamed corneas (keratoconus, Fuchs' corneal dystrophy, bullous keratopathy and non-vascularized corneal scars). In each of the corneas with acute or chronic inflammatory disease, HLA-DR positive Langerhans cells could be detected in varying numbers even in the central epithelial region. CD1 positive HLA-DR positive Langerhans cells could be detected in the epithelium of 15 out of 62 corneal buttons studied.
-In the epithelium of five corneas with epidermalization subsequent to severe alkali burns the largest amount of CD1 positive HLA-DR positive Langerhans cells was found at a concentration almost equalling epidermal counts (300-500 cells/mm^2). Furthermore,CD1 positive HLA-DR positive Langerhans cells could be detected in
- 3/7 patients with chronic herpes keratitis,
- 2/4 patients with Zoster keratitis,
- 3/6 patients with chronic allograft rejection and
- 2/8 patients with bacterial corneal ulcers.

The amounts of CD1 positive HLA-DR positive Langerhans cells detected in these disease entities were lower than in lye burns. In corneal buttons with an accumulation of Langerhans cells in the central epithelium, mononuclear inflammatory cells were mainly found in the stromal and the epithelial layers. In the anterior stromal section of the corneas diseased from lye burns, cellular infiltrates consisted mainly of lymphocytes and macrophages. In these corneas further investigation of the lymphocyte subpopulations with monoclonal antibodies resulted in the detection of helper-inducer as well as cytotoxic-suppressor T cells. According to the severity and the stage of the disease, an enormous cellular variability of these infiltrates was observed. Corneal buttons with epithelial CD1 positive Langerhans cells usually exhibited dense mononuclear infiltrates in the anterior corneal stroma and in the epithelium. Corneal buttons with CD1 negative Langerhans cells expressed only few cellular infiltrates with only very few mononuclear cells in the anterior corneal stroma.

Discussion

The lack of expression of the CD1 antigen on corneal Langerhans cells of normal corneas is not known. Some workers suggest that the same unknown factors responsible for the absence of Langerhans cells in the central part of the cornea may also be responsible for the lack of CD1 antigen on these cells.

In this report we have shown that corneal Langerhans cells in certain diseases may express the CD1 antigen. CD1 positive Langerhans cells were usually detected in diseased corneas with dense mononuclear cell infiltrates particularly in the anterior stroma and epithelium, e.g. in chronic herpes keratitis, Zoster keratitis or allograft rejection. Most CD1 positive HLA-DR positive Langerhans cells, however, could be found in corneas with epidermalization due to alkali burns.

An easy explanation for the induction of CD1 antigen expression might be the production of multiple cytokines including interleukin-1 by the multitude of inflammatory cells such as macrophages and T cells detectable in diseased corneas. If epidermalization or keratinization of corneal epithelium may also influence the CD1 antigen expression of corneal Langerhans cells cannot be proven with this study, since a great number of mononuclear cells has been found in inflamed corneas. The induction of the CD1 antigen on corneal Langerhans cells may be an important event for the antigen presenting function of these cells in various corneal diseases including corneal allograft rejections. These cells may be able to invade a transplant - as has been shown in animal experiments - and cause rejection.

Further studies are necessary to clarify the factors responsible for the induction of the CD1 antigen on corneal Langerhans cells. In particular, investigations should center on cytokine-producing inflammatory cells and on other factors, e.g. the epidermalization of corneal epithelium.

Fibrinolytic Enzymes and Corneal Infection

Timo Tervo, Ahti Tarkkanen, Olli Saksela and Pentti Kuusela

Abstract. Plasmin levels in tear fluid are elevated during contact lens wear. With a mean of 1.2μg/ml (SD 0.2μg/ml) they are, however, lower than the plasmin levels found in the tear fluid of eyes with corneal ulcers.
We have recently shown that some microbes such as S.aureus adhering to contact lenses are capable of cleaving plasminogen to active plasmin. Such an activation on the surface of S.aureus shows analogy to the plasminogen activation on the surface of tumor

cells; the cell surface-bound plasmin is not inhibited by the large molecular weight plasmin inhibitors. Aprotinin, on the other hand, has been found to effectively inhibit plasmin at the surface of S.aureus.
We have now investigated the effect of plasmin on the staphylococcal adherence on glass coverslips coated with fibronectin on fibrinogen.
Treatment of coated surfaces with high plasmin concentrations (1μg/ml) decreased the adherence, whereas plasmin-treated bacteria showed enhanced adherence to intact proteins. Treatment of either the surface or bacteria with smaller plasmin concentrations (0.1-0.01μg/ml) had a coordinate decreasing effect on staphylococcal adherence.

Introduction

The inflamed ocular surface can be subjected to a number of proteolytic activities due to microbial proteases (13), leucocytes (19), cytokine-mediated mechanisms (10), and certain serine proteinases (4). Activation of plasminogen to proteolytically active plasmin has been described to take place during corneal infections (23,27), mechanical irritation of the ocular surface (31), type I allergic reactions (24), and during contact lens wear (28,32). Similar stimuli also cause liberation of the mast cell-derived proteases, chymase and tryptase (4). Excess of proteolytic activities on the ocular surface may not only lead to development of epithelial microlesions, but also to delayed healing of the epithelium probably due to proteolytic degradation of the adhesive glycoproteins such as fibronectin (2,28).

Staphylococcus aureus is a common pathogen in corneal ulcers, particularly in atopic patients (3,23). These patients have high plasmin-like activities in tear fluid (23, and unpublished observations by the authors) and the combination of a small molecular weight plasmin inhibitor, aprotinin, together with antimicrobial therapy seems to improve the clinical response in this patient group. Aprotinin has been shown to inhibit tear fluid plasmin activities both in vivo and in vitro (25).

S.aureus is known to interact with several plasma and serum proteins such as IgG, fibrinogen, fibronectin, and vitronectin via its surface components (5,8,15,21). In addition, the interaction of S.aureus with laminin and collagens mediate staphylococcal adherence to cells and extracellular matrix (15,17,26,33). S.aureus also produces several exoenzymes thought to play a role in the pathogenesis of staphylococcal infections (13). Besides the exoenzymes certain strains of S.aureus produce staphylokinase, a 15.5 kD protein, which can activate plasminogen (22).

The native form of plasminogen (glu-plasminogen according to glutamic acid as its aminoterminal residue) binds specifically to the surface of S.aureus (16). Plasminogen bound to staphylococcal surface can be activated to plasmin by tissue plasminogen activator, which is the principal eukaryotic plasminogen activator present in circulation and intercellular fluid. The bound (surface-associated) plasmin can further convert itself from glu-plasmin to the lys-form, which subsequently increases the affinity of the bound plasmin to bacterial surface. The surface-associated plasmin is protected against the high molecular weight plasma inhibitors, alpha$_2$-antiplasmin and alpha$_2$-macroglobulin. This physiologically important protection is explained by the binding of plasmin to the bacterial surface via the some lysine binding sites of the molecule also involved in the complex formation with plasmin inhibitors (16).

Proteolytic activity due to trypsin was recently reported to enhance the adherence of Pseudomonas aeruginosa to corneal epithelial cells (25). We therefore investigated whether plasmin might have a similar influence on the adhesion of S.aureus on surfaces coated with fibrinogen or fibronectin. This experimental set up is closer to the adhesion studies investigating the mechanism of foreign body infections (e.g. contact lens or intraocular lens infections) than to revealing the infection mechanisms of corneal surface. The other goal is to assess whether plasmin activity created by the host would be beneficial for detaching the microbes from fibrinogen/fibronectin-coated surfaces.

Material and Methods

Adherence Assay

Round-edged glass coverslips were coated with fibronectin, isolated from human plasma (7), human fibrinogen (Kabi, Sweden) and bovine serum albumin (Behringwerke, Marburg) by incubating 100μl of 10μg/ml stock solution overnight at 20°C on the coverslips. Finally, the coverslips were treated with phosphate buffered saline (PBS) containing 1% (w/v) of bovine serum albumin (BSA) for 3 hours at 37°C.

S.aureus, strain Cowan I, was maintained on sealed blood agar plates and transferred every 4 to 6 weeks. For the experiments bacteria were grown in Todd-Hewitt broth for 9-11h at 37°C on a shaker, harvested by centrifugation at 3300g for 15 min at 4°C, washed twice with PBS containing 0.02% (w/v) sodium acide and finally suspended in the same buffer. The concentration of bacteria was determined spectrophoto-metrically by using the Klett-OD 80 for 2x10^8 bacterial cells/ml. Bacteria were stored in the ice bath and were used within 1-3h.

Bacteria (4x10^8 bacterial cells in 1ml of PBS were treated with 10-1000ng/ml of plasmin (Kabi, Sweden) solution, washed once with PBS, and finally suspended in the original volume of PBS with BSA. Coated coverslips were treated with the same plasmin concentrations by administering 100μl of enzyme solutions on the coated coverslips and finally washed with phosphate buffered saline. Adherence assay was performed by incubating 100μl of treated or nontreated bacterial suspension on treated or nontreated coated coverslips for 1 hour at 20°C. Coverslips were than washed twice with PBS, rinsed with water, air-dried, and finally Gram stained. The number of adhered microbes was calculated on the photomicrographs.

Results

The results show that plasmin has only a minor effect on staphylococcal adhesion on glass coverslips coated either with fibronectin of fibrinogen (Fig.1). Treatment of fibronectin-coated coverslips with a high concentration of plasmin seems to slightly enhance the adherence of nontreated staphylococci, whereas lower plasmin concentration had a negligible effect (Fig.1A). Plasmin treatment of bacteria tends to decrease the adherence to coverslips coated with non-treated fibronectin, but the effect was not concentration dependent (Fig.1B). Treatment of both staphylococci and fibronectin-coated coverslips with plasmin decreases the adherence thoroughly by 50% (Fig.1C). Plasmin treatment of fibrinogen-coated coverslips, staphylococci or both had no effect on the staphylococcal adherence (Figs.1A-C).

Discussion

The present results show that plasmin seems to be rather ineffective in cleaving off staphylococci from the glass surfaces coated with fibronectin or fibrinogen. However, bacterial binding to glass surfaces may not completely imitate the clinically relevant binding of bacteria to contact lenses, and S.aureus may use other contact lens-adsorbed macromolecules than fibronectin or fibrinogen as adhesion ligands.

Our results do not directly support the findings by Singh and coworkers (25) who showed that trypsin treatment of cornea increased the adherence of P.aeruginosa to the corneal epithelial cells. In this study, on the other hand, living tissue instead of glass slides, trypsin instead of plasmin and P.aeruginosa instead of S.aureus was used. The trypsin effect was not concentration dependent.

Patients wearing contact lenses show plasmin activity in their tears more frequently than the control individuals (29). This change can be reversed by cessation of the contact lens wear (28,32). There seems to be a difference between the types of contact lenses; gas permeable hard lenses do not cause elevation of tear fluid plasmin activity whereas the extended and daily wear of soft lenses do (34). Interestingly, the risk of corneal infection during contact lens wear seems to be higher among individuals wearing soft contact lenses (6).

S.aureus strains isolated from conjunctival smears can activate plasminogen and proteolytic plasmin-like activity has been recovered from soft contact lenses (12). Therefore, patients using contact lenses infected with staphylococci or other proteinase-producing bacteria might have an increased risk for breakdown of the infection barrier consisting of intact corneal epithelium and tear film.

Epithelial microlesions are not infrequent in the corneas of contact lens users. The proteolytic activity in tears of vernal conjunctivitis patients or contact lens wearers is frequently high (1,23,30,32). One can postulate that increased proteolysis and the mild mechanical abrasive effect of either contact lenses or papillae in vernal conjunctivitis can lead to liberation of prostaglandins and histamine (11). This is likely to be followed by the formation of epithelial microlesions, which are rapidly coated by fibronectin and fibrinogen (18,20). We suggest that one reason for the high frequency of S.aureus in atopic or vernal corneal ulcers (9) might result from the proteolytic cascade revealing extracellular matrix components such as fibronectin, laminin or collagens, which probably serve as matrix for microbial adhesion (34,35). Subsequent colonization and penetration of the surrounding tissues by means of microbial proteinases or by surface-associated plasminogen activation may then take place.

Assuming that the events suggested above take place, we postulate that the treatment of such patients should consist of both include elimination of microbial growth by effective antibiotics and treatment of the basic allergic/atopic condition responsible for the excess proteolysis on the ocular surface. For this purpose, proteinase inhibitors might be of further assistance in preventation of the proteolytic tissue destruction accompanying infection.

Acknowledgements. This work was supported by grants from Suomen Silmäsäätiö, Silmä- ja kudospankkisäätiö, Paulo Foundation and the Academy of Finland.

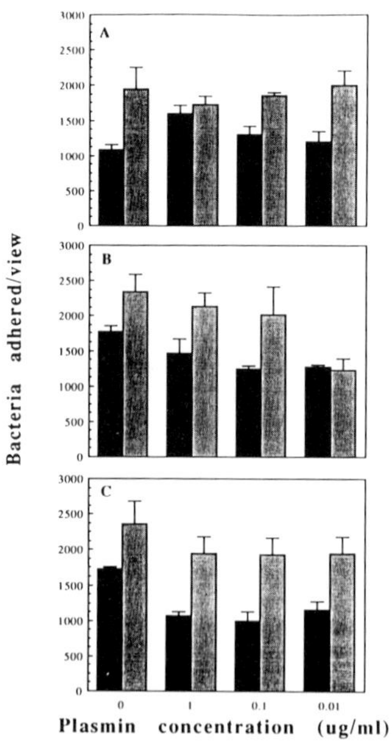

Fig.1. Adherence of S.aureus strain Covan I, to glass coverslips coated with fibronectin (dark bars) or fibrinogen (grey bars)
A. After pretreatment of the coverslips with plasmin.
B. After pretreatment of only the microbes with plasmin.
C. After pretreatment of both adhering staphylococci and the coverslips with plasmin.
The numbers indicate the plasmin concentrations used. The columns represent mean of two determinations and the range.

References

1. Barlati S, Marchina E, Quaranta CA et al (1990) Analysis of Fibronectin, Plasminogen Activators and Plasminogen in Tear Fluid as Markers of Corneal Damage and Repair. Exp Eye Res 51:1-9
2. Berman M, Kenyon K, Hayashi K et al (1988) The Pathogenesis of Epithelial Defect Formation and Stromal Ulceration. In: Cavanagh D (ed) The Cornea: Trans World Congr.Cornea III Raven Press New York pp.35-43
3. Buckley R (1988) Atopic Disease of the Cornea. In: Cavanagh D (ed) The Cornea: Trans World Congr.Cornea III Raven Press New York pp 435-437
4. Butrus SI, Ochsner KI, Abelson MB et al (1990) The Level of Tryptase in Human Tears - an Indicator of Activation of Conjunctival Mast Cells. Ophthalmology 97:1678-1683
5. Chatwall GS, Preissner KT, Muller-Berghaus G et al (1987) Specific Binding of the Human S Protein (Vitronectin) to Streptococci, Staphylococcus aureus and Escherichia Coli. Infect Immun 55:1878-1883
6. Dart JKG, Stapleton F, Minassian D (1991) Contact Lenses and Other Risk Factors in Microbial Keratitis. Lancet 338:650-653
7. Engvall E, Ruoslahti E (1977) Binding of Soluble Form of Fibroblast Surface Protein, Fibronectin to Collagen. Int Cancer 20:1-5
8. Forsgren A, Sjöqvist J (1966) Protein A from S.Aureus I. Pseudoimmuno-Reaction with Human yle-Globulin. Immunol 97:822-827
9. Foster CS, Calonge M (1990) Atopic Keratoconjunctivitis. Ophthalmology 97:992-1000
10. Girard MT, Matsubara M, Fini ME (1991) Transforming Growth Factor-Beta and Interleukin-1 Modulate Metalloproteinase

Expression by Corneal Stromal Cells. Invest Ophthalmol Vis Sci 32:2441-2454
11. Helleboid L, Khatami M, Wei Z-G et al (1991) Histamine and Prostacyclin. Primary and Secondary Release in Allergic Conjunctivitis. Invest Ophthalmol Vis Sci 32:2281-2289
12. Joutsimo L, van Setten GB, Renkonen OV et al (1990) On the Proteolytic Activity of Contact Lenses and Bacteria. Acta Ophthalmol (Copenh) 68:390-400
13. Kaplan MH, Tenenbaum MJ (1982) Staphylococcus Aureus: Cellular Biology and Clinical Applications. Am J Med 72:248-258
14. Kuusela P (1978) Fibronectin Binds to Staphylococcus aureus. Nature 276:718-720
15. Kuusela P, Vartio T, Vuento M et al (1985) Attachment of Staphylococci and Streptococci to Fibronectin, Fibronectin Fragments and Fibrinogen Bound to Solid Phase. Infect Immunol 50:77-81
16. Kuusela P, Saksela O (1990) Binding and Activation of Plasminogen at the Surface of Staphylococcus aureus. Increase in Affinity after Conversion to the Lys-Form of the Ligand. Eur J Biochem 193:759-765
17. Lauweryns B, van den Oord JJ, Volpes R et al (1991) Distribution of Very Late Activation Integrins in the Human Cornea. An Immunohistochemical Study Using Monoclonal Antibodies. Invest Ophthalmol Vis Sci 32:2079-2095
18. Leyden JJ, Maples RR, Kligman AM (1974) Staphylococcus aureus in the Lesions of Atopic Dermatitis. Br J Dermatol 90:525-530
19. Lopes JD, dos Reis M, Brentani RR (1985) Presence of Laminin Receptors in Staphylococcus aureus. Science 229:275-277
20. Nishida T, Ohashi Y, Awata T et al (1983) Fibronectin: a New Therapy for Corneal Trophic Ulcer. Arch Ophthalmol 101:1046-1048
21. Pfister RR, Haddox JL, Yuille-Barr D et al (1991) Amino Acid Composition of a Neutrophil Respiratory Burst Stimulant. Evidence for a Protein, Noncollagenous Source. Invest Ophthalmol Vis Sci 32:2112-2118
22. Phan T-MM, Foster CS, Boruchoff SA et al (1987) Topical Fibronmectin in the Treatment of Persistant Corneal Epithelial Defects and Trophic Ulcers. Am J Ophthalmol 104:494-501
23. Runehagen A, Schönbeack C, Hedner U et al (1981) Binding of Fibrinogen Degradation Products to S.Aureus and to Beta-Hemolytic Streptococci Group A, C and G. Acta Pathol Microbiol Scand Sect B 89:49-55
24. Sako T, Tsuchida N (1983) Nucleotide Sequence of Staphylokinase Gene from Staphylococcus aureus. Nucleic Acids Res 11:7679-7693
25. Salonen EM, Tervo T, Törmä E et al (1987) Plasmin in Tear Fluid of Patients with Corneal Ulcers: Basis for New Therapy. Acta Ophthalmol (Copenh) 65:3-12
26. Salonen EM, Lauharanta J, Sim P-S et al (1988) Rapid Appearance of Plasmin in Tear Fluid after Allergen Exposure. Clin Exp Immunol 73:146-148
27. Singh A, Hazlett L, Berk RS (1991) Characterization of Pseudomonal Adherence to Unwounded Cornea. Invest Ophthalmol Vis Sci 32:2096-2104
28. Speziale P, Raucci G, Visai L et al (1986) Binding of Collagen to Staphylococcus aureus. J Bacteriol 167:77-81
29. Tervo T, Salonen EM, Vaheri A et al (1988) Elevation of Tear Fluid Plasmin in Corneal Disease. Acta Ophthalmol (Copenh) 66:393-399
30. Tervo T, van Setten GB (1989) Aprotinin for Inhibition of Plasmin on the Ocular Surface: Principles and Clinical Observations. In: Beuerman RW, Crosson CE, Kaufman HE (eds) Healing Processes of

the Cornea. Portfolio Publ.Comp.Texas Inc.The Woodlands, TX, USA, pp 151-163
31. Tervo T, van Setten GB, Andersson R et al (1989) Contact Lens Wear is Associated with the Appearance of Plasmin in the Tear Fluid - Preliminary Results. Graefe Arch Clin Exp Ophthalmol 227:42-44
32. Tervo T, van Setten GB, Härkönen M et al (1991) Evaluation of Tear Fluid Plasmin Activity. Invest Ophthalmol Vis Sci 32(Suppl):740
33. van Setten GB, Salonen EM, Vaheri A et al (1989) Plasmin and Plasminogen Activator Activities in Tear Fluid During Corneal Wound Healing After Anterior Keratectomy. Curr Eye Res 8:1293-1298
34. van Setten GB, Tervo T, Andersson R et al (1990) Plasmin and Epidermal Growth in the Tear Fluid of Contact Lens Wearers: Effect of Wearing Different Types of Contact Lenses and Association with Clinical Findings. Ophthalm Res 22:233-240
35. Vaudaux P, Suzuki R, Waldvogel FA et al (1984) Foreign Body Infection: Role of Fibronectin as a Ligand for the Adherence of Staphylococcus Aureus. J Infect Dis 150:546-553
36. Westerlund B (1991) Interaction of Escherichia Coli with Mammalian Extracellular Matrix. M D Thesis, University of Helsinki, Helsinki
37. Zieske JD, Bukusoglu G (1991) Effect of Protease Inhibitors on Corneal Epithelial Migration. Invest Ophthalmol Vis Sci 32:2073-2078

Quantitation of Inflammation in Anterior Uveitis and the Clinical Use of the Laser Flare Cell Meter

J. Strobel

Abstract. The Laser Flare Cell-Meter is a new instrument to measure the pro-tein and cell concentration in the anterior chamber of the eye like a slit-lamp.
Utilising this device, it has become possible to detect subclinical inflammation in eyes after an iritis, posterior chamber lens implantation, differences in intraocular lenses with different styles, and differences in the location of the intraocular lense fixation. Differences in the inflammatory activities with respect to follow-ups of anterior and posterior chamber lens implants, secondary lens implants, eyes operated on with Phaco or extracapsular cataract extraction, different postoperative treatment regimens using Flurbiprofen or Indometacin, are reported. The effects of subconjunctival injections and the importance of an early detection of a fibrin reaction are shown.

Introduction

The Laser-Flare-Cell-Meter was developed by the Kowa Company in Japan. It was made for the detection of an anterior uveitis. Our institution was the first to use this instrument in the follow-ups of intraocular lens implants. Depending on the concentration of protein in the anterior chamber of the eye a flare is produced by a Helium-Neon-Laser-Beam. The Laser-Flare-Cell-Meter is a modified slitlamp. The outcoming light of the flare is detected with a photomultiplier. Special cells in the anterior chamber of the eye reflect the light like stars in the skies. It is possible to measure the flare and make counts of the reflecting cells.

Thus, the concentration of protein in the center of the anterior chamber of the eye and the number of cells per volume may be determined.

Normal Postoperative Values

In normal eyes, a range of cells between zero and two and a mean of three to six counts/0.075 mm^2 is found.

The first measurements were performed in eyes with posterior chamber lenses that had been longer than one year in place. Different cases were sought with a high range of flare and cells. We have concluded that posterior chamber lenses are not equal in their elicitation of inflammation requiring a differential approach.

Lenses were selected, which had been implanted four years ago into the ciliary sulcus (three-piece lenses). These lenses were compared with one-piece lenses that were implanted 9 months previously and the first differences were observed. Other lens types were studied having remained in an eye for more than one year and distinct pictures of flare concentrations were found.

In detail, a randomized double-blind study was performed using lenses implanted into the ciliary sulcus versus lenses implanted in the bag. The mean values of flare and cells showed significant differences. The differences were caused by the maximum amount of flare and cells.

Follow-ups of distinctly different intraocular lenses showed that depending on the patient special postoperative treatment was indicated. Distinct differences were found in two patients of the same age when a secondary intraocular posterior chamber lens was implanted in one and a secondary intraocular anterior chamber lens implant in the other. Secondary intraocular lens implantation using a posterior chamber lens shows less cells and less inflam-mation postoperatively than the lens implantation in the anterior chamber of the eye.

A prospective randomized international study focussing on phacoemulsification versus extracapsular cataract extraction showed significant differences in postoperative flare counts. The phaco cases showed less inflammation than the cases with extracapsular cataract extractions.

Fibrin Reaction

These results did not include cases with fibrin reaction. Patients with very little fibrin reaction, i.e. not more than one clinically seen fibrin filament have flare values between 20-90 counts.

Eyes with a visible fibrin reaction have flare values of more than 600 counts. In our studies we were able to follow the fibrin reactions in three eyes. All of these eyes remained uninflamed up to a certain time point: One eye up to 8 hours, the second eye up to one day and the third eye up to three days postoperatively. Between the surgery and the particular time point of the fibrin reaction the eyes had normal counts. Suddenly the flare increased up to more than 350 counts and a fibrin reaction could be clinically recognized. The borderline of 350 counts was well out of the 35-limit range of the mean of normal eyes postoperatively.

Postoperative Treatment

The use of the Laser-Flare-Cell-Meter was also helpful in the decision to use special therapeutics. Subconjunctival injection of corticosteroids after cataract extraction with intraocular lens implantation is a common procedure. In a randomized study we did this subconjunctival injection at the end of the operation was not done and the mean flare value was found to increase to about 100 counts. This value was much closer to the borderline of fibrin reaction than the cases in whom a subconjunctival injection was used. In those cases values of only 25 counts were measured.

Another problem encountered was the measurement of efficacy of non-steroidal antiinflammatory drugs such as Indometacin or Flurbiprofen. In a prospective double-blind randomized study both drugs were used and no significant differences in cell concentrations were found, however, at a p value of less than 0.01 a significant difference in flare in favor of Indometacin was noted.

Comment

In conclusion we may state that a lot of clinical decisions can be facilitated by using the Laser-Flare-Cell-Meter and are better defined than by using clinical impression alone.

Chemotherapy of Bacterial Infections of the Eye

Dieter Adam

Introduction

The eyeball and ocular adnexa are uniquely predisposed to infection by a variety of microorganisms. The principal routes are exogenous, endogenous, hematogenous, and by spread from adjacent tissue. As for other infectious diseases, control of morbidity and preservation of function require prompt recognition of the clinical site of infection, utilization of proper techniques of laboratory investigation, familiarity with the most likely responsible microorganisms, and initiation of effective antibiotic therapy.

The principal methods of ocular tract delivery are topical and depend on the severity of infection. Topical therapy of the lids, conjunctiva, and cornea should not be determined solely by standard antibiotic susceptibility testing, as the definitions of "susceptible" and "resistant" are arbitrarily determined by the concentration of antibiotic readily achieved in serum. Topically administered ointments and drops of antibiotics generally produce higher concentrations of drug in the preocular tear film. The volume of the preocular tear film is about 7μl.

Periocular injection of antibiotics is reserved for suppurative keratitis or endophthalmitis. This method produces concentrations of antibiotics in cornea, aqueous and vitreous greater than can be achieved by topical application or systemic administration. Penetration of ocular tissue and fluid is through the limbal zone and sclera and by way of preocular tear film through the cornea. The preferred technique is transconjunctival injection into the subconjunctival space. This produces higher intraocular levels than transcutaneous injection into the anterior or posterior periocular spaces. Systemic administration of antibiotics is utilized primarily for infections of the ocular adnexa and soft tissue of the lids, certain types of conjunctivitis, severe keratitis and endophthalmitis. Dosages in general are the same as for the other severe infections. Nevertheless intraocular penetration of antibiotics following systemic administration is limited by anatomic and physiologic barriers within the retinal and choroidal vasculature.

Intraocular inflammation alters permeability and enhances penetration of certain antibiotics. Also, low dosages of certain antibiotics can be safely injected directly into the aqueous or vitreous, this method being reserved for bacterial and fungal endophthalmitis.

Bacterial Conjunctivitis

The most common causes of bacterial conjunctivitis in adults are S.aureus, S.pyogenes, S.pneumoniae and the Hemophilus spp. Pretreatment bacterial cultures and Gram stains are recommended to assist in identifying a specific bacterial passaging.

Antibacterial treatment: Untreated bacterial conjunctivitis is usually self-limiting, lasting ten to fourteen days. Adequate topical antibiotic therapy usually shortens the course of illness.

The generally recommended antimicrobials are Neomycin alone or in combination with Polymyxin and/or Bacitracin. The combination therapy provides greater coverage (including S.aureus and P.aeruginosa) but also exposes the patient to the increased risk of a local allergic reaction to Neomycin which may be interpreted wrongly as an ongoing infection. Penicillin should not be used topically because of high risk of inducing hypersensitivity.

Systemic antibiotics are generally not indicated, unless one is dealing with highly pathogenic organisms, such as N.gonorrheae or Pseudomonas spp. or unless the conjunctivitis is only one aspect of a more extensive bacterial infection, such as an acute preseptal cellulitis or orbital cellulitis. Also, the use of corticosteroids in combination with antimicrobials is controversial. The generally recommended antimicrobials are listed in Tab.1.

Chlamydia trachomatis is an obligate intracellular parasite that is being recognized as a common cause of infections. Eye infections of newborns acquired in the birthcanal have been shown to be more frequent than was previously recognized; these are discussed in the chapter ophthalmia neonatorum. Adult inclusion conjunctivitis is an acute follicular conjunctivitis that is acquired by direct exposure to infective genital tract discharge. Treatment with oral

Erythromycin or Tetracycline daily for three weeks results in good response.

Neonatal Conjunctivitis (Ophthalmia Neonatorum)

Infectious conjunctivitis in the first ten days of life is usually the result of contamination of the infant's eye during passage through the birthcanal, and is usually due to Chlamydia, Staphylococcus, Gonococcus, and occasionally Pneumococcus.

Currently, most countries require an agent to be used to prevent purulent conjunctivitis. The common available agents include a 1% solution of silver nitrate, Erythromycin or 1% Tetracycline ointment or drops. Erythromycin ointment is effective in preventing chlamydial conjunctivitis and is well tolerated. Since chlamydial infections are much more common than gonococcal infections and since Erythromycin may be more effective than silver nitrate in preventing gonococcal infections, many hospitals are now using Erythromycin ophthalmic drops or ointment as their prophylactic agent for neonatal conjunctivitis.

Inclusion conjunctivitis due to Chlamydia trachomatis is the most common cause of ophthalmia neonatorum. Credé's prophylaxis (1% silver nitrate in the eye of a newborn) fails to protect against this organism. Oral Erythromycin (50-60mg/kg/d) for 10 to 14 days is effective and well tolerated.

Neisseria gonorrheae is the most serious cause of ophthalmia neonatorum, and it commonly occurs in the second to fifth days after birth. Treatment with aqueous Penicillin G (50000 IU/kg/d) intravenously, divided in two doses for 7 days plus instillations of saline should be initiated without delay.

S.aureus infection can result in an acute purulent conjunctivitis and is diagnosed by culture and Gram stain. Topical Neomycin (Bacitracin or Erythromycin or Ofloxacin) is generally effective. For more serious infections intravenous Oxacillin or another Isoxazolypenicillin is recommended for 7 days (Tab.2).

Corneal Infections

Infectious inflammation of the cornea (keratitis) is an ophthalmological emergency because of the risk of vision loss. These infections may be acute (Adenovirus) or chronic (fungi), relatively indolent (Herpes simplex virus) or rapidly destructive (Pseudomonas spp.). Many of the bacteria that cause conjunctivitis may invade the cornea. The most common bacterial causes of keratitis are S.aureus, S.pneumoniae, M.liquefaciens, and alpha-Streptococcus. Gram negative infections are increasing. Commonly, minor corneal trauma precedes infection, thus allowing bacterial penetration. Most bacterial corneal ulcers present acutely with pain and marked deep conjunctival hyperemia.

When a diagnosis of bacterial keratitis is suspected, there should be an emergency ophthalmological reversal for immediate corneal cultures and initiation of broad-spectrum topical antibiotic therapy, while the results of these cultures are pending. Because of the rapid progression of Pseudomonas infection, in particular, Polymyxin B or Gentamicin should be included in the initial topical/local therapy.

Many different fungi, often soil saprophytes, have been described as causing keratitis. The incidence of these conditions is increasing, presumably as a consequence and complication of topical antibiotic and steroid usage. Corneal trauma and preexisting dendritic keratitis also are common predisposing factors. Topical antifungal therapy should be administered (Tab.3).

Infectious Uveitis

A purulent uveitis is the most urgent and severe of any primary ocular infection. It is a relatively rare, painful, suppurative infection of the uveal tract which rapidly extends to the vitreous with abscess formation (endophthalmitis). Most commonly it results from exogenous seeding of intraocular contents, for example through surgery, trauma, penetrating corneal ulcer, but it may be a metastatic manifestation of systemic infection by pyogenic bacteria or occasionally also by fungi.

Septicemic patients may have a secondary uveitis. This entity appears to be increasingly common. There is usually other evidence of disseminated disease, such as cutaneous lesions, pulmonary infiltrates, or meningitis. The most common causative organisms are S.aureus, S.pneumoniae, and S.pyogenes. In previously debilitated patients, especially those who are immunologically compromised or on antibiotics, systemic candidiasis may present initially as a purulent uveitis.

Endophthalmitis is generally unilateral and results in intense local pain, marked chemosis and lid edema, intensive hyperemia of the globe, vitreous and corneal clouding with rapid opacification due to purulence in the anterior chamber (hypopyon), and occasional rupture of the globe. Extension to the outer ocular coats and surrounding orbital tissues (periorbital cellulitis) is common.

Treatment: Until a causative organism is identified, broad-spectrum antibiotic coverage should be instituted to obtain high intraocular concentrations of antibiotics. Semisynthetic penicillins (Oxacillin, Flucloxacillin), 2g intravenously every 4 hours, and an aminoglycoside are often recommended in adults. Substitution of a cephalosporin (for example Cefotiam, Cefazolin, Cefamandol) for penicillins in the patient allergic to penicillins is also recommended. One of the broad-spectrum penicillins for example Piperacillin, Mezlocillin or Azlocillin may be used in combination with an aminoglycoside (Gentamicin, Tobramycin, Netilmicin or Amikacin) to achieve synergy against certain Gram-negative bacteria. In severe cases, if S.aureus, enterococci or other Gram-positive microorganisms cannot be excluded Vancomycin or Teicoplanin are drugs of choice as well. Also, if anaerobes of S.aureus or S.pyogenes are suspected, Clindamycin should be drawn into account.

In view of the likelihood of systemic disease, patients with candida endophthalmitis should be treated as having disseminated candidiasis. However, the blood-eye barrier is highly resistant to the passage of Amphotericin B, and the addition of 5-Flucytosin may be helpful, because of its greater ocular penetration. Trials with newer antifungals as for example Itraconazol or Fluconazol must be done in the future.

In postoperative endophthalmitis the most common bacteria are S.aureus and S.epidermidis, Enterobacter spp., and

P.aeruginosa. If enterobacter and/or P.aeruginosa are isolated or suspected, systemic broad-spectrum antibacterial chemotherapy is necessary with either Ceftazidime plus an aminoglycoside (Tobramycin, Netilmicin, Amikacin) or Imipenem also in combination with an aminoglycoside. The third generation cephalosporins as for example Cefotaxime, Ceftriaxone and Ceftizoxim as well as Cefmenoxim are very important agents in the treatment of severe bacterial intraocular infections, because of their broader activity and improved penetration into the eye (Tab.4).

Orbital Cellulitis

Orbital phlegmonous inflammation is a rapidly progressive, potentially life-threatening infection involving the extraocular contents of the osseous orbit; it carries a high risk of permanent vision impairment. It occurs most commonly in children and young adults. In most cases the infection spreads from an adjacent infected ethmoid or frontal sinus (70 to 80% of cases), but it may also occur following penetrating injuries or eye surgery. Rarely, it may be secondary to otitis media, dental infections, facial cellulitis, or a bacteremic state such as endocarditis.

These infections are most commonly due to the major sinuses. Pathogens are S.pyogenes, S.aureus, H.influenzae, and anaerobic bacteria (especially in chronic sinusitis). Posttraumatic orbital cellulitis may follow any injury that penetrates the orbital septum. S.aureus is the most likely pathogen, but almost any organism may be involved, and these infections frequently are polymicrobial.

Treatment: After initial cultures, high-dosed intravenous antibiotic therapy should be initiated without delay. The initial choice of antibiotics will depend on the pathogenesis of the infection and the Gram stain of any purulent discharge. Intravenous Cefotaxime, Ceftriaxone, Cefmenoxime, Ceftizoxime or any other third generation cephalosporin will be active against S.pneumoniae and the majority of H.influenzae. The dosage for Cefotaxim should be 150-200mg/kg/d in children and 4-6g/d in adults divided in two to three dosages. If S.aureus cannot be excluded, one of the isoxazolylpenicillins (Oxacillin, Flucloxacillin) or Vancomycin or Teicoplanin should be administered. The third generation cephalosporins show high activity against S.pneumoniae as well as against H.influenzae and they are likely to be shown useful because of their broad activity and penetration into the cerebrospinal fluid. Also, adequate sinus drainage should be carried out. If anaerobic bacteria are isolated Clindamycin as well as Metronidazole are drugs of choice. Postoperative or trauma-related infections require broad coverage, and administration of a penicillinase-resistant penicillin, or a combination of a penicillin with a penicillinase inhibitor and an aminoglycoside (Gentamicin or Tobramycin) usually are recommended. In the patient allergic to penicillins Vancomycin, Teicoplanin or a cephalosporin may also be useful (Tab.5).

Cavernous Sinus Thrombosis

Although a septic thrombosis of the cavernous sinus may occur after trauma or neurosurgical procedures, it is most commonly due to infections of face, nasal cavity, paranasal sinuses and ear, that result in extension of septic thrombophlebitis into the cavernous sinus. Rarely, cavernous sinusthrombosis may complicate orbital cellulitis, resulting in bilateral eye-signs. When orbital cellulitis, which is almost always unilateral is complicated by rapid visual impairment, retinal changes, or meningeal signs, cavernous sinusthrombosis should be suspected. Cavernous sinus thrombosis secondary to extention from periorbital cellulitis should be treated in a manner singular to orbital cellulitis, i.e. with massive parenteral antibiotics. If the cerebrospinal fluid is involved, one must use antibiotics that penetrate into the cerebrospinal fluid well. Therefore one of the third generation cephalosporins should be used.

The use of anticoagulants and corticosteroids is controversial.

Adnexal Infections

Eyelids

These are acute suppurative infections of the glands of the eyelids or result from acute inflammation and swelling of the Meibomian glands, which are located in deeper, tough fibrous tissues of the tarsal plate rather than the skin (chalazions). These localized abscesses are most commonly due to S.aureus infections. The treatment as with most abscesses consists of the application of local warm compresses and local antibiotic ointment (Bacitracin, Erythromycin, or Neomycin) to the lid every four hours.

If there is no response to the above conservative therapy, these local abscesses may require incision and drainage. Coexisting blepharitis commonly occurs and should be treated as described below.

Blepharitis

The term blepharitis refers to a diffuse inflammation of the lid or its margins. Marginal blepharitis is a common, bilateral inflammation of the lid margins and should be treated with local ophthalmic antibiotic ointment (e.g. Bacitracin, Neomycin, or Erythromycin). Acute infectious blepharitis is generally a unilateral infection that involves the entire lid and surrounding tissues where S.aureus and Streptococcus pyogenes are the most common pathogens.

Treatment should be directed against S.aureus and S.pyogenes. Systemic isoxazolylpenicillins (Oxacillin, Flucloxacillin) or a parenteral cephalosporin of the second generation, Cefotiam, Cefuroxime or Cefamandole are recommended. In cases where Hemophilus infection is suspected, Cefotaximeshould be administered.

Dacryocystitis

Dacryocystitis is an infection of the lacrimal sac that may be acute or chronic and that is generally limited to infants and to adults over 40 years of age. In most cases, the infection is unilateral and secondary to obstruction of the nasolacrimal duct. S.aureus, S.pyogenes, and S.pneumoniae are the primary pathogens in acute dacryocystitis.

Treatment of acute dacryocystitis should consist of applications of frequent warm compresses and systemic antibiotics, initially directed against penicillinase producing staphylococci (Isoxazolylpenicillin, Flucloxacillin). Also, a cephalosporin of the second generation, e.g. Cefotiameor Cefamandole, are recommended.

Prevention of Neonatal Ophthalmia

At present, 1% silver nitrate, 0.5% Erythromycin and 1% Tetracycline given topically are equally acceptable for the prophylaxis of ocular gonorrhea in newborn infants. Silver nitrate may still be the best agent in areas where the incidence of penicillinase producing N.gonorrheae is appreciable as published data on the efficacy of Erythromycin prophylaxis against penicillinase producing N.gonorrheae are not available, and only one study has demonstrated effectiveness of prophylactic Tetracycline in an area with a high incidence of penicillinase producing N.gonorrheae infections.

In areas, where chlamydial infection is common and is of greater concern than gonococcal infections, Erythromycin or Tetracycline ointment might be preferable. The effectiveness of 0.5% Erythromycin ophthalmic ointment in the prevention of neonatal chlamydial conjunctivitis has been demonstrated in one single study, but other studies have given conflicting results.

Chlamydia organisms also are susceptible to Tetracyclines, but studies of the clinical efficacy of Tetracycline ointment in the prophylaxis of chlamydial conjunctivitis are also limited and have given conflicting results. Recent data indicate that either topical Tetracyclines or silver nitrate reduces the incidence of chlamydial conjunctivitis. Both Erythromycin and Tetracycline ointment are available also in single-dose tubes.

Therefore, the choice of drugs for prophylaxis of gonococcal ophthalmia neonatorum is a 1% silver nitrate solution in single- dose ampules, single-use tubes of ophthalmic ointment containing 0.5% Erythromycin, or 1% Tetracycline. For penicillin-sensitive gonococcal ophthalmia, intramuscular Penicillin G, 50000 IU for full-term infants and 20000 IU for low birth weight infants also is effective for prophylaxis. Neonatal chlamydial ophthalmia, although not as severe as gonococcal conjunctivitis is common in several Western countries. In many areas its frequency equals or surpasses that of gonococcal ophthalmia, but an optimized regimen for the prevention of chlamydial conjunctivitis has not yet been determined. Therefore, topical silver nitrate, Erythromycin and Tetracyclines are each considered equally acceptable, although silver nitrate may cause more chemical conjunctivitides.

Table 1: Chemotherapy of Bacterial Infections of the Eye

I. Bacterial Conjunctivitis

Infectious Agent	Treatment of Choice	Alternative
S.aureus	Topical Bacitracin	Topical Erythromycin or Topical Ofloxacin
S.pyogenes S.pneumoniae Haemophilus spp.	Topical Erythromycin	Topical Tetracyclin or Topical Ofloxacin
Gram-negative bacilli	Topical Neomycin-Polyxin B	Topical Gentamicin
N.gonorrhoeae	Parenteral Penicillin G	Oral and Topical Tetracyclin (Topical Penicillin in newborn)
P.aeruginosa	Topical Gentamicin or Ofloxacin (with or without parenteral aminoglycoside)	
Chlamydia trachomatis	oral Erythromycin or Tetracyclin	Topical Ofloxacin

Table 2: Chemotherapy of Bacterial Infections of the Eye

II. Neonatal Conjunctivitis (Ophtalmia neonatorum)

Infectious Agent	Treatment of Choice	Other Measurements (Comments)
Chlamydia trachomatis	Topical Erythromycin	Oral Erythromycin (50-60 mg/kg/day)
S.aureus	Topical Neomycin/Erythromycin/ Bacitracin	i.v. Oxacillin in severe cases
N.gonorrhoeae	i.v. Penicillin G	normal saline instillation
S.pneumoniae	Topical Erythromycin or Ofloxacin	Topical Tetracyclin

Table 3: Chemotherapy of Bacterial Infections of the Eye

III. Corneal Infections

Infectious Agent	Treatment of Choice	Other Measurements/ (Comments)
S. aureus S. pneumoniae M. liquefaciens alpha-Streptococcus	Broad-spectrum topical antibiotic therapy: Polymyxin B/ Gentamicin/Neomycin	Topical Ofloxacin
Gram-negative Bacilli	Topical Neomycin-Polymycin B	Topical Ofloxacin
Fungi	topical antifungal therapy (natamycin)	Eventually systemic antifungal therapy

Table 4: Chemotherapy of Bacterial Infections of the Eye

IV. Purulent Uveitis (Endophthalmitis)

Infectious Agent	Treatment of Choice Systemic (i.v.)
Septicemic patients:	
S. aureus	Isoxazolylpenicillin, Vancomycin/Teicoplanin
S. pneumoniae S. pyogenes	Cefotaxim or other 3rd generation Cephalosporin (+ Ofloxacin)
Candida	Amphotericin B + 5 Flucytosin (Fluconazole/Itraconazole?)
Posttraumatic patients:	
S. aureus	Isoxazolylpenicillin, Vancomycin/Teicoplanin
Postoperative:	
S. aureus S. epidermidis	Vancomycin/Teicoplanin
Enterobacter P. aeruginosa	Ceftazidime + Aminoglykoside or Imipenem + Ofloxacin

Table 5: Chemotherapy of Bacterial Infections of the Eye	
V. Orbital cellulitis (phlegmona)	
Infectious Agent	Treatment of choice systemic (i.v.)
S. aureus	Isoxazolylpenicillin or Vancomycin/Teicoplanin
S. pyogenes } H. influenzae }	Cefotaxim, Ceftriaxone or Ofloxacin
Anaerobic bacteria	Clindamycin, Metronidazole

Table 6: Chemotherapy of Bacterial Infections of the Eye		
VI. Adnexal Infections		
Diagnosis	Infectious Agent	Treatment of Choice
Eyelid Abscess		
Styes and Hordeolums	S. aureus	Local antibiotic ointment (Erythromycin/Bacitracin/ Neomycin) Topical Ofloxacin
Chalazion	S. aureus	
Blepharitis I. Marginal	S. aureus/ S. pyogenes	
II. Acute Infections	S. aureus S. pyogenes	Systemic penicillin + + penicillinase inhibitor (i.v.) e.g. Angmentin, Unacid
	H. influenzae	Cefotaxim, Mezlocillin, Piperacillin (i.v.)
Dacryocystitis	S. aureus S. pyogenes S. pneumoniae	Systemic Isoxazolyl-penicillin (Oxacillin, Flucloxacillin) or Cefotiam or Cefamandole + Systemic Ofloxacin

References

1. Behrens-Baumann W (1990) Chinolone in der Augenheilkunde. Eine Literaturübersicht. Fortschr. Antimikrob.Antineoplast Chemother S.4-9
2. Edwards JE (1986) Infections of the Eye. In: Yoshikawa TT, Chow AW, Guze LB (eds) Infectious Diseases - Diagnosis and Management. Houghton Mifflin Professional Publishers, Boston p.63-68
3. Jones DB (1980) Ocular Infections. In: Kagan BJ (ed) Antimicrobial Therapy, 3rd ed. W.B.Sanders, Philadelphia, London,Toronto p.422-437
4. Meyers BR (1983) Antimicrobial Prescribing. Inc. Princeton, New Jersey p.92-95
5. Riley GJ (1988) Eye Infections. In: Reese RE, Douglas RG Jr, Valenti WM (eds) A Practival Approach to Infectious Diseases. Little, Brown & Co., Boston, Toronto p.307-326
6. Wolfson JS, Hooper DC (1990) Quinolone Antimicrobial Agents and Ophthalmologic Infections. In: Wolfson JS, Hooper DC (eds) Quinolone Antimicrobial Agents. Am Soc Microbiol, Washington p.243-248

Benefit-Risk Evaluation of Antibiotics in Ophthalmology

Alfred Wegener, Ursula Müller-Breitenkamp and Otto Hockwin

Abstract. Antibiotic therapy in Ophthalmology is based on substances developed and registered in part more than 30 years ago. There is no doubt about their beneficial effects also demonstrated by the amount of prescriptions of 69000000 daily dosages in West Germany in 1988. Effective drugs have the risk of undesired effects which holds also true for topical ophthalmic antibiotics. Data from clinical as well as experimental studies are compiled according to the route of administration. Recently introduced topical quinolones have broadened the antibiotic spectrum in ophthalmic therapy. A few compounds deriving from nalidixinic acid caused cataracts in beagle dogs after systemic application of high dosages. A possible subliminal cocataractogenic effect of quinolones of the second and third generation was tested in experimental cataract models. Lens transparency measured by Scheimpflug photography and multilinear microdensitometry did not show an increase in density for Ciprofloxacin, Ofloxacin and Fleroxacin after systemic application as well as for topical Norfloxacin over a limited period of time.

Introduction

The introduction of antibiotics into Ophthalmology enables the specific and effective therapy of infectious eye diseases. The increasing variety of antibiotic substances and products complicates the knowledge of microbiological and pharmacological properties of the drugs in question. Nowadays, topical ophthalmic antibiotics comprise Aminoglycosides, Polypeptide antibiotics, Tetracyclines, Erythromycin, Chloramphenicol and Sulfanilamides. Newly available on the pharmaceutical market are topical Quinolones for ophthalmic use. Penicillin eye drops have been abandoned, due to their high sensitization rate and the ocular discomfort following topical application.

Antibiotics act by interfering either with the biosynthesis of the bacterial cell wall and cytoplasmic membrane or with the ribosomal protein synthesis (2,8,14).

Antibiotics, which are not systemically resorbed, thus not causing a systemic sensitization, are recommended for the therapy of conjunctival infections. Bacterial infections of the cornea, the subconjunctival tissue or the inner eye need therapy with those antibiotics that can be resorbed. Sometimes, an additional systemic antibiotic therapy is necessary to achieve effective intraocular drug concentrations via high blood levels (5). Apart from the obvious benefit of topical antibiotics in Ophthalmology, a number of drug induced side-effects have been reported during the last decades (4,6,7,9,10,16,23). Ocular side-effects following topical application of antibiotics occur more often than systemic side-effects, however, the latter can be very serious and sometimes life-threatening. The manifestation of side-effects is not mandatory, they depend on the patient's individual sensitivity, the drug concentration as well as the duration of therapy.

In this review, only the most frequent and clinically relevant side-effects following topical application of antibiotic drugs are presented. In the recent literature, no clinical data on ocular side-effects following topical Quinolone application have been available, probably due to a lack of experience since their recent registration.

Local Side-Effects Following Topical Application

Each of the topical ophthalmic antibiotics are able to induce local ocular irritation and allergic reactions of the eye lids and conjunctiva. Clinical manifestations are
- allergic blepharoconjunctivitis,
- dermatitis,
- chemosis and erythema of the eye lids,
- hyperplasia of the glands of the lid margins as well as nonspecific signs of inflammation.

Beside Atropin and Proparacain, it is Neomycin, which has a particularly high allergic potential.

All of the topically applied antibiotics can
- modify the local bacterial spectrum, resulting in
- bacterial shift,
- selection of pathogens or
- bacterial resistance.

The effect of antibiotics on epithelial regeneration of the cornea has often been studied experimentally. Most antibiotics cause a significant delay of corneal wound healing, which has been documented by histopathological methods. Chloramphenicol, Gentamicin and Tobramycin have been shown to be more toxic to the corneal epithelium than Neomycin, Gramicidin and Polymixin B. The use of the commercially available drug concentrations over a limited period of time usually does not interfere significantly with the corneal wound healing, however, the prolonged use of topical ophthalmic antibiotics may cause a chronic toxic keratoconjunctivitis. It is important to know about this side-effect, because an increase in the concentration, application interval or a change of the antibiotic substance would damage the corneal tissue even more (3,19).

The neuromuscular blocking activity of various antibiotics has been proven by in-vivo and in-vitro studies. Subconjunctivally applied Gentamicin has been reported to cause reversible mydriasis and conjunctival paresthesia. This effect is a rather rare ocular neurotoxic effect from local Gentamicin (1).

Corneal edema, uveitis as well as cataract development following the intraocular application of antibiotics are clearly related to the oculotoxic potential of antibiotics. Aminoglycosides are known to be retinotoxic, several case reports have described atrophies of the optic nerve following intraocular application of Gentamicin. To minimize severe complications it is recommended to carefully select the respective antibiotic substance, dosage height as well as drug concentration for intraocular application (15,17).

Systemic Side-Effects Following Topical Application

Topically applied ophthalmic antibiotics may induce not only ocular side-effects, but also systemic side-effects. After instilling one eye drop, only 20% remain in the conjunctival sac whereas 80% are drained through the lacrimal outflow system and are absorbed by the nasal mucosa. Systemic side-effects following topical antibiotic use are similar to those seen after systemic application of the drug in question. Topical ophthalmic antibiotics can induce systemic allergic reactions. Topical Tetracyclines may lead to photosensitization and dermal discoloration. Topical use of Sulfanilnamides may be complicated by the development of Stevens-Johnson Syndrome. Chloramphenicol eye drops are known to be able to cause bone-marrow-depression and aplastic anemia.

Little has been published on the use of topical ophthalmic antibiotics in pregnant or nursing women (18). Since ophthalmic drugs are highly absorbed systemically, the clinician must consider the adverse effects of the drug itself as well as its potential for teratogenicity (Tab.1,2). On the basis of available data, Erythromycin and Polymixin B appear to be the safest antibiotics.

Ophthalmic Antibiotics Affecting Lens Transparency

Among the various ocular side-effects described, several antibiotics have been recognized to cause cataracts, if applied intraocularly at toxic concentrations or over a prolonged period. With respect to the new type of antibiotics, the Quinolones, the situation has changed. Their pharmacological design and development, based on the structure of the nalidixinic acid, has been accompanied by reports on (co-)cata-ractogenic effects, when the respective compound was applied systemically. Rosoxacin, a non-fluorinated Quinolone for example, was found to be directly cataractogenic, when applied to Beagle dogs. Studies were initiated to clarify if this side-effect might be a characteristic of all variations of this molecular structure.

Preclinical Drug Safety Evaluations

The actual state-of-the-art in preclinical research, investigating the different aspects of co- and syncataractogenic mechanisms, however, allows an active resolution of these problems in many cases. A variety of well established animal cataract models, combined with reliable and reproducible in-vivo monitoring and documentation techniques (slit-lamp microscopy, Scheimpflug photography) complemented by a detailed post-mortem (PM) biochemistry after the treatment period, provide a wealth of information to analyse the direct or subliminal effects that alter the transparency of the lens (11,12,13,20,21).

Five Fluoroquinolones have been tested by these methods to investigate if Quinolones usually exhibit co- or syncataractogenic side-effects (22). Ciprofloxacin, Pefloxacin, Ofloxacin and Fleroxacin were tested in systemic application, Pefloxacin and Norfloxacin additionally as eye drops. Two cataract models of the Brown-Norway rat have been employed, the true diabetic cataract (type 1, juvenile diabetes, Streptozotocin-induced) and the naphthalene cataract. For a 6 weeks application period the following treatment scheme and examinations have been designed:

Group	Trmnt	SLM	SPP	PMB
control	none	w	III	enz, coenz, sub, red, prot
d	i	w	III	as in control group
n	2	w	III	as in control group
d + n	i + 2	w	III	as in control group
td	dy	w	III	as in control group
td + d	dy + i	w	III	as in control group
td + n	dy + 2	w	III	as in control group
td+d+n	dy+i+2	w	III	as in control group

Trmnt: treatment;
SLM: slit-lamp microscopy;
SPP: Scheimpflug photography;
PMB: post-mortem biochemistry;
w : weekly;
III : 3 examinations, baseline, middle examination, final examination;
i : diabetes induction;
2 : treatment every other day;
d: diabetes;
n : naphthalene;
td: test drug;
dy : daily;
enz : enzyme activities;
coenz: coenzyme concentrations;
sub : substrate concentrations;
red : redox potential;
prot : protein patterns.

Systemic Application: Three monofluorinated compounds and one trifluorinated Quinolone were studied. When in vivo monitoring of cataract as well as data of

post-mortem biochemistry were evaluated, only Pefloxacin had a cocataractogenic potential in combination with diabetes. Pefloxacin not only accelerated the formation of diabetic cataracts, it also lowered the activities of several key enzymes of the carbohydrate metabolism that are already compromised due to the diabetic metabolic situation. Ciprofloxacin, Ofloxacin and Fleroxacin did not show cocataractogenic effects.

Topical Application: Pefloxacin and Norfloxacin as eye drops (3x daily, both eyes) were tested in a comparable treatment group setting, with the omission of the model combination group. All documentation techniques were the same.

The results from this test clearly showed that the cocataractogenic potential of Pefloxacin was markedly decreased, but did not disappear completely. Norfloxacin demonstrated no such risk potential when applied as eye drops.

The results support the hypothesis that co-cataractogenicity is not a general characteristic of Fluoroquinolones, but may be associated with specific functional groups of the molecular structure. The differentiation between related compounds with respect to their co- or syncataractogenic risk potential is possible already during preclinical safety evaluation. This safety evaluation, however, calls for the application of relevant measuring devices and modern methods of documentation for the anterior segment of the eye including the lens.

Table 1. Topical Ophthalmic Antibiotics in Pregnancy

Drug	Toxicity in pregnancy	Recommendations
Aminoglycosides	Ototoxicity (?)	Caution
Chloramphenicol	Neonatal Gray-Syndrome	Contraindicated
Sulfanilamides	Hemolysis in G6P-deficiency	Caution
	Skeletal malformations	(animals)
	Kernicterus	
Tetracyclines	Growth suppression	Contraindicated
	Dental staining	
Erythromycin	No data available	Probably safe
Polymixin B	No data available	Probably safe

Table 2. Topical Ophthalmic Antibiotics in Lactation

Drug	Toxicity in lactation	Recommendations
Aminoglycosides	Ototoxicity (?)	Contraindicated
Chloramphenicol	Bone-marrow depression (?)	Contraindicated
Sulfanilamides	Diarrhea, Rash	Probably safe
Tetracyclines	Growth suppression	Contraindicated
	Dental staining	
Erythromycin	Modification of bowel flora	Caution
Polymixin B	No data available	Probably safe

References

1. Awan KJ (1985) Mydriasis and Conjunctival Paresthesia from Local Gentamicin. Am J Ophthalmol 99:723-724
2. Baum JC (1989) Antibiotic Use in Ophthalmology. In: Duane TO (ed) Clinical Ophthalmology vol 4, chapter 26, Lippincott, Philadelphia
3. Burstein NC (1980) Corneal Cytotoxicity of Topically Applied Drugs, Vehicles and Preservatives. Surv Ophthalmol 25:15-30
4. Fraunfelder FT (1982) Drug-Induced Ocular Side-Effects and Drug Interactions. 2nd edit. Lea & Febinger, Philadelphia.
5. Fraunfelder FT, Roy FH (1985) Current Ocular Therapy 2, W.B. Saunders Co. Philadelphia. pp 3-63
6. Fraunfelder FT, Meyer SM (1989) Ocular Toxicology. In: Duane TD (ed) Clinical Ophthalmology, vol 5, chapter 37, Lippincott, Philadelphia

7. Grant WM: Toxicology of the Eye. Charles C.Thomas, Springfield.
8. Havener WH (1978) Ocular Pharmacology. The CW Mosby Co, St.Louis pp.114-185
9. Hockwin O, Koch HR (eds) (1977) Arzneimittelnebenwirkungen am Auge. Gustav Fischer Verlag Stuttgart
10. Hockwin O, Koch HR (eds) (1982) Unerwünschte Arzneimittelwirkungen am Auge. Ein Ratgeber für die Praxis. Gustav Fischer Verlag Stuttgart
11. Hockwin O, Dragomirescu V, Laser H et al (1987) Measuring Lens Transparency by Scheimpflug Photography of the Anterior Eye Segment. Instrumentation and Application to Clinical and Experimental Ophthalmology. J.Toxicol-Cut. & Ocular Toxicol. 6(4): 251-271
12. Hockwin O, Wegener,A (1987) Syn- and Cocataractogenesis. A System for Testing Subliminal Lens Toxicity. In: Hockwin O (ed) Drug-Induced Ocular Side-Effects and Ocular Toxicology. Concepts Toxicol, Karger Basel.4:241-249
13. Hockwin O, Green K, Rubin L (to be published) Manual of Oculotoxicity Testing of Drugs. Gustav Fischer Verlag Stuttgart, New York
14. Leopold IH (1989) Chemotherapy of Infections. In: Duane TD, Jaeger EA (eds) Biomedical Foundations of Ophthalmology vol 3, chapter 36, Lippincott, Philadelphia.
15. McDonald HR, Schatz H, Allen AW et al (1986) Retinal Toxicity Secondary to Intraocular Gentamicin. Ophthalmology 93:871-877
16. Müller-Breitenkamp U, Hockwin O (to be published) Ophthalmica. In: Ammon HPT (ed) Arzneimittelneben- und -wechselwirkungen. Wissenschaftliche Verlagsgesellschaft mbH Stuttgart
17. Peyman GA, May DR, Ericson ES et al (1974) Intraocular Injection of Gentamicin, Toxic Effects and Clearance. Arch Ophthalmol 92:42-47.
18. Samples JR, Meyer M (1988) Use of Ophthalmic Medications in Pregnant and Nursing Women. Am J Ophthalmol 106:616-623
19. Stern GA, Schemmer GB, Farber MD et al (1983) Effect of Topical Antibiotic Solutions on Corneal Epithelial Wound Healing. Arch Ophthalmol 101:644-647
20. Wegener A, Hockwin O (1987) Animal Models as a Tool to Detect the Subliminal Cataractogenic Potential of Drugs. In: Hockwin O (ed) Drug-Induced Ocular Side-Effects and Ocular Toxicology, Concepts Toxicol. Karger Basel 4:250-262,
21. Wegener A, Hockwin O (1990) Arzneimitteltestung und Risikoabschätzung am Tierauge. Deutsche Apothekerzeitung 130 (2): 61-70.
22. Wegener A (1990) Oculäre Arzneimittelsicherheitsprüfung mit Kataraktmodellen der Ratte am Beispiel der Quinolone. Habil.-Schrift Med.Fak.Universität Bonn.
23. Zingler D (1990) Unerwünschte Arzneimittelwirkungen am Auge. Diss. Med. Fak. Universität Bonn.

- Bacterial Infections

Pathogenicity of Pseudomonas aeruginosa in Keratitis

Adolf Bauernfeind

Abstract. The majority (about 80%) of corneal ulcers are caused by S.aureus,

S.pneumoniae and Pseudomonas spp. P.aeruginosa is by far the most frequent and most malignant ocular pathogen within the genus Pseudomonas. It may cause corneal perforation within three days. Thus pathogen-specific virulence factors have been postulated for P.aeruginosa. Among the products synthesized by this organism, various proteolytic enzymes (e.g. elastase, exotoxin A) degrade corneal stroma. Thus, keratitis and corneal ulcers caused by P.aeruginosa demonstrate pathogen-specific characteristics necessitating rapid diagnosis and effective therapy. Protease inhibition may open a new perspective in the treatment of corneal infections caused by P.aeruginosa.

Microbiology of Keratitis

In human keratitis, the majority of human pathogens causing infections at other body sites may be involved (Fig.1 (6)). However, only a few of them are frequently associated with keratitis. These are mainly non-fastidious organisms growing in normal atmosphere.

Aerobic organisms predominate both among Gramnegatives and Gram- positives. The incidence of anaerobes in keratitis is mostly restricted to the Grampositive organisms like Peptostreptococcus spp., C.perfringens, and C.tetani.

Aerobic pathogens of keratitis are predominantly staphylococci and glucose nonfermenting bacilli (P.aeruginosa, Acinetobacter spp.).

Fastidious bacteria associated with keratitis grow on blood-supplemented media (chocolate agar, blood agar), which may be used for culture of non-fastidious organisms as well.

In rare cases mycobacteria may be involved in keratitis and diagnostic efforts for their culture have to be performed when no other etiologic agent has been identified. Growth of many mycobacterial species is slow and takes 3 to 6 weeks. However, the time necessary for the identification of mycobacteria has been shortened dramatically by molecular procedures developed recently. Specific parts of the genome amplified by Polymerase Chain Reaction allow an exact identification within one day (3).

Time-saving molecular procedures identifying specific parts of the genome may as well be used for the identification of chlamydia.

Various fungal species are associated with keratitis. Therefore the material should be streaked out on appropriate media (e.g. Sabouraud agar).

Acanthamoeba may cause chronic keratitis (7). Acanthamoeba grows on blood-supplemented media, however, a minimal medium with an overlay of Escherichia coli killed by heat is preferred.

Microbiological diagnosis of human keratitis should be performed by techniques, procedures and media appropriate for identification of the relevant organisms (8). The results of microbiological diagnosis are determined by the initial step, that is how the material is obtained. This should be performed by an ophthalmologist. A Kimura spatula may be used to scrape multiple areas of infection and to transfer the material directly onto agar media or slides. Separate samples have to be taken for each medium.

"Corneal smears obtained by a cotton swab are worthless!" (8).

Significance of Bacteriological Data for Keratitis

Microorganisms identified in material collected from the conjunctiva may represent the normal conjunctival flora. The majority of the organisms present on the conjunctiva of patients not suffering from keratitis may, however, as well play a role as causative organisms of keratitis (e.g. S.aureus). The significance of these opportunistic pathogens in an individual case of keratitis may be determined both by their high concentration and their proportion among other organisms as well as by signs and symptoms of infection. These are, however, not specific enough to assign the keratitis to a specific microorganism.

P.aeruginosa is the dominating corneal pathogen in contact lens associated keratitis. It was detected in 5/6 cases of corneal keratitis of patients wearing soft contact lenses (6). P.aeruginosa has been shown to adhere by its fimbriae to deposits on the surface of lenses (1). Corneal isolates of P.aeruginosa seem to weakly adhere more (25%) than isolates from other body sites (9). There is, however, no dominant O-serotype of P.aeruginosa among adhering strains (9, Tab.1). The distribution of P.aeruginosa O-serotypes found in keratitis shows about the same pattern as in other clinical isolates except for serotype O6 which seems to be less frequent in human keratitis (2). This would, however, have to be confirmed by further investigations.

Adherence of P.aeruginosa to contact lenses is mediated by fimbriae. This has been shown by stronger adherence of P.aeruginosa pregrown under conditions favoring fimbriation (growth at 37°C without shaking which leads to coadherence and pellicle formation caused by fimbriation) in comparison with growth of P.aeruginosa at 26°C with shaking (reduced fimbriation). Growth of P.aeruginosa at 37°C without shaking increases the hydrophobicity of its surface and favours adherence while treatment of contact lenses by Triton X-100 reduces the adherence to contact lenses significantly (9).

Adherence and growth of P.aeruginosa on contact lenses may facilitate the formation of surface deposits on contact lenses as well as preexisting lens deposits may favour the adherence and growth of P.aeruginosa (5). The close relationship between the number of deposits on contact lenses and the number of colony forming units of P.aeruginosa per lens has been demonstrated (1).

Factors Influencing Formation of Lens Deposits with Growth of P.aeruginosa

It has been shown that major factors favoring the adherence of P.aeruginosa are extended wear of contact lenses as well as the amount of tear components (albumin, lysozyme, lactoferrin). On the other hand, sialic acid (1%) or mucin, which contains sialic acid, reduce the adherence of P.aeruginosa to contact lenses. Efforts to reduce adherence like surfactant cleaning by papain, pork pancreatin or neuraminidase are unsuccessful. Enzymatic cleaning of worn extended wear contact lenses does not reduce further adherence of P.aeruginosa.

Various lens materials have been investigated to explore their influence on adherence. No one lens had a decisive advantage over another, because all, both new and worn, can bind amounts of P.aeruginosa that may potentially elicit bacterial keratitis in predisposed eyes (10).

Corneal ulcers are frequently caused by pathogens contaminating solutions. Preservation may select specific organisms e.g. S.marcescens or P.aeruginosa (11, Tab.2).

Therapy of P.aeruginosa Keratitis

Topical application of compounds killing P.aeruginosa has been the major therapeutic approach to P.aeruginosa keratitis. Systemic antibiotic therapy is insufficient as the concentrations achievable at the site of infection are too low in order to inactivate the pathogen.

Aminoglycosides have been the first-line antibiotic treatment of P.aeruginosa keratitis. The susceptibility of P.aeruginosa to the five most important aminoglycosides is shown in Tab.3 (Bauernfeind,A, unpublished data). So far, Tobramycin is the most potent aminoglycoside against P.aeruginosa.

Recently, betalactams with antipseudomonal activity of therapeutic relevance (as shown for cephalosporins in Tab.4, Bauernfeind,A, unpublished data) have been explored successfully in a rabbit keratitis model ((e.g. Imipenem, (13)).

The new generation of quinolones, the fluorol piperazinyl-4-quinolones demonstrate high in vitro activity against P.aeruginosa. The most active compound, so far, is Ciprofloxacin (Tab.5, Bauernfeind,A, unpublished data). In a rabbit model (12) the effect achieved by Ciprofloxacin is superior to Norfloxacin or Tobramycin.

Damage to corneal tissue may be caused by the pathogen directly e.g. by release of bacterial elastase or indirectly by an increased release of destructive host-derived enzymes like corneal or synovial collagenases or by elastase from polymorphonuclear leucocytes (14). Efforts to differentiate between keratogenic or non-keratogenic strains have not been successful (14). As with other infections it appears that a local or systemic defect of host defense is decisive for an infection with P.aeruginosa.

Most recent perspectives in the therapy of P.aeruginosa keratitis include dual enzyme inhibitors active both against P.aeruginosa elastase and corneal collagenase (not, however, polymorphonuclear leucocyte elastase). Initial investigations have shown promising results (4). Possibly, high concentrations of anti-P.aeruginosa antibodies or combinations with antibodies and appropriate inhibitors of pathogenetically relevant enzymes may improve therapy of P.aeruginosa keratitis.

Conclusions

The relevance of microbiological diagnosis in keratitis depends both on the appropriate collection of probes and appropriate microbiological techniques.

Interpretation of the results as to their pathogenetic relevance has to consider the physiological flora of the respective area and the fact that keratitis is an opportunistic infection and not caused by specific keratogenic pathogens (e.g. a specific sero- or virulence type of P.aeruginosa).

Adherence of the opportunistic pathogens to the susceptible cornea is the initial event. Measures to prevent opportunistic pathogens from adhering to the cornea (e.g. by contaminated wetting solutions) reduce the risk of keratitis. Extended wear soft contact lenses highly increase the risk of Pseudomonas aeruginosa keratitis.

Therapy of bacterial keratitis is based on the topical application of antibacterials, mainly of antibiotics active against the pathogen causing the respective keratitis. The treatment of keratitis caused by P.aeruginosa may be successful with an aminoglycoside (e.g. Tobramycin, the most active aminoglycoside against P.aeruginosa), a betalactam active against Pseudomonas aeruginosa (e.g. Imipenem, Ceftazidime) or a fluoropiperazinyl-4-quinolone (e.g. Ciprofloxacin).

In the future, antibiotic therapy may be supplemented by inhibitors of pathogenetically relevant enzymes and polyclonal antibodies against P.aeruginosa.

Table 1. O-Serotypes of P.aeruginosa from Keratitis

	O-Serotypes				
Soft CL users	4	5	8	10	16
No CL	1	4	5	7	10

No dominant P.aeruginosa O-serotype in keratitis (Klotz,1989)

Table 2. Infectious corneal ulcers reviewed in 1986

Type of lens[1]	Ethiological agent	Contaminated solution: Type	Preservative[2]	Dominant organism
RGP	S.marcescens	Wetting solution	BC	S.marcescens
RGP	S.marcescens	Wett.& soak.sol.	CXE	S.marcescens
None	S.marcescens	Steroid solution	BC	S.marcescens
SEW	P.aeruginosa	Lens case sol.	None	P.aeruginosa
		Irrigating saline	None	P.maltophilia
SEW	P.aeruginosa	Lens case sol.	None	P.aeruginosa
SDW	P.aeruginosa	Lens case sol.	None	P.aeruginosa
		Preserved saline	S	P.maltophilia
		Distilled water	None	P.cepacia
SEW	P.aeruginosa	Home-prepared sal.	None	Mixed gram-neg.
		Lens case sol.	None	P.aeruginosa

[1] RGP = Rigid, gas-permeable; SEW = soft, extended wear; SDW = soft, daily wear

[2] BC = Benzalkonium chloride; CXE = chlorhexidine; S = sorbic acid (Mayo,1987)

Table 3. Antibiotic Susceptibility of Pseudomonas aeruginosa to Aminoglycosides

	Compound	MIC (mg/l)		
		Range	50%	90%
P.aeruginosa	Gentamicin	1 - >64	4	64
(n = 30)	Tobramycin	0.13 - 32	0.5	4
	Netilmicin	4 - >64	8	32
	Amikacin	2 - 16	8	16
	Isepamicin	1 - 16	4	8

(Bauernfeind,A, to be published)

Table 4. Antibiotic Susceptibility of Pseudomonas aeruginosa to Betalactams

	Compound	MIC (mg/l)		
		Range	50%	90%
P.aeruginosa	Ceftazidime	0.25 - >64	2	8
(n = 70)	Cefpirome	0.5 - >64	16	64
	Cefoperazone	0.25 - >64	8	64
	Imipenem	0.13 - 32	2	8

(Bauernfeind,A, to be published)

Table 5. Antibiotic Susceptibility of Pseudomonas aeruginosa to 4-Quinolones

	Compound	MIC (mg/l)		
		Range	50%	90%
P.aeruginosa	Ciprofloxacin	0.03 - 8	0.5	4
(n = 70)	Ofloxacin	0.13 - 32	4	16
	Tosufloxacin	0.03 - 16	1	8
	Temafloxacin	0.13 - 32	4	16
	Sparfloxacin	0.03 - 16	1	8

(Bauernfeind,A, to be published)

Fig.1. Corneal Microbial Isolates (Dart, 1988, adapted)

	Numbers			Other
		Contact lens		
	SCL[1]	HCL[2]	TCL[3]	
Bacterial monoinfections				
Gram-negative				
- Pseudomonas spp.				
P.aeruginosa	4			
P.fluorescens			1	
Unidentified sp.				1
- Moraxella lacunata		1		2
- Unidentified Gram negative bacilli	1			1
- Serratia marcescens		1		
- Klebsiella oxytoca			1	
- Proteus mirabilis				1
Gram-positive				
- Staphylococcus aureus				2
- Staphylococcus epidermidis				1
- alpha-hemolytic streptococci				1
- beta-hemolytic streptococci				3
- Streptococcus pneumoniae			1	2
- Diphtheroids			1	1
Mixed bacterial infections				
Gram-negative				
- P.aeruginosa + Gram negative rods	1			
Gram-positive and Gram-negative				
- Moraxella + Micrococcus				1
Gram-positive				
- beta-hemolytic + alpha-hemolytic Streptococci				1
- S.epidermidis + alpha-hemolytic streptococci + diphtheroids				1
Fungal infections				
- Candida albicans				1
- Aspergillus fumigatus				1
Subtotals	6	2	5	19
Total				32

1 Soft contact lenses (all cosmetic daily and extended wear)
2 Hard contact lenses (aphakia and keratoconus daily wear)
3 Therapeutic contact lenses (hard daily and soft extended wear)

References

1. Aswad MI, John T, Barza M et al (1990) Bacterial Adherence to Extended Wear Soft Contact Lenses. Ophthalmology 97:296-302
2. Bauernfeind A, Przyklenk B (1987) Spectrum of Pseudomonas aeruginosa O-Serotypes from Hospitalized Patients and Content of Antibodies in Sera of Volunteers and in Immunoglobulins. Serodiagn Immunother 1:287-295
3. Böttger EC (1991) Systematik, Differenzierung und Nachweis von bakteriellen Infektionserregern - die Familie Mycobacteriaceae. Immun Infekt 19:143-152
4. Burns FR, Paterson CA, Gray RD et al (1990) Inhibition of Pseudomonas aeruginosa Elastase and Pseudomonas Keratitis Using a Thiol Based Peptide. Antimicrob Agents Chemother 34:2065-2069
5. Butrus SI, Klotz SA, Misra RP (1987) The Adherence of Pseudomonas aeruginosa to Soft Contact Lenses. Ophthalmology 94:1310-1314
6. Dart JKG (1988) Predisposing Factors in Microbial Keratitis: The Significance of Contact Lens Wear. Brit J Ophthalmol 72:926-930
7. Donzis PB, Mondino BJ, Weissmann BA et al (1989) Microbial Analysis of Contact Lens Care Systems Contaminated with Acanthamoeba. Am J Ophthalmol 108:53-56
8. Jones DB, Liesegang TJ, Robinson NM (1981) Laboratory Diagnosis of Ocular Infections. Cumulative Techniques and Procedures in Clinical Microbiology.13:1-27
9. Klotz SA, Butrus SI, Misra RP et al (1989) The Contribution of Bacterial Surface Hydrophobicity to the Process of Adherence of Pseudomonas aeruginosa to Hydrophilic Contact Lenses. Current Eye Res 8:195-202
10. Lawin-Brussel CA, Refojo MF, Leong FL et al (1991) Pseudomonas Attachment to Low-Water and High-Water, Ionic and Nonionic, New and Rabbit-Worn Soft Contact Lenses. Invest Ophthalmol Vis Sci 32:657-662
11. Mayo MS, Schlitzer RL, Ward MA et al (1987) Association of Pseudomonas and Serratia Corneal Ulcers with Use of Contaminated Solutions. J Clin Microbiol 25:1398-1400
12. Reidy JJ, Hobden JA, Hill JM et al (1991) The Efficacy of Topical Ciprofloxacin and Norfloxacin in the Treatment of Experimental Pseudomonas Keratitis. Cornea 10:25-28
13. Sawusch MR, O'Brien TP, Valentine J et al (1988) Topical Imipenem Therapy of Aminoglycoside-Resistant Pseudomonas Keratitis in Rabbits. Am J Ophthalmol 106:77-81
14. Steuhl KP, Döring G, Thiel HJ (1989) Die Bedeutung bakterieller Wirtsfaktoren bei Hornhautinfektionen durch Pseudomonas aeruginosa. Fortschr Ophthalmol 86:283-286

Pseudomonas Keratitis: Clinical Features

Hans-Jürgen Thiel

Abstract. Pseudomonas infections of the cornea constitute a special class of external infections of the eye. Numerous complications follow the migration of this bacterium into corneal tissues. In most cases, injury to the cornea initiates the cascade of infection and subsequent problems. Fortunately this situation is not common. As a first step the detection of bacteria in corneal tissues and superficial conjunctiva is important.

Treatment of corneal infections involving Pseudomonas aeruginosa calls for the immediate application of antibiotics; these should be administered locally and also systemically if there are clear signs of an adjunct intraocular inflammation. A combination of ß-lactam antibiotics with aminoglycosides has also proven useful. If no improvement is achieved by such a therapeutic regimen, emergency keratoplasty (keratolasty à chaud) should be considered, requiring, however, close follow-ups and eventually resulting in rejection of grafts in more than 50% of cases.

Introduction

The course of severe external infectious diseases of the eye is still uncertain; corneal involvement may lead to scarring, uneven surface, vascularization and reduction of visual acuity. Therefore, this disease entity should be diagnosed and vigorously treated as early as possible.

Substantial progress has been made in the microbiological diagnosis of infections. The spectrum of pathogens causing corneal infections is much broader than has previously been assumed and may comprise bacteria, fungi and parasites. Corneal infections by P.aeruginosa are most feared by ophthalmologists; fortunately, however, they are not very frequent. The clinical course is dramatic and treatment, medical as well as surgical, may not prevent a reduction of vision.

We still discuss the causes (etiology), the mechanisms of development of a P.aeruginosa keratitis (pathogenesis) and the course of the disease, since infections should be interpreted from the pathobiological and not the phenomenological (i.e. clinical description) standpoints.

Defense Mechanisms of the Outer Eye

Specific defense mechanisms prevent an invasion of pathogens into tissues of the outer eye, particularly the cornea. Protective factors are

- the lid reflex,
- the precorneal tear film and flushing action involving a reflex mechanism of the lacrimal glands,
- the epithelial surface with tight junctions between superficial cell layers preventing the invasion of bacteria, and probably
- the indigenous flora of the outer eye.

The conjunctiva also provides structural (47) and functional (45) characteristics for the defense against microbes. The regulatory mechanisms of the Conjunctiva Associated Lymphoid Tissue initiate an immunizing event after contact with antigens on the corneal surface has been established (9,10). Lacrimal gland-secreted lysozyme may join in the defense mechanisms by destroying cell walls and microbial cell membranes of Gram positive and Gram negative organisms (13).

The organ "eye" may be presumed to have a surface devoid of microbes or to have developed regulatory mechanisms preventing an invasion of microbes. However, bacterial growth has been detected on the conjunctiva and cornea. Therefore, an indigenous flora of the conjunctiva may be proposed. An indigenous flora has been found in many other sites of the body as well and may be regarded, as specific for certain locations (42). If such an indigenous flora exists, a specific function may possibly be ascribed to this microbial localisation. This hypothesis is supported by the finding that fungal infections of the outer eye have been observed after destruction of the normal indigenous flora caused by a long-term application of topical antibiotics and/or in immunodeficient patients. Therefore, the indigenous flora may conserve function and structure in order to prevent the spread of pathogens. Previous studies have shown that certain staphylococcal species are able to produce substances with inhibitory effects resembling antibiotics (16). Thus, it may be proposed that the saprophytic flora on the ocular surface plays an important role in the defense mechanisms of infection control of the outer eye (19,52), considered as being effective in a concerted action with the other protective mechanisms.

As with other bacteria, virulence factors of P.aeruginosa are influenced by environmental signals (12,31). These virulence factors are comparable with regulatory mechanisms of other bacterial species, whereby osmolality, temperature, pH, Ca^{++} supply, and aerobic or anaerobic conditions may be of importance. In so far, the saprophytic flora may play a significant role and therefore, the composure of the normal flora of the outer eye is of utmost importance. These problems have been elucidated by numerous investigations, e.g. by Hahn in 1982 (15) and recently by Schumacher in 1990 (41).

However, these studies have not differentiated the spectrum and incidence of bacteria according to age groups. We think that this aspect must be taken into account since Pseudomonas infections usually occur in the elderly.

Study

One hundred and thirty five subjects with asymptomatic outer eyes (age 3-90 yrs.) were studied (41). Ninetysix percent of all isolated bacteria were Gram positive, with
- Staphylococci,
- Corynebacteria and
- Propionibacteria

being most frequent with an overall incidence of 80% of specimens.

Eleven percent of probes contained bacterial strains commonly grown from animal samples.

The average number of strains from one subject was 4.1. The range of bacterial strains increased with age (3 to 5 strains per subject). Simultaneously, an increase in colony counts was noted, associated with a qualitative change of the conjunctival flora. Conventional pathogenic agents, e.g. S.aureus or Enterobacteriaceae could only be isolated in 10% of subjects, and a mean of 2.3 potentially pathogenic agents could be detected per person.

These data show that the bacterial colony counts of different species increases with age, a fact which might be due to a change of the precorneal tear film, e.g. a dry eye. A broader spectrum of agents has been isolated concurrent with the finding of an increased amount of conjunctival organisms in the elderly. On the other hand, conventionally pathogenic organisms could be found in only 10% of subjects. Certainly, causes for corneal infections are multifactorial. These may be (1):
- lid factors,
- altered precorneal tear film,
- external factors,
- corneal lesions,

- medical immunosuppression.

With respect to the limited percentage of P.aeruginosa among the potentially pathogenic agents in the conjunctiva, certain prerequisites must be fulfilled to elicit a clinical infection. Consensus has been met that a corneal infection can only develop in a compromised surface. Only very few organisms possess the enzymes needed for breaking up the corneal epithelial layer. With a corneal lesion as a prerequisite, it has to be clarified how an infection develops.

Etiology and Pathogenesis of Pseudomonas Keratitis

Among the more than 30 different strains of Pseudomonas, only P.aeruginosa has been recognized as a significant pathogen for the development of keratitis. This organism is ubiquitous, but requires specific conditions for replication on epithelial cells, e.g. the cornea. Pseudomonas may quickly change its virulence within a changing environment. Therefore, the amount of potential virulence factors produced during the course of an infection is substantial. Despite this fact, P.aeruginosa is an opportunistic organism causing an infection only under certain circumstances (40).

Adherence characteristics of the bacterium to certain corneal structures definitely marks the first step in the etiopathogenesis of Pseudomonas keratitis. Since P.aeruginosa cannot adhere to intact epithelium (36), compromised epithelial cell layers must play a key role in this process (32,37). In addition, defense mechanisms of the outer eye, e.g. blinking, normal tear secretion and the flushing effect may inhibit adherence. Therefore, specific structural and biological dysregulation must exist at the cellular receptor level in order to facilitate bacterial adherence to surface structures of the cornea, replication and invasion into the deep stromal layers.

In 1982, Stern and coworkers demonstrated Pseudomonas adherence to compromised corneal epithelium in a mouse model and invasion by this epithelial route and not via epithelial-free stromal surface. This finding demonstrates the decisive role of the corneal cellular components against the spreading of infections. Ellen and Gibbons (11) have already hinted at this association and have emphasized that pathogenicity of an organism is closely connected with the ability to adhere to epithelial structures. On the other hand, this statement is not a set rule, since different species bind differently to different receptors. According to recent investigations, different binding sites for staphylococci and streptococci exist.

An important role is played by trauma or microlesions,where surface epithelium produces mediators for a rapid closure of the epithelial defect, but at the same time offering binding sites for pathogens by expression of specific receptors, e.g. plasmin and plasminogen (28). Further investigations comparing binding sites for different species are necessary.

Corneal lesions play the most significant role as a predisposing factor for microbial adhesion, and Stern and coworkers (44) were able to demonstrate experimentally this process to be restricted to traumatized epithelial cells, but not to stroma devoid of epithelial cells. The flushing effect of the normal and reflex tear secretion carries away all of the non-adherent microbes.

These conclusions drawn from the experimental approach are in accordance with the clinical observations whereby infections of the cornea mostly occur in elderly patients with an altered precorneal tear film. In contrast, lye burns of the outer eye with a delayed epithelialization in young persons are rarely associated with secondary infections.

From the clinical standpoint, an association of the three factors
- old age,
- deficient precorneal tear film and
- infection

seems conclusive.

Clinical Features of Pseudomonas Keratitis

The beginning of a bacterial infection pathogenesis is marked by the
- adherence of organisms to traumatized corneal epithelium,
- replication and
- invasion into the corneal stroma.

Clinical disease characteristically begins with a mostly centrally located greyish epithelial and stromal infiltrate spreading quickly horizontally and vertically with an accompanying epithelial defect (Fig.1). Stromal and epithelial opacity of the cornea is caused by edema and advancing infection. The ulcer contains a putrid yellowish material (1,8), which may also be found on the conjunctiva. Gram negative organisms usually demonstrate disease progression (22), and only sporadically are slowly progressive ulcers due to bacterial strains with a low density of enzymes, e.g. proteases, etc. (20).

Six to 8 hours after infection involving an epithelial lesion, micro-infiltration of the epithelium and adjacent stroma may be evident.

Eighteen to 24 hours later, the infection spread centrifugally and deeper into the stromal layers succeeded by a marked anterior chamber reaction with a hypoypon (21). The corneal infiltration is symmetrical and ring-shaped with an adjacent epithelial edema.

Forty-eight to 96 hours after infection, untreated cases may present with a ring ulcer (Fig.2). Without the institution of a rigorous and effective treatment, corneal (Fig.3) and scleral (Fig.4) melting may be observed two to five days after infection (35). Perforation and endophthalmitis can follow and the eye is irreversibly doomed. Lid edema with a narrow fissure, often accompanied by conjunctival hyperemia, chemosis as well as pain may round off the clinical picture.

In moderate climates, Pseudomonas keratitis is less frequently found than in Mediterranean areas and subtropical regions; Pseudomonas, however, is one of the most frequent causative agents of corneal infections (30). Aside from these meteorological aspects, Pseudomonas keratitis may occur more frequently in
- elderly persons with insufficient wetting, "dry eyes" of various etiologies,
- imbeciles or
- derelict persons who cannot be integrated into social life, and
- contact lens wearers.

Also daily wear contact lenses pose a risk for Pseudomonas keratitis (14,20), primarily, these complications occur with extended wear lenses (2,14,17,26,39).

Sources of infection are contaminated solutions for contact lenses (cleansing, storage (56)), mascara (37,55) or fluorescein solutions in offices (53). Saliva or nosocomial infections (20,39) are rare, but lend support to the importance of meticulous contact lens hygiene in order to prevent the transmission of infections. From the clinical standpoint P.aeruginosa keratitis are particularly severe infections and may often lead to a loss of the globe. This progressive destruction is due to enzymes secreted by the microbes, e.g. proteases, elastases and exotoxins (22). According to some authors, P.aeruginosa may produce proteases destructive for the corneal stroma (7,18,24,25,27). In addition, exotoxin A may be important for an inhibition of protein synthesis and is similar in action to diphtheria toxin (3,34). Experimentally, exotoxin A has a concentration-dependent destructive effect on the epithelium, stromal keratocytes and the endothelium, an effect, which may be antagonized by an appropriate antitoxin. In conclusion, the destructive and ulcerative process of Pseudomonas keratitis is initiated and maintained by enzymes and toxins of the bacteria even when the bacteria have been killed by a specific and effective antibiotic regimen.

In this conception, however, bodily defense mechanisms and their significance for this biological process have not been considered yet. After the first hints of the destructive potential of lysosomal enzymes and oxydative products of metabolism of epithelial cells, keratocytes and particularly attracted leukocytes had been published (6,24), Steuhl and coworkers investigated the role of extracellular virulence factors of P.aeruginosa (45,46). Bacterial virulence factors were excluded by an active immunization of animals. The course of the disease was then followed using proteolytic and non-proteolytic strains of Pseudomonas in immunized and non-immunized animals. In this model, the host leukocytic lysosomal enzymes were more important for tissue destruction than the bacteria or bacterial enzymes.The investigators could demonstrate that a severe destruction of corneal stroma occurred adjacent to activated leukocytes. These data have shown that invading leukocytes produce enzymes at a high rate which may substantially influence the inflammatory reaction. Thus, the leukocytic infiltrate is responsible for corneal melting of bacterial corneal infections.

Destructive effects of bacterial exoenzymes should not be ignored, although their relevance may be limited to the first few hours of an infection until polymorphonuclear leukocytes invade the lesion and start the melting process.

Treatment of Pseudomonas Keratitis

The usual devastating course of Pseudomonas keratitis demands an immediate and effective treatment regimen.

Prior to treatment, conjunctival smears and specimens from the corneal lesion should always be obtained to identify the pathogen.

Antibacterial Medical Treatment

Many factors may indicate the pathogenic organism of corneal inflammation:
- history,
- course until presentation,

- history,
- course until presentation,
- spread of the infection,
- infiltration of tissue,
- intraocular reaction (cells,fibrin etc.) and
- complications (corneal melting, secondary glaucoma).

In each case of P.aeruginosa infection, immediate treatment with a broad-spectrum antibiotic, topically and subconjunctivally or parabulbar, should be instilled until the results of an antibiotic sensitivity test are obtained. These results will determine further treatment. In the most severe cases with a marked intraocular involvement, additional systemic application of broad-spectrum antibiotics should be considered. In cases with an inconclusive antibiotic sensitivity test the antibiotic will be adapted to the clinical course of the disease. Once or twice daily examinations are important to access the previous clinical impressions and to follow the course of the disease.In addition to antibiotics, mydriasis is indicated and pain relief may be necessary.

The application mode of specific antibiotics must be discussed: drops or ointment, subconjunctival or parabulbar injections or systemic adjuvant therapy. Only general nonspecific recommendations may be given, since the development of the disease is a continuous spectrum. A prerequisite for treatment are experience in the interpretation of clinical features and a reflective institution of therapeutic regimens. The severity of an infectious entity may be estimated by localization, size and extension into the deeper corneal layers and the involvement of iris and ciliary body. These observations are criteria for the application of appropriate medication.

Usually, the application of topical antibiotics - commonly aminoglycosides, e.g. gentamycin - is adequate for a localized infiltration of the anterior stromal layers of the cornea, which should be given at least 3x daily up to 2-hourly. Toxic reactions of the corneal or conjunctival epithelium may occur and therefore, more pronounced hyperemia may not necessarily indicate a worsening of the disease.

For infiltrates, which are deep-seated or extensive subconjunctival injections of a broad-spectrum synthetic penicillin or cephalosporin (or aminoglycoside) are indicated in addition to topical treatment, particularly when a marked intraocular inflammatory reaction with fibrin is present. If a hypopyon is present, subconjunctival and parabulbar injections may be recommended. If the vitreous is involved, systemic treatment must be considered. Although this or another therapeutic strategy may seem obvious, the application modes of antibiotics in corneal ulcers or keratitis have been controversially discussed in the recent past (3,4,5). It is undisputed that systemic antibiotic treatment is ineffective for a localized corneal lesion and that in these conditions topical application may certainly render better results. It must be considered, however, that an intact epithelium may be a barrier to topically instilled antibiotics. Epithelial defects may allow an unhindered antibiotic penetration into the stromal layers of the cornea. Subconjunctival or parabulbar injections of antibiotics is advantageous in that they may achieve higher concentrations in the structures adjacent to the injection sites. Antibiotic concentrations can be anticipated to be higher in the cornea as well as all of the tissues of the anterior segment of the eye. If action is observed, this therapeutic approach should be preferred.

Recently, corticosteroids in combination with antibiotics for the treatment of infectious corneal diseases have been controversially discussed (44). The application of corticosteroids may be considered appropriate,

- if a pathogenic organism has been correctly identified,
- if effective antibiotics are available and
- if the enforced antimicrobial regimen is effective.

The progressive corneal melting process, which is characterized by a cellular infiltration with leukocytes, collagenases and elastases may be limited by the application of corticosteroids (with the subconjunctival route probably being the most effective). This kind of treatment may only be done with an established rationale under continuous supervision and may prevent the most severe corneal lesions.

Surgery for Pseudomonas Keratitis

Medical treatment of Pseudomonas keratitis with antibiotics requires considerable time and patience. In most cases, the inflammatory process can only be brought under control after several weeks when a functional improvement may be observed depending on the localization of the infectious lesion (Figs.4-7).

We have successfully utilized a technique, keratoplasty à chaud, which has been described in previous literature (50,54). In our experience, this intervention may be indicated after an unsuccessful two or three day enforced antibiotic regimen with imminent intraocular invasion. After a perforating keratoplasty à chaud, recovery is usually rapid. After only a few days the inflammatory reaction quickly diminishes, particularly in the anterior chamber, and visual function improves markedly. A disadvantage of this procedure is the high incidence of graft rejections: approximately two thirds of patients have one graft rejection within 6 months; longterm irreversible rejections occur in 50% of the patients(49). This result may be improved by shortening the intervals between check-ups. Despite the high rejection rate, keratoplasty à chaud in our experience is a reasonable and valuable measure to speed up visual rehabilitation.

Comment

Corneal infections by P.aeruginosa must always be taken seriously since severe lesions and even the loss of the globe can occur in untreated cases. Trauma or epithelial abnormalities represent decisive predisposing factors for the development of the disease. Adherence of Pseudomonas to traumatized epithelial cells is followed by replication of the organism and corneal invasion initiating the spread of infection. The clinical features begin with a central greyish epithelial and stromal infiltrate spreading into the corneal periphery and in the deeper stromal layers. An epithelial defect quickly develops and subsequently an ulcer with involvement of the anterior chamber, e.g. a hypopyon, may be seen. It is most probable that corneal melting is caused primarily by enzymes (e.g.collagenases, elastases) of the attracted granulocytes, and exotoxins of the organisms are of lesser importance. Exotoxins may probably play a more important role at the are of lesser importance. Exotoxins may probably play a more important role at the beginning of infection. Treatment is primarily medical using antibiotics. Immediate application of a broad-spectrum antibiotic is indicated and dependent upon the clinical features subconjunctival, parabulbar or systemic antibiotics applications should be considered. In some cases, keratoplasty à chaud is indicated; however, a high incidence of graft rejections must be taken into account.

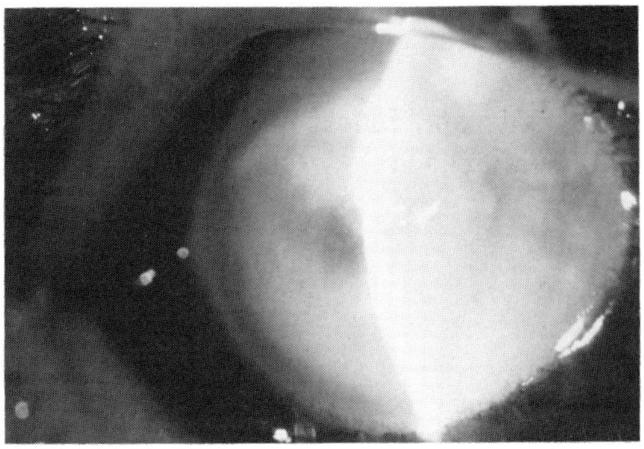

Fig.2 Corneal infection with ring ulcer

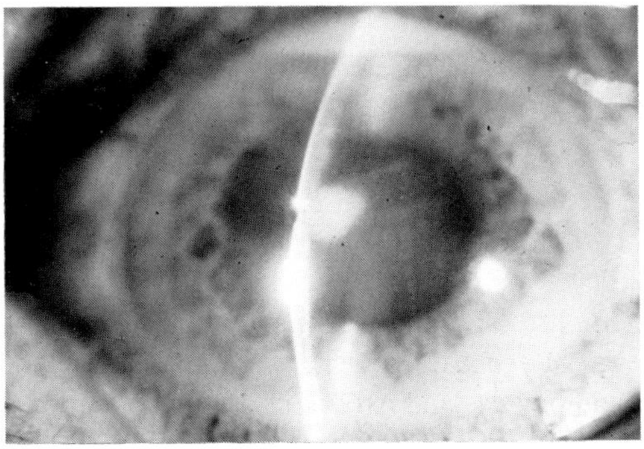

Fig.1 Central corneal infiltrate with circumscript epithelial defect and hypopyon

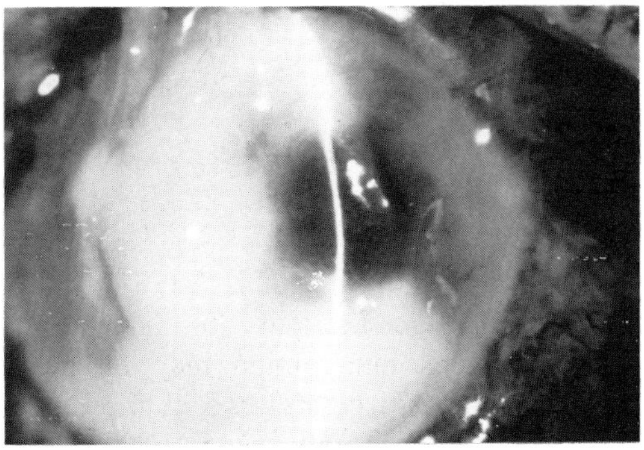

Fig.3 Severe corneal infiltration with epithelial and stromal defects

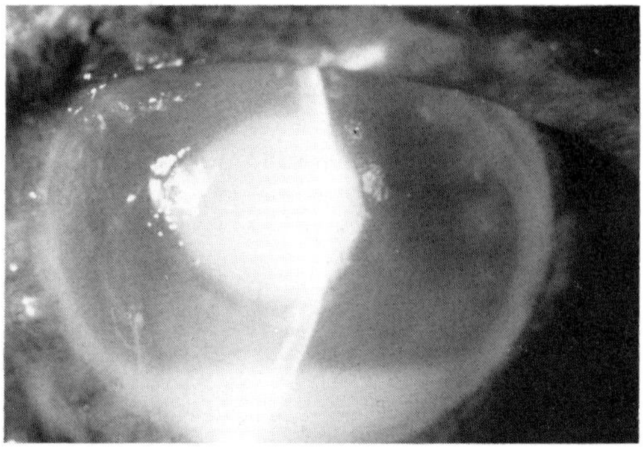

Fig.4 Corneal infiltration with ulcer and hypopyon; subconjunctival injections of Mezalocillin and Gentamycin

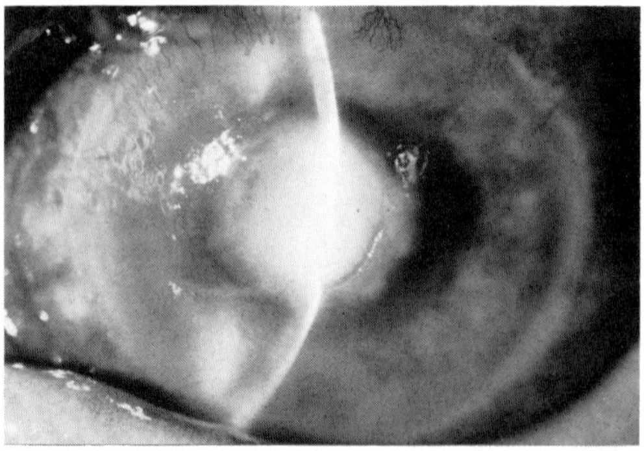

Fig.5 Pat. from Fig.4 one week after beginning of therapy; still marked corneal infiltration and epithelial defect.

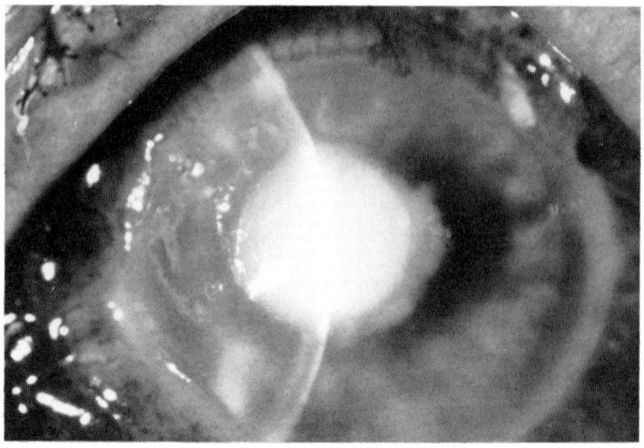

Fig.6 Pat. from Fig.4 two weeks after initiation of therapy; persistent epithelial defect

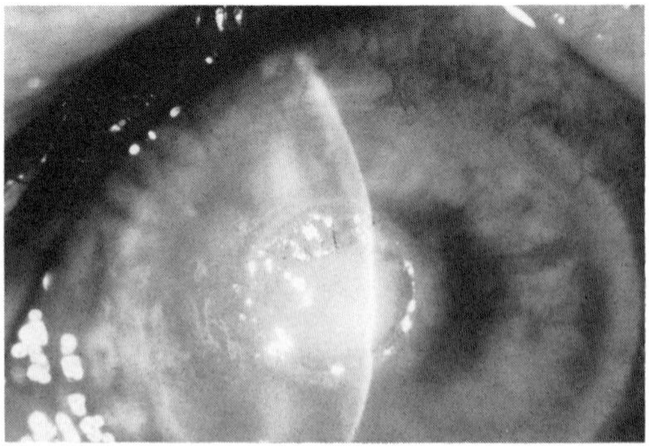

Fig.7 Pat from Fig.4 four weeks after beginning of treatment: delayed healing, still visible epithelial defect

References

1. Abbott RL, Abrams MA (1986) Bacterial Corneal Ulcers.In: Tasman W, Jaeger EA (eds) Duane's Clinical Ophthalmology, Vol.4, Chapt 18, Harper & Row, New York pp.1-34
2. Adams CP Jr, Cohen EJ, Laibson PR (1983) Corneal Ulcers in Patients with Cosmetic Extended-Wear Lenses. Am J Ophthalmol 96:705-709
3. Baum JC, Barza M, Weistein L (1973) Preferred Routes of Antibiotic Administration in the Treatment of Bacterial Ulcers of the Cornea. Int Ophthalmol Clin 13:31-37
4. Baum JC, Jones DB (1979) Initial Therapy of Suspected Microbial Corneal Ulcers. Surv Ophthalmol 24:97-116
5. Baum J, Barza M (1983) Topical vs Subconjunctival Treatment of Bacterial Corneal Ulcers. Ophthalmology 90:162-168
6. Blowsey JJ, Nisbet RM, Swedo JL et al (1976) Corneal Collagenolytic Activity in Rabbit Polymorphonuclear Leucocytes. J Ultrastruct Res 57:10-21
7. Brown SI, Bloomfield SE, Tam WI (1974) Corneal Destroying Enzyme of Pseudomonas Aeruginosa. Invest Ophthalmol Vis Sci 13:174-180
8. Burns RP (1969) Pseudomonas Aeruginosa Keratitis: Mixed Infections of the Eye. Am J Ophthalmol 67:257-262
9. Chandler JW, Axelrod AJ (1981) Conjunctiva-Associated Lymphoid Tissue: A Probable Component of the Mucosa-Associated Lymphoid System. In: O'Connor GR (ed) Immunologic Diseases of the Mucous Membranes. Masson, New York, pp.63-70
10. Chandler JV, Gillette TE (1983) Immunologic Defense Mechanisms of the Ocular Surface. Ophthalmology 90:585-591
11. Ellen RP, Gibbons RJ (1974) Parameters Affecting the Adherence and Tissue Tropisms of Streptococcus Pyogenes. Infect Immun 9:85-91
12. Finlay BB, Falkow S (1989) Common Themes in Microbial Pathogenicity. Microbiol Rev 53:210-230
13. Friedland BR, Anderson DR, Forster RK (1972) Non-Lysozyme Antibacterial Factors in Human Tears. Am J Ophthalmol 74:52-59
14. Galentine PG, Cohen EJ, Laibson PR (1984) Corneal Ulcers Associated with Contact Lens Wear. Arch Ophthalmol 102:891-894
15. Hahn H (1982) Bakteriologie von Erkrankungen des Auges. Ophthalmothek 1, Dr.Mann Pharma
16. Halbert SP (1972) Inhibitory Properties of the Ocular Flora. In: Locatcher-Khorazo D, Seegal BC (eds) Microbiology of the Eye. Mosby, Saint Louis, pp.24-40
17. Hassmann G, Sugar J (1983) Pseudomonas Corneal Ulcer with Extended-Wear Soft Contact Lenses for Myopia. Arch Ophthalmol 101:1549-1550
18. Hazlett LD, Berk RS, Iglewski BH (1981) Microscopic Characterization of Ocular Damage Produced by Pseudomonas Aeruginose Toxin A. Infect Immunol 34:1025-1035
19. Hsu C-Y, Viseman GM (1967) Antibacterial Substances from Staphylococci. Can J Microbiol 13:947-955
20. Hutton WL, Sexton RR (1972) Atypical Pseudomonas Corneal Ulcers in Semi-Comatose Patients. Am J Ophthalmol 73:37-39
21. Hyndiuk RA (1981) Experimental Pseudomonas Keratitis (Thesis). Trans Am Ophthalmol Soc 79:541-624
22. Hyndiuk AR, Nassif KF, Burd EM (1983) Infectious Diseases.In: Smolin G, Thoft RA (eds) The Cornea. Little, Brown & Comp. Boston/Toronto, pp.147-167
23. Iglewski BH, Burns RP, Gibson IK (1977) Pathogenesis of Corneal Damage from

Pseudomonas Exotoxin A. Invest Ophthalmol Vis Sci 16:73-76
24. Kessler E, Mondino BJ, Brown SI (1977) The Corneal Response to Pseudomonas Aeruginosa: Histopathologic and Enzymatic Characterization. Invest Ophthalmol Vis Sci 16:116-125
25. Kessler E, Kennah HE, Brown SI (1977) Pseudomonas Protease Purification, Partial Characterization, and its Effect on Collagen, Proteoglycan, and Rabbit Corneas. Invest Ophthalmol Vis Sci 16:488-497
26. Krachmer JH, Purcell JJ (1978) Bacterial Corneal Ulcers and Cosmetic Soft Contact Lens Wearers. Arch Ophthalmol 96:57-61
27. Kreger AS, Gray LD (1978) Purification of Pseudomonas Aeruginosa Protease and Microscopic Characterization of Pseudomonal Protease-Induced Rabbit Corneal Damage. Infect Immunol 19:630-648
28. Kuusela P, Ullberg M, Kronvall G et al (to be published) Binding and Activation of Plasminogen by Tissue-Type Plasminogen Activator (t-PA) on Staphylococci and Streptococci. Wound Healing of the Ocular Surface. Symposium of the XXX Nordic Congress of Ophthalmology, Helsinki
29. Lemp MA, Balckman HJ, Wilson LA et al (1984) Gram Negative Corneal Ulcers in Elderly Aphakic Eyes Extended Wear Lenses. Ophthalmology 91:60-63
30. Liesegang TJ, Forster RK (1980) Spectrum of Microbial Keratitis in South Florida. Am J Ophthalmol 90:38-47
31. Miller JF, Mekalandos JJ, Falkow S (1989) Coordinate Regulation and Sensory Transduction in the Control of Bacterial Virulence. Science 243:916-922
32. Ofek I, Beachey EH (1980) Bacterial Adherence. Adv Intern Med 25:503-532
33. Pavlovski OR, Iglewski BH, Pollack M (1978) Mechanism of Action of P.aeruginosa Exotoxin A in Experimental Mouse Infections: Adenosine Diphosphate Ribosylation of Elongation Factor 2. Infect Immun 19:29-33
34. Pollack M, Taylor HS, Callahan CT III (1977) Exotoxin Production by Clinical Isolates of Pseudomonas Aeruginosa. Infect Immun 15:776-780
35. Raber IM, Laibson PR, Kurz GH (1982) Pseudomonas Corneal-Scleral Ulcers. Am J Ophthalmol 92:353-362
36. Ramphal R, McNeice MT, Polack F (1981) Adherence of P.Aeruginosa to the Mouse Cornea: A Step in the Pathogenesis of Corneal Infections. Ann Ophthalmol 13:421-425
37. Reed WP, Williams RC (1978) Bacterial Adherence: First Step in Pathogenesis of Certain Infections. J Chronic Dis 31:67-72
38. Reid FR, Wood TO (1971) Pseudomonas Corneal Ulcers, the Causative Role of Contaminated Eye Cosmetics. Arch Opthalmol 97:1640-1641
39. Rosenkranz L (1983) Pseudomonas Keratitis. Am J Ophthalmol 94:556
40. Sabath DE (ed) (1980) Pseudomonas Aeruginosa, the Organism, Disease, Its Causes and Their Treatment. Hans Huber Publ Bern
41. Schumacher U (1990) Untersuchungen zur bakteriellen Besiedelung normaler menschlicher Bindehäute. nauguraldissertation Mediz. Fakultät Klin. Medizin Tübingen
42. Skinner FA, Carr JG (1974) The Normal Microbial Flora of Man. Academic Press,New York
43. Stern GA, Weitzenkorn D, Valenti J (1982) Adherence of Pseudomonas Aeruginosa to the Mouse Cornea. Arch Ophthalmol 100:1956-1958
44. Stern GA, Buttross B (1991) Use of Corticosteroids in Combination with Antimicrobial Drugs in the Treatment of Infectious Corneal Disease. Ophthalmology 98:847-853
45. Steuhl KP, Rohen JW (1984) Cellular Structure of the Conjunctival Epithelium of Rabbits. Graefe's Arch Clin Exp Ophthalmol 221:265-271

46. Steuhl KP, Döring G, Heni A et al (1987) Relevance of Host-Derived and Bacterial Factors in Pseudomonas Aeruginosa Corneal Infections. Invest Ophthalmol Vis Sci 28:1559-1568
47. Steuhl KP (1989) Ultrastructure of the Conjunctival Epithelium. In: Straub W (ed) Developments in Ophthalmoloy, Karger, Basel
48. Steuhl KP, Döring G, Thiel HJ (1989) Die Bedeutung bakterieller und Wirtsfaktoren bei Hornhautinfektionen durch Pseudomonas Aeruginosa. Fortschr Ophthalmol 86:283-286
49. Szymankiewicz M, Weidle EG, Thiel HJ (1987) Klinik, Verlauf und Ergebnisse der Keratoplastik à chaud. Fortschr Ophthalmol 84:506-509
50. Thiel HJ (1978) Keratoplastik bei akuten infektiösen Hornhautprozessen. Klin Mbl Augenheilk 173:171-181
51. Thiel HJ, Manthey KF (1980) Die Häufigkeit von Immunreaktionen nach perforierenden Keratoplastiken. Klin Mbl Augenheilk 177:274-283
52. van der Vaaij D, Berghuis-De Vries JM, Lekkerkerk-van der Vees JEC (1971) Colonisation Resistance of the Digestive Tract in Conventional and Antibiotic-Treated Mice. J Hyg 69:405-411
53. Vaugh DG Jr. (1955) The Contamination of Fluorescein Solutions (with Special Reference to Pseudomonas Aeruginosa). Am J Ophthalmol 39:55-61
54. Weidle EG, Thiel HJ (1984) Keratoplastik à chaud als therapeutische Maßnahme bei akuten Infektionen. Klin Mbl Augenheilk 184:520-528
55. Wilson LA, Ahearn DG (1977) Pseudomonas-Induced Corneal Ulcers Associated with Contaminated Eye Mascara. Am J Ophthalmol 84:112-119
56. Wilson LA, Schlitzer RL, Ahearn DG (1981) Pseudomonas Corneal Ulcers Associated with Soft Contact Lens Wear. Am J Ophthalmol 92:546-554

- Fungal Infections

Laboratory Diagnosis of Domestic Visceral Mycosis

Reinhard Rüchel

Abstract. Deep-seated mycosis can be diagnosed by microscopic examination of biopsies, culture, skin test and by monitoring antibodies and antigens, or fungal metabolites in body fluids. Candidiasis, the most important domestic mycosis, is preferentially diagnosed by culture and by antigen tests.
Aspergillosis is diagnosed by microscopy and culture. An Aspergillus antigen test has recently become available.
The rare Zygomycosis and Fusariosis have mostly been diagnosed by culture; serological tests are not available.
Cryptococcosis, which is very often associated with the acquired immunodeficiency syndrome, can be diagnosed by antigen tests, by microscopy and by culture using selective media.
The systemic mycoses of the Americas (Blastomycosis, Histoplasmosis, Coccidioidomycosis, Paracoccidioidomycosis) may be diagnosed by microscopy and biopsy, culture, serological tests, and, away from endemic areas, by skin tests.

Introduction

In the recent decades, an increasing incidence of deep-seated or systemic mycoses due to yeasts (Candida species and Cryptococcus neoformans), or moulds (Aspergillus species, and Zygomycetes of the family Mucoraceae) has been observed (1,8). In the course of hematogenous dissemination or even by continuous growth, these mycoses may affect the eye.

Deep-seated fungal infections are much feared because of their lack of typical clinical signs, as well as the difficulties with the treatment of an established infection. Many cases of such mycoses are misdiagnosed and are recognized only upon autopsy.

Consequently, many attempts have been made to improve the diagnosis of such life-threatening infections. For an in-depth review, the reader is referred to the references 5 and 9. This brief review will highlight only some points of practical diagnostic importance:

1. The diagnosis of deep-seated mycoses requires the recognition of predisposing factors and typical underlying conditions as has repeatedly been emphasized. Important predisposing factors are listed in Tab.1. Persistent fever of unidentified origin in these patients is often caused by visceral mycosis.
2. Isolation and cultures of fungi must be attempted. Candida albicans isolates may represent an irrelevant colonization of mucosal sites. They need to be interpreted according to the site of recovery, the number of colony forming units, and the prophylactic use of antimycotics. Unlike C.albicans, other candidal species, cryptococci, and moulds (aspergilli, zygomycetes) do not belong to the normal mucosal flora. Their isolation should always arouse attention. However, mould isolates may represent air-borne contamination of the specimens or media.
3. Specific antibody titers should be monitored, and fungal antigens or metabolites should be traced in the body fluids, provided that appropriate tests are available.

The results of these three lines of evidence need to be evaluated synoptically. According to the "majority rule", deep-seated mycosis may be assumed, if at least two lines of evidence are in favor of the diagnosis.

Laboratory Diagnosis - Candidiasis

Candidiasis (Candida mycosis, Candidosis) accounts for approximately 90% of the cases of deep-seated mycoses in Germany.

Particularly neutropenic patients are endangered by Candidiasis when the granulocytes drop below 500 cells/mm^3. Due to the known risk of such patients to acquire candidiasis, prophylactic measures including topical or systemic antifungal therapy are popular.

Candidiasis in severely compromised patients, particularly during neutropenia, proceeds at the pace of bacterial septicemia, thus necessitating fast action. In immunocompetent patients with regular bone marrow function, Candidiasis develops slowly, leaving ample time for diagnostic measures. This applies particularly to surgical patients during a prolonged stay in intensive care units.

Procedures for the diagnosis have been reviewed recently (5,6).

Candida is rarely isolated from blood cultures. The poor yield of blood cultures in invasive candidiasis may be improved by arterial punctures or lysis procedures. Fungemia often reflects infection of an intravenous line. Antigen testing may aid in the differentiation of the true fungemia from catheter-borne infection.

Candida counts exceeding 10^5 colony forming units per ml urine may reflect renal Candidiasis or thrush of the bladder.

Again, antigen testing may aid in the detection of the visceral type of urinary tract mycosis.

Intestinal thrush plays an important role as a cause of deep-seated Candidiasis. Fungal overgrowth as a first step of such infections can be detected by microscopy of fecal smears and by quantitative culture. In neutropenic patients, intestinal thrush may spread to the liver via the portal vein.

A selectively elevated alkaline phosphatase and fever well beyond the neutropenic phase are also possible signs of hepatic Candidiasis, which can be substantiated by sonography, computed tomography, or magnetic resonance imaging.

C.albicans accounts for approximately 75% of the clinical yeast isolates, and C.tropicalis for approximately 10%. The latter does not belong to the normal microbial flora as does C.albicans, but it is equally pathogenic as an opportunistic agent. C.glabrata, which used to be called Torulopsis glabrata, C.parapsilosis and C.krusei occur less frequently and are less pathogenic but may be particularly resistant to some of the antifungal agents.

Serological tests are a useful aid in the diagnosis of Candidiasis. However, it has to be kept in mind, that antibodies against C.albicans are present in virtually all healthy individuals reflecting the high rate of asymptomatic carriage of this yeast. Therefore, low titers of such antibodies are considered as a sign of general humoral immunodeficiency.

Monitoring of antibody titers can be helpful for the diagnosis of infection in immunocompetent patients, provided sequential serological specimens are available. Detection of a specific IgM response is an additional argument for a recent infection. However, even invasive thrush causes an immune response; and only truly epidermal candidiasis is usually experienced without a rise of antibody titers. Antibody-directed serodiagnosis is also unreliable in severely immunosuppressed or neutropenic patients who may not be able to mount an immune response, or who react in a retarded fashion. Since these patients are particularly prone to an overwhelming mycosis, they should be subjected to surveillance with antigen tests.

Antigen tests may give a direct impression of the stage of Candidiasis. However, antigen titers can change quickly, and daily testing in high-risk patients with fever of unknown origin may be advisable.

Among the candidal antigens, which have been proposed for diagnostic use monitoring of an intracellular 47kD protein, (enolase), and heterogeneous mannoproteins (mannan) of the fungal cells can be performed using commercial test kits (Tab.2). Most experience, though, has been gathered with a Cand-Tec^R latex agglutination test (Ramco.Inc., Houston,TX,USA). Despite the fact that the antigen detected by the Cand-Tec^R test has not yet been identified the test has proved useful as an aid in the diagnosis of deep-seated candidiasis. It will detect any type of candidiasis, which has turned invasive, e.g. by penetrating into the lamina propria of the mucosa.

The test does not allow for the differentiation of invasive thrush from truly deep-seated Candidiasis. Antigen titers are low in cases of Candidiasis, which is confined to the peritoneal or pleural cavities, and no antigen is detectable in massively infected urine. The Cand-Tec^{R} antigen may be a stress protein, or neo-antigen, which is produced by phagocytes processing ingested fungal cells. Thus, in neutropenic patients, low titers may already indicate visceral Candidiasis (Fig.1).

The Cand-Tec^{R} test may be affected by rheumatoid factor. Certain false-positives in the Cand-Tec^{R} test can be identified by pretreating the serum sample for 15 min. at 56°C. Antigen, which is not drastically reduced by the treatment, is discarded. The only group, which is often difficult to interpret in the Cand-Tec^{R} test includes patients who have undergone major thoracic surgery. Among these, we have often observed cases with serum titers of 1:>16 lacking any clinical evidence of Candidiasis.

The enolase antigen test (Directigen-Candida^{R}, Becton-Dickinson, Heidelberg, Germany) is more specific, but has proven less sensitive in our hands. It should only be applied to fresh sera of granulocytopenic patients. Enolase antigen may be neutralized by specific antibody leading to false-negative results (11).

The latex agglutination test for mannan antigen (Pastorex Candida^{R}, Pasteur Diagnostics) is likewise specific, but in our hands it has also lacked sensitivity. In this test, blocking antibody can be eliminated by a dissociation step.

Laboratory Diagnosis - Aspergillosis

Aspergillosis is an infection of the respiratory tract, which may disseminate. Aspergillosis accounts for approximately 10% of the deep-seated mycoses. Aspergillosis is largely due to A.fumigatus. Other species encountered in patients are A.flavus and A.niger, the latter being a mere saprophyte, which is often found in cerumen (2).

The diagnosis of deep-seated Aspergillosis is more difficult than the diagnosis of deep-seated Candidiasis, since serology is of little use for reasons outlined below, and, hence, every other case of disseminated Aspergillosis is only detected by the pathologist.

There are patients, who are at risk of developing invasive pulmonary aspergillosis. Among them, patients suffering from pancytopenic leukemia or bone marrow transplant recipients are particularly endangered by this infection. In such patients, chest X-rays often remain inconclusive until the granulocytes return. Aspergillosis in these patients disseminates quickly with metastases often involving the central nervous system.

Likewise, patients under long-term immunosuppression, e.g. lupus erythematodes, myasthenia or Wegener's granulomatosis, may develop disseminating Aspergillosis.

In some patients, cultivation of A.fumigatus from sputum may give a first hint of Aspergillosis. Direct microscopy of such specimens or broncho-alveolar lavage fluids occasionally allows the detection of typical conidophores, which prove the infection to be in those parts of the lung, which are still ventilated (Fig. 2). Aspergillosis is also seen in patients following polytrauma or major surgery and who have been kept on the respirator for a prolonged period of time. Likewise, chronic alcoholics are at risk for invasive pulmonary Aspergillosis.

The typical aspergilloma (fungus ball) is rarely seen these days. Its association with a history of cavernous pulmonary tuberculosis is well-known.

The serodiagnosis of Aspergillosis is still unrewarding. The available antibody tests are more likely to identify patients with allergic bronchopulmonary Aspergillosis than patients with life-threatening invasive mycoses. Recently, a first antigen test for the fast diagnosis of invasive Aspergillosis became available (Pastorex Aspergillus^{R}, Pasteur Diagnostics). This latex agglutination test detects galactomannan from the fungal cell wall. The antigen can be dissociated from blocking antibody prior to testing. In our hands, the test has proven sufficiently specific, but the sensitivity needs to be improved. In the future, monitoring of this antigen in urine may become possible.

Laboratory Diagnosis - Mucormycosis:

Mucormycosis, also called Zygomycosis, is caused by species of Rhizopus, Mucor or Absidia. Generally, this is a rare disease. Typically, there are two types of Mucormycosis. The rhinocerebral type evolves from colonized paranasal sinuses occurring preferentially in diabetics or in patients under deferoxamine therapy (3,7). The infection may mimic paresis of the facial nerve. Likewise, the infection may cause orbital cellulitis and subsequent blindness due to occlusion of the central artery. The second type of Mucormycosis involves the lungs with a preference for the arteries. Arterial perforation or obliteration by pseudothrombi may lead to a rapid fatal outcome.

No reliable serological tests are presently available for the diagnosis of the Zygomycoses. Therefore, cultures should be tried on these fast-growing moulds. Tissue biopsies can quickly be examined microscopically after maceration in 10% potassium hydroxide and subsequent staining with an optical brightener, e.g. Fungiqual^{R}, Citifluor^{R} and Calcofluor^{R} (8). Typical non-septate hyphae with a large diameter and bizarre structures are indicative of a zygomycete (Fig.3).

Laboratory Diagnosis - Cryptococcosis

Cryptococcosis has been very rare before the advent of the acquired immunodeficiency syndrome, which has become the typical underlying disease for this yeast infection (4). Aside from the well-known involvement of the central nervous system, Cryptococcosis in patients with the acquired immunodeficiency syndrome tends to spread systemically.

The infection first affects the lungs and hence, C.neoformans may be cultured from respiratory secretions. Later on, it can be retrieved from cerebrospinal fluid, blood or urine. For culture, Staib agar may be used. It allows the detection of C.neoformans by virtue of its brown color, which reflects the ability of the fungus to produce melanin.

Specific antibodies play only a minor role in the diagnosis of Cryptococcosis. However, capsular polysaccharide antigen (glucuronoxylomannan) of the fungus after proteolytic unmasking can be detected with high sensitivity and specificity by latex agglutination. Test kits are commercially available, e.g. from Immuno-Mycologics, Inc., Norman, OK, USA.

The test may produce low titers, if the cryptococcal strain produces little capsular antigen. However, in most cases, the capsular layer is that massive it can be even recognized by the time-saving method of microscopy with India ink contrasted smears.

Conclusions

The diagnosis of deep-seated mycoses requires the synoptical evaluation of cultures, clinical conditions and serological data. In the case of Candidiasis, I consider these three aspects to be equally important. According to majority rule, a deep-seated Candidiasis may be assumed, if two aspects are in favor of the disease. It may be conceded that probably some cases of Candidiasis will never be fully proven, and that this diagnostic approach may generate patients who are over-treated with systemic antifungal agents. However, the risks of systemic antifungal combined therapy have been reduced, and new antimycotics may further alleviate the problem of undesirable side-effects. Our diagnostic approach has clearly reduced the incidence of lethal deep-seated Candidiasis among our patients.

The situation is worse with deep-seated Aspergillosis, the diagnosis of which is still largely based on cultures of the organism. An association of Aspergillosis with pancytopenia may be observed, but fatal cases can also occur in other compromised patients and often go unnoticed. The first antigen test for Aspergillosis is presently being tested for routine diagnosis.

Deep-seated Mucormycosis (Zygomycosis) is mostly fatal, since an early diagnosis, which is still exclusively based on culture or microscopy, is rarely established in time.

Only the diagnostic tools for the detection of Cryptococcosis are satisfying, since a highly reliable antigen test and selective culture media are available. The diagnosis of Cryptococcosis is facilitated by the significant association of this mycosis with the acquired immunodeficiency syndrome.

Table 1. Major predisposing factors for deep-seated mycosis

Candidiasis:	Neutropenia, major abdominal surgery, intravenous drug abuse
Cryptococcosis:	Acquired Immunodeficiency Syndrome (AIDS)
Aspergillosis	Neutropenia, alcoholism, corticosteroids, organ transplant, tuberculosis
Zygomycosis:	Diabetes mellitus, deferoxamine therapy

Table 2. Commercial test kits for Candida antigen testing

Cand-Tec[R]	latex agglutination	Ramco Inc.
LA-Candida[R]	latex agglutination	Immuno-Mycologics
Pastorex Candida[R]	latex agglutination	Pasteur Diagnostics
Directigen[R1]	dot blot	Becton-Dickinson

[1] The Directigen test has been discontinued by the manufacturer in Jan.1992

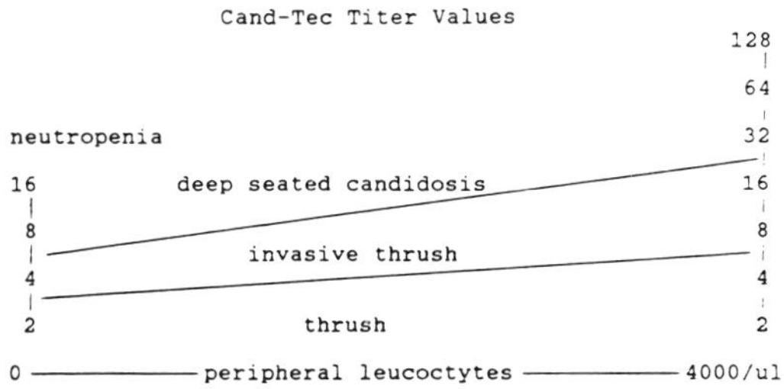

Fig.1. Empirical relationship between Candida antigen (Cand-Tec[R]) titer values and the peripheral white blood cell count. Borderline positive titers are suggestive of invasive candidiasis only if the white blood cell counts are low. With normal white blood cell counts, higher titers can be tolerated. (Invasive thrush is exemplified by candida esophagitis in AIDS).

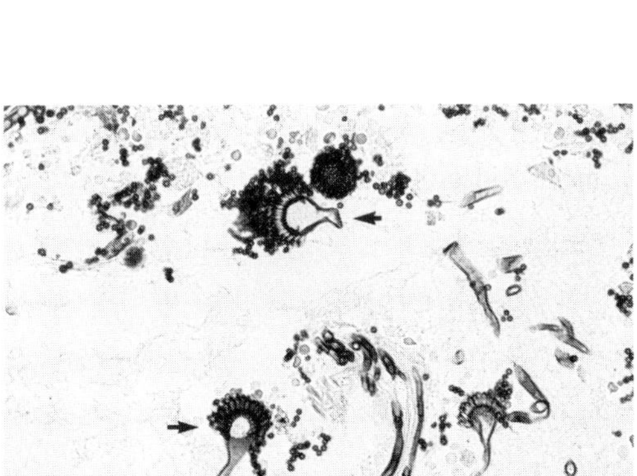

Fig.2. Elements of Aspergillus fumigatus in bronchial secretions of a patient who died of invasive aspergillosis. Hyphae, conidiophors (arrow) and numerous conidia can be seen. The presence of conidiophors is indicative of the disease. It suggests the invasion of the ventilated parts of the lung. (Gomori-Methenamine-Silver (GMS) stain, bar=20microns).

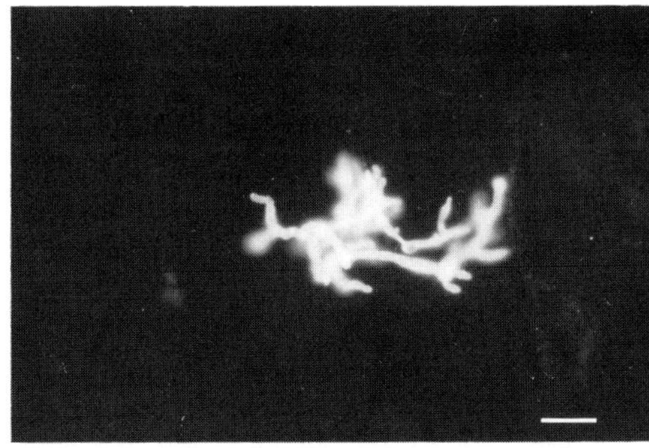

Fig.3. Mycelium of a zygomycete (Rhizopus microsporus) as detected in the sinusoidal mucosa of a patient who developed orbital cellulitis during treatment with deferoxamine. (Fungiqual[R] staining after maceration of the tissue with potassium hydroxide, fluorescent microscopy, bar=20microns). (From R. Rüchel, Mycoses, 1993, in press).

References

1. Bodey GP (1986) Fungal Infection and Fever of Unknown Origin in Neutropenic Patients. Am J Med 80/5C:112-119
2. Bodey GP, Vartivarian S (1989) Aspergillosis. Eur J Clin Microbiol Infect Dis 8:413-437
3. Boelaert JR, Fenves AZ, Coburn JW (1989) Deferoxamine Therapy and Mucormycosis in Dialysis Patients: Report on an International Registry. Am J Kidney Dis 18:660-667
4. Chuck SL, Sande MA (1989) Infections with Cryptococcus neoformans in the Acquired Immunodeficiency Syndrome. New Engl J Med 321:794-799
5. Jones JM (1990) Laboratory Diagnosis of Invasive Candidiasis. Clin Microbiol Rev 3:32-45

6. Lew MA (1989) Diagnosis of Systemic Candida Infections. Ann Rev Med 40:87-97
7. Sugar AM (1990) Agents of Mucormycosis and Related Species. In: Mandell GL, Douglas RG, Bennett JE (eds) Principles and Practice of Infectious Diseases. 3rd ed.Churchill,Livingstone, New York pp.1962-1972
8. Monod M, Baudraz-Rosselet F, Ramelet AA et al (1989) Direct Mycological Examination in Dermatology: A Comparison of Different Methods. Dermatologica 179:183-186
9. Musial CE, Cockerill FR, Roberts GD (1988) Fungal Infections of the Immunocompromised Host: Clinical and Laboratory Aspects. Clin Microbiol Rev 1:349-364
10. Repentigny L de (1989) Serological Techniques for Diagnosis of Fungal Infections. Eur J Clin Microbiol Infect Dis 8:362-375
11. Walsh TJ, Hathorn JW, Sobel JD et al (1991) Detection of Circulating Candida Enolase by Immunoassay in Patients with Cancer and Invasive Candidiasis. New Engl J Med 324:1026-1031

Keratomycosis: The European Standpoint

Wolfgang Behrens-Baumann

Abstract. The diagnosis and therapy of keratomycosis commonly present many problems due to the fact that there is a discrepancy between early invasion of fungi into the deep corneal stroma and late ulceration of the cornea. Swabs taken for microbiological and microscopic diagnosis are often negative, because intact epithelium may cover the organisms.

Keratomycosis clinically shows some characteristics, which are helpful in differentiating the inflammation from bacterial infections of the cornea: (a) geographical configuration and (b) non-delineated margins of the corneal infiltration, (c) satellites, (d) epithelium often intact, (e) elevated corneal areas and (f) tenacious, convex hypopyon.

The poor therapeutic response to most antimycotic agents can be explained by (a) deep infiltration of the fungi, (b) almost intact epithelium, (c) high molecular weight of many substances, so that the antimycotics will not come in contact with the organisms. Repeated debridements are helpful for diagnostic and moreover therapeutic reasons especially when Amphotericin B is used topically. With respect to the new antimycotics, Fluconazole is the most promising candidate for candidal keratomycosis derived from experimental results in the rabbit model.

Introduction

Diagnosis and management of keratomycosis is more difficult than that of bacterial keratitis. This is due to the fact that fungi penetrate early into the corneal stroma without a major superficial defect. Therefore, a simple swab for microbiologic or microscopic diagnosis is usually negative. In addition, since the drug must penetrate into the deep stromal layers in order to reach the fungi, therapy is often long-lasting and frustrating.

Clinical Diagnosis

There are several clinical characteristics of keratomycosis that differ from bacterial keratitis (Tab.1). The corneal infiltrates frequently have a geographical configuration (Fig.1), the borderlines are soft and fluffy and radiating stripes (branching hyphae) may be seen (Fig.2). At the beginning there is no visible or only a minor defect of the epithelium. In addition, the satellite phenomenon is not always present, but, if this is the case, it is rather pathognomonic. Furthermore, the infiltrates are sometimes elevated (26, Fig.3). Finally, the early liquid and horizontal hypopyon becomes viscous and gets a pyramidal and convex shape (6, Fig.3-5).

However, these characteristics of keratomycosis are not always present. Frequently only one or two signs may be observed. In cases with an underlying different primary pathology of the anterior segment of the eye (e.g. Herpes simplex, ocular pemphigoid), keratomycosis may exhibit a totally different aspect (Fig.6).

Microscopic Diagnosis and Microbiology

To confirm the clinical diagnosis, specimens containing hyphae have to be obtained. As has been already pointed out, a simple swab from the conjunctiva is usually negative, because the fungi are located in the corneal stroma. Therefore, a debridement of the epithelium and the anterior stroma is necessary (9). This should be repeated if the result is negative (27). In some cases, keratectomy must be done for successful sampling (21).

The specimens should be placed into a transport medium. In the mycologic laboratory the cultures are incubated for 3-6 days, with some organisms needing several weeks to grow. It is therefore more practicable to examine a part of the specimen under a microscope. Moreover, positive results are more frequently obtained using microscopic techniques than using cultures. Staining can be done by the Gram or Giemsa methods or with 10% potassium hydroxide mixed with ink 9:1 (1). Alternatively, methenamine silver staining may be used; this method requires about one hour to get results (14). Staining with Calcofluor 0.1% and Evans Blue 0.1% and reading under a fluorescence microscope is faster (two minutes) (1,30). Lactophenol Blue solution (Merck, Darmstadt, FRG) is also suited for that purpose, and fungi react with this solution in a few minutes at room temperature.

If keratoplasty material must be evaluated, the host button should be cut in two pieces: one half can be used for microbiologic and the other for histopathologic studies (2).

Therapy

Keratomycosis should be treated medically if the process is not too advanced.

Alternatively, surgical treatment may be indicated.

Medical Therapy

Topical administration is recommended, because in the anterior segment of the eye the bioavailability is better than with systemic therapy (18). In rare events, additional systemic chemotherapy may be indicated. Several antimycotics are currently available.

The molecular weight of these substances is of particular interest, because the epithelium can hardly be penetrated by agents with a molecular weight of more than 500000 D (31). In Tab.2, the molecular weights of several antimycotics are listed.

Differences in the incidences of fungi are known to exist with respect to geographic locations. Selecting an antimycotic should take this fact into account. In temperate climates (Central Europe, England, Northern part of the USA, San Francisco) Candida is the most frequent fungus followed by Aspergillus (10,19,24,42). In South Florida, South America, Japan, Nigeria and South Africa, Fusarium dominates (11,13,16,20,-22,28,44,45). In India, Aspergillus is more frequent than Fusarium (8).

Amphotericin B: In mycosis due to Candida, Amphotericin B 0.5% is the drug of choice (7,40). For topical administration, eye drops have to be custom-made using injection systems for systemic use (6). Due to its high molecular weight of 924.11 D, Amphotericin B can hardly penetrate the epithelium (5). Therefore, a debridement (36) is recommended.

Miconazole 1% may be used alternatively as well as Flucytosine 1% or Nystatin. Miconazole has been administered subconjunctivally (35).

Pimaricin (Natamycin) at a concentration of 5% is more effective in keratomycosis due to Fusarium and Aspergillus than Amphotericin B (24,29). This concentration, however, is not available in Germany.

Fluconazole: This new drug is very promising due to its high bioavailability (34,39). It is effective against Candida species. In the rabbit aqueous, the concentration of Fluconazole is higher without debridement than the concentraion of Amphotericin B after corneal abrasion (6). For keratomycosis caused by Candida, the therapeutic regimen listed in Tab.3 is recommended. The eye drops can be used from the solution for infusion, ointments may be prepared by the pharmacist (6).

Corticosteroids: These substances are believed to be one of the risk factors for the development of a keratomycosis. Therefore, corticosteroids should be used with caution (23). The patient must be immunocompetent to avoid systemic spread of the infection (33). However, topical low-dose corticosteroids applied additionally to antimycotics are valuable in reducing secondary inflammatory reactions of the anterior segment of the eye. The benefit of corticosteroids in keratomycosis has been studied experimentally (4,32) and has been confirmed clinically (33,37). Probably, the time factor is important: in the early stages of keratomycosis, corticosteroids have a negative effect, after about two weeks they may be beneficial (6).

Surgical Treatment

In rare instances, a lamellar corneal graft (38) may be indicated. However, in most cases a penetrating keratoplasty is recommended (3,13,15,17,41,43). The advantage of a penetrating graft includes the elimination of fungi simultaneous with the secondary inflammatory reaction, which affects both the cornea and the anterior chamber. In addition, reactive corneal neovascularization may be avoided, which is important for the prognosis of the graft (3).

If medical treatment fails and there is no regression of the inflammatory process, an early penetrating keratoplasty may save the integrity of the globe and may lead to visual rehabilitation.

Table 1. Clinical Characteristics of Keratomycosis

* Geographical corneal infiltrates
* No visible or only minor epithelial defect
* Satellite phenomenon
* Soft and fluffy borders of the infiltrates
* Infiltrates sometimes elevated (26)
* Pyramidal viscous hypopyon (6)

Table 2. Molecular Weights of Antimycotics

Amphotericin B	924.11 D
Clotrimazole	344.84 D
Econazole	381.68 D
Fluconazole	306.30 D
5-Fluocytosine	129.09 D
Ketoconazole	531.44 D
Miconazole	416.12 D
Nystatine	926.11 D
Natamycin	665.75 D

Table 3. Medical Treatment Regimen for Candida Keratomycosis

Topical:	Amphotericin B eye drops 0.5%
*	after corneal debridement
	or
	Fluconazole eye drops 0.5%
	or
	Miconazole eye drops 1%
	or
	Nystatine eye drops 100000 I.U.
Subconjunctival:	Miconazole 5-10mg
Systemic:	
	Fluconazole 2 x 200mg
*	or
	Ketoconazole 2 x 200mg

* Eye drops hourly during the day, ointments for the night.

** Additional systemic treatment is not imperative with respect to pharmakokinetic data.

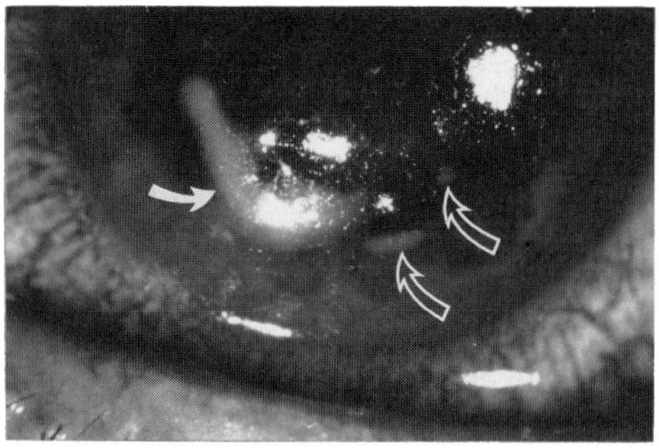

Fig. 1. Geographic corneal infiltrate with satellites (from 6).

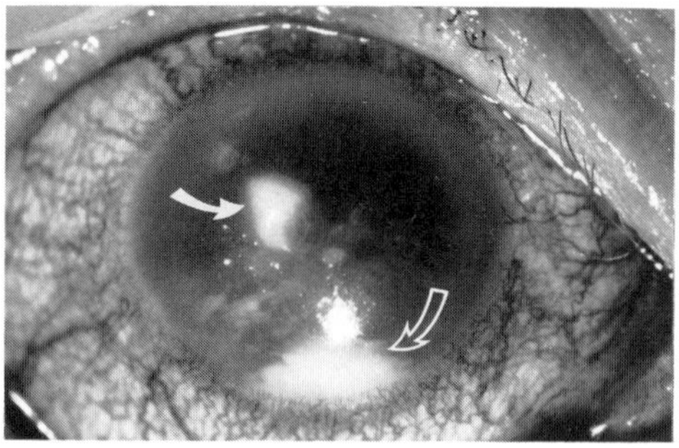

Fig. 3. Prominent infiltrate, satellite phenomena, pyramidal hypopyon (from 6).

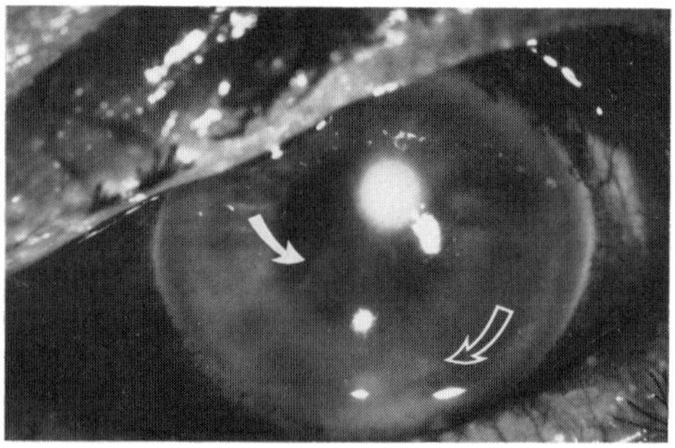

Fig. 2. Candida keratomycosis with radiating infiltrates (hyphae). Pyramidal, convex hypopyon (from 6).

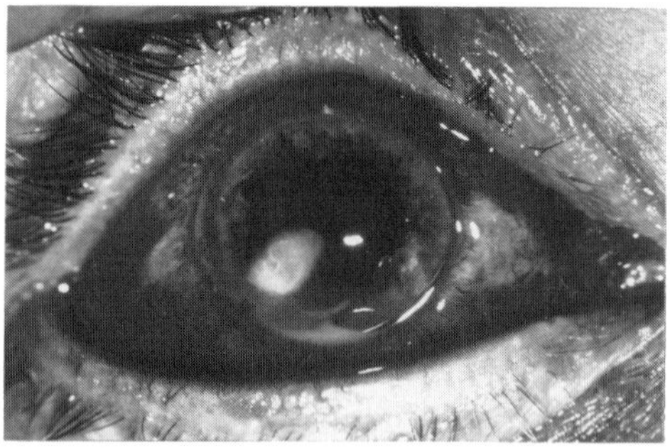

Fig. 4. Aspergillus fumigatus keratitis with small hypopyon (from 6).

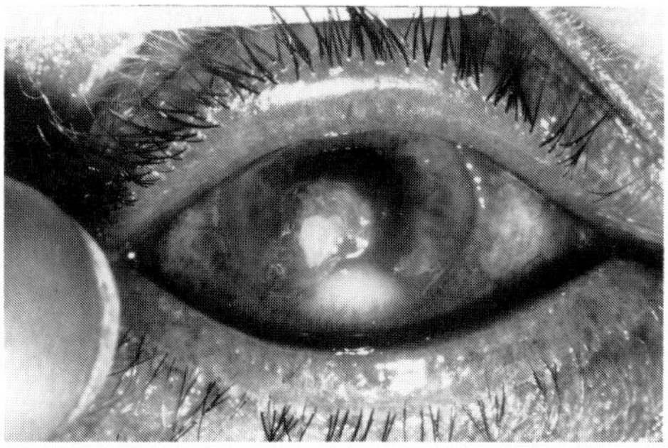

Fig.5. Same patient as in Fig.4; three weeks later presenting with a pyramidal, convex hypopyon (from 6).

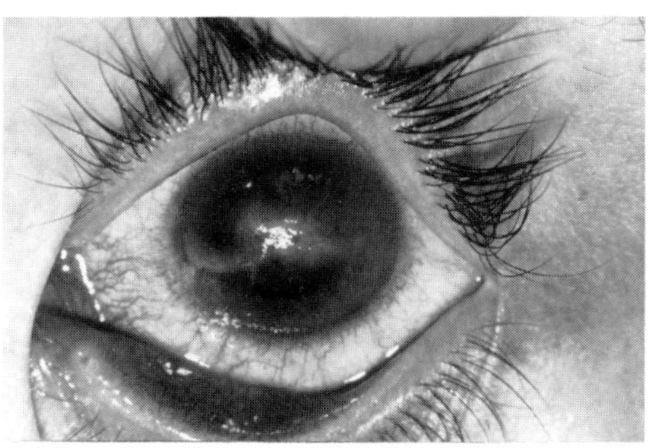

Fig.6. Secondary keratomycosis by Trichophyton rubrum in chronic Herpes simplex virus keratitis (from 6).

References

1. Arffa RC, Avni I, Ishibashi Y et al (1985) Calcofluor and Ink-Potassium Hydroxide Preparations for Identifying Fungi. Am J Ophthalmol 100:719-723
2. Arora R, Venkateswarlu K, Mahajan VM (1984) Keratomycosis: A Retrospective Histopathologic and Microbiologic Analysis. Ann Ophthalmol 20:306-315
3. Behrens-Baumann W (1984) Ergebnisse der Keratoplastik à chaud. Klin Mbl Augenheilk 185:25-27
4. Behrens-Baumann W, Küster M (1987) Der Einfluß von Kortikosteroiden bei der antimykotischen Therapie der Candida-Keratitis. Klin Mbl Augenheilk 191:222-225
5. Behrens-Baumann W, Uter W, Ansorg R (1987) Experimentelle Untersuchungen zur lokalen Therapie der Candida Keratomykose mit Amphotericin B. Klin Mbl Augenheilk 91:125-128
6. Behrens-Baumann W (1991) Pilzerkrankungen des Auges. Bücherei des Augenarztes, Enke Verlag, Stuttgart
7. Clayton YM (1970) Antifungal Drugs for Oculomycosis. II. Sensitivity of Certain Fungi to Antifungal Drugs. Trans Ophthal Soc UK 89:837-844
8. Dasgupta LR, Gupta AK, Gosh Ray B et al (1973) Mycological Studies in Keratitis. Indian J Med Res 61:165-168
9. Dieckhues B (1966) Die Behandlung der Keratomykose mit Nystatin und Pimaricin. Klin Mbl Augenheilk 148:895-896
10. Doughman DJ, Leavenworth NM, Campbell RC et al (1982) Fungal Keratitis at the University of Minnesota: 1971-1981. Trans Am Ophthal Soc 80:235-247
11. Fitzsimons R, Peters AL (1986) Miconazole and Ketoconazole As a Satisfactory First-Line Treatment for Keratomycosis. Am J Ophthalmol 101:605-608
12. Forster RK, Rebell G (1975) Therapeutic Surgery in Failures of Medical Treatment for Fungal Keratitis. Brit J Ophthalmol 59:366-371
13. Forster RK, Rebell G (1975) The Diagnosis and Management of Keratomycosis. I.

Cause and Diagnosis II. Medical and Surgical Management. Arch Ophthalmol 93:975-978
14. Forster RK, Wirta MG, Soli M et al (1976) Methenamine Silver Stained Corneal Scrapings in Keratomycosis. Am J Ophthalmol 82:261-265
15. Gracner B (1987) Therapeutische Möglichkeiten bei mykotischen Hornhautprozessen. Fortschr Ophthalmol 84:245-246
16. Gugnani HC, Talwar RS, Njoku-Obi ANV et al (1976) Mycotic Keratitis in Nigeria. A Study of 21 Cases. Brit J Ophthalmol 60:607-613
17. Hallermann W (1975) Keratoplastik aus akuter Indikation. Klin Mbl Augenheilk 167:345-352
18. Havener WH (1983) Pharmacokinetics: Routes of Administration. In: Havener WH (ed) Ocular Pharmacology. C.V.Mosby, St.Louis pp.18-43
19. Hollwich F, Dieckhues B (1970) Die Keratomykose - eine Spätkomplikation der Hornhautentzündung. Klin Mbl Augenheilk 156:395-401
20. Ishibashi Y (1982) Keratomycosis in Japan Reported from 1976-1980. Nippon Ganka Zasshi 86:651-656
21. Ishibashi Y, Kaufman HE (1986) Corneal Biopsy in the Diagnosis of Keratomycosis. Am J Ophthalmol 101:288-293
22. Ishibashi Y, Hommura S, Matsumoto Y (1987) Direct Examination vs. Culture of Biopsy Specimens for the Diagnosis of Keratomycosis. Am J Ophthalmol 103:636-640
23. Johns KJ, O'Day DM (1988) Pharmacologic Management of Keratomycosis. Surv Ophthalmol 33:178-188
24. Jones DB, Richards AB, Morgan G (1969) Direct Fungal Infection of the Eye in Britain. Trans Ophthalmol Soc UK 89:727-741
25. Jones DB, Sexton R, Rebell G (1969) Mycotic Keratitis in South Florida: A Review of Thirty Nine Cases. Trans Ophthalmol Soc Uk 89:781-797
26. Kaufman HE, Wood RM (1965) Mycotic Keratitis. Am J Ophthalmol 59:993-1000
27. Lemp MA, Blackman HJ, Koffler BH (1990) Therapy for Bacterial and Fungal Infections. Int Ophthalmol Clin 20:135-147
28. Liesegang TJ, Forster RK (1980) Spectrum of Microbial Keratitis in South Florida. Am J Ophthalmol 90:38-47
29. Malik SRK, Mitter S (1979) Medical Treatment in Keratomycosis. Indian J Ophthalmol 27:190-192
30. Marines HM, Osato MS, Font RL (1987) The Value of Calcofluor White in the Diagnosis of Mycotic and Acanthamoeba Infections of the Eye and Ocular Adnexa. Ophthalmology 94:23-26
31. Maurice DM (1960) The Permeability of the Cornea. In: Duke-Elder S, Perkins ES (eds) The Transparency of the Cornea. Blackwell Scientific Publications, Oxford, pp.67-71
32. Newmark E, Ellison AC, Kaufman HE (1971) Combined Pimaricin and Dexamethasone Therapy of Keratomycosis. Am J Ophthalmol 71:718-722
33. O'Day DM, Moore TE, Aronson SB (1971) Deep Fungal Corneal Abscess. Combined Corticosteroid Therapy. Arch Ophthalmol 86:414-419
34. O'Day DM, Foulds G, Williams TE et al (1990) Ocular Uptake of Fluconazole Following Oral Administration. Arch Ophthalmol 108:1006-1008
35. Pflugfelder SC, Flynn HW, Zwickey TA et al (1988) Exogenous Fungal Endophthalmitis. Ophthalmology 95:19-30
36. Polack FM (1973) Diagnosis and Treatment of Keratomycosis. Int Ophthalmol Clin 13:75-91
37. Roberts SS (1957) Nystatin in Monilia Keratoconjunctivitis. Am J Ophthalmol 44:108-109

38. Sanitato JJ, Kelley CG, Kaufman HE (1984) Surgical Management of Peripheral Fungal Keratitis (Keratomycosis). Arch Ophthalmol 102:1506-1509
39. Savani DV, Perfect JR, Cobo LM et al (1987) Penetration of New Azole Compounds into the Eye and Efficacy in Experimental Candida Endophthalmitis. Antimicrob Ag Chemother 31:6-10
40. Smolin G, Tabbara K, Whitcher J (1984) Fungal Infections. In: Infectious Diseases of the Eye. Williams and Wilkins, Baltimore, pp.102-131
41. Thiel HJ (1978) Keratoplastik bei akuten infektiösen Hornhautprozessen. Klin Mbl Augenheilk 173:171-181
42. Thygeson P, Okumoto M (1974) Keratomycosis: A Preventable Disease. Trans Acad Ophthalmol Otolaryngol 78:433-439
43. Weidle EG, Thiel HJ (1984) Keratoplastik à chaud als therapeutische Maßnahme bei akuten Hornhautinfektionen. Klin Mbl Augenheilk 184:520-528
44. Zapater RC (1980) The Genus Fusarium as Agent of Keratomycosis in Argentina. In: Kuttin ES, Baum GL (eds) Human and Animal Mycology. Proceedings of the 7th International Congress of ISHAM. Excerpta Medica, Amsterdam, pp.35-38
45. Zapater RC, Arrechea A (1975) Mycotic Keratitis by Fusarium. A Review and Report of Two Cases.Ophthalmologica 170: 1-12

Fungal Keratitis: The American Standpoint

Eduardo C. Alfonso

Abstract. Fungal keratitis is often a difficult management problem and is compounded by a delay in making the correct diagnosis.
This survey discusses the incidence, etiology, pathogenesis, clinical features, complications, laboratory diagnosis, histopathology, and management.
The incidence of fungal keratitis has increased significantly because of the higher rate of recognition by ophthalmologists as well as the greater number of immunocompromised patients. Approximately 40 species of fungi are known to cause keratitis in man. Predisposing factors are primarily trauma with vegetable matter in rural settings, and altered corneas with surface and/or systemic immunosuppression. The organisms are commonly divided into the filamentous (e.g. Fusarium) and yeast forms (e.g. Candida). The clinical features include stromal keratitis with a hypopyon, which can rapidly progress to scleritis and endophthalmitis.

The laboratory diagnosis is made by corneal scrapings for smears and cultures. Corneal biopsy may be required in difficult cases. Smears should be stained with Giemsa, Calcoflor, and Gomori methenamine silver stain.

Initial therapy is begun upon identification of the organism on a smear. Commercially available topical 5% Natamycin is used on an hourly basis. Other topical and/or systemic antifungals (polyenes, imidazoles, and pyrimidines) may be used. Corticosteroids should be avoided unless careful follow-up is given to the patient. Surgical therapy may be necessary if there is progression of the process. Recurrences may occur.

Introduction

Fungal corneal ulceration is a difficult management problem often compounded by a delay in making the correct diagnosis. The disease process has gained interest because of the improved laboratory techniques used to make the correct diagnosis and the availability of antifungal agents for treatment.

Historically, the first reported case of fungal corneal ulceration appeared in 1879 (5). Up to 1951, only 53 cases had appeared in the literature (4). Since then, numerous case reports and series have appeared.

Natamycin, the first commercially available topical antifungal in the United States did not appear until 1979, almost one hundred years after the first reported case of fungal keratitis (13).

Clinical Presentation

Patients developing fungal keratitis have been typically exposed to one of the known risk factors. The majority have sustained ocular trauma with plant or agriculture material. Other risk factors include: ocular surface disorders, previous corneal surgery such as keratoplasty and keratotomies, use of contact lenses and use of contaminated medications.

Fungal keratitis has been described in the past as a seasonal disease occurring primarily in the Spring and Fall, this being related possibly to agriculture activity (11). Today, the seasonal incidence is less marked, due to the number of patients presenting after home gardening activities. There is a geographic predilection for tropical and subtropical climates, but the disease is widespread, the only difference that geography makes being the species of organisms cultured.

Patients with ocular surface disorders may be at a higher risk of developing fungal keratitis because of the damaged surface epithelium's inability to form a barrier against invading organisms and possibly enhancing the ability of the organism to attach to injured cells. There may also be a weakness in the surface immune system in protecting against and fighting the infection. Patients who have undergone corneal surgery such as penetrating keratoplasty and keratotomies are also more vulnerable to infection for the reasons already stated and also because they usually require long-term treatment with topical corticosteroids, which weakens the immune system and enhances fungal growth.

Although fungal keratitis has been reported in patients using contact lenses, in most series of contact lens related corneal ulcers, the incidence of fungal etiology is markedly reduced compared to those cases of patients not wearing contact lenses (2)

Use of contaminated topical medications has recently received increasing attention as a risk factor for developing fungal keratitis (17). Although Gram-negative organisms are more frequently implicated in the contamination of topical ocular medications, fungal species can also contaminate these, and if trauma occurs with the tip of the dispenser during application of the drops and contamination is present, then an infectious keratitis is likely to develop.

Pain and discomfort are usually presenting symptoms. The pain may be intense initially, sometimes becoming only a discomfort if the surface epithelium has healed. Patients with pre-existing corneal diseases which have reduced corneal sensation such as herpetic and neurotrophic keratitis and/or a recent corneal transplant may have very little symptoms.

Slit-Lamp Characteristics

A definite diagnosis cannot be made by the slit-lamp appearance of the keratitis, only by isolation and identification of the organism in the microbiology laboratory. Nevertheless, cases of fungal keratitis often present with somewhat characteristic clinical findings (10).

The conjunctiva is often injected and a mucopurulent discharge may be present. In cases where topical corticosteroids have been used or immunosuppression is present, these findings may not be evident. Patients with chronic ocular surface disease may not show a marked change in findings once infected with fungi when compared with their baseline signs and symptoms and in these cases, the clinicians have to be observant to subtle anatomic changes that may herald the beginning of an infection.

There is usually an epithelial defect present in the cornea, but sometimes because of the indolent nature of the keratitis, the epithelium overlying the infectious infiltrate may have healed. The infiltrate may be central or peripheral in the stroma. The border of the infiltrate is often ill-defined, sometimes with radiating feathery edges. Satellite infiltrates may be present. Often, the depth and width of the infiltrate is similar, although fungal infiltrates may be quite deep as compared to bacterial infiltrates. The surface of the cornea may be raised and rough. The infiltrate usually has a dirty grey color, but with some pigment producing species, a brown or black tinge may be present. An immune ring may surround the infiltrate as well as an inflammatory endothelial plaque and hypopyon. Some cases may present with an adjacent scleritis or more advanced with perforation and associated endophthalmitis.

Pathogenesis

Fungal species accounting for most cases of human keratitis can be divided into yeast and filamentous by their morphology (14). The filamentous forms may be further divided into non-pigmented and pigmented varieties. Most of the filamentous species that invade the human cornea are septated. The most important nonseptated filamentous fungi that cause ophthalmological disease is Rhizopus (Mucormycosis) species (Tab.1).

In South Florida, where 20% of microbial keratitis is of fungal etiology, Fusarium solani comprises 50% of the isolates, and this resembles the findings reported from most tropical areas.

In temperate regions, Aspergillus is more commonly isolated than in tropical areas. In both climatic areas, a significant number of the isolates are of the Candida species. The clinical setting may also influence the organism isolated with Candida favored in immunocompromised (15) and diseased ocular surface, post surgery and in the use of contaminated ocular medications.

Microbiologic Isolation

Fungi have been difficult to isolate in the past because of the difficulty in obtaining adequate material from the ulcer and the fastidious nature of growth of the organisms in culture media (1). In order to obtain the best material possible from the ulcer, magnification should be available either by using an operating microscope or the slit-lamp biomicroscope. Topical anesthesia is necessary, and a lid or retrobulbar block may be considered but usually patients are sufficiently cooperative making these unnecessary. In small children, general anesthesia or intramuscular sedation may be necessary. (3)

To scrape the ulcer, a platinum spatula (Storz Instruments Co.) may be sterilized with an alcohol burner or a sterile surgical blade (Beard-Parker #15) may be used. In cases where the stromal infiltrate is deep with overlying intact epithelium and stroma, it may be difficult to obtain an adequate specimen unless a deep puncture is made with a 6-0 silk suture on a cutting needle, which is then passed through the infiltrate. Another alternative is to use a blade or a 2 to 3mm trephine to perform a corneal biopsy.

Once an adequate specimen is obtained, it is submitted for microbiologic and/or pathologic studies. Specimens should be submitted for Gram, Giemsa and an additional glass slide for other possible stains such as a Calcofluor white. An albumin coated slide may be used for staining with the Gomori methenamine Silver method.

Our protocol for culturing all microbial keratitis is to use blood agar at 25°C and 37°C; the latter is placed in an 10% CO_2 container. A chocolate agar plate is also placed at 37°C in the 10% CO_2 jar. A CDC-ANA plate is placed in an anaerobic container. We use trypticase soy broth as liquid media. A Sabouraud's plate is placed at room temperature. For better recovery, it should not contain cycloheximide but rather gentamicin. Additional plates containing other media may be used depending on level of suspicion of other organisms. The solid media is plated using the C-streak technique, each row of C's representing a new scraping with resterilization of the spatula.

Table 3 shows the percentage of recovery of organisms from the different media plated. Additional steps may be taken to enhance fungal growth. The media should be fresh and used at room temperature. The media should be in petri dishes and not in a test tube since this allows wide plating of the specimen and dispersion of any growth inhibiting substances present in the ocular discharge. Placing the plates inside plastic bags with a moist gauze may also enhance growth. Sometimes a corneal biopsy may be necessary, specially in deep keratitis or chronic cases. A piece of the tissue obtained should be submitted to the pathology laboratory for examination (12).

Treatment: Choice of Antifungal

Once appropriate cultures are obtained, treatment should be started. Antifungals are not used as broad-spectrum antimicrobial coverage routinely in cases of ulcerative keratitis. Even though a high index of suspicion for fungal keratitis may be present based on the history and slit-lamp appearance, it is prudent to hold antifungals until the Gram and Giemsa stain are performed. If fungal elements are not present, and one has a high index of suspicion, the treatment should be started with a topical antifungal.

The only currently commercially available antifungal in the United States is Natamycin in a 5% suspension.

Other formulations of topical antifungals are made by taking the intravenous or oral preparation and making into a topical form. The classification and availability of the major antifungals are listed in Table 4. The dosages and possible routes of administration are presented in Table 5.

Eventhough sensitivity data may be obtained, it is often impractical because of the delay in obtaining this information and the variability in the behaviour of the organisms to a particular antifungal.

Initial treatment may be chosen based on the likely organism to be encountered. For example, agriculture trauma in South Florida is very likely to yield Fusarium as the causative organism, where as a deep ulcer in a patient using topical corticosteroids following a corneal transplant is likely to be due to Candida. We have developed sensitivity data for organisms isolated at the Bascom Palmer Eye Institute from cases of ulcerative keratitis and this information is presented in Table 6. This information helps us select the best possible agent. Antimicrobial activity of antifungal agents based on published reports is included in Table 7. Of course, this sensitivity data is in vitro laboratory information not taking in consideration bioavailability and sensitivity in a clinical environment.

Treatment: Routes of Administration

Topical administration appears to deliver the fastest, easiest, and highest concentration of antifungal to the involved site.

Subconjunctival injections may be given and experience is available with some of the antifungals. For the most part, these may be quite painful and do not seem to enhance the concentration of the topical agent alone.

Oral and intravenous administration as concomitant therapy of keratitis has been tried. It appears that oral Ketoconazole is well-tolerated and may enhance the topical therapy (8). Intravenous Amphotericin and Miconazole may be used with a greater risk of systemic toxicity (9). Newer antifungals not yet available commercially such as Itraconazole offer new horizons for better bioavailability both as a topical and systemic preparation (4). Sufficient clinical experience is not available with these newer antifungals, which are listed in Table 4.

Treatment: Other Medical

Besides the use of topical antifungals, frequent topical lavage with sterile saline may be necessary to remove the inflammatory debris from the ocular surface as well as residual nonactive medication such as happens when a suspension of Natamycin is used.

Cycloplegic drops may help reduce some of the pain caused by ciliary spasm and prevent the formation of iris synechiae by keeping the iris moving.

The use of topical corticosteroids is controversial since they are known to enhance fungal growth. They can be used to control the destructive inflammatory response but this must be done with great caution. They should not be started until evidence is available that the isolated fungi respond clinically to the antifungal being used.

Treatment: Surgery

Surgical therapy is often used concurrently with the medical treatment (16):

Debridement of the surface, especially in the first few days of treatment, helps increase the contact between the organisms and the antifungals. Some authors have developed considerable experience with the use of conjunctival flaps for the treatment of keratomyosis. The thought is that increasing the vascular supply to the area may inhibit growth of the fungi. A drawback of this therapy, as well as performing a lamellar keratoplasty, is that the infected area is being further shielded from topical therapy.

The use of cryotherapy has been reserved for cases in which there is involvement of the sclera. It seems that once the organism has invaded the sclera or an endophthalmitis has developed, with rare exceptions, the eye will be lost.

Penetrating keratoplasty is used when there is progressive disease unresponsive to medical treatment or impending or frank perforation (7).

In our institution, 7% of keratoplasties were done for management of microbial keratitis and in 24% of these, the etiology was fungal. The graft should be large enough to encompass all areas of involvement. Any intraocular tissue such as iris, lens and vitreous that appears to be involved is removed. Postoperative treatment is continued with antifungals and the situation is carefully monitored for recurrences. Since the goal is to eradicate the organism and to tectonically preserve the globe, corticosteroids are used with great caution. Topical Cyclosporin A may also be used in hopes of preventing a rejection. In our series of therapeutic keratoplasties, 95% of the grafts had opacified within one year.

Conclusions

Despite the enormous progress in the last 30 years in the diagnosis and treatment of fungal keratitis, it continues to be one of the most feared infectious diseases of the eye.

It is hoped that with prevention of corneal trauma and better antifungals much progress will be achieved in the future.

Table 1. Fungi Causing Human Keratitis

Yeasts:		
	Candida albicans	
		parapsilosis
		krusei
		tropicalis
Filamentous septated:		
Non-pigmented:		
	Fusarium solani	
		oxysporium
		moniliforme
		episphaesia
	Aspergillus fumigatus	
		flavus
		acremonium (cephalosporium)
		paecilomyces
Pigmented:		
	Curvularia senegalensis, verruculosa	
	Lasiodiplodia theobromae	
	Cladosporium	
	Colletotrichum	
Filamentous Non-septated:		
	Rhizopus (Mucormycosis)	

Table 2. Percentage of Positive Identification of Fungi Using Different Staining Methods with Light Microscopy

	Percentage Positive
Gram	55%
Giemsa	66%
Gomori Methenamine Silver	86%

Table 3. Percentage of Recovery of Fungal Organisms from Different Culture Media

	Percentage
Sabouraud's Agar (25°C)	80%
Blood Agar (25°C)	70%

Table 4. Classification of Antifungals

Standard:			
Polyenes	Imidazoles	Pyrimidines	
Amphotericin B (2,4)	Clotrimazole (4)	5-Fluorocytosine	(1)
Amphotericin B methyl ester(2)	Miconazole (2,4)		
Natamycin (3)	Econazole(4)		
	Ketoconazole(1,4)		
	Thiabendazole(1)		
	Fluconazole(1,2)		
	Itraconazole (5)		
Others:			
Pradicimicins			(5)
Cispentacin			(5)
Jasplacinolide			(5)
Terbinafine			(5)
Nystatine			(4)

Commercial availability:
- oral (1),
- intravenous (2),
- ocular (3),
- dermatologic (4),
- not available (5).

Table 5. Antifungal Dosages

Antifungal Agent	Topical	Subconjunctival	Intravitreal	Intravenous	Oral
Amphotericin B	2.5-10 mg/ml	750 μg/ml every other day	5-10μ	Maitenance dose 1.0 mg/KG/day refrigerated	
Clotrimazole	1% suspension 1 % solution	5-10 mg (0.5-1 ml)			60 - 100 mg/kg/day adults 60 - 150 mg/kg/day children
Econazole	1 % suspension 1 % ointment			30 mg/kg/day	200 mg tid
Ketoconazole	1 % suspension				200-400mg day
Miconazole	1 % suspension 1 % solution	5-10 mg (0.5-1 ml)	0,25 mg	600-3600 mg/day divided into 3 doses	
Natamycin	50 mg/ml				
Nystatin	Ointment 100,000 units/gm				
Thiabendazole	4% suspension				25 mg/kg/day
5-Fluorocytosine	10 mg/ml				50-150 mg/kg/day 6-hr intervals

Table 6. Ten Year Summry of Sensitivity Testing of Clinical Isolates at the Microbiology Laboratory of the Bascom Palmer Eye Institute.

Antifungal (μg/ml)	FUSARIUM SP (40)	CANDIDA SP (10)	ASPERGILLUS SP (15)	CURVULARIA (6)
Amphotericin				
range	0.078 - 5	0.08 - 5	0.01 - 2,5	0.04 - .31
mean	1.2 (S)	2.7 (S)	1.0 (S)	0.16 (S)
Natamycin				
range	0.15 - 5	0.31 - 5	0.62 - 25	0.62 - 2.50
mean	1.5 (S)	2.5 (S)	2.0 (S)	1.4 (S)
Ketoconazole				
range	0.78 - 50	0.10 - 1.6	0.78 - 1250	0.20 - 12.50
mean	10.9 (I)	0.71 (S)	4.0 (S)	2.7 (S)
Miconazole				
range	0.78 - 50	0.78 - 62	0.20 - 3.10	0.05 - 3.1
mean	14.21 (I)	2.0 (S)	1.2 (S)	1.3 (S)
5-FC				
range	0.05 - 100	0.05 - 3.10		25 - 100
mean	921 (R)	1.2 (S)		68 (R)

Table 7. Antimicrobial Activity of Antifungal Agents Based on Published Reports

Antifungal agent	Alter-naria	Asper-gillus	Candida	Cephalo-sporium	Clado-sporiu,	Curvu-laria	Fusarium	Paecilo - myces	Penicil-lium
Polyenes									
Amhotericin	S	S	S		S		S	R	S
Nystatin		S	S						S
Natamycin		S	S	S	S		S	R	
Imidazoles									
Clotimazole	S	S	S		S	S	I	S	
Miconazole		S	S		S		I	I	
Econazole		S	I		S		S	I	
Ketoconazole		I	S		S		S		S
Fluconazole		S	S						
Pyrimidines									
5-Fluorocyto-sine		R	S		S		R	R	I

S = susceptible; I = variable susceptibility; R = resistant.

References

1. Al-Doory YU (1980) Laboratory Medical Mycology.Philadelphia: Lea & Febiger
2. Alfonso E, Mandelbaum S, Fox MJ et al (1986) Ulcerative Keratitis Associated with Contact Lens Wear.Am J Ophthalmol 101:429-433
3. Cruz OA, Sabiz SM, Capo H., Alfonso EC (1993) Microbial Keratitis in Childhood. Ophtalmology 100: 192 - 196
4. Dupont B, Drouhet E (1987) Early Experience with Itraconazole in Vitro and in Patients: Pharmacokinetic Studies and Clinical Results. Rev Infect Dis 9:571-576
5. Forster RK, Rebell G (1975) The Diagnosis and Management of Keratomycosis: I Arch Ophthalmol 93:975-978
6. Forster RK, Rebell G (1975) The Diagnosis and Management of Keratomycosis: II Arch Ophthalmol 93:1134-1136
7. Guilford JH, Alfonso E, Roussel TJ et al (1988) Large Therapeutic Keratoplasty in Microbial Keratitis. Inv Ophthalmol 105/3S:330
8. Ishibashi Y (1983) Oral Ketoconazole Therapy for Keratomycosis. Am J Ophthalmol 95:342
9. Ishibashi Y, Matsumoto Y, Takei K (1984) The Effects of Intravenous Miconazole on Fungal Keratitis. Am J Ophthalmol 98(4):433-437
10. Jones DB (1978) Fungal Keratitis. In: Duane TD (ed) Clinical Ophthalmology. Harper & Row, Hagerstown, MD Vol.4,pp.1-13
11. Liesegang TJ, Forster RK (1980) Spectrum of Microbial Keratitis in South Florida. Am J Ophthalmol 90:38-47
12. Naumann G, Green WR, Zimmerman LE (1967) Mycotic Keratitis. Am J Ophthalmol 64:668-682
13. Newmark E, Kaufman HE, Polack FM et al (1971) Clinical Experience with Pi-

maricin Therapy in Fungal Keratitis. South Med J 64:935-941
14. Okumoto M: Infectious Agents: Fungi. In: Thoft R, Smolin G (eds) The Cornea
15. Parrish CM, O'Day DM, Hoyle TC (1987) Spontaneous Fungal Corneal Ulcer as an Ocular Manifestation of AIDS. Am J Ophthalmol 104:302-303
16. Sanitato JJ, Kelley CG, Kaufman HE (1984) Surgical Management of Peripheral Fungal Keratitis (Keratomycosis) Arch Ophthalmol 102:1506-1509
17. Song DY, Alfonso E, Holland SP et al (1990) Contaminated Eye Drops and Ocular Infections. Invest Ophthalmol Vis Sci 31S:452

Keratomycosis in a New England Referral Center: Spectrum of Pathogenic Organisms and Predisposing Factors

Lisa D. Kelly, Deborah Pavan-Langston, Ann S. Baker

Abstract. Causative organisms and predisposing factors in keratomycosis vary significantly according to geography. To date, however, there have not been any published series reviewing fungal keratitis in the New England region of the United States. We reviewed the complete records of all patients with culture-proven keratomycosis over a five year period at the Massachussetts Eye and Ear Infirmary for a total of 25 cases. Forty-eight percent (=12) were caused by Candida species. The filamentous fungi Aspergillus, Penicillium and Fusarium accounted for 20% (=5), 12% (=3) and 8% (=2) respectively. As well there was one case each of Pseudoallescheria boydii, Chrysosporium and Wangiella.
Four categories of patients appear to be at risk for keratomycosis in this region: post-penetrating keratoplasty 44% (=11), post-organic trauma 28% (=7), prior ocular surface disease 20% (=5), and extended wear contact lens use 8% (=2).

Introduction

Keratomycosis continues to be a difficult diagnostic and management problem in ophthalmology. Much of the success in recognizing and treating this disease depends on accurate knowledge of epidemiologic patterns in fungal keratitis. Fungi are distinct among infectious etiologies of keratitis in that the epidemiology is influenced not only by host factors, but also by the geographic location of the population studied. Large series of keratomycosis cases reported from Florida, California, New York, and the Midwestern United States suggest that the distribution of pathogenic organisms, predisposing factors and the significance of prior corticosteroid use vary according to geographic locale (1,3,4,8,10,12). The epidemiology of keratomycosis in New England is less clear. Although there have been case reports from this region (6), there have not been any large published series. We reviewed the complete records of all patients with culture proven keratomycosis treated over a five year period at the Massachusetts Eye and Ear Infirmary.

The 25 cases of this report represent the largest published series of fungal keratitis from the New England region of the United States.

Materials and Methods

The logbook of the microbiology laboratory of the Massachusetts Eye and Ear Infirmary for the period from October 1, 1983 to October 1, 1988 was reviewed to identify all patients with corneal scrapings positive for fungal isolates.

Corneal scrapings were stained with Gram, Giemsa or Calcofluor reagents and inoculated onto blood, chocolate, modified Sabouraud's agar, and meat broth. The Sabouraud's agar was incubated at 25°C; all other media were incubated at 37°C. Fungal cultures in our laboratory are routinely held for three weeks before read as negative.

For the purpose of this study, cultures were considered positive if the isolate grew in more than one medium or was present in one medium and identified by appropriate fungal stain.

Patient Criteria

Twenty-five patients met the criteria for positive corneal scraping for fungus. The complete medical records of all 25 cases were reviewed to evaluate possible predisposing factors for acquiring fungal keratitis. In each case the patient age, sex, eye involved, date of presentation, contact lens use, history of trauma, prior ocular disease or surgery, history of corticosteroid use, and therapeutic outcome were evaluated. In addition to clinical data, microbiologic information including Gram and Giemsa smear, culture results and pathogenic organism were documented.

Results

A total of 25 patients met the predetermined criteria for a diagnosis of fungal keratitis. There were 10 females and 15 males; the average age was 53.7, with a range from 18 to 82 years. Keratomycosis was more likely to occur in the summer and fall months with 72% of infections occurring between June and November.

The microbiological profile revealed that 12 cases were infected with yeast and 13 cases were infected with filamentous fungi. Candida species were the most frequent isolates with six cases of C.albicans, four of C.parapsilosis, and two of C.tropicalis. Aspergillus species were the most frequent filamentous pathogen, present in five cases. Next in frequency were Penicillium (3 cases), Fusarium (2 cases), and one case each of Chrysosporium, Pseudoallescheria boydii and Wangiella. Gram, Giemsa or Calcofluor white stains identified fungal infection in 64.0% of cases.

There were four categories of predisposing factors for acquiring keratomycosis in this population:
- following penetrating keratoplasty,
- organic ocular trauma,
- pre-existing ocular surface disease, and
- extended-wear contact lens use.

The largest group, which included 11 cases (44%), consisted of patients who became infected after penetrating keratoplasty. Candida species were the causative organisms in nine of the eleven cases in this group; there was one case each of Aspergillus and Fusarium. The onset of keratomycosis ranged from five days to 23 months postoperatively. Unlike those patients with organic trauma, prior ocular surface disease or extended-wear contact lens use, patients with keratomycosis following penetrating keratoplasty had a significant history of prior corticosteroid use. Ten of the eleven patients with post-penetrating keratoplasty keratomycosis had a history of steroid use at the time of infection; the one patient who was not using corticosteroids had a chronic Fusarium dacryocystitis that was the presumed source of inoculation. In five of the eleven patients the infection was a suture-related abscess; in the remainder of the cases there was either no association with sutures or the infection had advanced too far at the time of presentation to determine its origin.

Seven of the 25 cases occurred in patients who had sustained ocular trauma, which in most cases was clearly related to organic material. The average age of these seven patients was 33.9; significantly younger than those patients in the other categories with an average age of 62.1 ($p < .01$). Those patients with keratomycosis following trauma were also significantly more likely to be male than patients in the other categories of fungal keratitis; six of the seven patients were male ($p < .001$).

Five of the twenty-five patients had a history of prior ocular surface disturbance: Two patients had retinal detachment repair but were not on steroids, one patient had pre-existing neovascular glaucoma, one patient had Stevens-Johnson syndrome with ocular involvement and one was a moribund patient with exposure keratitis.

The smallest group included two aphakic patients who developed Aspergillus keratitis in association with extended-wear soft contact lens use. Neither of these patients were using topical steroids at the time of infection. The contact lens hygiene in these patients prior to infection is not known.

Management

Because of the retrospective nature of this investigation, patients were treated by various physicians and management was not uniform. This makes it impossible to compare various medical and surgical therapies and the clinical outcome; however, a few general observations are possible.

Two of the twenty-five patients developed endophthalmitis; both were patients that were post penetrating keratoplasty. Of the remaining 9 post-corneal transplant cases, six developed irreversible graft rejection following fungal infection.

In the post-traumatic keratomycosis group final visual acuity, which in three cases involved optical corneal grafting, ranged from 20/25 to 20/60.

In patients with prior ocular surface disease, discussion of visual outcome is less relevant. However, in this group there were no cases of endophthalmitis and all globes were salvaged.

Comments

Fungi are eukaryotic organisms that cause infectious keratitis following organic corneal trauma or opportunistic disease in patients with pre-existing ocular surface compromise. More than 70 genera of fungi have been identified as pathogens in human keratitis, and these pathogens are generally divided into two categories; filamentous fungi (moulds) and yeasts. Filamentous fungi, such as Fusarium, Aspergillus or Penicillium species have been most closely asssociated with corneal infections following organic trauma. Yeasts, of which Candida species are most common, are more often associated with opportunistic infection.

Any discussion of the epidemiology of fungal keratitis must address the geographic location of the source of the data, since both the distribution of the organisms encountered and of the population acquiring the disease varies with climate (1,3,4,8,10,12). Liesegang and Forster found in a Florida population keratomycosis was a disease primarily affecting young males with a history of ocular organic trauma, and that Fusarium was the most commonly encountered pathogen.

In our series we had a subpopulation that parallels this Florida population. Seven of the twenty-five cases occurred after organic trauma. Six of these seven patients were male and their age was statistically significantly lower than the remainder of the population studied. The isolates in this group were again primarily filamentous; only one of the seven was positive for yeast. This difference in the filamentous fungi isolated may reflect differences in fungal ecology based on climate. Liesegang found no significant history of steroid use in his trauma population; similarly there was no history of topical or systemic steroid use in this subpopulation of our series.

In contrast, Thygeson in a northern California population found that Candida species were the most frequent pathogens in fungal keratitis. Although some of Thygeson's patients had a history of organic trauma, a significant proportion had a history of Herpes simplex ocular surface disease and antecedent corticosteroid use (12). We did not find a population of keratomycosis patients with a history of Herpes simplex keratitis. Our subgroups of patients with prior ocular surface disease and prior penetrating keratoplasty, however, share some characteristics with Thygesons's population in that these patients frequently had large areas of exposed corneal stroma and Candida species were the most frequent isolates. Unlike Thygeson's group, our five patients with ocular surface disease did not have a history of chronic topical corticosteroid use.

Early and late postoperative fungal keratitis in patients following penetrating keratoplasty has been described by other investigators (5,7,9,13). Of those patients who developed keratomycosis following penetrating keratoplasty in this series, all except one used topical corticosteroids and antibiotics at the time of infection. In five of the eleven post-keratoplasty patients, the infiltrate was associated with a suture-related breach in the epithelium.

These findings suggest that while chronic corticosteroid and or antibiotic use are not significant risk factors in patients with trauma, they may be risk factors associated with fungal keratitis, mainly Candida, in the post-keratoplasty period (12,14). It is of note that the one keratoplasty patient who developed keratomycosis and did not use topical corticosteroids had Fusarium keratitis subsequent to Fusarium dacryocystitis.

The smallest group were two patients with contact lens related fungal keratitis. Similarly, in all published series of keratomycosis or of contact lens related infection, this is an infrequent category (2,11). In both cases the patients wore soft contact lenses and in both cases the isolate was Penicillium species.

The series presented in this publication documents the pattern of fungal keratitis in a New England based referral center. In this region of the United States, Candida species are the most frequent, followed by the filamentous fungi, Aspergillus and Penicillium. There were four groups of patients at risk for disease: post penetrating keratoplasty, post organic trauma, preexisting ocular surface disease and extended wear soft contact lens use.

Table 1. Pathogens in Keratomycosis

Candida albicans		6
Candida parapsilosis		4
Candida tropicalis	2	
Aspergillus		5
Penicillium		3
Fusarium	2	
Chrysosporium		1
P. boydii	1	
Wangiella		1
TOTAL		25

Table 2. Predisposing History for Keratomycosis

Post penetrating keratoplasty	11	
Post organic trauma		7
Prior ocular surface disease	5	
Extended wear contact lens use		2
TOTAL		25

Table 3 Age in Keratomycosis Patients

Average of series (years)		53.7
Post penetrating keratoplasty	64.3	
Post trauma		33.9
Ocular surface		51.0
Contact lens		71.0

TABLE 4

	Age/Sex	Organism	Mecical Therapy Topical	Surgical Therapy	Ocular Hx	Theraputic Outcome
OCULAR SURFACE DISEASE						
1)	60/M/OS	Candida albicans	Natamycin	none	exposure heratitis	death not related to ocular disease
2)	42/M/OS	Wangiella	Natamycin Miconazole	PK at 7 weeks	S/P retinal detach x3	no graft recurrence
3)	66/M/OS	Pseudoaller-echeria boydii	Amphotercin B 5-Flucytosine	none	S/P retinal detach xl	CF acuity
4)	65/F/OD	Aspergillus	Natamycin Miconazole	none	proliferative diabetic retinopathy	lost to follow/up
5)	22/M/OS albicans	Candida	Natamycin	none	Stevens-Johnson syndrome	PED-L.P. acuity
EXTENDED WEAR CONTACT LENS						
6)	82/M/OD	Penicillium	Amphotericin B (topical + IV)	cyanoacrylate glue	aphakic EWSCL	N/A
7)	60/F/OS	Penicillum	Miconazole Natamycin Ketoconazole	thermal cautery	aphakic EWSCL	20/200
OCULAR TRAUMA						
8)	31/M/OD	Aspergillus	Amphotericin B Ketoconazole (p.o.)	PK at 5 weeks	landscaper-organic trauma	20/50-no graft recurrence
9)	40/M/OS	Chrysosporium	None	PK at 5 days	farmer-organic trauma	20/70
10)	57/M/OD	Aspergillus	Amphotericin B	none	sanitation worker-organic trauma	20/30+
11)	18/F/OS	Aspergillus	Amphotericin B (topical + IV) Miconazole	PK at 8 weeks limbal cryo	organic trauma at the beach	20/40
12)	18/M/OD	Candida tropicalis	Amphotericin B	none	auto accident	20/40
13)	54/M/OD	Fusarium	Amphotericin B 5-Flucytosine	PK at 3 days	sanitation worker	20/40
14)	19/M/OS	Penicillium	Miconazole Ketoconazole (p.o.)	none	auto accident	lost to follow up
POST PENETRATING KERATOPLASTY						
15)	71/F/OS	Fusarium	Natamycin	PK at 4 days	S/P PK 14 mo not suture related	phthisical
16)	62/M/os	Candida parapsilosis	Amphotericin B	none	S/P PK 19 mo. not suture related	irreversible graft rejection
17)	76/M/OD	Candida	Amphotericin B	PK at 1 wk	S/P PK 5 mo	lost to followup
18)	18/M/OS	Aspergillus	None	at one day	PK/ant vit	enucleation for fungal endophthalmtis
19)	80/F/OD	Candida albicans	Miconazole Flucytosine	none	S/P PK 2 mo	LP 20/fungal endophthalmitis
20)	71/F/OS	Candida parapsilosis	Miconazole Flucytosine	none	S/P PK 13 mo	graft rejection
21)	78/F/OS	Candida albicans	none	PK at 1 day	S/P PK 8 mo	20/70
22)	66/F/OD	Candida tropicalis	Amphoterican B Flucytosine	none	S/P PK 5 mo	20/70
23)	80/F/OS	Candida albicans	Amphotericin B	none	S/P PK 10 days	20/70
24)	67/F/OD	Candida parapsilosis	Miconazole	none	S/P PK 35 mo	HM
25)	39/M/OD	Candida parapsilosis	Miconazole Flucytosine	none	S/P PK 17 mo	lost to follow-up

References

1. Asbell P, Stenson S (1982) Ulcerative Keratitis: Survey of 30 Years Laboratory Experience. Arch Ophthalmol 100:77
2. Berger RO, Streeten BW (1981) Fungal Growth in Aphakic Soft Contact Lenses. Am J Ophthalmol 91:630-633
3. Chin GN, Hyndiuk RA, Kwasny GP et al (1975) Keratomycosis in Wisconsin. Am J Ophthalmol 79:121-126
4. Doughman DJ, Leavenworth NM, Campbell RC et al (1982) Fungal Keratitis at the University of Minnesota: 1971-1981. Trans Am Ophthalmol Soc 80:235-247
5. Fong L, Gladstone D, Casey TA (1988) Corneo-Scleral Rim Cultures: Donor Contamination - A Case of Fungal Endophthalmitis Transmitted by K-Sol Stored Cornea. Eye 2:670-676
6. Foster CS (1981) Miconazole Therapy for Keratomycosis. Am J Ophthalmol 91:622-629
7. Harris DJ, Stulting RD, Waring GO et al (1988) Late Bacterial and Fungal Keratitis After Corneal Transplantation: Spectrum of Pathogens, Graft Survival, and Visual Prognosis. Ophthalmology 95:1450-1457
8. Jones DB, Sexton R, Rebell G (1969) Mycotic Keratitis in South Florida: A Review of Thirty-Nine Cases. Tr Ophth Soc UK 89:781
9. Leavenson JE, Duffin RM, Gardner SK et al (1984) Dematiaceous Fungal Keratitis Following Penetrating Keratoplasty. Ophthalmic Surg 15:578-582
10. Liesegang TJ, Forster RK (1980) Spectrum of Microbial Keratitis in South Florida. Am J Ophthalmol 90:38-47
11. Palmer E, Ferry A, Safir A (1975) Fungal Invasion of a Soft Contact Lens. Arch Ophthalmol 93:27
12. Thygeson P, Okumoto M (1974) Keratomycosis: A Preventable Disease. Tr Am Acad Ophthalmol Otolaryngol 78:433-439
13. 13.Weiss JL, Parker WT (1987) Candida albicans Endophthalmitis Following Penetrating Keratoplasty. Arch Ophthalmol 105:173
14. 14.Williamson J et al (1968) Fungal Flora of the Conjunctival Sac in Health and Disease. Influence of Topical and Systemic Steroids. Br J Ophthalmol 52:127

Antifungal Sensitivity Testing of Keratitis Isolates at Moorfields Eye Hospital 1975-1990: Therapeutic Implications

Michael F.P. Griffiths, Yvonne M.Clayton, John K.G. Dart

Abstract. Fungal keratitis is rare in the United Kingdom and may be difficult to manage. Isolation and antimicrobial sensitivity testing takes several days. First line treatment must therefore be based on the expected antimicrobial sensitivity of common fungal pathogens; these may differ from region to region.

We present sensitivity data from 31 consecutive cases seen at Moorfields Eye Hospital between 1975 and 1990. Most (15/31) were Candida sp.; Aspergillus sp. being the next largest group (6/31). Fusarium sp. were isolated in only 4 cases. Nutrient solutions were sterilised by membrane filtration. 2ml aliquots were placed in 11 tubes and serial dilutions of drugs from 50.0mg/l to 0.10mg/l or 64.0mg/l to 0.125mg/l added. One tube without drug was used as a control. The tubes were inoculated with the fungus and incubated at 37°C for 48 hours for yeasts and Aspergillus or at 26°C for 5 days for filamentous fungi. The minimum inhibitory concentration is the lowest concentration of drug in which there is no visible growth after incubation.

From our sensitivity data, Econazole (as a 1% topical suspension) is the best first line treatment for all cases of fungal keratitis.

Introduction

Fungal keratitis is rare in the United Kingdom and may be difficult to manage. Isolation and antimicrobial sensitivity testing takes several days. First-line treatment must therefore be based on the expected antimicrobial sensitivity of common fungal pathogens; these may differ from region to region.

Other authors have made various recommendations as to first-line treatment, but the case selection (occupational and geographic) should be born in mind when seeking to extrapolate ((1), Tab.1).

As part of a reappraisal of our clinical management of fungal keratitis we reviewed sensitivity data from 31 consecutive cases seen at Moorfields between 1975 and 1990. The most common isolate was candida sp. (15/31), aspergillus sp. being the next largest group (6/31). Fusarium sp. were isolated in only four cases.

Aliquots of fungal isolate in nutrient medium were added to serial dilutions of antifungal agent and the minimum inhibitory concentration established.

Our sensitivity data shows Econazole to be the best agent overall in that it does not have a "therapeutic gap" in its spectrum of activity against any of the fungi cultured in this series (Fig.1). We are now using this agent (as a 1% topical suspension in Arachis oil) routinely as our first line treatment for all cases of fungal keratitis.

Materials and Methods

Sensitivity to antifungal agents was carried out using Sabouraud's dextrose broth for filamentous fungi. For yeast, when Flucytosine or Fluconazole were tested, a yeast nitrogen base medium was used.

The solution was sterilised by membrane filtration and provided a 10x concentrate which was diluted 1:10 in sterile distilled water (11). 2ml volumes of media were dispensed into 11 tubes. Two-fold serial dilutions of drug ranging from 50 to 0.10mg/l or 64 to 0.125mg/l were made in 10 tubes. One tube without drug was used as control. Tubes containing diluted drug were inoculated with $1x10^3$ cells/ml for yeasts or $5x10^3$ viable units/ml (or 1:100 dilution for 48 h broth culture homogenised by shaking with glass beads) for filamentous fungi. Yeasts and aspergilli were incubated at 37°C for 48 h, other filamentous fungi at 26°C for five days.

Minimal Inhibitory Concentration is defined as the lowest concentration of drug in which no visible growth is observed after incubation.

Results

The results of sensitivity testing are summarised in Fig.1. It would seem that Econazole has good activity against candida, aspergillus and fusarium (the most common fungal pathogens), as well as against less common fungi, which nonetheless made up a sizable proportion of our series (Tab.2). It is at least as active against Fusarium as Natamycin and better than Amphotericin B, Natamycin or Ketocconazole for aspergillus. It does not seem to have a "therapeutic gap" in its spectrum of activity and overall, would appear to be the best choice as first-line, single agent, "blind" antifungal (Tab.3).

Discussion

Making the diagnosis of fungal keratitis is difficult. There is often an indolent course and long history complicated by prior treatment with topical corticosteroids. Fusarium however, can be rapidly progressive.

Geographical location and some aspects of the history such as previous ocular surface disease or injury sustained while gardening or outdoors may be helpful not only in raising the question of fungal keratitis but also in suggesting an organism. Fusarium is more common in tropical and subtropical regions, Candida more common in eyes with preexisting ocular surface disease, and filamentous fungi (for example Aspergillus) would be more likely pathogens in an agricultural or gardening injury.

A culture result can be obtained in 48-72 hours. Sensitivity testing however, takes about one week. It is usually necessary therefore to make a clinical judgement of the most likely fungus and start "blind" treatment with an antifungal. Response to treatment is slow and can lead to multiple changes in therapy.

We reviewed all cases of fungal keratitis at Moorfields over a fifteen year period in order to establish which antifungal agents were most effective. Against the panel of agents tested, Econazole emerged as the most effective overall. There are such differences in antifungal sensitivity even within species that we feel sensitivity testing has an important part to play in the management of fungal keratitis.

As our present choice of first-line agent, we therefore use Econazole as a 1% solution in Arachis oil administered hourly (day and night) for three days, then hourly (day only) for two days and thereafter as clinically indicated. Our initial clinical impression is that it is well tolerated and of low toxicity.

Table 1.

Recommended Agent	Reference
Miconazole	2, 10
Miconazole and Ketoconazole	1
Natamycin	3,4,6,7,12
Natamycin and Amphotericin B	9
Econazole	8

Candida sp	45% [14/31]
Candida albicans	29% [9/31]
Aspergillus sp	19% [6/31]
Fusarium solani	13% [4/3
Others[1]	23% [7/31]

[1] Cladosporium cladosporiodes
Pseudoallescheria boydii (2)
Paecilomyces lilacinus
Sphaeropsos subglobosa
Trichosporon beigelii
Alternaria sp

Table 3. Antifungals According to Sensitivity Testing

	First or First=	MIC>2
Itraconazole	57% [8/14]	21% [3/14][1]
Econazole	48% [15/31]	19% [6/31]
Flucytosine	45% [10/22]	41% [9/22][1]
Clotrimazole	35% [11/31]	39% [12/31]
Miconazole	35% [11/31]	42% [13/31]
Amphotericin B	32% [10/31	39% [12/31]
Ketoconazole	25% [6/24]	50% [12/24][1]
Natamycin	4% [1/24]	83% [20/24][1]
Fluconazole	0% [0/7]	43% [3/7][1]
Nystatine	0% [0/6]	100% [6/6][1]

1Not tested against all fungi

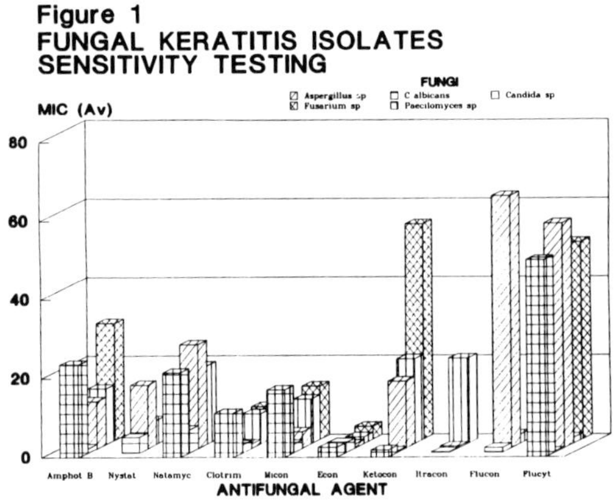

Fig. 1: Fungal keratitis isolates sensitivity testing

References

1. Fitzsimmons R, Peters AL (1986) Miconazole and Ketoconazole as a Satisfactory First-Line Treatment for Keratomycosis. Am J Ophthalmol 101:605-608
2. Forster CS (1981) Miconazole Therapy for Keratomycosis. Am J Ophthalmol 91:622-629
3. Forster RK, Rebell G (1975) Therapeutic Surgery in Failures of Medical Treatment for Fungal Keratitis. Br J Ophthalmol 59:366-371
4. Forster RK, Rebell G (1975) The Diagnosis and Management of Keratomycoses. Arch Ophthalmol 93:975-978
5. Jones DB, Wilson L, Sexton R and al (1969) Early Diagnosis of Mycotic Keratitis. Trans Ophthalmol Soc UK 89:805-813
6. Jones BR (1975) Principles in the Management of Oculomycosis. Am J Ophthalmol 79:719-751
7. Jones DB (1981) Decision-Making in the Management of Microbial Keratitis. Ophthalmology 88:814-820
8. Jones BR, Clayton YM, Oji EO (1979) Recognition and Chemotherapy of Oculomycosis. Postgrad Med J 55:625-628
9. O'Day DM (1987) Selection of Appropriate Antifungal Therapy. Cornea 6:238-245
10. Pettit TH, Ehrlich M (1990) Fungal Keratitis. In: Fraunfelder FT, Roy FH (eds) Current Ocular Therapy. Saunders, Philadelphia, pp.445-448
11. Shadomy S (1969) In Vitro Studies with 5-Fluocytosine. Applied Microbiology 17: 871-877

- Viral Infections

Management of Herpetic Keratitis

Herbert E. Kaufman

Abstract. Oral acyclovir may be especially useful in children and the disabled. Its role in stromal disease and iritis is now being studied in a National Institutes of Health (NIH)-sponsored national study. New drugs that specifically inhibit viral thymidine kinase have no effect on the multiplication of virus but will probably prevent recurrences of viral infection. Studies in monkeys indicate that recurrences are suppressed even by drugs that are not ideal. The use of both corticosteroids and antiviral agents has dramatically improved the prognosis of keratoplasty after herpes, but since herpes latency is so common in man, the use of steroids after keratoplasty may reactivate otherwise unexpected herpes, producing disease that is difficult to diagnose.

Introduction

Herpes simplex keratitis is the most common corneal infection in the United States. The virus is ubiquitous; more than 90% of adults are likely infected with herpes simplex virus type 1 (HSV-1), which remains latent in the trigeminal ganglia after the primary infection. The virus reactivates from the ganglia in response to a number of triggers, including stress, temperature, fever, neural sectioning and probably a host of other so far unidentified signals. The reactivated virus travels from the ganglia, where it has been quiescent, to the end organ, in this case the cornea, where it multiplies and causes a variety of herpetic syndromes which require different approaches to treatment.

Dendritic Keratitis

Dendritic keratitis is caused by virus multiplying rapidly in the corneal epithelial cells. The characteristic branching "dendritic" lesions result when the virus overload destroys the infected cells, spilling the virus into the nearby cells, where the process is repeated. If the ulcer remains untreated, the branches coalesce, forming a map-shaped or "geographic" ulcer. The treatment for dendritic keratitis is a topically applied antiviral that interferes selectively with replication of the virus without killing the uninfected corneal epithelial cells with which it comes in contact.

In the United States, the drug of choice for epithelial herpes infection is trifluridine (trifluorothymidine). In the earliest clinical trials, 97% of patients with dendritic keratitis were healed within 2 weeks using trifluridine (11). Trifluridine is also used in patients with geographic ulcers, but healing requires more time. Older antivirals, including idoxuridine and vidarabine, are less effective, but are still used in cases where trifluridine is unsatisfactory, such as allergic reactions or virus resistance.

Topical acyclovir has been found to be equally effective for dendritic keratitis, and the toxicities of acyclovir and trifluridine are similar. However, the development of acyclovir-resistant virus is relatively easy; therefore, the widespread use of topical acyclovir is considered to carry an unacceptable risk of creating a pool of resistant virus that could jeopardize the treatment of patients requiring systemic treatment and the ointment is only available in the United States on a compassionate need program. Orally administered acyclovir is shed in the tears, however, and can be used to treat patients for whom the frequent application of topical drugs presents a problem, including children and disabled adults.

Disciform Keratitis

A later phase of herpetic corneal infection involves corneal swelling and clouding, with loss of vision and pain, which often lasts for months, and frequently results in scarring and vascularization. The area of clouding assumes a round or ovoid shape, hence the name disciform edema or disciform keratitis. This condition is not caused by multiplying virus and cannot be treated successfully with topical antivirals alone.

Disciform keratitis is considered to be a hypersensitivity reaction to the virus and its products (probably one or more glycoproteins); the symptoms of pain and inflammation can be treated with topical corticosteroids. However, the steroids create an environment in which epithelial herpes can undergo massive recrudescence. Thus, effective treatment for disciform keratitis requires both corticosteroids to suppress the inflammatory disease and a topical antiviral, such as trifluridine, to prevent the resurgence of surface herpetic disease. The two drugs must be given in relatively large doses on the same dosage schedule, usually for a period of about three months. By that time, the disciform disease has generally resolved and both drugs can be tapered with little risk of epithelial recurrence.

For the same reasons that topical acyclovir is not used for dendritic keratitis, it is not used in combination with steroids for the treatment of disciform keratitis. Here, even longer term use is required and the risk of resistant virus would be greatly enhanced. A multicenter controled study sponsored by the National Eye Institute is underway in the United States to determine whether oral acyclovir is beneficial to patients with stromal keratitis or iritis, but to date the results have not been published.

Necrotizing Keratitis

Ultimately, a few herpes patients develop white necrotic lesions in the corneal stroma, characterized by a combination of the hypersensitivity reaction typical of disciform keratitis and the presence of multiplying virus. The virus, however, is located deep in the stroma and the rate of virus multiplication appears to be very slow. For these reasons, topical antiviral treatment is largely ineffective and the benefits of oral acyclovir are uncertain. However, the combination of a topical antiviral and corticosteroids can be used to treat the hypersensitivity component, and some patients respond successfully although a therapeutic result is not a certainty.

Metaherpetic Keratitis - Post-Infectious Ulcers

Another aspect of the post-herpetic syndrome is a chronic, recurrent ulceration that was originally thought to be a result of ongoing virus multiplication but was refractory to topical antiviral therapy. Often these ulcers were treated with a succession of antivirals in the hope of finding one that worked. In fact, however, this condition, called metaherpetic keratitis, occurs after the multiplying virus is eradicated from the corneal epithelium. It is believed to be the result of a damaged basement membrane to which the healing epithelium is unable to form a permanent attachment (6). When the epithelium migrates and spreads to cover the areas denuded by the herpes infection, new hemidesmosomes must form to anchor the basal cells to Descemet's membrane. If the basement membrane/stromal surface has been severely damaged by the previous infection, these attachment complexes do not form successfully and the epithelium is repeatedly wiped off the corneal surface by the action of the lids. The application of topical antivirals, which provide some irritation, only adds to the toxicity.

Metaherpetic keratitis is treated wih preventative measures, including ointments, a patch, and/or a bandage soft contact lens, to reduce friction between the eyelids and the epithelium.

Strain Specificity of Herpes Simplex Virus and Disease

Characteristics

Clinically, some infections are far more virulent than others. Some cases of epithelial herpes resolve with treatment and some patients suffer recurrences more often than others. Only some develop disciform or necrotizing keratitis. Additionally, treatment is more effective in some patients.

We were among the first to show that virulence is a property of the genome encoding the HSV-1 strain and that differences in the infecting strain can account for a number of the characteristics of the resulting ocular disease (1-4,9,10). We found that the shape of the dendritic ulcer was determined at a specific locus on the HSV genome, relatively independently of virulence and host factors, and that epithelial disease and stromal disease segregate separately on the viral genome.

We also found that, for a given individual, the primary infecting virus strain colonizes the ganglia essentially for life. Additionally, the colonizing strain prevents superinfection, even with a more virulent strain. Thus, the genome of the initial infecting strain determines to a great extent the character of the disease that an individual will experience, from mild or even nonexistent lesions perhaps once in a lifetime to recurrent and/or potentially blinding stromal invasion.

Other studies have shown that virus multiplication may occur at different rates in different tissues, with factors such as temperature resulting in slowed rates of replication and hence, a reduced opportunity for effective antiviral drug activity. This idea is interesting and may have bearing on the problems of treating stromal disease, but the investigation of this phenomenon is early and incomplete.

Recurrent Ocular Herpes and the Future of Antiviral Research

From my initial discovery of idoxuridine as the first effective antiviral (5) and the elucidation of the various forms of ocular herpetic disease and their appropriate treatment regimens, as described previously (7), to today's improved understanding of the molecular mechanisms of drug activity, the development of effective chemotherapy for ocular herpes has so far spanned approximately 30 years. During this time, several useful antiviral drugs have become available. However, despite our increased knowledge of basic mechanisms and considerable investment in basic and clinical research, we still have no means of preventing recurrent ocular disease and the blinding consequences thereof.

Although oral acyclovir has been shown to prevent recurrences of genital and skin herpes, it probably does not prevent recurrent ocular herpes. It may be that the amount of reactivated virus reaching the end organ from the sacral ganglia is small, so that considerable viral multiplication is needed to cause genital lesions. In this situation, acyclovir is effective because it prevents viral multiplication at the end organ. In the eye, however, the virus arriving from the trigeminal ganglia may be sufficient to produce a corneal epithelial lesion, so there is little local replication and chronic oral administration of acyclovir cannot prevent the development of new disease.

We are studying a new class of compounds that may be more useful for preventing recurrences. These compounds selectively inhibit viral thymidine kinase, which is essential for virus replication. Since there is little or no thymidine kinase in the central nervous system, the virus cannot replace the inhibited viral enzyme with cellular enzyme from the ganglionic cells, and thus cannot replicate and travel to the end organ to cause disease. In preliminary studies, one of these compounds (5'-ethynylthymidine) appears to reduce the risk of recurrences in the eye of primates previously infected and subject to spontaneous recurrences (8). Other compounds with a similar mechanism of action are under study.

Acknowledgements

This work was supported in part by US Public Health Service grant EY02672 from the National Eye Institute, National Institutes of Health, Bethesda, Maryland.

References

1. Centifanto-Fitzgerald YM, Kaufman HE (1981) Herpes Simplex Virus Strain Specificity and Ocular Disease. In: Sundmacher,R (ed) Herpetische Augenerkrankungen. Bergmann.Verlag, Munich, pp.19-24,
2. Centifanto-Fitzgerald YM, Fenger T, Kaufman HE (1982) Virus Proteins in Herpetic Keratitis. Exp Eye Res 35:425-441
3. Centifanto-Fitzgerald YM, Varnell ED, Kaufman HE (1982) Initial Herpes Simplex Virus Type 1 Infection Prevents Ganglionic Superinfection by Other Strains. Infect Immun 35:1125-1132
4. Centifanto-Fitzgerald YM, Yamaguchi T, Kaufman HE et al (1982) Ocular Disease Pattern Induced by Herpes Simplex Virus is Genetically Determined by a Specific Region of Viral DNA. J Exp Med 155:475-489
5. Kaufman HE (1962) Clinical Cure of Herpes Simplex Keratitis by 5-iodo-2'-deoxyuridine. Proc Soc Exp Biol Med 109:251-252
6. Kaufman HE (1964) Epithelial Erosion Syndrome: Metaherpetic Keratitis. Am J Ophthalmol 57:983-987
7. Kaufman HE, Martola EL, Dohlman CH (1962) The Use of 5-iodo-2'-deoxyuridine (IDU) in the Treatment of Herpes Simplex Keratitis. Arch Ophthalmol 68:235-2398.

   Kaufman HE, Varnell ED, Cheng YC et al (1991) Suppression of Ocular Herpes Recurrences by a Thymidine Kinase Inhibitor in Squirrel Monkeys. Antiviral Res 16:227-232
9. Smeraglia R, Hochadel J, Varnell ED et al (1982) The Role of Herpes Simplex Virus Secreted Glycoproteins in Herpetic Keratitis. Exp Eye Res 35:443-459
10. Wander AH, Centifanto-Fitzgerald YM, Kaufman HE (1980) Strain Specificity of Clinical Isolates of Herpes Simplex Virus. Arch Ophthalmol 98:1458-1461
11. Wellings PC, Awdrey PN, Bors FH et al (1972) Clinical Evaluation of Trifluorothymidine in the Treatment of Herpes Simplex Corneal Ulcers. Am J Ophthalmol 73:932-942

Management of Herpes Simplex Virus Disease in the Anterior Segment of the Eye

Rainer Sundmacher

Abstract. Due to a better pathologic understanding of herpes simplex virus ocular disease, and due to major medical (acyclovir, interferon) and surgical advances (keratoplasty, intraocular lenses), most clinical situations in herpes patients can nowadays be treated very sufficiently.
The clinician has to distinguish true viral disease from metaherpetic (nonviral, postherpetic) and pseudoherpetic disease. True viral disease must be separated into superficial (epithelial) forms, in which immunology plays a positive part and in which corticosteroids are strictly prohibited, and in deep forms, in which immunology plays a dubious, mostly deteriorating part. Superficial forms must be treated with antivirals (plus interferon) only. These types of therapy have been developed on the basis of multiple well-controlled clinical studies. Deep forms must be treated with a combination of acyclovir plus corticosteroids. Based on uncontrolled clinical experience, it is inefficient or dangerous to treat these forms with either acyclovir or corticosteroids alone.
Different regimens for antiviral-corticosteroid combinations are currently evaluated in prospective studies in the USA. All intraocular types of herpes simplex virus disease are most efficiently treated by a combination of high-dosed systemically administered acyclovir plus moderately dosed corticosteroids. This is especially true for all cases with secondary glaucoma (trabe-culitis).
Systemic acyclovir is also the most efficient prophylactic and therapeutic measure for eliminating the virus-related problems with herpes keratoplasty, and its availability even allows for relatively safe implantation of intraocular lenses in herpes eyes, which had been impossible in the pre-acyclovir era.

Introduction

Management of Herpes simplex virus keratitis has considerably changed and improved during the past 15 years. Our group has contributed to some of the therapeutic progress. Even the more we have continously been working on improving the diagnostic criteria and practical guidelines for a successful medical and surgical therapy. These guidelines have been presented many times in courses at the yearly Convention of German Ophthalmologists in Essen.

Whilst many of the different pathophysiological and practical aspects have been published in scattered papers - mostly in the German literature - no update review of my experiences and teaching has ever been written. It has been in the intention of the organizer of this symposium to make me deliver such a personal review. Herb Kaufman will elaborate on his experiences and philosophies. I will try the same for my personal experiences and philosophies. I will do so in a very simple and simplified manner in an attempt to give a pathophysiological, diagnostic and therapeutic framework but also to give at hand some kind of a cook book with short paragraphs for every day's herpes problems.

Such kind of presentation would neither benefit from vast citations from the literature nor from balanced discussions of the various disputable problems. As I was asked to make my personal points clear, I rather restrict myself to some citations from our own work - and beg the international research community's pardon for that!

This is my personal "credo". With "credos" everybody understands that it means we do not know for sure and errors are likely to be included. To stimulate critical reading and discussion I would dare to expose myself and predict that no big errors are contained in this presentation. The great lines will hold true. Details, of course, are always apt to modifications, which have served and will further serve for practical progress in the herpes field.

1. Available Therapy

The available therapy is mostly the same in the USA and in Germany. However, one difference exists (Tab.1):
Topical antiviral therapy in the USA is restricted to only trifluorothymidine (TFT) eye drops, whereas in Germany we can take additional advantage of acyclovir ointment and interferon eye drops. All three drugs are useful and needed. None serves optimally in all situations. Rather, one should exploit their advantages and avoid their disadvantages (Tab.2) in different therapeutic situations (see below). Whatever the reasons may have been for no interest in and nonapproval of acyclovir ointment and interferon eye drops in the USA, it cannot have been lack of proven action. Both drugs have been tested in a multitude of well controlled clinical studies outside the USA and have unanimously been found active and virtually free from side-effects. Thus, from the German point of view I must say that withholding acyclovir ointment and interferon eye drops from the US ophthalmologists means to burden them with a therapeutic handicap, which they certainly do not deserve.

2. Clinical Classification and Basic Principles of Therapy

Successful management must be based on safe pathophysiological grounds. To serve this purpose we have suggested a simplified diagnostic classification of herpes simplex virus anterior segment ocular diseases which we evolved from our clinico-virologic correlation studies (11, Fig.1). First, a decisive distinction has to be made between true viral disease and metaherpetic disease. True viral disease goes along with replicating herpes simplex virus in the different tissues and cell layers of the anterior segment or the lids (Fig.1, no. 1-10, left side of the scheme). Viral disease, of course, calls primarily for antiviral therapy. Metaherpetic diseases (Fig.1, no. 11-14, right side of the scheme) are secondary to viral diseases, viral replication plays no role in their ongoing pathophysiology (7), and consequently antiviral therapy is of no use for metaherpetic diseases.

This vertical separation line in the scheme must be supplemented by a horizontal separation line, which is especially meaningful and necessary for viral diseases (Fig.1, no. 5-10, group II). Making this distinction is extremely important because of the different role that immunology plays in these two groups of viral diseases. In superficial viral diseases immunity is very helpful. The more potent immunity reacts the quicker healing is achieved without notable side effects. Ideally the epithelial defects are quickly filled in by invading healthy cells with full functional restitution. Thus, superficial herpes simplex virus diseases must be vigorously treated with antivirals, they benefit from stimulating immunity, and corticosteroids are to be avoided.

Things are much more complicated and different with deep herpetic diseases. If we would treat deep diseases like superficial ones we would again achieve healing somewhen, but we would loose a considerable percentage or all of function by immunologic destruction. What we see in terms of infiltration or what we realize as secondary sequelae (e.g. acute secondary glaucoma) is mostly brought about by immunologic reactions to cells harbouring herpes simplex virus and expressing herpes simplex virus antigens on their surface. Viral replication and viral cytolysis play only a minor quantitive part in the destruction of cells and tissues that are vital for the eye. Most of the destructions are brought about by immune reactions to antigen expressing cells. Consequently, with deep viral diseases - as with superficial ones - basic therapy has to consist of an effective antiviral therapy. However, this antiviral therapy must be combined and supplemented by an intelligently adjusted corticosteroid therapy. Treating deep viral diseases with an antiviral monotherapy means slow healing and great functional losses. Treating deep viral diseases with a corticosteroid monotherapy - as was still done a decade ago - often meant quicker healing and preservation of a good deal of function in many cases but a considerable risk of herpes simplex virus reactivation and herpes simplex virus persistence in also many cases. Combining both drugs intelligently is the solution of the problem. Unfortunately, no data from controlled studies are up to now available which would help us making the required intelligent decisions. I am confident that the results of a large collaborative study, which is just underway in the USA, will bring us a good step forward on safer grounds.

In table three a summary is offered of the basic principles to treat the four classes of herpetic eye diseases (Fig.1).

Although it is common sense, I would like to stress at this point that "schemes" and "principles" are only tools to simplify a very complex world and make life easier. In clinical practice we often do not deal with just one defined clinical entity but with a continously varying mixture of entities. This calls for detailed analysis, compromises in the therapeutic regime and frequent reevaluations and readjustments of therapy (Tab.4).

I also regret that - on the pages allowed here - I cannot elaborate in detail on our practical diagnostic criteria for diagnosis of the different herpes simplex virus diseases. One or the other item that may be of central interest will be shortly touched in subsequent paragraphs dealing with special therapeutic questions.

3. Treatment of Superficial (Epithelial) Viral Disease

Before coming to the typical corneal epithelial herpes simplex virus disease, i.e. dendritic keratitis (Fig.1, no. 4), I would shortly mention that in herpes simplex virus blepharitis (Fig.1, no. 1) and intermarginal blepharitis (Fig.1, no. 2) topical therapy has no significant effect. If at all, therapy of blepharitis has to be by systemic acyclovir. But this means mostly overdoing it, because - except for the primary variant of blepharitis and except for blepharitis in atopic patients - spontaneous healing in blepharitis is quick and without sequelae. Limbitis (Fig.1, no. 3) is a very special event which is only seen in some cases of primary infection. It calls for systemic acyclovir therapy, which I recommend for all kinds of primary infection.

Dendritic keratitis and its variants (stellate, geographic keratitis) nearly always represent endogenously recurrent herpes simplex virus disease. This is also true for the great majority of first clinical attacks. The antecedent primary infection, which is mostly atypical or subclinical, normally escapes our notion.

Dendritic keratitis must primarily be treated with a synthetic antiviral. Both available antivirals, trifluorothymidine and acyclovir, given as a monotherapy lead to healing in about six days with some cases taking protracted courses up to two weeks. In so far they are about equal in spite of their differing molecular action. This difference could therapeutically offer a chance for a better antiviral action by combining both antivirals. However, I know of no controlled study showing that such a combination would have increased the velocity and quality of healing.

On the other hand, it has been shown many times in well controlled clinical studies that a combination of either trifluorothymidine or acyclovir with interferon eye drops accelerates healing considerably to about three days. Even more important, it eliminates virtually all prolonged courses (4,5,15,18). Thus the optimal therapy of dendritic keratitis is a fully dosed topical antiviral plus one drop of a sufficiently high-titered interferon per day. The interferon can be stopped as soon as the epithelium has closed, whereas the synthetic antiviral should be given some days longer. The basis for this somehow intriguing interferon action has remained widely obscure. An antiviral acitivity of interferon, which should already work at much lower doses, does not sufficiently explain its action in this combination therapy. An immunomodulating effect, i.e. triggering of immune and nonimmune defence mechanisms, may explain a good deal more. However, I suspect that there may be still other unknown activities of interferon in this special situation.

We still prefer trifluorothymidine as first choice drug in the combination with interferon because of its broad antiviral activity, lack of viral resistance and good patient's compliance (Tab.2). If deep viral disease is primarily coexistent or develops in the course of superficial viral disease, we prefer acyclovir instead of trifluorothymidine because of better penetration of acyclovir into the corneal stroma and into the anterior chamber of the eye. Acyclovir is also preferred with primarily coexisting or developing epithelial healing disorders because of its lesser potential for epithelial toxicity. For the same reason acyclovir is recommended instead of trifluorothymidine in all cases where a safe differential diagnosis between viral and metaherpetic disease cannot be made (see paragraph 5).

Debridement has widely come out of use, not because it is bad, but mostly because it is thought to annoy patients and it takes time, two reasons for a busy modern doctor to forget about it. But it still has a definite place in treatment of dendritic keratitis, especially in uncooperative children and mentally deficient adults whom one cannot treat topically several times a day. Debridement is done in short general anesthesia. Afterwards, it is tried to give acyclovir ointment as often as possible. If post-debridement therapy can be done only once a day, interferon eye drops are a very good solution to the problem (6). If no topical therapy at all can be exerted, one should know that systemic acyclovir is also active in dendritic keratitis. Some of these adults may accept tablets. Normal patients also benefit from "minimal wiping debridement" prior to subsequent topical antiviral therapy, especially with acyclovir ointment. This is common practice in Britain.

4. Treatment of Deep Viral Disease

Deep viral diseases are the major threat to vision. They destroy the optical clarity of the anterior segment - especially of the cornea - and lead to severe glaucoma. Treatment consists of a combination of antivirals plus corticosteroids as outlined in paragraph two. However, principal agreement on such a regime does not help us very much in selecting the appropriate mixture for the individual case. No randomized controlled clinical studies have been finished that could help us in making a decision. For the time being we must rely on guidelines that we have evolved for our own use on the basis of pathophysiologic understanding and clinical experience with its continuous feed-back. These are my current guidelines for management of deep Herpes simplex virus diseases:

I. The antiviral substances must exert good activity at the deep sites of disease. The only drug approved to date with these characteristics is acyclovir. It should initially be dosed maximally and kept continously at this maximal level throughout therapy as long as more than minor amounts of corticosteroids are needed and added.

II. Corticosteroids must be dosed case-adjusted. To know that dose is the real problem. At the moment it can only be solved by sufficient personal experience. It is mandatory never to give a large dose of corticosteroids. It suffices to apply the minimal dose that is effective in stopping and gradually eliminating destructive reactions. As soon as the corticosteroid effect is notable and immunology calms down, one can start to slowly taper out with the corticosteroids, while acyclovir is still kept on its maximal level until the corticosteroids fall below a "safe" level. What this "safe" corticosteroid level is, nobody knows for sure. We assume it at the moment at 20mg triamcinolone orally per day and at two drops of 1% prednisolone-21-acetate per day.

III. Acyclovir can be administered as an ointment, as tablets, or as an infusion. Corticosteroids can be given topically (preferably as drops), subconjunctivally as a crystalline depot, or as tablets. Which combination fits the therapeutic requirements of a special case best differs from patient to patient and needs frequent reevaluation (Tab.4).

To work out the principles a little better, in Tabl.5-6 examples and proposals are given for three different groups of deep herpes simplex virus disease.

For interstitial herpes simplex virus keratitis and low grade herpes simplex virus endotheliitis (Tab.5) it mostly suffices to combine acyclovir ointment (5 times daily continuously) with topical corticosteroids (initially 3 times daily, reduced to 2 times daily when inflammation has considerably calmed down, not further reducing before all biomicroscopically visible inflammation has gone, than tapering out for some time on 1 drop daily; at this level no further antiviral shield is needed and acyclovir can be withdrawn). If more antiviral activity is wanted one may add 5 times 400mg acyclovir orally, and if more baseline corticosteroid activity is needed, one may inject subconjunctivally a small dose of a crystalline corticosteroid (e.g. 2-mg dexamethasone-21-acetate) and repeat that measure as is judged necessary. Crystalline corticosteroids may have negative side effects, especially may they promote subconjunctival localized scarring. The pros and cons of their application must therefore always be carefully weighed.

Most uncertainty exists as to when one can start to taper corticosteroids, and most mistakes are made in this respect when endotheliitis is treated. Endotheliitis is characterized by endothelial cells harboring replicating herpes simplex virus and expressing herpes simplex virus antigens on their surface. These antigens attract immune cells which attack the endothelial cells and destroy them leading to leaks in the endothelial cell layer with endothelial edema visible with specular microscopy and frank corneal edema visible by the slitlamp biomicroscopy. The endotheliitic immune cells aggregate on the endothelium in a typical strictly edema-associated manner which is totally different from the distribution of iritic precipitates (16). These endotheliitic precipitates serve as a marker for tapering out with the corticosteroids. If they persist - and be it only one or two precipitates! - one has to carry on with a sufficiently high-dosed combination therapy. Only after all precipitates have gone and one or two weeks more have elapsed one can dare to finally taper. If one does not follow this experience, local disease is likely to flare up again. Unfortunately, many patients experience such a relapse-back. Many of them several times. Doctors use to say that a recurrence took place every time they tried to lower the therapeutic dose. That is wrong from the pathophysiological point of view. In such cases we do not deal with neuronally transmitted recurrences. In all probability the ophthalmologist did not treat long and efficiently enough to eradicate viral replication in the cornea. That allowed the establishment of peripheral viral persistence. From this "subclinical" inflammatory resource the flare-up of the disease originates as often as the corticosteroids fall below a critical level and their "masking" action is no longer operative. Knowing about this pathophysiological background and the indicative importance of endotheliitic precipitates helps a good deal not to step into a very common therapeutic trap.

One of the most difficult cases to treat is ulcerative interstitial herpes simplex virus keratitis (Tab.6). If perforation threatens one would anyway consider keratoplasty à chaud. However, if there is no urgent need for keratoplasty it may be preferable first to try to heal the cornea by medical means and thereafter think about keratoplasty. I would primarily use a combination of full-dose acyclovir systemically (5x400mg tablets) and for the corticosteroid part try to get along with subconjunctivally injected small doses of crystalline corticosteroids in order not to compromise the healing epithelium. In addition I would give acyclovir ointment, whilst more corticosteroid activity - if needed - should only be brought about by adding corticosteroids systemically. I would not recommend corticosteroid drops or ointment in this situation.

Finally, we turn to the most dangerous cases in which so much virus is present in the aqueus humor that it can easily be cultivated from it (8,9). These are severe endotheliitis, focal iritis, and trabeculitis (Tab.7). Focal iritis is characterized by focal disease of the iris pigment epithelium with subsequent focal defects, which transilluminate. It is further characterized by relatively large, often pigmented iritic precipitates, and mostly by an associated rise in intraocular pressure (13). This pressure rise is also existent, but to a much more pronounced effect in trabeculitis. If these diseases are diagnosed, either singly or in combination, a vigorous systemic acyclovir therapy must immediately be instituted (5x400-800 mg/d, acyclovir infusion in the most severe cases) and corticosteroids systemically (e.g. 30mg triamcinolone per day). Additional acyclovir and corticosteroid action may be brought about by topical therapy. It has been my experience, however, that systemic therapy is the decisive one. It can be supplemented but not substituted by topical therapy. For most cases systemic therapy is needed for about two weeks duration before one is allowed to start to taper. Some cases may take some weeks more, raising the question whether some kind of relative viral resistance against acyclovir is operative in such patients. However, following consequently the above outlined principles we will finally be successful even in the most difficult cases, i.e. in the cases with trabeculitis and associated severe acute glaucoma (19).

Acute glaucoma in herpes simplex virus patients is a vision-threatening event that calls for immediate therapeutic action. From history - which is only ten years ago - we know that symptomatic antiglaucomatous therapy has rarely been effective without antiviral therapy in such cases. Fortunately enough, the sign of acute glaucoma also tells us what is going on in the eye. It has been found that acute glaucoma is regularly associated with massive intraocular herpes simplex virus replication (9). By knowing this pathophysiologic background and taking the appropriate therapeutic measures, acute glaucoma in herpes simplex virus patients has lost most of its previously ominous signs.

5. Treatment of Superficial (Epithelial) Metaherpetic Healing Disorder

Epithelial metaherpetic healing disorder is a common event. The pathogenesis is complex and not well investigated. Destruction of the "anterior corneal membrane" (basement membrane and Bowman´s), an altered tear film, and a reduced regeneration rate of the corneal epithelium become operative to a varying extent and lead to reduced epithelial stability. These negative influences may further be aggravated by undesired medical side-effects (e.g. by benzalconiumchloride and higher doses of trifluorothymidine over a prolonged period of time). Mostly we deal only with chronic superficial punctate keratopathy. However, some cases may show slowly healing erosions or even progress to persistent or recurrent erosions.

As prophylaxis is always better than therapy, we generally prescribe artificial tears prophylactically together with topical antivirals. If the corneal epithelium looks primarily rather compromised, we prescribe acyclovir ointment instead of trifluorothymidine drops and artificial tears without preservatives. These have become available in single dose packages.

In case of rather prolonged healing or non-healing one should also suspect some persistent low-grade viral activity underneath the zone of epithelial alteration. In such cases we apply only acyclovir ointment for a prolonged period of time. Acyclovir will slowly bring down viral activity, it has no remarkable negative effect on epithelial regeneration, and the ointment base in itself serves to smoothen and shield the vulnerable corneal epithelium.

Some cases of persistent or recurrent metaherpetic erosion call for a therapeutic soft lens therapy. It is mandatory that all viral activity has stopped before a contact lens is fitted. The lens has to move freely, and it has to be rehydrated at hourly or two-hourly intervals with balanced salt solution or saline (preferably without preservatives). This brings about healing in a few days, and the lens can be removed after some more days. Conventional dry eye therapy must be reinstituted after removal of the lens. Recurrence of an epithelial viral keratitis while the soft lens is on the cornea poses a real danger. Such recurrences never express in the typical picture of dendritic keratitis. They present as atypical, enlarging erosions! Thus, if under a well fitted contact lens a preexisting erosion enlarges and inflammatory signs gradually increase, the most likely diagnosis is recurrence of an epithelial viral keratitis. The soft lens must be removed immediately and the keratitis treated as outlined in section three.

6. Treatment of Deep Metaherpetic Disease

Deep metaherpetic diseases comprise a rather heterogenous group of conditions that involve mainly the corneal stroma, the endothelium, and the trabecular meshwork. Viral replication is no longer a matter of concern. We deal with chronic corneal ulcers that heal slowly or not at all (metaherpetic ulcers). We further deal with a chronic loss of corneal endothelium as a consequence of endotheliitis resulting in bullous keratopathy, and finally we deal with chronic secondary glaucoma, which may become a problem after multiple attacks of herpes simplex virus trabeculitis.

With the exception of glaucoma, which should as long as ever possible be treated conservatively, deep metaherpetic disease has become a domaine for rehabilitating surgery (section 7). Only those patients are treated medically who refuse surgery or who are judged to have too little compliance and cannot adequately be controlled after surgery.

The following arguments speak in favor for a early surgery:

- Healing by conservative treatment takes a long time (metaherpetic ulcer) or cannot sufficiently be brought about at all (bullous keratopathy).
- After finally "calming down" the eye by medical means there is still a profound and permanent loss of function and still a constant need for further therapy and control.
- Not rarely such unoperated eyes have become corticosteroid-dependent to an extent of 1-2 drops per day. This may go along with a continuous slow deterioration of an otherwise still relatively clear lens.
- Keratoplasty with or without combined cataract surgery in herpes simplex virus eyes has become extremely successful during the past 5-10 years, provided the ophthalmologist's knowledge and the patient's compliance are good.
- In the medium run the therapeutic efforts of the patient are less worthwhile without surgery, and functional rehabilitation is possible only with surgery.

7. Surgery in Herpes Simplex Virus Disease

Only two decades ago surgery in herpes simplex virus eyes often meant mutilating surgery. Eyes were enucleated for blindness and intractable secondary glaucoma, or corneas were covered with conjunctiva to get rid of non-healing ulcers. No enucleation of a herpes simplex virus infected eye has taken place in our institution during the past five years. Only two conjunctival flaps were necessary in very old patients who refused keratoplasty or were not able to be done in.

All other operations were rehabilitating surgery (Tab.8) with penetrating keratoplasty at the outstandingly first place, with triple procedures coming up more and more, and with glaucoma surgery (trabeculectomy) or rotating auto-keratoplasty remaining relatively rare events (1). Having become a referral center for both, keratoplasty and herpes simplex virus diseases, we did 207 perforating keratoplasties in 1991. Thirtyfour (16.4%) of these were done for herpes simplex virus disease. Seventy five percent were perforating keratoplasties, 23.5% triple procedures, and 6% rotating autokeratoplasties.

These large numbers are a consequence of the general progress in management of herpes simplex virus diseases as outlined above, and also a consequence of general progress in the management of keratoplasty problems (which cannot be discussed here).

The one important difference between herpes simplex virus eyes and all other eyes is the constant threat of relapsing endogenous herpes simplex virus disease. Recurrences may be triggered by medical means, or may come "spontaneously". If one succeeds in eliminating this special threat, then herpes simplex virus eyes behave "normally" and have a similarly good prognosis as any other comparable keratoplasty eye. This approach has been made possible with the availability of systemically applicable acyclovir. One may therefore accentuate that the key for successful surgery of herpes simplex virus eyes is the availability of acyclovir (Tab.9).

We use acyclovir in two dosages depending on the situation. If we want to act prophylactically in order to inhibit endogenous recurrences we give 5x200mg acyclovir for the time period of increased risk of recurrences. Two such identifiable situations exist: first perioperatively, and second in the special situation of high-dosed corticosteroid treatment of immune reactions. If acyclovir is needed for therapeutic purpose (during keratoplasty à chaud or for treatment of intraocular herpes simplex virus recurrences after keratoplasty) we give 5x400mg acyclovir together with moderately dosed systemic corticosteroids and other measures as outlined in paragraph four. One may double the acyclovir dosages for safety reasons, but I have rarely found this necessary.

Implanting artificial lenses into eyes with the potential danger of endogenously recurring intraocular herpes simplex virus disease requires some explanation. Such surgery is certainly still controversial in most eye centers around the world. However, one has to accept that in a considerable proportion of patients keratoplasty alone is no sufficient solution to the functional problem. Often a cataract exists or deteriorates in the course of the necessary postoperative treatment. Some of these patients even become blind from a "white" cataract. Doing an extracapsular procedure in such a situation is again no functional solution because aphakia contact lenses are mostly not well tolerated on keratoplasty eyes and furthermore they may mean an additional risk for herpes simplex virus recurrences (17). Finally, as most herpes simplex virus disease is unilateral, there is also no way of binocular vision by means of spectacles. Intraocular lenses are the only functionally satisfying solution.

Well aware of our therapeutic possibilities and limitations we have implanted posterior chamber lenses for four years now (2) and meanwhile probably follow the largest number of these patients. A recent evaluation has shown, that 28 out of 29 such patients could be functionally rehabilitated by triple procedures in the medium run (20). These good results do not come by themselves. Dangerous complications had to be overcome in the postoperative treatment. One third experienced intraocular herpes simplex virus recurrences, another third experienced immune reactions against donor endothelium (12). Both complications would have resulted in loss of the graft and more severe sequelae if one would have not succeeded in rapid diagnosis and effective therapy. It highlights that this kind of surgery bears considerable risks under undue conditions and therefore can currently not be recommended as an easy everyday procedure.

8. Prevention of Recurrences

Simple and efficient prevention of herpes simplex virus recurrences has been a dream of ophthalmologists and will stay a dream for some more time. A valid discussion of the recurrence topic is beyond the scope of this article. I restrict myself to some practical remarks.

Recurrences are brought about by "stress", whatever that means in the individual case. It may be fever, it may be psychic upset and professional overstress, it may be undue sunburn, it may be medical immuno-suppression, it may be unknown - and that is the majority of cases.

As outlined above, with systemic acyclovir we have a means of preventing recurrences reliably as long as we give it. The possible time period is limited by the individual's tolerance of acyclovir, which is normally good. Nonetheless, I would not recommend to overdo it. I would tend to reduce such a systemic acyclovir prophylaxis to a couple of weeks. These will be mostly surgical patients with the rare exception of patients who know for sure from their experience that they will react with an endogenous recurrence to a given trigger stimulus (e.g. respiratory infections with fever). For such patients it may be helpful to know that clinical disease usually flares up some three days after the trigger stimulus (17). This helps us estimating for what period of time a general acyclovir prophylaxis may be meaningful. If nothing has happened three days after the stimulus has gone there would be no more great sense to continue with systemic acyclovir.

Giving acyclovir ointment as a prophylactic measure in times of higher risk of recurrence is a good means to inhibit dendritic recurrences, as has been shown for trifluorothymidine eye drops (10). It eliminates the epithelial recurrence problem. However, it is very doubtful, that acyclovir ointment can have the same beneficial activity within the cornea, and it is quite certain, that trifluorothymidine has no inhibitory effect on intracorneal or intraocular recurrences.

Interferon was formerly thought to bring a solution. This was wrong. Systemically applied interferon reduces endogenous recurrences but does not totally eliminate them. Above all, systemic interferon injections are not well tolerated in the long run and may bring about serious side effects. Topically applied interferon drops, on the other hand, have proven to be totally inefficient (3). This is presumably because interferon does not penetrate the superficial epithelial cell layer and does not reach the basal cell layers where endogenous recurrent virus is "injected" from the nerve endings and where dendritic keratitis starts flaring up.

Thus, for the "normal" herpes simplex virus patient we have not much more to offer for reduction of recurrences than a general discussion about "stress" as the only known trigger. It has been my experience, though, that many patients appreciate that very well. They agree and admit that they too have been pondering about such a causative relationship and that they would try to eliminate at least part of their private and professional overstress. This makes me hope that such explanations and talks are not totally useless. They may, in fact, help in reducing the general incidence of herpes simplex virus recurrences.

Table 1. Available Therapy in the USA and in Germany

Available Therapy	Germany	USA
antivirals		
1. Trifluorothymidin (TFT) eye drops	X	X
2. Interferon (IF) eye drops	X	-
3. Acyclovir (ACV) ointment	X	-
4. Acyclovir tablets, intravenous	X	X
Steroids topically/systemically	X	X
Dry eye therapy	X	X
Glaucoma therapy	X	X
Corneal surgery	X	X

Table 2. Advantages and Disadvantages of the Topical Antivirals Approved in Germany

topical antiviral	advantages	disadvantages
TFT eye drops -	potent "broad spectrum" antiviral, practically no resistance, good compliance	potential epitheliotoxicity, limited corneal penetration, limited intracorneal and intraocular activity
acyclovir ointment*	fair corneal penetration, very low toxicity, safe use in the transition phase between viral and metaherpetic disease	occasionally resistant strains, interferes with vision, may interfere with patient's compliance
IF eye drops*	accelerate healing of viral dendritic keratitis in combination with either TFT or ACV	no disadvantages, practical limitations: handling and prize

* not approved in the USA

Table 3. Basic Principles for Management of Herpetic Disease (Groups I-IV Refer to the Basic scheme in Fig.1)

Disease	Principles	Therapy
I. superficial (epithelial) viral disease	1. treat viral disease 2. stimulate immunology 3. help resurfacing	ACV topically IF topically artifical tears etc
II. deep viral disease	1. treat viral disease 2. supress adverse immunology 3. treat acute glaucoma 4. don´t await perforation	ACV top/ syst full steroids top/sc/syst as low as possible medical therapy kerastoplasty à chaud if necessary
III. superficial (epithelial) metaherpetic healing disorder	1. eliminate adverse therapy 2.protect surface	eliminate TFT, if viral persistance is suspected give ACV top, all kinds of dry eye therapy, sofr lenses may become necessary (caution!)
IV. deep metaherpetic disease	1. treat chronic glaucoma 2. estimate visual function after healing 3.evaluate cataract	surgery if medication fails consider early keratoplasty for visual rehabilitation consider cataract surgery with IOL

Table 4. Practical management of herpes simplex virus keratitis

1. Analyze pathophysiological background of individual disease. Most diseases present a combination of problems.
2. Determine the - may be divergent - therapeutic requirements.
3. Establish a combination therapy, which should be the currently possible optimal compromise.
4. Frequently reevaluate the pathophysiological background and readjust the therapy adequately.

Table 5. Combination Therapy of Interstitial Herpes simplex Keratitis and/or Lower Grade Herpes Simplex Endotheliitis ("disciform edema")

	ACV top	ACV syst
Steroids top	+++	
Steroids sc		(add)
steroids syst		

Table 6. Combinatioan Therapy of Ulcerating Interstitial Herpes simplex Virus Keratitis

	ACV top	ACV syst
Steroids top		
Steroids sc		+++
Steroids syst	(add)	

Table 7. Combination Therapy of Severe Intraocular Herpes simplex Virus Disease: Severe Endotheliitis, Iritis, Trabeculitis

	ACV top	ACV syst
Steroids top		(add)
Steroids sc		
Steroids syst	+++	

Table 8. Rehabilitating Surgery in Herpes simplex Virus Disease

1. perforating homo-keratoplasty
2. cataract surgery plus IOL
3. glaucoma surgery
4. rotating perforating auto-keratoplasty

Table 9. The Key for Successful Surgery in Herpes simplex Virus Eyes

1.	for therapy of intraocular herpes simplex virus disease 5 x 400 (-800)mg/d
2.	for prophylaxis of herpes simplex virus recurrences during periods of increased risk 5 x 200 (-400)mg/d

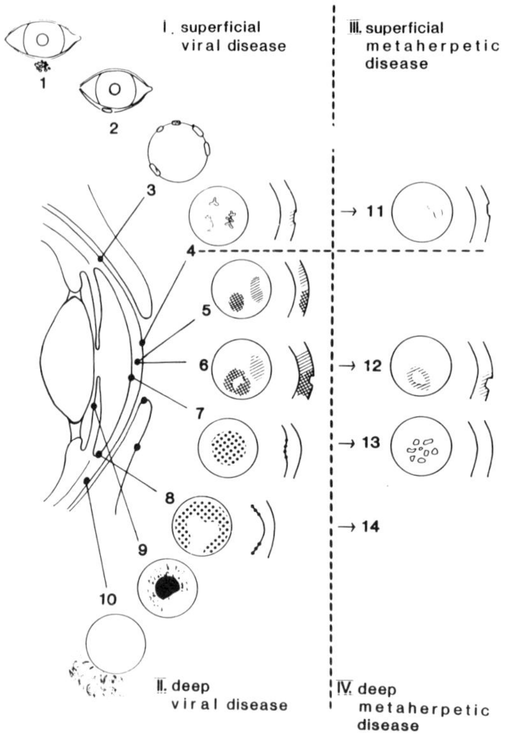

Figure 1. Basic Scheme for Classification of Herpes simplex Virus Anterior Segment Disease

I. superficial (epithelial) viral disease
1. blepharitis
2. intermarginal blepharitis
3. limbitis
4. dendritic keratitis (stellate, geographic keratitis)

II. deep viral disease
5. interstitial keratitis
6. ulcerating interstitial keratitis
7. endotheliitis
8. trabeculitis
9. focal serous iritis
10. scleritis/episcleritis

III. superficial (epithelial) metaherpetic healing disorder
11. (recurrent, persistent) erosion

IV. deep metaherpetic disease
12. deep metaherpetic ulcer
13. bullous keratopathy
14. chronic secondary glaucoma

References

1. Meiser S, Sundmacher R, Greber H (1991) Keratoplastiken im Säuglings- und Vorschulalter unter besonderer Berücksichtigung der Autorotationstechnik. Fortschr Ophthalmol 88:363-367
2. Sundmacher R, Ameye C (1989) Keratoplastik und Kapselsacklinseneinpflanzung bei Herpes-Patienten. In: Lang,GK et al. (eds) 2. DGII-Kongreß, Enke Verlag, Stuttgart, pp.106-109
3. Sundmacher R, Cantell K, Haug P et al (1978) Interferon-Prophylaxe von Dendritica-Rezidiven bei lokaler Steroidtherapie. Ber Dtsch Ophthalmol Ges 75:569-570
4. Sundmacher R, Cantell K, Mattes A (1984) Combination Therapy for Dendritic Keratitis. High-Titer Alpha-Interferon and Trifluorothymidine. Arch Ophthalmol 102:554-555
5. Sundmacher R, Cantell K, Neumann-Haefelin D (1978) Combination Therapy of Dendritic Keratitis with Trifluorothymidine and Interferon. Lancet II:687
6. Sundmacher R, Neumann-Haefelin D, Cantell K (1976) Interferon Treatment of Dendritic Keratitis. Lancet I:1406
7. Sundmacher R, Neumann-Haefelin D (1976) Keratitis metaherpetica. Klinische und virologische Befunde. Klin Mbl Augenheilk. 169:728-737
8. Sundmacher R, Neumann-Haefelin D (1979) Herpes Simplex Virus-Positive and Negative Keratouveitis. In: Silverstein A, O'Connor R (eds) Immunology and Immunopathology of the Eye, Masson, New Yorks/Paris, pp.225-229
9. Sundmacher R, Neumann-Haefelin D (1979) Herpes simplex-Virus-Isolierung aus dem Kammerwasser bei fokaler Iritis, Endotheliitis und langdauernder Keratitis disciformis mit Sekundärglaukom. Klin Mbl Augenheilk 175:488-501
10. Sundmacher R (1978) Trifluorothymidinprophylaxe bei der Steroidtherapie herpetischer Keratouveitiden. Klin Mbl Augenheilk 173:516-519
11. Sundmacher R (1981) A Clinico-Virologic Classification of Herpetic Anterior Segment Diseases with Special Reference to Intraocular Herpes. In: Sundmacher R (ed) Herpetic Eye Diseases, Bergmann, München. pp.203-208
12. Sundmacher R (1981) Differential Diagnosis of Post-Keratoplasty complications in Herpes Patients. In: Sundmacher R (ed) Herpetic Eye Diseases, Bergmann, München. pp.439-444
13. Sundmacher R (1981) Die fokale Iritis durch Herpes-simplex- und Varizellen-Zoster-Virus. Ber Dtsch Ophthalmol Ges 78:73-76
14. .Sundmacher R (1983) Orale Acyclovir-Therapie virologisch nachgewiesener intraokularer Herpes simplex Virus-Infektionen. Klin Mbl Augenheilk 183: 246-250
15. Sundmacher R (1984) The Role of Interferon in Prophylaxis and Treatment of Dendritic Keratitis. In: Blodi FC (ed) Contemporary Issues in Ophthalmology, Vol.1, Herpes Simplex Infections of the Eye, Churchill Livingstone, New York, pp.129-146
16. Sundmacher R (1984) Endotheliitis corneae, Begriffsbestimmung und klinische Abgrenzung. Klin Mbl Augenheilk 184: 163-167
17. Sundmacher R (1984) Trauma und Herpes. Fortschr Ophthalmol 81:409-415
18. Sundmacher R (1990) Interferon in der Augenheilkunde. In: Niederle N, v. Wus sow P (eds) Interferone, präklinische und klinische Befunde. Springer Verlag, Berlin/Heidelberg, pp. 395-405
19. Weber U, Sundmacher R (1988) Die systemische Acyclovirtherapie herpetischer Sekundärglaukome. Fortschr Ophthalmol 85:85-87

20. Wolff M, Reinhard T, Sundmacher R (1991) 4 Jahre Erfahrung mit Keratoplastik und Intraokularlinsenimplantation in Herpesaugen.89. Tagung der Deutschen Ophthalmologischen Gesellschaft, Leipzyig

Acyclovir in Herpes Zoster: A Reexamination of its Effect on Postherpetic Neuralgia and Ocular Involvement

James McGill

Abstract. Oral Acyclovir at a dose of 800mg five times a day for seven days significantly reduced acute pain, rash development and progression in 38 immunocompetent patients compared to 36 control patients receiving placebo.
At six months and five years, post herpetic neuralgia was also significantly reduced in the treated group. Those in the treated group with trigeminal involvement developed fewer ocular problems and none had any progression of the disease, compared to controls.

Introduction

Herpes zoster infection is a common clinical problem, particularly in the elderly and leads to much morbidity, with post herpetic neuralgia being the most common problem. Ocular involvement can be severe, causing long-term visual problems often necessitating treatment for considerable time.

Post-herpetic neuralgia is usually defined as pain persisting for more than a month after the original Herpes zoster infection. Its incidence varies greatly in the reported works from 6%-70% (10) and is age-related with 16% under 60, 47% over 60 (11). It is variable in intensity and type, and is difficult to evaluate, can resolve spontaneously from a few months to years after the initial attack so that many alternate means of recording and measuring it have been devised which may, in part, explain the different rates and severities which have been recorded in reported trials.

Until the advent of Acyclovir, there was no specific antiviral treatment for this condition.

Of the many trials on the effect of Acyclovir on Herpes zoster (9), only two have shown an effect on post-herpetic neuralgia and this was when high doses of 800mg of the drug were used (3,8). However, in these two trials, different criteria for measurements of post-herpetic neuralgia were made and different age groups included in the trial.

A large multicenter United Kingdom trial of 364 patients was carried out (6), which showed a significant effect on the acute skin rash and pain, but overall analysis failed to show any significant effect on post-herpetic neuralgia (7).

The question arises as to why the United Kingdom trial did not show any such effect when the others did. One of the difficulties of a multicenter trial is of standardization of the recording of clinical signs and symptoms, especially in the recording of post-herpetic neuralgia. Also, as post-herpetic neuralgia can recur unless patients are followed up for some time after the first time pain has subsided, the final incidence of post-herpetic neuralgia may be underestimated, because in many cases there is a recurrence of the pain after patients are discharged following the first cessation of pain, giving a lower incidence of post-herpetic neuralgia if patients are not followed up for long enough. This may therefore explain why, in the United Kingdom trial, no significant effect of the drug on post-herpetic neuralgia was noted. The reason though why there was a difference between the outcome of the United Kingdom trial and the other two trials, which showed an effect on post-herpetic neuralgia is not clear, but in the United Kingdom trial, treatment continued for 7 days but in the United States trial (3) for 10 days. In the United Kingdom trial the lower age limit was 60 years, in the United States 18 years.

It would therefore seem that a way around this dilemma, to determine the incidence of post-herpetic neuralgia, is to evaluate the number of patients pain-free on long-term follow-up, in other words, when the patient was finally pain-free.

Study

Recently we re-examined the clinical data (McGill and White, to be published) not only from the first six months continuous follow-up of the placebo controlled trial of oral Acyclovir (800mg five times a day for 7 days) on immune competent patients over 60, from a single centes, namely Southampton, taking part in the large United Kingdom trial (6), taking as the end point of post-herpetic neuralgia the time when the patient was finally pain free as opposed to the time of first cessation of pain. Also, the patients in the original trial from this center were followed up for five years to determine the long-term effect of Acyclovir on reducing post-herpetic neuralgia (McGill and White, to be published). This took into account any recurrence of pain.

For the five year follow-up of patients, patients were either seen in the clinic or communication was by telephone or by writing. The patients were asked to record on a trial sheet whether they still had pain, whether the pain was mild, medium or severe, and did it keep them awake at night, and they were also asked to score it on a 0-10 basis.

For the 74 patients entered into the trial from the single center, Southampton, for acute Herpes zoster skin involvement duration of pain was significantly less in the treated group (Tab.1). Re-analysis of the Southampton figures showed that, taking as an endpoint the final time pain-free or complete cessation of pain, Acyclovir had a significant effect on post-herpetic neuralgia, with 93,75% of the treated group being pain-free compared to 30.3% of the control group at six months (Tab.2).

For the five year follow-up, there was a high rate of patient recall of those in the original trial, 27 in the Acyclovir group (71%), 24 in the placebo group (67%), only one of the Acyclovir group had post-herpetic neuralgia at the five year follow-up compared to 7 out of 24 in the placebo group (Tab.2) the difference being statistically significant.

This is the first time that any Herpes zoster trial of Acyclovir has followed up the patients for 5 years and it takes into account those patients who may have prolonged post-herpetic neuralgia or have a recurrence of their pain. The results show that in the five year follow-up, oral Acyclovir had a significant effect in preventing post-herpetic neuralgia when assessed using the parameter of being finally pain free. This finding that Acyclovir had a significant effect on post-herpetic neuralgia is in agreement with those of Huff and coworkers (3) and Morton and coworkers (8) but in these trials follow-up was only until pain had ceased and was not prolonged after this time, so that they may have missed patients who had a late recurrence of this pain.

The fact that oral Acyclovir at 5 years follow-up had a significant effect on reducing post-herpetic neuralgia and that one third of the surviving patients in the placebo group had some form of post-herpetic neuralgia, is of clinical and economic significance in the long-term treatment of such patients with analgetics and the quality of life after Herpes zoster.

Ocular Involvement

For ocular involvement no specific treatment was available until the development of Acyclovir. Corticosteroid treatment, whilst suppressing the ocular signs has been associated with prolonged treatment and, in some cases it was very difficult to wean patients completely off corticosteroids.

Topical Acyclovir though, has been shown to be effective in the treatment of the ocular involvement (4) and superior to corticosteroids, for in a controlled trial comparing topical corticosteroids with topical Acyclovir, topical Acyclovir treatment was effective and associated with a shorter course of treatment with fewer recurrences (5).

Since that time, oral Acyclovir has been shown to be effective in reducing the ocular complications of Herpes zoster and protecting the eye during the acute attack (1,2). In a recent re-evaluation of their trial of oral Acyclovir in acute Herpes zoster, McGill and White (to be published) have shown that oral Acyclovir 800mg five times a day protects the eye from the development of the disease as Acyclovir treated patients with ocular signs at initial presentation fared much better than the placebo controlled patients. Over 90% of the patients with trigeminal involvement treated with Acyclovir were either protected from the development of ocular signs if they were not present at the initial examination, or the disease regressed on oral Acyclovir treatment, whereas only 20% of the placebo controlled patients failed to develop ocular signs.

Of those with acute trigeminal involvement in the original trial, seven in the Acyclovir group and 6 patients in the placebo group had ocular involvement on presentation with the acute rash. Of these, only one in the Acyclovir group progressed after oral treatment had been started when conjunctival injection progressed to an epithelial ulcer. Seven out of 15 did not develop any ocular signs.

However, in the placebo group, nine patients developed ocular signs later, i.e. were not present on the initial examination. Seven developed corneal signs of an epithelial ulcer with stromal involvement in six cases and three with uveitis. A further two cases developed uveitis or scleritis. Of the whole group, only three of 18 failed to develop any ocular signs.

Ocular involvement was more severe in the placebo group, with only one patient in the Acyclovir having anything more severe than an epithelial ulcer - but 8 of the placebo group had deep corneal stromal or uveitic involvement.

Conclusion

It would therefore appear that, for those patients with acute Herpes zoster infection, oral Acyclovir is effective in treating not only the acute rash but also in preventing long-term post-herpetic neuralgia, and ocular involvement in those that have developed trigeminal forms of Herpes zoster infection.

Table 1. Evaluation of Post-Herpetic Neuralgia

	No.		
Acyclovir	38	2.44	mean
Placebo	36	3.59	
	p = 0.005		

To demonstrate duration in weeks of post-herpetic neuralgia after oral placebo or Acyclovir 800mg 5 times a day for 7 days.

Table 2. Post-Herpetic Neuralgia - % pain free

	6 months	5 years
Acyclovir	93.7	92.4
Placebo	41.5	71

2 tailed t-test p = 0.073
Fisher Exact test = 0.006

To demonstrate percentage incidence of patients pain free at 6 months and 5 years follow-up after trial of oral Acyclovir 800mg 5 times a day for 7 days. There is a statistically significant difference in the incidence of post-herpetic neuralgia between the treated and control groups.

Table 3. Numbers of Patients Contacted 5 Years After Orignial Trial of Acyclovir in Herpes zoster Infection

Post-herpetic Neuralgia	5 Year Follow-Up	
	Acyclovir	Placebo
No. in Original Trial	38	36
Contacted	27	24
Pain	1	7

2 tailed t-test p = 0.073
Fisher Exact test = 0.006

Table 4. Effect of Acyclovir on the Development of Ocular Involvement

	No signs developed No.	i.e.protected	After treatment started developed signs	Eye signs present with rash
Acyclovir	15	7	1	7
Placebo	18	3	9	6

To show the effect of Acyclovir on the development of ocular involvement.

References

1. Cobo M (1988) Reduction of the Ocular Complications of Herpes Zoster Ophthalmicus by Oral Acyclovir. Am J Med 85:90-93
2. Cobo M, Foulks FN, Liesegang T et al (1986) Oral Acyclovir in the Treatment of Acute Herpes Zoster Ophthalmicus. Ophthalmology 93:763-770
3. Huff JC, Bean B, Balfour HH et al (1988) Therapy of Herpes Zoster with Oral Acyclovir. Am J Med 85:84-89
4. McGill J, James C, Hiscott P et al (1979) Drug Treatment of Herpes Zoster. Trans Ophthalmol Soc UK 101:3-5
5. McGill J, Chapman C (1983) A Comparison of Topical Acyclovir with Steroids in the Treatment of Herpes Zoster Kerato-Uveitis. Br J Ophthalmol 67:746-750
6. McKendrick MW, McGill JI, White JE et al (1986) Oral Acyclovir in Acute Herpes Zoster. Br Med J 293:1529-1532
7. McKendrick MW, McGill JI, Wood MJ (1989) Lack of Effect on Post-herpetic Neuralgia. Br Med J 298:431
8. Morton P, Thompson AN (1989) Oral Acyclovir in the Treatment of Herpes Zoster in General Practice. New Zealand Med J 102:93-95
9. O'Brien J, Campoli-Richards DM (1989) Acyclovir: An Updated Review of its Antiviral Activity, Pharmacokinetic Properties and Therapeutic Efficacy. Drugs 37:233-309
10. Ragazzino MW, Malton LJ, Kurland LT et al (1982) Population-Based Study of Herpes Zoster and its Sequelae. Medicine 61:310-316
11. Russell K, Portenoy RK, Duma C et al (1986) Acute Herpetic and Post-herpetic Neuralgia-Clinical Review and Current Management. Ann Neurol 20:651-656

Acute Herpes Zoster Ophthalmicus: Prevention of Severe Ocular Complications by Adequate Acyclovir Therapy

Carl P. Herbort, Francois X. Borruat, Ernest R. Büchi

Abstract. 238 herpes zoster ophthalmicus patients were divided into three groups and analysed for the incidence of severe ocular complications. 164 patients without any antiviral therapy were analysed retrospectively from 1950-1978; 48 patients with adequate Acyclovir therapy analysed prospectively from 1984-1990 and 26 patients treated inadequately with Acyclovir analysed retrospectively from 1985-1990. Patients with inadequate Acyclovir treatment or none at all showed similar rates of severe complications 27% (7/26) and 21% (34/164) respectively). In contrast, when adequate Acyclovir therapy was given, severe ocular complications occurred in only 4% (2/48) of patients. Our study emphasizes the necessity for early and adequately dosed Acyclovir therapy to prevent severe ocular Herpes zoster ophthalmicus complications.

Introduction

Acute herpes zoster ophthalmicus is caused by reactivation of latent Varizella-Zoster Virus in the trigeminal ganglion and infection of the dermatoma of the first division of the trigeminal nerve (5). Ocular involvement occurs in approximately 65% of cases (6,9,10) and can lead to severe ocular complications (6). Acute signs and symptoms are directly caused by replicating virus (6). In contrast to ocular herpes simplex virus recurrences, the disease is usally more explosive with abundant viral replication, viral spread along perineural and perivascular routes and a strong antibody response (3). Post-zoster neuralgia, as well as severe ocular complications which occur in up to 20% of cases are the major problems found associated with Acute Herpes Zoster Ophthalmicus.

The introduction of acyclovir, an antiviral drug active against varicella zoster virus has fundamentally changed the outcome and morbidity of acute herpes zoster ophthalmicus. Because of the widespread viral replication and the systemic components of the disease, systemic rather than only topical therapy should be given (2). At the oral dose of 5x800mg daily of acyclovir, the plasma level is sufficient to inhibit most varicella zoster virus strains (8). To be effective, Acyclovir should be given early in disease, within 3 days of skin eruption, at the time of maximal viral replication (6). Consequently, at present, the recommended oral dose of Acyclovir is 5x800mg daily (5). The body of clinical evidence available at present indicates that this therapy is extremely efficient (2,5,8).

We have previously shown in a prospective study including 48 patients that had received 5x800mg oral Acyclovir and topical Acyclovir 5x daily within three days of skin eruption that the rate of severe complications decreased from 21% in a historical control group to 4% in the adequately treated patient group (3). No patient went on to suffer from chronic or recurring disease and no patient needed corticosteroid therapy.

The aim of this study was to analyse retrospectively the outcome of Acute herpes zoster ophthalmicus in patients seen at our clinic in the subacute stage that had received inadequate Acyclovir therapy, as defined thereafter.

Patients and Methods

Patients: A total of 238 immunocompetent herpes zoster patients were analysed and subdivided into three groups (Tab.1):

1. One hundred and sixty-eight patients having received no antiviral therapy, analysed retrospectively from 1950 to 1978.
2. Forty-eight patients having received adequate Acyclovir therapy: oral Acyclovir 5x800mg + Acyclovir ointment 5x daily given within three days after skin rash for at least 7 days, analysed prospectively from 1984-1990.
3. Twenty-six patients, seen later than three days after skin eruption, having received inadequate Acyclovir therapy (insufficient dosis of oral Acyclovir or too late treatment, or only local treatment) were analyzed retrospectively in the time period from 1984-1991.

The study populations are detailed in Tab.1. There were no significant differences for sex and age distribution. A distinction was made between "ocular involvement" defined as ocular participation in the acute phase of the disease and "ocular complications" defined as severe ocular sequelae or persistence of ocular signs beyond the acute phase. It is important to note that there was no difference in incidence of ocular involvement between the groups indicating that our third group was not biassed towards more severe cases. This group of patients was recruited during the years when Acyclovir was already available and because of the referral nature of our center might have concentrated a greater proportion of complicated cases.

Methods

In all three groups the percentage of severe ocular complications was reported. The following conditions were considered as severe ocular complications:

- persistent (>3 months) or recurrent uveitis,
- persistent or recurrent disciform keratitis,
- neurotrophic keratitis,
- lid scarring and exposure keratitis,
- ocular perforation,
- sectorial iris atrophy,
- persistent oculomotor palsy and
- loss of visual acuity of more than three Snellen lines due to zoster.

In the Acyclovir and inadequate Acyclovir groups we further analyzed the types of therapy used, the mean total duration of ocular treatment and the mean numbers of office visits in patients with ocular involvement. Adequate Acyclovir therapy was defined as oral Acyclovir therapy at the dosage of 5x800mg daily given within three days of skin rash for at least 7 days with or without topical Acyclovir. Inadequate Acyclovir therapy, on the other hand, was defined as an oral Acyclovir dosage of less than

5x800mg/day or/and oral Acyclovir given later than three days after skin rash, or only topical Acyclovir therapy. Intravenous Acyclovir therapy was considered an adequate therapy, but is presently rarely used in immunocompetent patients for practical reasons.

Results

The incidence and types of ocular complications are listed in Tab.2 for each group. In the Acyclovir group it is important to note that no patient presented with ocular involvement after day 7 and no patient developed chronic disease.

Comparison of disease durations and type of therapy needed in the Acyclovir and inadequate Acyclovir groups are summarized in Tab.3. Follow-up has been more than two years in all patients treated with Acyclovir. In the inadequate Acyclovir group follow-up is more than two years in 20/26 patients, 12 months or less in 3/26 and 6 months or less in 3/26 patients. It is noteworthy that corticosteroids were not necessary in any of the Acyclovir-treated patients.

Discussion

We have recently shown that adequate oral Acyclovir therapy drastically reduced severe ocular complications (3).

In the present retrospective study analysing the outcome of patients having received insufficient Acyclovir therapy, we found the disease pattern to be similar to untreated patients. The group of 26 patients that received inadequate Acyclovir therapy as defined earlier showed a rate of severe ocular complications identical to non-treated patients. It has to be noted that the inadequate Acyclovir treatment group is very small reflecting increasingly early and adequate management of Acute Herpes Zoster Ophthalmicus by the general practitioners of our area who usually see the patients first. Despite the unequal sizes of our groups, the similar rates of ocular involvement indicates that they are probably comparable, taking into account that results from studies with historical control groups should be interpreted cautiously. Regarding the participation of the eye in herpes zoster, it is important to distinguish between "ocular involvement" and "ocular complications", as defined above, Acyclovir has probably no effect on ocular involvement, as this is determined by the pattern of viral reactivation, whereas ocular complications are positively influenced by systemic Acyclovir.

Despite several reports on the effectiveness of early systemic Acyclovir in Acute herpes Zoster Ophthalmicus, there is still a lot of confusion on how to manage properly this condition (1,2,5). Systemic Acyclovir therapy has clearly divided ocular zoster patients into two different disease cathegories:

1. Patients who were treated adequately with Acyclovir in their acute phase. These patients are rarely ever going to develop chronic and recurrent inflammatory disease (0/48 patients in our study). As shown earlier, neither topical nor systemic corticosteroids are necessary in this situation (3). In particular, zoster uveitis, analysed by laser flare-cellmetry is self-limited without corticosteroid treatment (4).

2. Patients who reached the subacute stage without any antiviral therapy. In this study, we have shown that patients who had received inadequate Acyclovir treatment tend to evolve in a similar fashion than those without any treatment at all. About 20% of these patients develop chronic and/or recurrent inflammatory disease, often leading to severe ocular complications.
In the latter group the role played by viral replication is probably minimal. Immune mechanisms possibly of an autoimmune type are thought to play a major role for disease morbidity, and therapy should be adapted accordingly.

As treatment has clearly been established for acute disease, treatment for subacute or chronic zoster has yet been less well-defined. Most of these cases need individually dosed topical steroids, which are usually tapered over long periods. Additional topical Acyclovir seems to have a beneficial effect by possibly lowering the recurrence rate of inflammatory episodes (7).

Conclusions

In conclusion, it is reemphasized that early and adequate dosages of oral Acyclovir should be given in Acute Herpes zoster Ophthalmicus. This approach shortens total treatment duration, simplifies treatment, prevents severe ocular complications and is well-tolerated. On the basis of our findings, we suggest the following therapeutical attitude in Acute Herpes zoster Ophthalmicus, knowing that there will be an "overtreatment" of about 30% of patients:
1. Treat all cases of Acute Herpes Zoster Ophthalmicus with 5x800mg oral Acyclovir (and topical Acyclovir) within three days of skin rash for 7 days.
2. Reapprise the situation after 7 days; stop all antiviral therapy if there is no ocular involvement and if skin lesions are disappearing; treat for another 3-5 days if there is ocular involvement or if the skin lesions are progressing in the absence of ocular involvement.

Table 1. Study Populations

	No ACV retrospective	ACV (5x800) prospective	ACV inadequate retrospective
Number	164	48	26
Men	98 (60%	21 (44.%)	12 (46%)
Women	66 (40%)	27 (56%)	14 (54%)
Age (mean)	58 +/-17	62 +/-15	64 +/-18
Ocular involvement	96 (59%)	32 (67%)	16 (62%)

No significant differences for parameters between groups

Table 2. Severe Ocular Complications (Number of Cases)

	No ACV retrospective	ACV (5x800) prospective	ACV inadequate retrospective
Number of patients (%)	34/164 (21%)	2/48 (4%)[1]	7/26 (27%)[NS]
Recurrent uveitis	11	-	4
Recurrent disciform KEatitis	24	-	1
Upper lid scarring	5	-	-
Sectorial iris atrophy	5	1	1
Perforation	1	-	-
Encephalitis	1 (lethal)	1 (no sequels)	-
Loss of VA > 3 Snellen	-	1	1
AION [2]	-	-	1
Persistent oculomotor palsy	-	-	1

Total of complications can be greater than number of patients as some patients had more than one complication.

[1] Significantly less severe complications than no ACV and inadequate ACV
[2] AION = Anterior ischemic optic neuropathy

Table 3. Disease Course and Management in ACV and Inadequate ACV Groups

	ACV-group	inadequate ACV-group
Number of patients with ocular involvement	32/48 (67%)	16/26 (62%)
Mean total ttt duration	23 ±15 days[2]	90±68 days[2]
Mean office visits (n)	5.5±0.88[2]	10.1±3.2[2]
Type of therapy:		
Local ACV (%patients)	82%	93%
Mean ttt duration	21±16 days[2]	68±57 days[2]
Mydriatics (%)	22%[3]	81%[3]
Mean ttt duration	8+3.6 days[1]	37±37 days[1]
Hypotensive drops (%)	15%	44%
Mean ttt duration	4.8±2 days[1]	71±62 days[1]
Corticosteroids (%)	0%	31%
Mean ttt duration	0[2]	86±64 days[2]

[1] $P < 0.05$ (Student's t test)
[2] $P < 0.0001$ (Student's t test)
[3] $P < 0.0001$ (chi square test)

References

1. Büchi ER, Herbort CP, Ruffieux C (1986) Oral Acyclovir in the Treatment of Acute herpes Zoster Ophthalmicus. Am J Ophthalmol 102:531-532
2. Cobo LM, Foulks GN, Liesegang TJ et al (1986) Oral Acyclovir in the Treatment of Acute Herpes Zoster Ophthalmicus. Ophthalmology 93:763-770
3. Herbort CP, Büchi ER, Piguet B et al (1991) High-Dose Oral Acyclovir in Acute Herpes Zoster Ophthalmicus: The End of the Corticosteroid Era. Curr Eye Res 10:171-175
4. Herbort CP, Bigar F, Pittet N (1991) Usefulness of the Laser Flare-Cell Meter (LFCM, Kowa FC-1000) in Clinical Practice. Klin Mbl Augenheilk 198:470-473
5. Liesegang TJ (1991) Diagnosis and Therapy of Herpes Zoster Ophthalmicus. Ophthalmology 98:1216-1229
6. Liesegang TJ (1985) Corneal Complications from Herpes Zoster Ophthalmicus. Ophthalmology 92:316-324
7. Marsh RJ, Cooper M (1991) Double-Masked Trial of Topical Acyclovir and Steroids in the Treatment of Herpes Zoster Ocular Inflammation. Br J Ophthalmol 75:542-546
8. McKendrick MW, McGill JI, White JE et al (1986) Oral Acyclovir in Acute Herpes Zoster. Br Med J 293:1529
9. Womack LW, Liesegang TJ (1983) Complications of Herpes Zoster Ophthalmicus. Arch Ophthalmol 101:42-45
10. 10.Yamada K, Hayasaka S, Yamamoto Y et al (1990) Cutaneous Eruption with or without Ocular Complications in Patients with Herpes Zoster Involving the Trigeminal Nerve. Graefe's Arch. Clin. Exp. Ophthalmol.228:1-4

- Contact-Lens Associated Infections

Epidermal Growth Factor in the Tear Fluid During Corneal Disease and Contact Lens Wear

Gysbert-B.van Setten, Timo Tervo and Ahti Tarkkanen

Abstract. Epidermal growth factor (EGF) is potentially involved in the maintenance of the corneal integrity and processes of corneal wound healing. EGF has been detected in the tear fluid of both healthy individuals and patients with corneal disease. Recently we investigated the effects of contact lens wear on the presence of EGF in tear fluid. Although the concentration of EGF was not significantly altered by contact lens wear, the interaction with the EGF receptors at the ocular surface and with other systems, such as the fibrinolytic system has to be considered, too. The present article highlight current knowledge of the presence and significance of EGF in tear fluid with special reference to the effects of contact lens wear.

Introduction

The protection mechanisms of the cornea include the eyelid movements, a continuous flow of tear fluid, its adequate composition and its proper distribution over the ocular surface as well as the continuous regeneration of the epithelial cells covering the cornea and conjunctiva. If the integrity of the ocular surface is weakened or disturbed, microbes on the ocular surface may invade the corneal stroma leading to severe corneal disease. The accumulation of polymorphonuclear leucocytes in the wound area further retards corneal reepithelialization. This, together with proteolytic degradation of corneal tissues (11) allows the infection to spread into the cornea with the risk of severe ocular complications. One of the principal functions of tear fluid is immunological defense against corneal disease. This is achieved in part by the presence of antibodies like IgE, IgA, and IgG and of antimicrobial substances such as lysozyme and ß-lysin in tear fluid (13).

However, these physiological defense mechanisms are often insufficient and therapeutic application of various substances is required for restitution and maintenance of corneal integrity. Growth factors are a group of proteins that appear to be the most powerful drugs currently available (2). Recently, Epidermal Growth Factor has been detected in the tear fluid of both healthy individuals and patients with corneal disease (7,14,15,16).

This suggests that Epidermal Growth Factor might be of importance for both the normal turnover of corneal epithelial cells and for the promotion of corneal wound healing. The present article highlights current knowledge of the presence and significance of Epidermal Growth Factor in tear fluid.

General Actions of Epidermal Growth Factor

Of the numerous growth factors identified thus far, Epidermal Growth Factor is the best known. In human body fluids Epidermal Growth Factor occurs in two forms. This paper focusses on the smaller form of Epidermal Growth Factor, the "low molecular weight human Epidermal Growth Factor". This is a 6kD polypeptide that is very stable energetically and consists of 53 amino acids. The primary structure and biological effects show great homology between different species (4).

Epidermal Growth Factor molecules influence the cellular metabolism of their target cells via binding to specific receptors at their surface. The binding of Epidermal Growth Factor to the extracellular domain of the Epidermal Growth Factor receptors lead to the formation of Epidermal Growth Factor-receptor complexes and results in activation of protein kinase activity. The formation of Epidermal Growth Factor-receptor complexes is followed by their aggregation (clustering) and endocytosis which finally induces changes in the cellular metabolism.

Effects of Epidermal Growth Factor on Corneal Tissue

The earliest observed effects of Epidermal Growth Factor on corneal cells include the induction of epithelial cellular hypertrophy and the enhancement of cell division. Furthermore, application of topical Epidermal Growth Factor leads to an increased number of epithelial cell layers. The resulting enhancement in corneal reepithelialization led to great interest in the possibility of local application of this growth factor and to the initiation of numerous studies (2).

Investigations have also shown that Epidermal Growth Factor increases the production of fibronectin by corneal tissue. Like other extracellular matrix proteins, fibronectin is very important during the initial steps of corneal wound healing (6).

On the other hand, Epidermal Growth Factor also increases the production of plasminogen activator by various cells, suggesting interactions with the fibrinolytic system. The proteolytically active part of the fibrinolytic cascade, plasmin, proved to have an elevated activity during corneal disease and it interferes with corneal wound healing by cleaving extracellular matrix proteins (11). Accordingly, the most recent approaches evaluating the therapeutic potency of Epidermal Growth Factor in the enhancement of corneal wound healing suggest the combined use of Epidermal Growth Factor together with fibronectin and/or enzyme inhibitors (9). The external application of Epidermal Growth Factor requires, however, a good knowledge of the natural presence of this growth factor at the ocular surface.

Epidermal Growth Factor in Human Tear Fluid of Healthy and Diseased Eyes

Epidermal Growth Factor has proved to be a natural constituent of tear fluid (7,8,14). Although both low and high molecular weight forms have been found in tear fluid (8), the smaller one (Low Molecular Weight Epidermal Growth Factor) predominates (van Setten and coworkers, 1991 unpublished data).

Immunohistochemical investigations indicate that the main lacrimal gland would be the source of Epidermal Growth Factor in tear fluid (17). This has been supported recently by biochemical studies on the content of mRNA for Epidermal Growth Factor in the lacrimal gland (19). Hence, the anatomical integrity of the lacrimal gland and the physiology of tear fluid secretion have a major influence on the presence of Epidermal Growth Factor in the tear fluid and its availability to the ocular surface (16). However, the mechanisms of Epidermal Growth Factor secretion from the lacrimal gland are still only poorly understood. Its constant presence in tear fluid implies that it might be of importance for the natural turnover of epithelial cells and for maintenance of corneal integrity.

Like other components of tear fluid derived from the lacrimal gland, the presence of Epidermal Growth Factor also has to be evaluated in relation to the actual secretion rate of tear fluid (7,15,16).

- Tear fluid collected with a minimum of stimulation (tear fluid flow rate of 50-60nl/s) contains an average of 6-7ng Epidermal Growth Factor/ml (15).
- After stimulation of reflex tearing (flow rate about 500nl/s) the concentration decreases to a mean of 2.7ng Epidermal Growth Factor/ml (15).
- Elevation of the tear fluid secretion rate over a longer period due to corneal disease led to a further decrease of Epidermal

Growth Factor concentrations to levels of around 0.8-1.0 ng Epidermal Growth Factor/ml at tear fluid flow rates around 400nl/s (15,16).

This decrease in tear fluid Epidermal Growth Factor concentration during corneal disease has to be seen together with simultaneously elevated activities of collagenolytic proteases, plasminogen activators, and plasmin (10). Although plasmin does not degrade Low Molecular Weight Epidermal Growth Factor, the possible influence of plasmin or other proteolytic enzymes on Epidermal Growth Factor receptors and their interactions is not known. On the other hand, ligands with specific receptors have the ability to modulate the level of their own receptor. Hence, just as an abundance of Epidermal Growth Factor might decrease the number and activity of Epidermal Growth Factor receptors, a notable, prolonged decrease of Epidermal Growth Factor levels in tear fluid may explain the observed increase of Epidermal Growth Factor receptors during healing of corneal wounds. These interactions are considered in models evaluating the alterations of tear fluid Epidermal Growth Factor concentrations during corneal wound healing (van Setten and coworkers, 1991 unpublished data). They also have to be understood in considering the external application of Epidermal Growth Factor.

The system regulating the presence of Epidermal Growth Factor in tear fluid appears to be rather sensitive to external influences since even minor external stimuli such as collection of the tear fluid from the fellow eye may alter the concentration of Epidermal Growth Factor in the tear fluid of healthy eyes. Even contact lens wear may affect the concentration of Epidermal Growth Factor in tear fluid by leading to a slight, reversible decrease during contact lens wear (18). Other contact lens wear associated changes in tear fluid composition include the elevation of plasmin activity (12) and reduced pH in tear fluid and the increase in the conjunctival flora of contact lens wearers (3). The attachment of enzyme producing bacteria to contact lenses may further increase proteolytic activity in tears.

Therefore, the decreased availability of Epidermal Growth Factor due to impaired tear fluid exchange under the contact lens (especially in the case of extended wear soft contact lenses) combined with other factors (1) may predispose to corneal complications caused by contact lens wear (Fig.1).

Comments

- Epidermal Growth Factor is a normal component of the tear fluid and probably derives from the lacrimal gland.
- Like other proteins of the same origin its presence in tear fluid depends on the actual secretion rate of the lacrimal gland.
- The concentration of Epidermal Growth Factor is significantly decreased in eyes with diseases of the ocular surface or the lacrimal gland.
- The improvement of corneal wound healing frequently observed after external application of topical Epidermal Growth Factor may result from a decreased availability of Epidermal Growth Factor to the ocular surface together with an increased number of receptors during wound healing.

- The failure to demonstrate any wound healing promoting effects of Epidermal Growth Factor in other studies (5), however, underlines the complexity of growth factor actions on the ocular surface.
- The possible involvement of growth factor deficiency in the development of corneal complications associated with wearing of contact lenses together with the activation of the fibrinolytic system deserve further investigation.

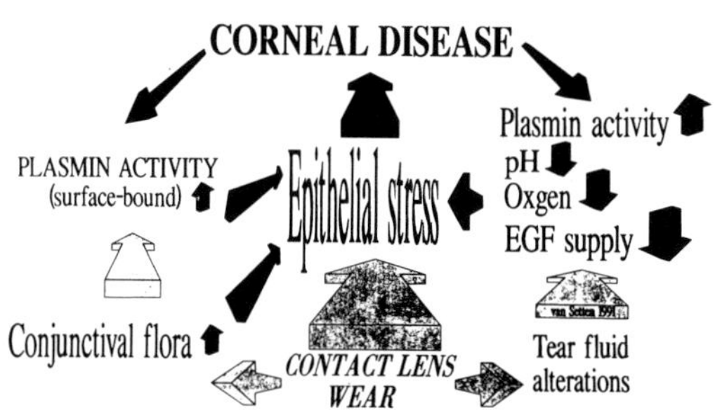

Fig.1. The possible involvement of various factors in the development of corneal complications associated with wearing of contact lenses and their interaction.

References

1. Bruce AS, Brennan NA (1990) Corneal Pathophysiology with Contact Lens Wear. Surv Ophthalmol 35:25-58
2. Burstein NL (1987) Review: Growth Factor Effects on Corneal Wound Healing. J Pharmacol 1:263-277
3. Callender MG, Tse LSY, Charles AM et al (1986) Bacterial Flora of the Eye and Contact Lens Cases during Hydrogel Lens Wear. Am J Optom Physiol Optics 63:177-180
4. Cohen S, Carpenter G (1975) Human Epidermal Growth Factor: Isolation and Chemical and Biological Properties. Proc Nat Acad Sci USA 72:1317-1321
5. Kandarakis A, Page C, Kaufman HE (1984) The Effect of Epidermal Growth Factor on Epithelial Healing After Penetrating Keratoplasty in Human Eyes. Am J Ophthalmol 98:411-415
6. Nishida T (1988) Role of Fibronectin in Corneal Epithelial Wound Healing. In: Cavanagh, HD (ed) The Cornea: Transactions of the World Congress on the Cornea III. Raven Press, New York pp.619-625
7. Ohashi Y, Motokura M, Kinoshita Y et al (1989) Presence of Epidermal Growth Factor in Human Tears. Invest Ophthalmol Vis Sci 30:1879-1882
8. Pesonen K, Viinikka L, Koskimies A et al (1987) Size Heterogenity of Epidermal Growth Factor in Human Body Fluids. Life Sci 40:2489-2494
9. Schultz GS, Davis JB, Eiferman RA (1988) Growth Factors and Corneal Epithelium. Cornea 7:96-101
10. Tervo T, Salonen EM, Vaheri A et al (1988) Elevation of Tear Fluid Plasmin in Corneal Disease. Acta Ophthalmol 66:393-399
11. Tervo T, van Setten GB (1989) Aprotinin for Inhibition of Plasmin on the Ocular Surface: Principles and Clinical Observations. In: Beuerman RW, Crosson CE, Kaufman HE (eds) Healing Processes of the Cornea. Portfolio Publ Co of Texas, The Woodlands pp.151-160
12. Tervo T, van Setten GB (1991) Plasmin-Like Activity in Tear Fluid and Contact Lens Wear.The Contact Lens J 19:142-152

13. van Haeringen NJ (1981) Clinical Biochemistry of Tears. Surv Ophthalmol 26:84-96
14. van Setten GB, Tervo T, Tarkkanen A et al (1989) Epidermal Growth Factor is a Constant Component of Normal Human Tear Fluid. Graefes Arch Clin Exp Ophthalmol 227:84-87
15. van Setten GB (1990) Epidermal Growth Factor in Human Tear Fluid: Increased Release but Decreased Concentrations during Reflex Tearing. Curr Eye Res 9:79-83
16. van Setten GB, Pesonen K, Tervo T et al (1991) Ocular Disease Leads to Decreased Concentrations of Epidermal Growth Factor in the Tear Fluid. Curr Eye Res 10:523-527
17. van Setten GB, Tervo T, Virtanen I et al (1990) Immunohistochemical Demonstration of Epidermal Growth Factor in the Lacrimal and Submandibular Glands of Rats. Acta Ophthalmol (Copenh) 68:477-480
18. van Setten GB, Tervo T, Andersson R et al (1990) Plasmin and Epidermal Growth Factor in the Tear Fluid of Contact Lens Wearers: Effect of Wearing Different Types of Contact Lenses and Association with Clinical Findings. Ophthalmic Res 22:233-240
19. Wilson SE, Lloyd SA, Kennedy RH (1991) Epidermal Growth Factor Messenger RNA Production in Human Lacrimal Gland. Cornea 10:519-524

Contact Lens-Associated Infections: Epidemiology and Therapeutic Considerations

Oliver D. Schein

Abstract. Contact lens use is now the leading risk factor for ulcerative keratitis in many centers. The increasing prevalence of this condition has paralleled the growth in the population of contact lens wearers, particularly hydrophilic daily and extended wear lens users. In the United States, it is estimated that ulcerative keratitis occurs at a rate of approximately one per 2500 users of soft daily wear and one per 300-500 extended wear soft lens users per year. Thus, in a given year in the United States, about 12000 cases of contact lens-associated ulcerative keratitis are anticipated.

The principal risk factors appear to be the extent of overnight use and microbial contamination of lens paraphernalia. Lesser risk factors include smoking and lens care frequency. Pseudomonas is the predominant bacterium, followed in frequency by staphylococcal and streptococcal species. Treatment centers on aggressive antibiotic treatment for these organisms, pending corneal culture results, and vigilance for recalcitrant infections caused by acanthamoeba or other unusual microorganisms.

Industry, practitioners and patients all have important roles to play in the prevention and early recognition of lens-associated ulcerative keratitis.

Introduction

In 1987, it was estimated that 18.2 million Americans wore contact lenses. Of these, approximately 5 million were estimated to be hard or gas-permeable, 9.1 million were daily-wear soft, and 4.1 million were extended-wear soft lens users (8). More recent estimates have approximated 23 million contact lens users in the United States. The overall proportions of lens use are similar with the exception of an ongoing reduction in the number of Polymethylmethacrylate (PMMA) lens users and a rising market share, perhaps 10 percent, of disposable contact lenses.

Contact lens use is associated with a broad range of adverse effects. However, with the exception of ulcerative keratitis, most of these adverse effects are transient, responding to simple discontinuation of lens use. The term "ulcerative keratitis" refers to an ulceration of the corneal epithelium with underlying inflammation of the corneal stroma. In the presence of contact lens use, this process is presumed to be microbial and is usually bacterial. Before the explosion of contact lenses in the 1970s and 1980s, ulcerative keratitis occurred almost exclusively in the context of trauma or concomitant disease of the ocular surface. However, recent case series have shown that contact lenses have been associated with approximately 30 to 66 percent of all cases of ulcerative keratitis (1,2,4,12,15).

Pathophysiology and Microbiology

The most common bacterium isolated from the cornea in contact lens-associated microbial keratitis is pseudomonas aeruginosa (1,2,4,12,15). As will be discussed later in relation to treatment, awareness of the likelihood of this virulent organism should guide initial therapy for contact lens-associated keratitis. A wide variety of other organisms has been associated with this condition. Most commonly, staphylococcal species, both coagulase positive and negative, and various streptococci predominate. Additionally, a host of other Gram-negative bacilli, particularly other pseudomonas, serratia, and klebsiella species may be found. Fungal infection in the setting of contact lens use is very rare. This condition occurs more frequently in the setting of therapeutic contact lens use where chronic ocular surface disease and frequent corticosteroid use are concomitant. Vigilance for Acanthamoeba, with its unique clinical presentation, must also be maintained, despite the rarity of this condition.

Although the pathophysiology of contact lens-related infection is still incompletely understood, it appears that this disease requires a series of events acting in concert. These events include contamination of the contact lens care system including the lens itself, the lens case, and solutions. Additionally, infection with the common organisms requires a break in the corneal epithelium. The corneal surface is altered by contact lens wear, especially overnight wear. Holden (9) has demonstrated that contact lens wear, particularly overnight wear, suppresses aerobic metabolism of the corneal epithelium which likely compromises the epithelial barrier to infection.

Mounting evidence implicates the contact lens care system, particularly the contact lens case, as an important repository for pathogenic organisms (5,6). Contact lens cases are routinely contaminated with pathogenic organisms including pseudomonas and acanthamoeba. Such contamination is found frequently in the paraphernalia of asymptomatic contact lens wearers. Such contamination has not been shown to differ with rigid versus soft lens use or with chemical versus heat disinfection. Additionally, organisms found in lens care systems and isolated from the cornea in cases of microbial keratitis have been documented to be identical. For example, Mayo (11) documented identical antibiograms, serotypes, and plasmid profiles of P.aeruginosa from the cornea and saline of five patients.

Also acting in concert to predispose to infection is the avidity with which bacteria adhere to contact lenses, particularly hydrophilic lenses. Such adherence occurs with both new and worn contact lenses. Adherence may be enhanced by the presence of lens deposits, although this remains unsettled (3,10).

Epidemiology

Microbial keratitis has been reported in association with all types of contact lenses including PMMA, rigid gas-permeable, soft, daily, extended wear, and disposable contact lens use.

The population at risk for infection has increased dramatically with the introduction of soft contact lenses. Over the past decade, reports and interest in contact lens-associated infections have increased substantially. Although the majority of infections associated with contact lenses are secondary to bacteria, the first controlled study of lens-associated ulcerative keratitis was published in 1987 on infections limited to acanthamoeba (17). This study firmly implicated the use of home-made saline in the pathogenesis of amoebic keratitis. Additionally, use of contact lenses while swimming and a low frequency of lens disinfection were also associated with this condition. No specific predilection for daily versus extended or hard versus soft lenses was found.

Institutional case series of patients with lens-associated keratitis from a variety of centers in the 1980s (1,2,12,15) confirmed the microbiology of this condition and pointed towards extended-wear lens use as a potential risk factor. The first controlled study was reported in 1989 (14). This multicenter, prospective study enrolled 99 patients from six centers. Eligible cases were limited to wearers of cosmetic soft contact lenses. A standardized definition required a corneal epithelial defect, underlying stromal infiltrate, performance of a corneal scraping for culture, treatment with topical antibiotics, and case verification by a corneal specialist. Both hospital-based and community-based control groups were used. Hospital-based controls were recruited from the same clinical sources as the case patients. Community controls were selected from matched households based on random digit dialing.

The risk of ulcerative keratitis was found to be approximately four times greater in extended-wear as compared with daily wear soft lens users when subjects were divided by type of lens worn. This estimate of relative risk was similar for both population-based and hospital-based comparisons. However, these relative risks were based only on the type of lens used without regard to how the lens was actually worn. Specifically,

38% of those in the control groups who used extended-wear lenses wore them only during the day, and 11% of those who used daily wear lenses wore them overnight at least once in the two-week period before their hospital visit or telephone interview. Tab.1 shows relative risk estimates of ulcerative keratitis by lens type and overnight use. For daily wear soft contact lens users, occasional overnight wear had 9 times the risk of ulcerative keratitis compared with strict daily wear users. Extended-wear lens users who used their lenses overnight incurred a 10- to 15-fold greater risk. Tab.2 illustrates the effect on risk of keratitis of the number of consecutive days that extended-wear lenses were worn before removal for cleaning. This risk increased substantially with increasing extent of overnight wear. This risk also increased incrementally for each night of additional use of daily wear lenses.

The frequency of lens cleaning, rinsing, disinfection, enzymatic treatment, and cleaning of the case were also examined. These individual behaviors were not found to significantly affect risk. A lens care index based on these parameters was generated in order to examine the overall effect of lens care hygiene. This lens care index approached significance in the population control group. Cigarette smoking was also found to be independently related to disease conferring a three- to four-fold increased risk.

These data strongly indicated that the overnight use of soft lenses was a principal risk factor for disease. Although an effect of lens care hygiene was found, this effect paled in comparison to actual overnight lens use as a risk factor. For hygiene-related measures, the evidence of a protective effect was strongest for lens case cleaning, supporting the growing clinical evidence that contamination of the lens case may be important in the pathogenesis of this condition.

A similar project in London was recently reported by Dart and coworkers (4). This group found the lowest rate of ulcerative keratitis among users of rigid gas-permeable lenses. Using this group as the reference, they found an increasing risk of ulcerative keratitis with PMMA (relative risk, 1.3), daily wear soft contact lenses (relative risk, 3.6), and extended-wear soft contact lenses (relative risk, 20.8). These relative risks are analogous to those found in the New England study. Although there was a trend towards increased risk, the available data did not statistically confirm a difference in relative risk between daily wear rigid gas-permeable and daily wear soft contact lens use. Of further interest is the finding that the study from London also failed to confirm a significant role for lens-care hygiene as a risk factor for disease.

These relative risks and risk factors are best reviewed within the context of a study of the absolute incidence of disease (13). This project was based on the population of approximately 9 million persons in the New England region of the United States. Over a four-month period, all incident cases of ulcerative keratitis associated with contact lenses were enumerated by the region's ophthalmologists. This count provided the numerator for the rate. Random digit dialing to over 4000 households within the study area ascertained the distribution of lens wear within the population. These proportions were then applied to the United States Census Bureau counts to generate a denominator for the incidence rate. Annualized rates are shown in Tab.3. The rates of disease among extended-wear soft lens users were significantly higher ($p < 0.00001$) compared with daily wear soft lens users. The rate ratio of approximately 5 to 1 was consistent with the case-control study when risk was calculated strictly by lens type.

One may extrapolate by projecting incidence rate for the United States based on this study, with the understanding that this extrapolation assumes equal rates geographically and throughout the year. Such estimates approximate that 4000 daily wear lens users and 8000 extended-wear soft lens users will develop ulcerative keratitis annually in the United States. Additionally, one may estimate that strict daily wear use of soft lenses carries an incidence rate of approximately 2 to 3 per 10000 wearers per year whereas extended-wear lens users with overnight use have an incidence of approximately 20 to 30 per 10000.

The same data base was used to estimate risk of ulcerative keratitis for aphakic contact lens users (7). These rates are summarized in Tab.4. These rates are approximately 5 to 10 times the risk for cosmetic lens use. In particular, the risk of ulcerative keratitis for extended-wear soft aphakic contact lenses of approximately one in 80 per year is clinically quite significant and may serve to place in perspective the risk of secondary intraocular lens implantation or other surgical methods for correction of aphakia.

Clinical Presentation

Initial signs and symptoms of bacterial keratitis associated with contact lenses are nonspecific and resemble contact lens-induced abrasions. These findings include pain, reduced acuity, erythema, and photophobia. Contact lens practitioners should educate their patients to remove the lens and seek ophthalmologic consultation promptly for such symptoms. The keratitis associated with microbial infection characteristically involves a corneal epithelial defect with underlying stromal suppuration. These findings may occur anywhere on the cornea and be of any size.

Sterile infiltrates are known to occur with contact lens use, particularly with extended-wear lenses, and may represent an immunologic phenomenon, corneal hypoxia, or perhaps even the initial process predisposing to microbial keratitis. These sterile infiltrates typically do not involve an ulceration of the corneal epithelium. In the setting of contact lens use, any corneal infiltrate with an overlying epithelial defect should be considered microbial. Additionally, the infection should be considered to be caused by P.aeruginosa until proven otherwise.

Appropriate documentation includes a measurement of the size and depth of the infiltrate and its location in relation to the pupil and the limbus. Infections involving the sclera characteristically have a very poor prognosis.

Laboratory Diagnosis

Corneal scrapings for culture and microscopy should be performed using standard techniques. A Gram stain may also be helpful in guiding initial therapy. As previously discussed, P. aeruginosa is the most frequently isolated bacterium in the setting. This species is followed in frequency by staphylococci and streptococci. Consequently, initial antimicrobial therapy pending culture results should be tailored to cover these organisms.

Vigilance must also be maintained for the possibility of acanthamoeba or fungal keratitis, although these conditions comprise only a minor fraction of contact-lens related cases of ulcerative keratitis. Early recognition of acanthamoeba depends on a high index of suspicion. Raised epithelial lines, radial keratoneuritis, and ring infiltration should raise the possibility of an acanthamoeba infection. This diagnosis must be considered as well if a history of homemade saline use or a history of swimming with contact lenses in place is elicited. Once suspected, special stains (e.g. Calcofluor white) and culture media (E.coli-plated non-nutrient agar) should be used. Additionally, in the evaluation of lens-associated keratitis, whether bacteria or amoeba are suspected, it may frequently be helpful to confiscate patients' contact lens cases and solutions so that these may be cultured as well.

Treatment

The standard treatment for many years has been intensive topical treatment with fortified antibiotic drops, typically a first-generation cephalosporin and an aminoglycoside. For significant keratitis in the setting of contact lens use, one may presume the presence of pseudomonas and add Ticarcillin or Piperacillin (6mg per ml) empirically pending culture results. The advent of topical quinolone antibiotics may result in a gradual shift towards use of these agents in place of the current standard. However, a comparative study has yet to be performed.

Subconjunctival delivery affords no advantage over topical treatment.

Corticosteroids are not indicated for early treatment but should await clinical conviction that the primary infection has been contained and the cornea rendered sterile. At that junction, topical corticosteroids may favorably modify the host response to limit scarring. The principles of management of lens-associated ulcerative keratitis do not differ significantly from the management of keratitis associated with other predisposing factors. These management and therapeutic issues are discussed in detail in separate chapters.

Conclusion

Although contact lens use is certainly safe for the majority of users, the enormous size of the population at risk for keratitis mandates a careful consideration of factors predisposing to disease. This is particularly true since these eyes are otherwise healthy and alternative methods for refractive correction exist.

There are many questions yet unanswered about the epidemiology and risk factors for this disease. However, available knowledge does pinpoint a number of areas that may be exploited to reduce the incidence of disease. Based on the studies from New England described earlier, the Food and Drug Administration in the United States tightened its restriction on approval of extended-wear lenses from 30 to 7 days. Given that overnight wear appears to be the strongest predictor of ulcerative keratitis, this should reduce the incidence of disease. Some, however, feel that 7 days may still be too long (16). Increasing evidence has pointed to the lens case as a source of potential contamination (18). It is appropriate to begin to consider strategies directed at this possible source of infection. It is insufficient and inaccurate simply to blame lens users for inadequate hygiene since there is ample evidence that the majority of contact lens wearers (i.e. those not developing disease) do not follow recommended schedules either. Additionally, the only controlled studies to date (4,14) have failed to support hygiene as a major risk factor.

Limiting overnight use is therefore likely to be the best method at present to lower the incidence of disease. Future efforts directed at maintaining sterility of contact lens cases may prove to be helpful. This may be a more fruitful method of controlling the source of bacterial inoculum than attempting to modify bacterial adherence to the lens.

Although such methods of primary prevention are always preferable, it is also worthwhile to educate not only patients but general medical practitioners (who are frequently the first to see such patients) about the risk of ulcerative keratitis. Prompt removal of the contact lens for acute symptoms, prompt presentation, and early treatment will limit the extent of the disease once initiated.

Table 1. Estimated relative risks of ulcerative keratitis according to lens type and level of overnight use as compared with daily wear lenses not worn over night

Lens type and Overnight Use	Relative Risk (95% CI)[1] Case Patients vs Population-Based Controls	Case Patients vs Hospital-Based Controls
Daily wear		
No overnight use	1.00[2]	1.00[2]
Overnight use	8.96 (4.09-19.63)	9.55 (2.87-31.80)
P value	0.0001	0.0002
Extended-wear		
No overnight use	2.76 (1.06- 7.20)	2.57 (0.70- 9.51)
P value	0.038	0.156
Overnight use	10.17 (5.29-19.55)	15.04 (5.21-43.43)
P value	0.0001	0.0001

1 CI denotes confidence interval.
2 By definition, because risks are relative to the risk for daily wear lenses with no overnight use.

Table 2. Relative risks of ulcerative keratitis for extended-wear lenses as compared with daily wear lenses not worn overnight, according to the number of consecutive days extended-wear lenses are worn

Days[1]	Relative Risk (95% CI)[2] Case Patients vs Population-Based Controls	Case Patients vs Hospital-Based Controls
1	3.6 (1.3-9.7)	2.4 (0.7-0.9)
2-7	6.8 (3.3-14.0)	10.0 (3.1-31.9)
8-14	11.8 (4.7-30.0)	37.9 (3.4-423.2)
≥15	14.5 (5.6-37.9)	45.0 (4.3-467.3)

1 Value indicates number of consecutive days the lense were worn before cleaning
2 CI denotes confidence interval

Table 3. Estimated annualized incidence of ulcerative keratitis per 10000 cosmetic wearers and estimated relative risk of ulcerative keratitis[1]

Type of Lens	Incidence of Ulcerative Keratitis	Relative Risk[2]
Daily wear soft	4.1 (2.9-5.2)	1.00[3]
Extended-wear soft	20.9 (15.1-26.7)	5.15 (3.47-7.65)
Hard	2.0 (0 - 4.4)	0.50 (0.15-1.65)
Rigid gas-permeable	4.0 (0 - 8.2)	1.00 (0.34-2.89)

1 The figures in parentheses are 95 percent confidence intervals.
2 The risk shown is relative to the risk when using daily wear lenses.
3 The relative risk is by definition 1.00.

Table 4. Estimated prevalence of the use of specific lens types for aphakic correction and estimated incidence of ulcerative keratitis by lens type

Type of Lens for Aphakic Correction	Incidence of Ulcerative Keratitis (95% Confidence Interval)[1]
All lenses	52.0 (31.1-86.9)
Daily wear soft	25.9 (8.0-83.3)
Extended-wear soft	181.0 (75.1-436.5)
Hard	9.1 (2.2-37.7)
Rigid gas-permeable	11.3 (1.3-100.0)

1 Estimated annual incidence per 10,000 aphakic persons using this lens type

References

1. Adams CP, Cohen EJ, Laibson PR et al (1983) Corneal Ulcers in Patients with Cosmetic Extended-Wear Contact Lenses. Am J Ophthalmol 96:705-709
2. Alfonso E, Mandelbaum S, Fox MJ et al (1986) Ulcerative Keratitis Associated with Contact Lens Wear. Am J Ophthalmol 101:429-433
3. Dart JK, Badenoch PR (1986) Bacterial Adherence to Contact Lenses. CLAO J 12:220-224
4. Dart JK, Stapleton F, Minassian D (1991) Contact Lenses and Other Risk Factors in Microbial Keratitis. Lancet 338:650-653
5. Donzis PB, Mondino BJ, Weissman BA et al (1989) Microbial Analysis of Contact Lens Care Systems Contaminated with Acanthamoeba. Am J Ophthalmol 108:53-56
6. Donzis PB, Mondino BJ, Weissman BA et al (1987) Microbial Contamination of Contact Lens Care Systems. Am J Ophthalmol 104:325-333
7. Glynn RJ, Schein OD, Seddon JM et al (1991) The Incidence of Ulcerative Keratitis Among Aphakic Contact Lens Wearers in New England. Arch Ophthalmol 109:104-107
8. Herman CL (1987) An FDA Survey of U.S. Contact Lens Wearers. Contact Lens Spectrum 2:89-92.
9. Holden BA, Sweeney DF, Vannas A et al (1985) Effects of Long-Term Extended Contact Lens Wear on the Human Cornea. Invest Ophthalmol Vis Sci 26:1489-1501
10. Lawin-Brüssel CA, Refojo MF, Leong FL et al (1989) Pseudomonas Attachment to Various New and Worn Hydrogen Soft Contact Lenses. Sixteenth Cornea Research Conference September 23, p.41
11. Mayo MS, Cook WL, Schlitzer RL et al (1986) Antibiograms, Serotypes and Plasmid Profiles of Pseudomonas Aeruginosa Associated Corneal Ulcers and Contact Lens Wear. J Clin Microbiol 24:372-376
12. Ormerod LD, Smith RE (1986) Contact Lens-Associated Microbial Keratitis. Arch Ophthalmol 104:79-83
13. Poggio EC, Glynn RJ, Schein OD et al (1989) The Incidence of Ulcerative Keratitis Among Users of Daily Wear and Extended-Wear Soft Contact Lenses. New Engl J Med 321:779-783
14. Schein OD, Glynn RJ, Poggio EC et al (1989) The Relative Risk of Ulcerative Keratitis Among Users of Daily-Wear and Extended-Wear Soft Contact Lenses: A Case-Control Study. New Engl J Med 321:773-778
15. Schein OD, Ormerod LD, Barraquer E et al (1989) Microbiology of Contact Lens-Related Keratitis. Cornea 8:281-285
16. Smith RE, MacRae SM (1989) Contact Lenses - Convenience and Complications. New Engl J Med 321:824-826
17. Stehr-Green JK, Bailey TM, Brandt FH et al (1987) Acanthamoeba Keratitis in Soft Contact Lens Wearers. A Case-Control Study. J Am Med Ass 258:57-60
18. Wilson LA, Sawant AD, Ahearn DG (1991) Comparative Efficacies of Soft Contact Lens Disinfectant Solutions Against Microbial Films in Lens Cases. Arch Ophthalmol 109:1155-1157

Contact-Lens-Associated Infections: Clinical Features

H.W. Roth

Abstract. Severe corneal and conjunctival inflammations are the most common and most complicated side-effects of contact lens wear.
Data have revealed that the primary cause of these complications has been a lack in daily lens handling and disinfection and overwearing of the lenses. Besides, contact lenses are irritating chronic foreign bodies prediposing to infections.
The microbial spectrum of contact-lens related infections primarily involves pseudomonas, staphylococci, pneumococci and hemophilus suggesting a distinctly different microbial pattern than in non-wearers.
Careful patient selection, counseling and regular check-ups may decrease the high risk of infection.

Introduction

Contact lens wearers are prone to ocular infections compared to persons who do not use lenses. According to recent studies, contact lens wearers experience infections of the anterior segment approximately four times as frequent as wearers of glasses, and the factor by which a corneal ulcer is seen approximates 310x (6). Therefore, the question arises as to why infections of the anterior segment of the eye are facilitated by the use of contact lenses.

Data of 1920 wearers of contact lenses have been evaluated at our institution from 1981 to 1991 exhibiting signs of a bacterial infection of the lids, conjunctiva or cornea. Data of the etiologic spectrum and incidence of are listed in Tab.1. This overview demonstrates that any contact lens, whether hard or soft will compromise the normal physiology and immunologic defense mechanisms of the anterior segment of the eye and may therefore represent a risk factor for the development of infections of the lids, conjunctiva and cornea.

Epithelial Defects

Due to the mechanical actions, 57% of all patients suffered from an epithelial lesion of the cornea or conjunctiva before they developed overt infectious disease. On the one hand, the constant movement of the lens during blinking and eye motility had been the mechanical reason for superficial epithelial defects. With longer worn contact lenses, scratches, deposits and tears in the surface of the lens and marginal defects resulting in conjunctival and corneal lesions can be shown (Fig.1). Demarcated corneal epithelial lesions may be observed when a foreign body accidentally moves between the lens and the cornea. Overwearing also results in destruction of the corneal epithelium (Fig.2)(5). As the corneal sensitivity decreases during contact lens wear, any lesion of the anterior segment of the eye resulting from bad contact lenses or foreign bodies will only be detected late. This is also true for infections, since the hallmark of pain is missing and the patient presents to an Ophthalmologist late in the course of the disease.

Cleaning

Hygienic deficiencies in lens cleansing have been documented in up to 48% of all infections. Insufficient elimination of those deposits on the lens surface, which can also be seen in routine check-ups of contact lens wearers, has been a most frequent finding. Regular daily cleansing of the lens, however, is mandatory in order to eliminate deposits due to proteins or lipids of the tear film, foreign bodies and desquamated conjunctival and corneal epithelium. These deposits have been shown to be an ideal medium for pathogenic bacteria (3,4). For example, the contact lens of a 25 year old myopic patient presenting with bilateral blurred vision and recurrent bacterial conjunctival infections is demonstrated in Fig.3. As seen in the picture, the surface of the lens is covered almost completely with organic material, a fact that resulted in decreased visual acuity, photophobia and mechanical destruction of the superficial layers of the cornea and conjunctiva with a subsequent keratoconjunctivitis.

Incorrect Hygienic Measures

In 35% of the cases evaluated, faulty disinfection of the lens had been etiologic for the transmission of pathogenic agents to the eye. Another study has shown that a large percentage of contact lens wearers do not disinfect their lenses properly or totally omit cleansing (4), a fact reflected by the finding of 13% contaminated storage vessels during a routine screening in asymptomatic lens wearers. In all of the patients reporting to have carefully cleansed and disinfected their lenses, smears were taken from the disinfecting solution, the conjunctiva and the storage solution in order to evaluate for the antimicrobial effects of the disinfecting/storage solutions. In all of those cases with an isolation of identical organisms, sensitivity patterns were established using the solutions. All of these studies resulted in no growth of organisms in the presence of disinfecting/storage solutions. Thus it may be stated that many patients do not adhere to contact lens care guidelines obviously resulting in a higher incidence of infection (10).

Compromised Tear Secretion

Another reason for the high incidence of infections in 25% of contact lens wearers are qualitative and quantitative deficiencies of lacrimal secretion. Thus, it has been estimated that 5% of all complications in contact lens wearers may have been due to a relative lack of tears (11). An explanation for this deficit may be the increased need of wetting: a soft contact lens, as for example an aphakic lens with a water content of 65% will need one gram per day for maintenance of elasticity. Hard contact lenses need a certain amount of tears to avoid corneal lesions during wearing. Dry eyes facilitate infections - a circumstance that may become a problem particularly in elderly patients (2).

Local Immunologic Factors

In 25% of all patients wearing contact lenses who presented with a bacterial infection of the anterior segment of the eye, defense mechanisms were compromised (7). Primarily, giganto-papillary conjunctivitis, a disease with an increasing incidence in recent years has been found to be associated with contact lens wear related compromised immune reactions (1). The etiopathogenesis has been elucidated: Resulting from denatured tear film proteins by cleansing and storage solutions deposits on the surface of the lens may become immunogenic and elicit an antigen-antibody reaction. These antibodies may cover protein deposits on the surface of the contact lens and result in a mechanical as well as immunological decompensation of the tarsal conjunctiva with an ensuing papillary reaction. The respective typical morphology is shown in Fig.4.

Systemic immunocompromising diseases may also facilitate an infection of the anterior segment of the eye (12). In a study of 84 contact lens wearers we have found diabetes mellitus, leukemia and the acquired immunodeficiency syndrome predisposing factors for the development of corneal ulcers (6). During influenza or other acute infections at distant sites even smaller pertubations of the immune system may be associated with the development of infections in contact lens wearers (6).

Oxygen Deficit

Lack of corneal oxygen supply in contact lens wear is a further facilitating factor for infections (11). Studies using microachymetry have revealed that wear of any contact lens is associated with a certain lack of oxygen supply to the cornea, e.g. metabolic acidosis resulting in stromal edema. Any hard or soft contact lens will compromise the fluxes of the precorneal tear film; the extent to which damage is done depends on the form of the lens, the physical characteristics of the material and the oxygen permeability (DK) as well as the technique of fitting. Thus, misfits have been observed in 15% of patients suffering from infections in our study. Although oxygen permeability of modern plastics has been increased considerably, a quick decrease due to aging of the material and contamination of the lens surface can be stated when in use. In our study, long-term use of contact lenses of more than two years has been found associated with 81% of all infectious complications occurring with contact lens wear. A tight-lens syndrome being a typical complication of hydrophilic extended-wear soft contact lenses was associated with P.aeruginosa infections in 90% of bacterial keratitis, and in 18% of corneal ulcers (5).

Bacteria

In 92% of all cases of contact lens wear-related anterior segment infections pseudomonas, pneumococci, staphylococci and hemophilus were found (Fig.5,6). These organisms were detected in only 22% of a control population comprising 200 patients with anterior segement infections and no history of contact lens wear (8). Thus, it may be proposed that a shift in the spectrum of microbial colonization occurring with contact lens wear may be due to decreased defense mechanisms and oxygen supply. This may possibly be related to the contamination of cleansing/storage solutions, use of preservative-containing wetting ointments and the increased temperature of the anterior surface of the lens-wearing eye.

Conclusions

Published data show a comparably higher incidence of bacterial infections of the anterior segment of the eye in contact lens wearers than in non-weareres. Contact lenses are chronic foreign body inoculations causing alterations, which are mechanical, metabolic, microbiologic and immunologic in nature. Infections are facilitated by

- lack of proper hygiene and care of contact lenses,
- lack of awareness for substitution of old lenses,
- epithelial lesions and
- overwearing (Tab.2).

Therefore, further risks of infection must be excluded when fitting. No patients with acute or chronic anterior segment infections should be fitted. Patients suffering from immunocompromising diseases or diabetes should only be fitted after all other means of visual rehabilitation have been evaluated (3). Contraindications for fitting are

- chronic and recurrent infections (blepharoconjunctivitis, hordeyolosis, dacryocystitis, tear film deficiencies),
- non-compliance for adequate hygiene,
- non-compliance for proper handling and
- non-compliance for limited wearing.

This patient group is at the highest risk for severe infections and must be excluded from contact lens wear.

Table 1. Etiology of contact-lens wear related infections (n=1920)

Etiology	Incidence (%)[1]
Distinct microbial spectrum	92%
Epithelial defects	57%
Lack of proper cleansing	48%
Lack of proper disinfection	35%
Impaired tear film	25%
Immunocompromising disease	21%
Lack of adequate oxygen supply	15%

[1] more than one etiology possible

Table 2. Etiology of corneal ulcers during contact-lens wear

- compromised materials
- corneal epithelial defects/erosions
- lack of adequate cleansing or disinfection
- lack of proper handling
- overwearing
- deposits
- aging of materials
- underlying ocular disease
- underlying systemic compromising disease

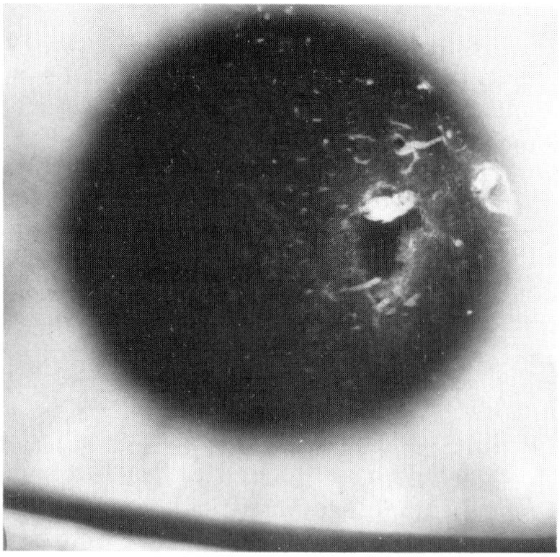

Fig.1. Paracentral deep corneal erosion due to improper handling of a hard contact lens.

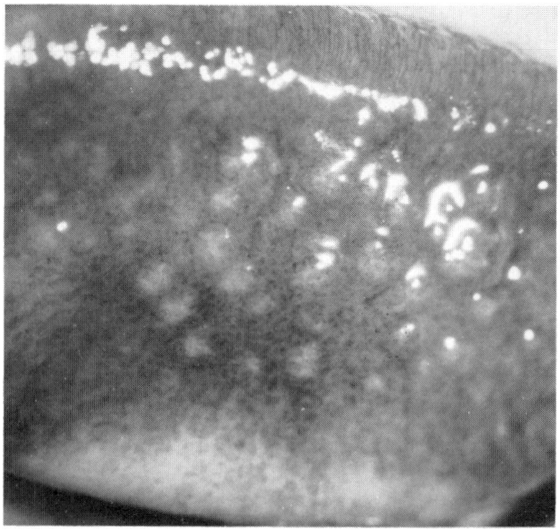

Fig.3. Gigantopapillary conjunctivitis due to a soft contact lens some months in use.

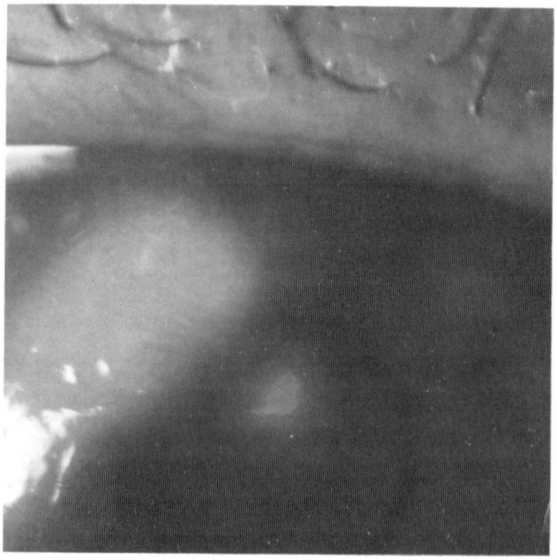

Fig.2. Corneal erosion and bullous epithelial lesions in overwear (contact lens wear during night sleep).

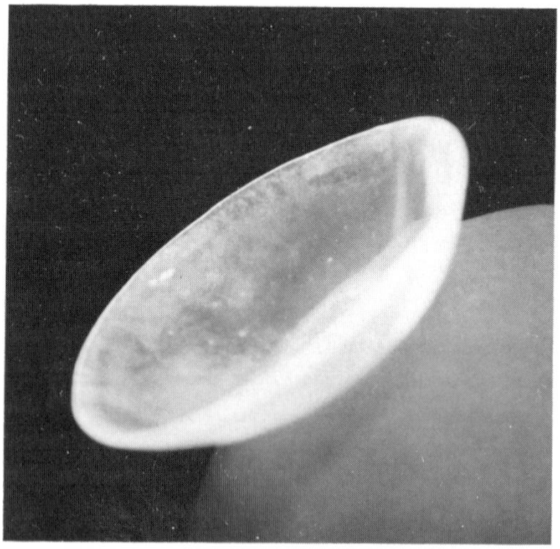

Fig.4. Inadequately cleaned soft contact lens. Staining with fluorescein factilitates visualization of deposits.

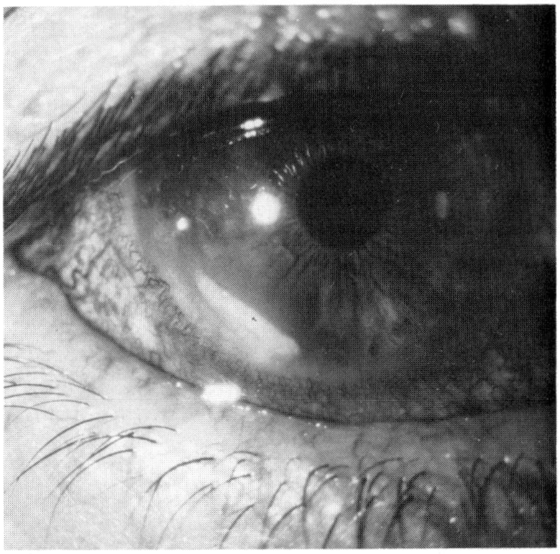

Fig.5. Corneal marginal ulcer after hard contact lens wear.

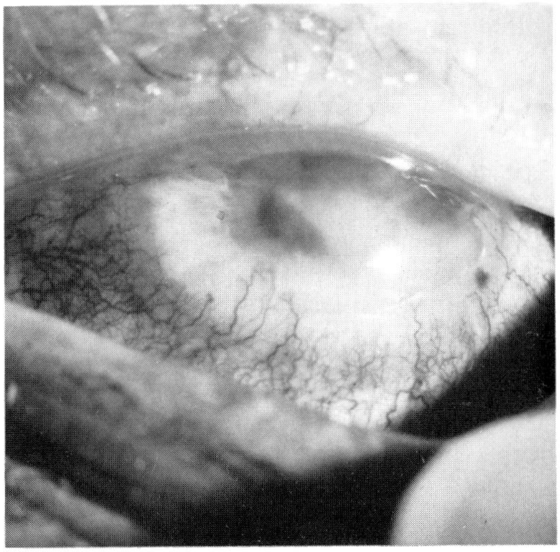

Fig.6. Central corneal ulcer after soft contact lens wear.

References

1. Allansmith MR, Korb DR, Greiner JV (1977) Giant papillary Conjunctivitis in Contact Lens Wearers. Am J Ophthalmol 83:697-700
2. Marquardt R, Lemp MA (1991) Das trockene Auge in Klinik und Praxis. Springer-Verlag, Heidelberg
3. Neuhann T, Blassmann K, Roth HW (1978) Pilzwachstum auf weichen Kontaktlinsen. Klin Mbl Augenheilk 73:648-653
4. Roth HW (1978) The Etiology of Ocular Irritation in Soft Lens Wearers: Distribution in a Large Clinical Sample. Contact and Intraocular Lens Medical J 2:38-47
5. Roth HW (1986) Das Tight-Lens Syndrom: Weitere Untersuchungen zur Ätiologie und Pathogenese. Contactologia 8:49-56
6. Roth HW (1990) Zur Ätiologie und Pathogenese des Hornhautulkus beim Kontaktlinsenträger. Contactologia 12:110-114
7. Roth HW (1991) Untersuchungen zur Ätiologie und Therapie der gigantopapillären Konjunktivitis beim Kontaktlinsenträger. Contactologia 13:112-116
8. Roth HW (to be published) Micropachometry of Normal, Diseased and Contact Lens Wearing Eyes. German J Ophthalmol
9. Roth HW, Leimbeck R, Anger CB et al (to be published) Zum antibakteriellen Wirkungsspektrum von Sulfacetamid. Klin Mbl Augenheilk
10. Vegh M, Nagy E, Matyi A (1988) Der klinische Fall: Hornhautulkus bei weichen Kontaktlinsen. Contactologia 10:194-195
11. Weinstock F (1990) Kontaktlinsenanpassung in der Klinik und Praxis. G.Fischer Verlag, Stuttgart
12. Wilson LA, Schlitzer L, Ahearn DG (1981) Pseudomonas Corneal Ulcers Associated with Soft Lens Wear. Am J Ophthalmol 82:546-554

Laboratory Diagnosis of Acanthamoeba Infections of the Cornea

H.M. Seitz

Abstract. Acanthamoebae are free-living protozoans with an ability for invasiveness. Reports on corneal involvement are getting more frequent. Many details of location, cycle, epidemiologic facts and the modes of infection are still unknown.
A survey on the parasitology of acanthamoebae will be provided as an introduction to the clinically oriented papers.

Introduction

According to our experience Acanthamoeba infections of the cornea can be diagnosed in two ways: by direct smear and microscopical examination or by culture. If possible, both methods should be used in parallel, since they supplement each other. In case that only very little material is available, culture is preferred.

Direct smear

Material scraped from the corneal lesion is smeared on a glass slide, dried, fixed in pure methanol, and stained with Giemsa working solution in the usual way. Principally, it is easy to distinguish Acanthamoeba from corneal cells: The conspicuous karyosome and the vacuoles within the amoebic cytoplasm identify the parasite cell. Certainly, it is difficult to find acanthamoebae if only few are present.

Culture

A number of media has been proposed for the culture of Acanthamoeba. We prefer a routine agar plate seeded evenly with bacteria, preferably Escherichia coli. Even plates taken from routine bacteriological diagnostics may be used if it takes too long to prepare them specifically. The specimen is placed on the agar. The Petri dish is kept at 26°C and examined daily under a microscope (preferably an inverted microscope) (Fig.1). Usually, acanthamoebae appear within one or two days, migrating out from the specimen to the periphery. If the amoebae multiply fast, the bacterial sheet is destroyed and a clear zone develops around the place where the specimen was introduced (Fig.3).

Beginning approximately at the fifth day of culture, vast numbers of cysts may appear in the plates. The cysts show the typical shape with a wrinkled cyst wall (Fig.2).

Sometimes the acanthamoebae or the cysts can be found in histological preparations from corneal tissue. The cysts can be embedded in the stroma without any inflammatory reaction in the surrounding tissue. No special stains are required for identification. A routine hematoxylin-eosin stain will be sufficient. Differentiation of the Acanth-amoeba species may be accomplished by immune peroxydase staining if specific sera are available.

Specimens and cultures with Acanthamoeba are potentially dangerous materials and should be handled with care. By some authors the use of safety cabinets and surgical masks is recommended together with the usual gloves and gowns.

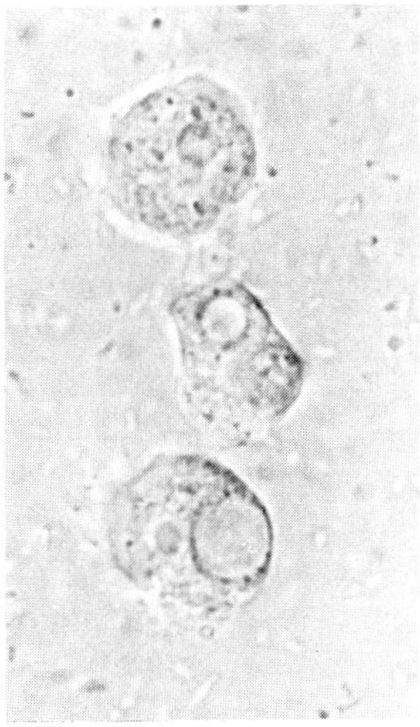

Fig.1. Acanthamoeba spec. Three trophozoites in a culture originating from scrapings of a corneal ulcer. The contractile vacuoles and the large karyosome are characteristic.

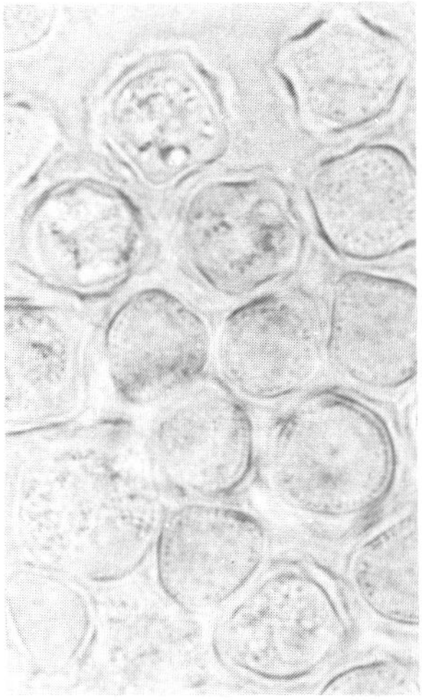

Fig.2. Acanthamoeba spec. A number of cysts in the same culture, but one week later. Note the wrinkled cyst walls.

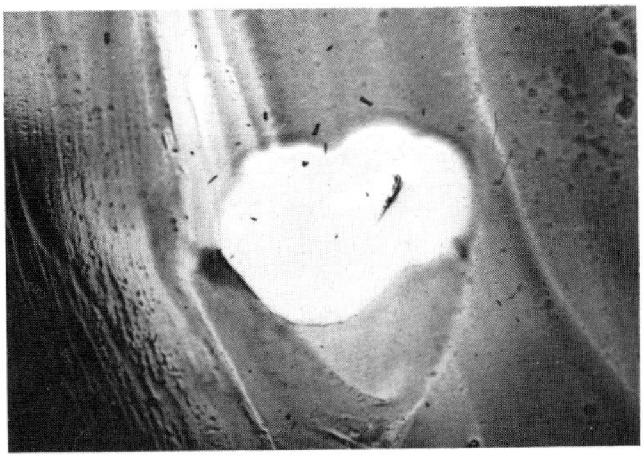

Fig.3. Agar plate covered with a carpet of Escherichia coli. The plate was inoculated with scrapings from a corneal ulcer. The developing amoebas have eaten away the bacteria, a clear zone around the application place of the material results.

References

1. Martinez AJ (1985) Free Living Amebas. CRC Press Inc, Boca Raton

Acanthamoeba Keratitis

James P. McCulley, Hassan Alizadeh, Jerry Y. Niederkorn

Abstract. Acanthamoeba keratitis has been found to be frequently associated with contact lens wear of all types with the consistent

factor being exposure to contaminated contact lens solutions or exposure to contaminated water sources. Our laboratory has extensively evaluated contact lens preservatives and care systems and found that some of the commercially available solutions are effective in killing trophozoites and cysts, whereas others are not; e.g. hydrogen peroxide, chlorhexidine, benzalkonium chloride, thiomersal and Polyaminopropyl biguanide effective, whereas ascorbates and quaternary ammonium products are not.
A combination of Brolene and Neomycin has been shown to be an effective therapy in many patients with this disease process. In an ongoing multicenter national trial in the United States, we are finding that treatment failure is not uncommonly being reported largely because of poor understanding of the course of this disease under therapy rather than medication failure.
In order to be able to evaluate risk factors for infection as well as therapy more effectively, it would be most helpful to have an animal model. To this end, we have evaluated corneas from multiple species in vitro for their ability to have Acanthamoeba attach to and penetrate the epithelial surface. We have found that in addition to human corneas, pig corneas are susceptible to infection. We have proceeded to develop an in vivo pig animal model of Acanthamoeba keratitis that parallels the disease process in man and that should allow us to understand and develop better therapy for this disease.

Introduction

Acanthamoeba keratitis is an uncommon, but devastating ocular infection that has become increasingly prevalent in recent years.

The first cases were diagnosed in the early 1970's with very few cases being recognized until approximately 1985, at which time the apparent incidence increased dramatically. The incidence remained at the increased levels through 1989.

It is no longer a reportable condition in the United States; therefore, we do not have data on current prevalence, however; it is the impression of many who deal with these patients that the prevalence has been declining. The most likely reasons for the initial increase in prevalence was multifactorial including: increased awareness by practitioners, increased numbers of contact lens wearers, insufficient instruction on lens care to contact lens wearers, ease of obtaining contact lenses without proper instruction and supervision, rapid diagnostic tests to confirm the diagnosis in those thought to have Acanthamoeba keratitis, and correct diagnosis of previous cases that had been misdiagnosed as Herpes simplex virus keratitis.

History

There are a number of characteristics of patients with Acanthamoeba keratitis that should be kept in mind, and that will in turn assist in making a timely correct diagnosis.

The patients are typically young, healthy individuals, who frequently are contact lens wearers (9). The most commonly infected contact lens wearers are those who are daily soft contact lens patients. Another frequently found association in the past was the use of nonpreserved saline made from bottled distilled water and salt tablets. These patients typically gave no antecedent eye trauma or surgery.

Fortunately, the disease most frequently is unilateral; however, bilateral cases have been diagnosed.

One of the most important features of the disease is that patients have severe pain far out of proportion to the clinical signs, at least in the early phases of the infection.

The earliest changes, if the patient is seen during this phase by an ophthalmologist, are characterized by mottled dendritiform epithelial defects. The corneal stroma can be involved in a variety of ways, which will be described subsequently. A characteristic form of stromal involvement that occurs later in the disease process is that of corneal ring infiltrate, which may or may not have overlying recurrent epithelial breakdown. A sign that is thought to be pathognomonic at this time is that of a radial corneal neuritis. Several of the more important of these findings will be discussed in greater detail.

There are several important risk factors associated with Acanthamoeba keratitis, with the vast majority of patients having at least one of these factors identifiable.

Exposure to contaminated water or soil has been found in a small number of patients with the largest number of patients having been contact lens wearers (10). No type of contact lens has been excluded from the association with Acanthamoeba keratitis. Daily wear soft contact lens patients in our series accounted for 75% of the patients, extended wear soft contact lens patients 14%, hard contact lens 6%, rigid gas permeable lenses 4%, and combined hardsoft lens wearers 1% (13).

We previously reported that Acanthamoeba did not adhere to unworn contact lenses (15); however, more recently we have found that Acanthamoeba will adhere not only to worn, but new contact lenses of all types (5, and unpublished data). The association with contact lenses would appear to be that the contact lens serves as a carrier for Acanthamoeba if it becomes exposed to the organism.

We have found that the common factor is exposure of contact lenses to contaminated fluids. In our series, 62% of the patients made saline at home using distilled water and salt tablets. We were unable to culture Acanthamoeba from distilled water as it was being purchased; however, we were able to culture bacteria from such water, as it is not required by law to be sterile and completely free of bacteria. We therefore, assume that the distilled water becomes contaminated over time with repeated use while making homemade saline.

The next most frequently associated fluid was that of tap water, with 16% of the patients apparently contaminating their contact lenses in this manner. It is well known that Acanthamoeba is a ubiquitous organism, and that it is frequently found in tap water around the world.

We have observed a limited association of Acanthamoeba keratitis with contamination from saliva, intravenous saline, and non-preserved bottled saline (10).

Therefore, it would seem that any contact lens is a potential carrier of Acanthamoeba to the ocular surface after being exposed to a contaminated fluid source.

It is not known whether an epithelial defect is required for invasion into the cornea for Acanthamoeba; however, we have shown that Acanthamoeba can adhere to and penetrate intact human corneal epithelium (16,23). It is, therefore, recommended that any patient who is a contact lens wearer who presents with keratitis be considered as potentially having Acanthamoeba keratitis. This should especially be true if there are other factors in the history such as the use of distilled water and salt tablets to make homemade saline, and excessive pain, relative to the clinical appearance of the cornea.

Diagnosis

Confirmatory laboratory tests are important in the diagnosis of Acanthamoeba keratitis. This is especially important considering the very long treatment that is required for patients with Acanthamoeba keratitis. It is, therefore, important to establish the accuracy of the initial diagnosis.

A number of diagnostic tests are available. The ones that we most frequently use include culturing of the specimen on a confluent lawn of Escherichia coli plated on non-nutrient agar. The E.coli serve as a food source for Acanthamoeba which will in effect produce identifiable tracks through the bacteria. The E.coli will not fill in these tracks, since the bacteria are plated on non-nutrient agar. Other methods of culturing the organism have been suggested, such as various types of blood agar; however, we find these to be more difficult to interpret and to be less reliable.

Scrapings of active lesions can be stained with either Giemsa or Wright stain and observed microscopically. It is possible to recognize both trophozoites and cysts in this manner. One can also stain the specimens with Calcofluor white, which stains the wall of cysts, but not trophozoites (18). This is an excellent stain, but requires access to a fluorescent microscope.

If there are no active epithelial lesions, but there are accessible stromal lesions, a biopsy is recommended. The biopsy specimens can be stained with hematoxylin and eosin, Calcofluor white, or be exposed to fluorescein labeled antibodies directed against Acanthamoeba. The latter two approaches require access to a fluorescent microscope for effective observation. It is much easier to recognize the characteristic cysts, as they are double walled, with the inner wall having a variety of polygonal shapes, depending on the species of the organism. Trophozoites can be somewhat more difficult for the untrained observer to identify unequivocally as the cysts can be confused with other cellular forms.

The diagnosis of Acanthamoeba keratitis is aided by a high degree of suspicion on the part of the ophthalmologist, as well as several characteristic clinical appearances that may or may not be present.

Acanthamoeba can mimic a number of types of keratitis. In the past, it most frequently was misdiagnosed as Herpes simplex virus keratitis because of the recurrent epithelial breakdown that not uncommonly was in a dendritiform pattern. Cultures taken from these lesions also showed apparent plaque forming units on cellular tissue culture plates. Most likely these were pseudoplaques, as the Acanthamoeba created the defects in the cell layer as it destroyed the individual cells.

In its earliest stage, Acanthamoeba is limited to the epithelium. The appearance varies from that of whitish elevated epithelium to a variety of patterns of epithelial defects, including a dendritiform pattern. These defects may come and go throughout the course of the disease, whether the disease process is being effectively treated or not.

The recurrent epithelial breakdown overlying ring infiltrates and abscesses lead to the frequent diagnosis of ring abscesses being caused by Herpes simplex virus. Most likely, the vast majority, if not all, of the previously misdiagnosed herpes ring abscesses were caused by Acanthamoeba.

Stromal involvement prior to the development of a ring abscess varies tremendously. There can be single or multiple anterior stromal infiltrates, a nummular keratitis appearance at one or all levels of the stroma, or the formation of dense single or multiple stromal infiltrates.

The most characteristic form of stromal disease occurs late and is characterized by a ring infiltrate or abscess that can consist of single, multiple, or overlapping rings. The explanation for the often dense ring infiltrate has been elusive in the past as pathological specimens have demonstrated few organisms and minimal inflammatory cells. We therefore suspected that Acanthamoeba might be producing substances that destroyed the normal collagen pattern and, therefore, created an opacity. We found that Acanthamoeba constitutively elaborated collagenolytic enzymes that produced characteristic ring infiltrates when injected into the cornea (3). Moreover, injection of purified collagenase into healthy rat corneas produced lesions characteristic of Acanthamoeba keratitis (3).

The stromal involvement can also present with an appearance exactly similar to that seen in herpes simplex disciform keratitis.

The differentiating point in these patients is that they typically have excessive pain when Acanthamoeba is the offending organism. A not uncommonly encountered sign is that of infiltration along the corneal nerves, creating what appears to be a radial neuritis. At this point, the radial neuritis would appear to be a pathognomonic sign for Acanthamoeba (11). We have found that Acanthamoeba has a great affinity for neural cells, and that it prefers them as a food source over most other eukaryotic cells. Acanthamoeba destruction of the nerves most likely accounts for the severe pain that these patients have.

Management

Brolene and Neomycin

Following the lead of Peter Wright from Moorfield's Eye Hospital and his suggestion, we have used a combination of Brolene and Neomycin as our favored treatment for Acanthamoeba keratitis. We have reported our initial success rate and therapeutic approach previously (12,14).

We initially treat with hourly instillation of both medications around the clock for approximately 48 hours, and then decrease the frequency of treatment to hourly instillation during awake hours. We continue this intensive therapy with medication toxicity being the dictator of when the intensity of therapy is decreased.

As toxicity becomes significant, we begin to taper therapy, with the goal of maintaining the patient on both medications topically 3-4 times a day for one year. It is not uncommon for patients to break through with activity while on maintainance therapy. This occurrence does not indicate treatment failure from a qualitative standpoint, but merely that inadequate amounts of drug are being delivered.

It is well known that medications are much more effective against the trophozoite form as compared to the cyst. It is our estimation that the initial therapy kills many of the organisms in trophozoite form while stimulating other trophozoites to encyst. In the encysted form the therapy is much less effective. Therefore, with the frequency of maintenance at 3-4 times a day, the cysts are apt to find the environment much more favorable and excyst leading to a burst of trophozoite activity and thus causing recrudescence. When this occurs, it is important to increase the frequency of the medications which to date with one exception, has resulted in reestablishment of therapeutic control and the ability eventually to cure medically the disease process and thereby withdraw topical therapy.

Clotrimazole/Polyhexamethylene - Biguanide

We have encountered one treatment failure in a patient with bilateral disease.

We followed the recommendation of Driebe and coworkers (2) and added topical Clotrimazole, which resulted in the disease process being brought under control in one eye.

In the contralateral eye, we followed the recommendation of Larkin (7) and added topical polyhexamethylene biguanide with resultant control of disease.

The ideal medical therapy of Acanthamoeba keratitis is yet to be adequately established. With the development of an effective animal model, it should be possible to determine the most appropriate therapy for Acanthamoeba keratitis.

Management of Pain

The pain that is often severe in these patients is best managed with oral Clinoril^{RX}, in its recommended therapeutic doses (6). We specifically recommend trying to avoid narcotics and resort to a retrobulbar alcohol block if Clinoril^{RX} is ineffective.

Patients often present having been misdiagnosed as Herpes simplex virus keratitis and are on topical corticosteroids in addition to antivirals. We withdraw the antivirals immediately and taper the patients completely off of corticosteroids as quickly as possible.

Corticosteroids

We do not use topical corticosteroids actively in therapy, and agree with those who have suggested that exposure of these patients to topical corticosteroids is a bad prognostic indicator.

There does, however, continue to be some controversy about the appropriateness or inappropriateness of the use of topical corticosteroids. Again, it is anticipated that this issue will be resolved with the development of an effective animal model.

Keratoplasty

There also is controversy about the timing of penetrating keratoplasty. It is our recommendation that penetrating keratoplasty not be done unless there is a medical cure of the infectious process, unless one must do the surgery as a globe-saving maneuver.

If the infection is not controlled and a penetrating keratoplasty is done, the infection often recurs in the donor with the greatest devastation in the area of the wound, which tremendously compromises the integrity of the globe and the potential for one being able to salvage useful vision or even the globe itself. We have not yet had a failure with a corneal transplant in any of these patients; however, we have not operated on any who have not had a medical cure.

It, therefore, continues to be our strong recommendation that one not do a penetrating keratoplasty unless forced until there is a medical cure as we have seen a number of globes that have been lost when penetrating keratoplasty has been done prematurely.

This issue will also be more effectively addressed once an animal model is developed.

Prevention

Considering the devastating nature of the disease process and the many problems that we still face with therapy, the most important consideration is to attempt to prevent the disease.

As indicated above, the disease frequently occurs in patients who are contact lens wearers. It would not appear that the contact lens per se is the culprit, but that its exposure to contaminated fluids is the major problem. The frequent association of disease with homemade saline made from distilled water and salt tablets has led to the voluntary withdrawal from the market by several companies of salt tablets.

It is our strong recommendation that distilled water and salt tablets not be used by anyone to make saline. It is unrealistic to expect that a person can use a large container of distilled water over time in making saline without running the risk of significant contamination of the distilled water. Additionally, patients typically keep the large container of distilled water in their kitchen or toilet area, neither one of which would be considered a very sterile environment. The use of large containers of intravenous fluids or buffering solutions commonly found in hospitals and laboratories run a similar risk for contamination, and therefore, should not be used for lens care.

It has been shown that the commercially available heat sterilization units are effective in killing both Acanthamoeba trophozoites and cysts. This, therefore, is an effective method of sterilizing contact lenses, so long as the lens is not contaminated after sterilization and prior to reinsertion onto the eye. We have found that hydrogen peroxide in its active state is effective in killing both trophozoites and cysts if the organism is exposed to the hydrogen peroxide for two hours.

Therefore, the hydrogen peroxide systems that are available that allow one to add the deactivating agent in a timed manner after the lens is placed into hydrogen peroxide can be used effectively to kill Acanthamoeba, providing that the hydrogen peroxide deactivator is not added before the Acanthamoeba have been killed (21,22). We have also examined the preservatives that are found in the various cold sterilization solutions. There is some variability in terms of time exposure required for those that are effective (19,20). It is more practical in our estimation, to simply remember that the cold sterilization preservatives that are effective require four hours of exposure for the Acanthamoeba trophozoites or cysts to be killed (19).

The preservatives that we found to be effective are benzalkonium chloride, thiomersal with EDTA, chlorhexidine, and polyaminopropyl biguanide (PAPB) when encountered in a concentration of 0.0015% but ineffective at a concentration of 0.00005%. We found that sorbate, sorbic acid, polyquaternium, thiomersal alone, and EDTA alone are ineffective in killing Acanthamoeba (19). It is our opinion that for an agent to be accepted as being effective, that it must kill both trophozoits and cysts.

The Future

It does appear that the prevalence of Acanthamoeba keratitis has declined. This decline is probably explained by the fact that the previously misdiagnosed cases have now been appropriately diagnosed and that the frequency of patients making homemade saline has declined significantly. Additionally, the need to educate patients in the care of their contact lenses and specifically the avoidance not only of homemade saline but tap water contamination of lenses have also contributed to this decline.

There will continue to be new infections and they will continue to represent a devastating problem.

It is therefore important to develop an animal model so that we can learn more about risk factors, host immunologic factors, and both medical and surgical therapy.

A suitable animal model must mimic the human disease, both in appearance and chronicity. In a quest for an animal model, we evaluated the possibility that rats might be susceptible, as has been reported by others (1,8). However, we have noted that rats develop a self-limiting, acute keratitis whether they are injected with live or heat-killed Acanthamoeba. We interpret this findings to indicate that the keratitis created in rats by injection of live or killed Acanthamoeba represents a foreign body reaction rather than a true infectious process.

Moreover, we have been consistently unsuccessful in creating an infectious keratitis in mice or rabbits and conclude that these species are unsatisfactory models for Acanthamoeba keratitis.

It is not uncommon for parasites to exercise host specifity. We, therefore, reasoned that the attachment and penetration of Acanthamoeba to intact human corneal epithelium might be used as a screening tool for selecting other potentially susceptible hosts. Accordingly, corneal organ cultures from a variety of mammals, including humans, were examined for susceptibility to Acanthamoeba infection. Acanthamoeba trophozoites adhered to and penetrated corneal epithelium from humans, pigs, and Chinese hamsters only, suggesting that these latter mammalian species would be attractive candidates to serve as animal models for the human counterpart (17).

Based on the previous in vitro results, the pig was selected for further study and evaluated as a potential animal model for Acanthamoeba keratitis. The similarity of the pig eye to the human eye made this model even more attractive for clinical studies. In order to establish the feasibility of the pig model, parasite-laden soft contact lenses were placed onto the corneas of pigs and secured by tarsorrhaphy that was left in place for five days to ensure that the contact lens was not lost. Controls consisted of hosts that were similarly treated with uncontaminated contact lenses. Pigs that received Acanthamoeba-laden contact lenses developed a keratitis that closely resembled human Acanthamoeba keratitis (4).

Three distinct disease stages were apparent. The first was a marked inflammatory diffuse keratitis followed by the formation of a ring abscess that ultimately progressed to a scarred vascularized cornea. Acanthamoeba was recoverable from the animals until they reached the scarred vascularized phase, after which all cultures were negative; however, cyst walls were discernible within the stroma. At no stage of the disease process were pathogenic bacteria recovered; only normal bacteria flora were detected. With further development, the pig model should permit the evaluation of risk factors and therapy. However, the pig is a cumbersome model for elaborate studies on the immunology of Acanthamoeba keratitis. Therefore, the Chinese hamster is currently being examined as a possible model for immunological studies.

By combining these animal models, it will be possible to evaluate, in a prospective setting, the pathophysiology, immunology, and risk factors involved in Acanthamoeba keratitis.

References

1. Badenoch PR, Johnson AM, Christy PE et al (1990) Pathogenicity of Acanthamoeba and Corynebacterium in the Rat Cornea. Arch Ophthalmol 108:107-112
2. Driebe WTjr, Stern GA, Epstein RJ et al (1988) Acanthamoeba Keratitis. Potential Role for Topical Clotrimazole in Combination Chemotherapy. Arch Ophthalmol 106:1196-1201
3. He YG, Niederkorn JY, McCulley JP et al (1990) In Vivo and in Vitro Collagenolytic Activity of Acanthamoeba castellanii. Invest Ophthalmol Vis Sci 31:2235-2240
4. He,YG, McCulley,JP, Alizadeh,H et al (1992) A pig Model of Acanthamoeba Keratitis: Transmission Via Contaminated Contact Lenses. Invest Ophthalmol Vis Sci 33:126-133
5. John T, Desai D, Sam D (1991) Adherence of Acanthamoeba Castellanii Cysts and Trophozoites to Extended Wear Soft Contact Lenses. Rev Inf Dis 13/S5:419
6. Koenig BS, Solomon MJ, Hyndiuk AR et al (1987) Acanthamoeba Keratitis Associated with Gas-Permeable Contact Lens Wear. Am J Ophthalmol 103:832
7. Larkin DFP, Dart JKG, Kilvington S et al (1991) Treatment of Acanthamoeba Keratitis with Polyhexamethylene Biguanide. Invest Ophthalmol Vis Sci 32S:1183
8. Larkin DFP, Easty DL (1990) Experimental Acanthamoeba Keratitis: I. Preliminary Findings. Br J Ophthalmol 74:421-424

9. McCulley JP (1991) Clinical Perspectives of Acanthamoeba Keratitis. Ophthalmology (Japan) 33:727-736
10. Moore MB, McCulley JP, Luckenbach M et al (1985) Acanthamoeba Keratitis Associated with Soft Contact Lenses. Am J Ophthalmol 100:396-403
11. Moore MB, McCulley JP, Kaufman HE et al (1986) Radial Keratoneuritis as a Presenting Sign in Acanthamoeba Keratitis. Ophthalmology 93:1310-1315
12. Moore MB, McCulley JP (1987) Letter to the Editor: Treatment of Acanthamoeba Keratitis. Am J Ophthalmol 104:310-311
13. Moore MB, McCulley JP, Newton C et al (1987) Acanthamoeba Keratitis: A Growing Problem in Soft and Hard Contact Lens Wearers. Ophthalmology 94:1654-1661
14. Moore MB, McCulley JP (1989) Acanthamoeba Keratitis Associated with Contact Lenses: Six Consecutive Cases of Successful Management. Br J Ophthalmol 73:271
15. Moore MB, Ubelaker J, Silvany RE et al (1991) Scanning Electron Microscopy of Acanthamoeba castellanii: Adherence to New and Used Contact Lens Surfaces and to Human Corneal Button Epithelium. Rev Inf Dis 13:423-424
16. Moore MB, Ubelaker J, Martin J et al (1991) In Vitro Penetration of Human Corneal Epithelium by Acanthameba castellanii. A Scanning and Transmission Electron Microscopy Study. Cornea 10:291-298
17. Niederkorn JY, Ubelaker J, McCulley JP et al (1992) Susceptibility of Corneas from Various Animal Species to in Vitro Binding and Invasion by Acanthamoeba castellanii. Invest Ophthalmol Vis Sci 33:104-112
18. Silvany RE, Luckenbach MW, Moore MB (1987) The Rapid Detection of Acanthamoeba in Paraffin Embedded Sections of Corneal Tissue with Calcofluor White. Arch.Ophthalmol. 105:1366-1367
19. Silvany RE, Moore MB, McCulley JP (1989) The Effect of Less than Four Hour Exposures of Thimerosal, Benzalkonium Chloride, and Chlorhexidine on Acanthamoeba castellanii and Acanthamoeba Polyphaga. Invest Ophthalmol Vis Sci 30:41
20. Silvany RE, Wood TS, Bowman RW et al (1988) The Effect of Contact Lens Solutions on Two Species of Acanthamoeba. Invest Ophthalmol Vis Sci 29 (suppl):253
21. Silvany RE, Dougherty JM, McCulley JP et al (1990) The Effect of Currently Available Contact Lens Disinfection Systems on Acanthamoeba Castellanii and Acanthamoeba Polyphaga. Ophthalmology 97:286-290
22. Silvany RE, Dougherty JM, McCulley JP (1991) The Effect of Contact Lens Preservatives on Acanthamoeba. Ophthalmology 89:854-857
23. Ubelaker JE, Moore MB, Martin J et al (1991) In Vitro Adherence of Acanthamoeba Castellanii to Human Corneal Epithelium: A Scanning and Transmission Electron Microscopy Study. Cornea 10: 299-304

- Surgery

Surgical Management of Ocular Infections

Eduardo C. Alfonso

Abstract. The goals of surgical therapy in microbial keratitis are to eradicate the responsible organisms and restore the integrity of the cornea and globe.

The incidence of therapeutic keratoplasty in bacterial keratitis is apfroximately 3% and for fungal keratitis is 24%.

Management consists of appropriate microbiologic studies in order to recover the offending microorganisms. Medical treatment is begun and if possible continued for 24 to 48 hours prior to instituting surgical therapy. In cases of scleritis, cryotherapy may be required for control of the scleral involvement. The surgical management consists of tissue glue, debridement, keratoplasty and in rare circumstances lamellar keratoplasty or conjunctival flap.

The keratoplasty technique needs to be modified from the conventional technique used due to the hypotonus and inflamed nature of the eye. Often, tissue glue must be used intraoperatively in order to restore intraocular tension. Large grafts are required to eradicate the process and thus donor tissue from a whole globe may be benefical. Intraocular surgery is often required due to the involvement of the iris, lens and vitreous.

Intraoperative and postoperative antibiotics are mandatory. The use of postoperative medications such as corticosteroids and systemic and topical cyclosporin will be discussed.

The main postoperative problems that arise are recurrences of the infection, glaucoma, and opacification of the graft.

Introduction

Ocular infections can usually be successfully managed medically without the need for surgical intervention. At times, because medical therapy alone is not sufficient, surgical interventions must be considered. Clinical entities that are likely to require surgical intervention are keratitis, scleritis, endophthalmitis, cellulitis and dacryocystitis.

In this survey, surgical options in the management of keratitis and scleritis are discussed.

Keratitis - Epidemiology

In keratitis, the role of surgical intervention is to control a progressive infection and/or to tectonically repair the globe. In a review of therapeutic penetrating keratoplasties performed at the Bascom Palmer Eye Institute, two-thirds were done to repair infected perforations, while one-third were done to control progression of the infection (2). The common reason for reaching this clinical situation is usually an improperly treated infection, with the exception of those caused by organisms known not to respond well to medical treatment.

The most common etiologic agent involved in a keratitis eventually requiring keratoplasty because of progression of the infection or perforation is Fusarium solanii. Even though this organism represents less than 10% of all cases of microbial keratitis seen at the Bascom Palmer Eye Institute, it represents a high percentage of the eyes requiring keratoplasty (3).

Fifty percent of eyes requiring keratoplasty have infections with Gram negative organisms. In the majority of these, Pseudomonas species is cultured. Other less common causes are Neisseria gonorrhoeae, acanthamoeba and mycobacteria.

Sampling

Before considering surgical intervention, appropriate scrapings for culture must be performed. If scrapings fail to yield an organism, consideration should be given to performing a corneal biopsy.

In our series of corneal biopsies performed for previously culture negative microbial keratitis, the biopsy recovered an organism in approximately 50 % of the cases (5). A biopsy may be difficult to undertake in an already perforated cornea and thus should only be performed if one is not considering a therapeutic keratoplasty.

Medical Treatment

Subconjunctival injections of antibiotics are given in cases of bacterial keratitis, if the organism is not known and therefore specific therapy cannot be given, then broad-spectrum antibiotics such as cephazolin 50mg and gentamicin 20mg are given. Because of their toxicity, subconjunctival antifungals are not used.

Systemic and fortified topical antibiotics are continued based on culture results. The use of topical corticosteroids is controversial. For cases of bacterial and acanthamoeba infections, if broad-spectrum or specific antibiotic therapy is being given, then the cautious use of topical corticosteroids may be indicated. In cases of fungal infections, topical corticosteroid therapy should be withheld and only non-steroidal topical antiinflammatory drops may be used. In both scenarios, topical cyclosporin A is used. In viral keratitis, topical antivirals as well as systemic acyclovir are continued as long as high dose topical corticosteroids are used.

Surgery

While one is waiting for tissue availability and operating room time, consideration should be given to application of tissue glue to the site of the perforation. During this time, antimicrobial coverage should be continued either broad-spectrum or specific based on culture results. Systemic antibiotics are also desirable in order to enhance intraocular concentration.

Because these eyes are often perforated and the amount of surgery to be done may be unpredictable, it is best to use general anesthesia.

If a perforation has occurred, a viscoelastic can be used through the site of the perforation to reform the anterior chamber, followed by liberal application of tissue glue to the site of perforation. This will make surgical manipulation easier in preparation for and during trephination.

A conjunctival peritomy should be done, especially in cases of extensive keratitis, since it is often necessary to perform a graft which includes the limbus and adjacent sclera.

A Flieringa ring helps maintain the rigidity of the globe.

Keratoplasty

Trephination of the host may be done first in cases of free-hand grafts or large grafts, otherwise, the donor should be prepared first in the usual fashion.

For trephination of the host, if the size of the tissue to be excised is encompassed by a 9 mm or smaller trephine, then this is done with a motorized trephine, which places no pressure on the globe. If the globe is too soft to trephine, then a mark can be made by placing methylene blue ink on the blade of the trephine and using this to mark the tissue. This same marking technique can be used for larger grafts using for reference a Flieringa ring. Other manual and vacuum trephines can be used at times, but difficulties may arise with the presence of hypotony and necrotic tissue. Free-hand grafts may be cut by using sharp corneal scissors or a diamond blade.

Inflammatory and necrotic tissue should be excised from the cornea, leaving a healthy border. Any tissues removed should be submitted in part to microbiology and pathology.

The donor corneal button should be sutured with interrupted sutures in most cases. This technique provides ease of selected suture removal in cases of recurrences, vascularization, or rejection. Scleral sutures are 9-0 nylon while corneal sutures are 10-0 nylon. All knots are buried.

Combined Procedures

The lens-iris diaphragm should be preserved, since this may prevent further spread of organisms into the vitreous.

If the clinical picture is such that an endophthalmitis is suspected, then a lensectomy, vitrectomy and injection of intraocular antimicrobials is recommended. In our experience, we rarely encounter cases of end-ophthalmitis, which have begun as infectious keratitis.

In cases where a lensectomy has been performed, we implant a posterior chamber intraocular lens based on the clinical response of the infection. This is typically done in cases where the infection has been controlled, but a perforation is present with an associated dense cataract. In contrast, we rarely implant a lens in cases of fulminant endophthalmitis.

Other Surgical Options

Other available surgical therapies include
- debridement,
- tissue glue,
- lamellar keratoplasty,
- conjunctival flap, and
- cryotherapy.

Debridement is useful to remove necrotic tissue and enhance antimicrobial penetration. Obviously it cannot be used if a perforation has occurred. The use of tissue glue is beneficial to seal a small perforation or near-perforation while it is attempted to medically control the infection or in some cases, until tissue for keratoplasty becomes available. Reports have indicated that tissue glue may be bacteriostatic (6).

A lamellar keratoplasty has the disadvantage that one may be protecting deep infected material from having an adequate concentration of antibiotic. Lamellar surgery may be useful in cases where no other means of sealing a perforation is available.

A conjunctival flap has been used for the management of peripheral and central keratitis, particularly those caused by fungi. The thought is that enhancing the vascular supply to the area with conjunctiva may decrease fungal replication (4). Limited reports are available in the U.S. literature to compare this form of therapy to currently available antimicrobials.

Cryotherapy has been advocated and used effectively in the management of bacterial corneoscleritis (1). Usually, retrobulbar anesthesia is required and a conjunctival recession is performed to expose the infected sclera. Using a retinal cryoprobe, two freeze-thaw cycles of several seconds are apllied primarily to the borders of the infection where presumably organisms are replicating and invading. The area is left exposed and subconjunctival antimicrobials are injected. These patients are usually continued on fortified topical antibiotics as well as systemic antibiotics.

A review of our cases of corneoscleritis shows that when this surgical and antibiotic intervention is used 82% of the eyes are cured, whereas when only medical therapy is used, the cure rate is only 25% (7).

Conclusions

In summary, surgical intervention should be considered when attempting to cure a microbial keratitis and scleritis.

Medical treatment should be optimized and surgery properly timed to enhance the recovery of visual functions.

References

1. Alfonso E, Kenyon K, Ormerod D et al (1987) Pseudomonas Corneoscleritis. Am J Ophthalmol 103(1):908
2. Forster RK (1988) The Role of Excisional Keratoplasty in Microbial Keratitis.In: Cavanagh HD (ed) The Cornea: Transactions of the World Congress on the Cornea III. Raven Press, New York
3. Guildford JH, Alfonso E, Roussel T et al (1988) Large Therapeutic Keratoplasty in Microbial Keratitis. Invest Ophthalmol Vis Sci 29S:6
4. Gunderson T (1958) Conjunctival Flaps in the Treatment of Corneal Disease with Reference to a new Technique of Application. Arch Ophthalmol 60:880
5. Haimovici R, Alfonso E, Miller D (1990) Corneal Biopsy in the Management of Refractory Microbial Keratitis. Invest Ophthalmol Vis Sci 31S:571
6. Hyndiuk RA, Seideman S (1978) Clinical and Laboratory Techniques in External Ocular Disease. In: Fedukowicz (ed) External Infections of the Eye (2nd ed). Appleton-Century-Crafts, New York Chap.5
7. Reynolds M, Alfonso E (to be published) Infectious Scleritis and Corneoscleritis.Am J Ophthalmol

The Role of Penetrating Keratoplasty in the Management of Microbial Keratitis: A Brief Review

Colin M. Kirkness, Linda A. Ficker

Abstract. Penetrating keratoplasty has an important role for anterior segment reconstruction in eyes severely disorganized by microbial keratitis. Although timing can be difficult, delay in surgery can be detrimental once perforation has occurred. Attention to minute detail regarding the health of the eye, particularly the ocular surface, is vital in the postoperative period. It is imperative, therefore, that patients understand this and can present themselves to the supervising surgeon immediately they are aware of the development of new symptoms. Though these cases are demanding of time, the results may be very rewarding for surgeon and patient alike.

Introduction

The prime aim of the management of microbial keratitis is to identify the infecting agent with the least delay and commence appropriate antimicrobial chemotherapy to minimize tissue damage and so restore visual function. To this end it is important to follow logical sequence in the investigation and appraisal of the efficacy of medical treatment (4). There are occasions, however, when inappropriate treatment has been instituted or the patient delays presentation so that the corneal abscess produces extensive tissue destruction or perforation. Even centers, which have a particular expertise in the investigation of ocular infections report that initial investigations are positive in only 75% of cases (6,8).

Some uncommon pathogens have unusual antibiotic sensitivities and delay in optimal treatment may be occasioned until these are identified. In the same way, some organisms are so fastidious that culture may be difficult again delaying ideal treatment until the disease process is advanced. In such circumstances, biopsy or excisional keratoplasty may be called for.

Surgery

For these reasons, it has been increasingly recognized that penetrating keratoplasty has a role to play in the active management of microbial keratitis. The generally accepted indications for keratoplasty are shown in Tab.1. Hill (7) adopted a slightly more liberal approach, including all cases, which appeared to have so much tissue disorganisation that penetrating keratoplasty would be necessary at a later date. This pragmatic approach was appropriate to the patient population with which he dealt but would not necessarily be accepted in a Western European setting.

Although Descemet's membrane acts as a barrier to the spread of infection, the risks of keratoplasty converting a sterile intraocular environment into endophthalmitis are small. Indeed, it is probable that delay in operating once perforation has occurred, is more likely to result in endophthalmitis.

The alternate approach of performing a deep lamellar keratoplasty, which at first sight may appear attractive in preserving the integrity of the globe, risks leaving viable organisms behind.

Nevertheless, its use has been advocated in combination with a conjunctival flap. It is suggested that the proximity of blood vessels permits better delivery of immune mediators (15).

Conjunctival flaps alone have been advocated both for the control of keratomycosis and for the control of peripheral perforations but it is difficult to gauge the outcome in such series (16).

Where the perforation is small and peripheral, the use of a sector keratoplasty or mini-tectonic grafts as advocated by Völcker and Naumann would seem preferable in being more predictable in its ability to control the situation as well as providing more tissue for histopathological and microbiological examination (17).

The use of tissue adhesives (cyano-acrylate) has also been advocated, but these are only useful if the perforation is not larger than 1 mm in diameter. Tissue adhesives may, however, have a useful role during surgery when the perforation may be sealed temporarily allowing the anterior chamber to be reformed prior to cutting the host bed. This is technically much easier and lessens the risks damaging the underlying tissues when the eye is formed (13).

Few authors have specially addressed the particular techniques, which need to be adopted in the presence of acute infections or perforations.

Weidle and Thiel (18) who broadly adopted the indications for keratoplasty described here, highlighted that these cases may prove difficult demanding special care. Iris bleeding was often a problem due to intensive hyperemia. They recommended irrigating the anterior chamber with antibiotic solution. This procedure may be superfluous (see below) and may cause toxic damage to the remaining endothelium and iris. They also recommended high doses of systemic corticosteroids in rapidly decreasing dosage postoperatively.

Behrens-Baumann was also concerned about blood clots in the anterior chamber and used sodium citrate to prevent clotting (2).

Pouliquen and coworkers recommended irrigation of the anterior chamber, removal of inflammatory debris as well as ensuring full excision of necrotic material (14). They did not use intracameral antibiotics. They used long-term corticosteroids postoperatively.

Hill (7) did not describe his technique in detail.

Kirkness and coworkers (10,11) indicated that attention to simple details might be important in producing a good outcome. Great care was taken to excise all infected tissue. This was sent for further culture and for microscopic examination. The wound edge was in healthy tissue (even if this meant having a graft considerably larger than the usual 7-8 mm - the range of sizes in this series is greater than the others published) to aid healing and prevent melting at the wound edge. At the same time, great care was taken to ensure that the donor button was large enough, bearing in mind that, in perforated eyes, a trephine may excise a block of tissue considerably larger than its nominal size. A whole eye stored in a moist chamber allowed much greater adaptibility at this point. When the graft had to be very large, part of the limbus was preserved, where possible, to aid re-epithelialization. This was achieved by siting the graft slightly eccentrically or by using a sector keratoplasty avoiding healthy limbal tissue.

The use of viscoelastic material was also helpful in delaminating the structures in the anterior chamber and so avoiding damage to the iris and underlying lens. Viscoelastic delamination was also helpful in opening up the angle and may have reduced the formation of anterior synechiae.

Clearance of inflammatory debris from the anterior chamber or vitreous was also attempted to speed visual rehabilitation and reduce postoperative inflammation.

The crystalline lens was not routinely removed unless there was an intumescent cataract.

In some eyes, which were very inflamed, prophylactic iridectomy was also performed to avoid a pupillary block even though synechiolysis and excision of anterior cyclitic membranes were attempted.

Interrupted sutures were always used, since suture loosening was common in inflamed eyes and it was easier to remove a single interrupted suture than to deal with a continuous suture. Surprisingly, this point has not been made widely by the other authors writing on this subject (Tab.2).

Postoperatively, antibiotics appropriate for the infecting organism were used. These were changed depending upon laboratory culture and sensitivity results and upon the clinical reponse. If the eye was sterile, chloramphenicol drops were employed.

Topical corticosteroids were given in high dosage beginning with a minimum of prednisolone 1% or equivalent gutt. every two hours (and often more) titrating the frequency and strength against the clinical response. Frequently patients were still taking gutt. prednisolone 1% four times a day at four months postoperatively and prednisolone 0.3% once a day at one year. This regimen was employed even when the infecting agent was known to be pseudomonas. This practice is justifiable on the basis that the infected tissue has been excised and corticosteroids are therefore unlikely to cause recrudescence.

Mydriatics (gutt. Atropine) were used where there was inflammatory activity. Systemic corticosteroids were not used regularly, neither were prophylactic antiviral drugs in the case of an eye with a history of Herpes simplex keratitis. Ancillary medications were employed where indicated.

Success of Sugery - Graft Survival

The only realistic way that the success of corneal grafting can be understood as far as graft clarity is concerned is to consider Kaplan-Meier survival curves (11). These allow different lengths of follow-up and different times of recruitment into a series to be weighted appropriately. Since graft survival is a dynamic parameter, survival probabilities avoid the use of meaningless statements such as "72% of grafts remained clear". This latter statement is very different from saying "at two years there was a survival proportion of 0.72". Apart from Kirkness and coworkers (11) no previous paper has produced survival curves. Weidle and Thiel (18), and Pouliquen and coworkers (14) did, however, report enough data for accurate survival curves to be constructed. Fig.1

shows the combined data from these three series. Although Kirkness' series does seem to be statistically superior at four years, there is no difference at two years and it is probable that the apparent difference is explainable purely on the basis of the size of the individual series involved.

Hill's (7) published results cannot easily be reproduced in the form of survival curves, but they are probably consistent with the others. Du's results cannot be so analyzed (3). The consistency of the results suggests that despite minor differences in management the main determinants of success is the underlying ocular condition. There is, however, considerable morbidity associated with emergency grafts and patients require many follow-up visits, often indefinitely.

In contrast to graft survival in cases performed à chaud, where the reported survival proportion at five years is 50% or less (Fig.1), eyes undergoing keratoplasty after successful medical therapy for microbial keratitis can expect a relatively good prognosis. Kirkness (11) indicated that these transplants might be expected to show a survival proportion of 90% at 5 years.

Complications

Several complications are seen regularly in published series, although the incidence does vary. Some are predictable and can be dealt with without undue difficulty. These include delayed re-epithelialization and secondary cataract. The latter may be extracted once the graft is secure, i.e. as minimum of 6 months after keratoplasty with a minimal risk of graft survival (5). Graft rejection, not surprisingly, is common and may account for more of the failures when the graft size is large (3). It is difficult, however, to obtain good statistical correlations, since the numbers involved in so many of the series are small. The relative frequency of this complication certainly justifies high-dose topical corticosteroid therapy, the place of systemic corticosteroids in corneal transplantation remains controversial.

There may be a role for the use of topical or even systemic Cyclosporin A in the long-term management of many of these eyes, but its value also remains to be demonstrated. Even if Cyclosporin A has a role, the results will not improve dramatically, since two of the major complications are likely to be unaffected.

Glaucoma may occur in 20% of eyes grafted à chaud (11). The reasons are multifactorial, but almost certainly involve obstruction of the drainage angle by peripheral anterior synechiae. Kirkness and coworkers (12) have demonstrated the importance of this sign for the development of post-keratoplasty glaucoma and also that this is more likely the longer the eye is left perforated (10). The intense intraocular inflammation producing hypopyon, fibrin clot, iris engorgement, that accompanies a microbial keratitis, however, may be sufficient per se to cause damage to the angle producing glaucoma. Following keratoplasty, the intraocular pressure in these eyes may be very difficult to control medically or surgically (2, 7, 10, 11, 13, 14, 17, 18). Trabeculectomy and subsequent silicone drainage surgery may be required to bring pressure control within acceptable limits (11). The present authors do not recommend cyclodestructive procedures for post-keratoplasty glaucoma because of its very poor prognosis.

The remaining complication is probably the most serious of all: Most series reliably report recurrences of ocular infections (2,7,10,11,14,18) following emergency keratoplasty at times up to several years, but 90% within the first ten months of keratoplasty. In the majority of cases, this is due to a different organism and is not due to failure to eradicate the original infection (exceptions have been documented). The reasons for reinfection have nearly always been due to an adverse ocular environment, e.g. cicatricial disease, such as pemphigoid or Stevens-Johnson syndrome, Sjögren's syndrome or Herpes simplex keratitis. These conditions are containable by medical treatment, but are not curable. Affected patients need scrupulous attention to detail with regard to the ocular surface. Lid hygiene with daily scrubs to the margin and local and/or systemic antibiotics are important. Maintenance of an adequate tear film using tear substitutes and/or punctal occlusion where indicated may be helpful. Urgent attention to epithelial defects and removal of loose sutures may help prevent reinfection. Unfortunately, there is no good evidence that the prophylactic use of topical antibiotics prevents infections in corneal grafts, and one series demonstrated that, in cases receiving antibiotic prophylaxis, 50% of pathogens isolated were sensitive to antibiotics being taken prophylactically (1). Several eyes reported by Kirkness and coworkers (11) underwent a second emergency keratoplasty. There may be some justification for combining repeat emergency keratoplasty with the formation of a full conjunctival flap where there is demonstrable conjunctival abnormality, e.g. Stevens-Johnson and where improvement is unlikely. This measure may preserve navigational vision and reasonable cosmesis. The authors feel that this procedure should only be performed if it is intended to be permanent. Because the stem cells are irretrievably damaged by the surgery, undoing the flap is unlikely to lead to a stable ocular surface.

It is worth considering in Kirkness' series (11) that only 20% of eyes had no serious complications at all and these were nearly all in the control group of patients who underwent keratoplasty after successful medical treatment for microbial keratitis. In other words, every patient should anticipate at least one major sight-threatening complication following this surgery.

Visual Acuity

In view of the complexity of the surgery and the numerous serious complications, which may be encountered, it is perhaps not surprising that the range of visual acuities encountered is wide. Reported figures vary between 20/20 to no perception of light (2,3,7,10,11,14,18). As many as a third of the eyes, however, are reported as achieving driving standard vision (11). It is perhaps unfair to use such criteria as a measure of success, since the alternative to penetrating keratoplasty in many cases would inevitably have been enucleation or evisceration.

Thus, in terms of preserving the globe, most published series are spectacularly successful, since less than 10% of all eyes have a visual acuity of no light perception (2,3,7,10,11,13,14,17,18).

Acknowledgements
This work originated form the Pocklington Transplant Unit & Corneal Clinic, Moorfields Eye Hospital, City Road, London.

Table 1. Indications for penetrating keratoplasty in microbial keratitis
- Perforation
- Threatened perforation
- Scleral invasion
- Threatened invasion
- Absolute failure to control the condition medically, esp. where there appear to be contradictory laboratory and clinical findings

Table 2. Key points in surgery for perforated eyes
- General anesthesia
- Ensure wound edge in healthy tissue and that all abscess is excised
- Ensure donor button large enough (whole eye allows greater flexibility)
- Preserve healthy limbus if possible (eccentric of sector keratoplasty)
- Restore anterior chamber if possible
- Use viscoelastic delamination of open up angle and prevent damage to iris and lens
- Remove all inflammatory debris including cyclitic membranes
- Peripheral iridectomy x2 or sector iridectomy
- Preserve the crystalline lens unless subluxated or intumescent
- If aphacic, consider open sky vitrectomy to remove debris
- Use interrupted 10/0 nylon sutrues wherever possible
- Send all excised material to laboratory

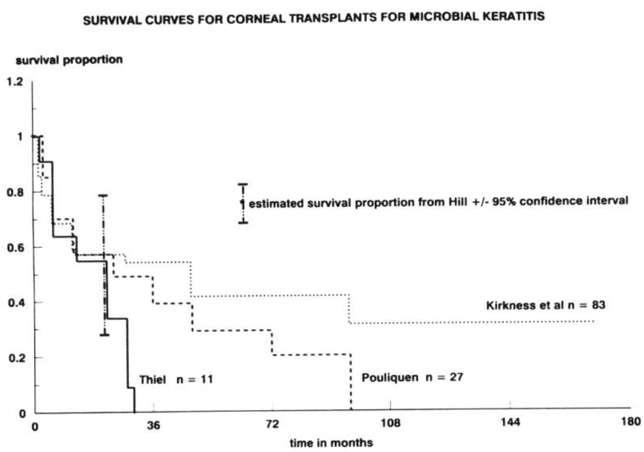

Fig.1. The survival curves from Kirkness and coworkers (11) and those derived from Weidle an coworkers (18) and Pouliquen and coworkers (14) are given. An estimation for the 24 months survival proportion from Hill (7) has been made.

References

1. Bates AK, Kirkness CM, Ficker LA et al (1990) Microbial Keratitis Following Penetrating Keratoplasty. Eye 4:74-78
2. Behrens-Baumann W (1984) Results of Keratoplasty à chaud. Klin Mbl Augenheilkd 815:25-27
3. Du NZ, Chen JQ, Gong XM et al (1979) Therapeutic Keratoplasty in the Management of Purulent Corneal Ulceration - Report of 100 Cases. Jpn J Ophthalmol 23:412-420
4. Ficker LA, Kirkness CM, Seal DV et al (to be published) Microbial Keratitis - the False Negative. Eye.
5. Ficker LA, Kirkness CM, Steele ADMcG et al (1990) IntraocularSurgery Following Penetrating Keratoplasty: The Risks and Advantages. Eye 4:693-697
6. Harris DJ, Stulting RD, Waring GO et al: Late Bacterial and Fungal Keratitis After Corneal Transplantation.
7. Hill JC (1986) Use of Penetrating Keratoplasty in Acute Bacterial Keratitis. Br J Ophthalmol 70:502-506
8. Jones DB (1981) Decision-Making in the Management of Microbial Keratitis. Ophthalmology 88:814-820
9. Kaplan E, Meier P (1958) Non-Parametric Estimation from Incomplete Observations. J Am Statist Assoc 53:457-481
10. Kirkness CM, Steele ADMcG, Rice NSC (1989) Penetrating Keratoplasty and the Management of Suppurative Keratitis. Dev Ophthalmol 19:172-175
11. Kirkness CM, Ficker LA, Steele ADMcG et al (1991) The Role of Penetrating Keratoplasty in the Management of Microbial Keratitis. Eye 5:425-431
12. Kirkness CM, Ficker LA (to be published) The Risk Factors for Post-Keratoplasty Glaucoma. Cornea
13. Maguen E, Nesburn AB, Macy Ji (1984) Combined Use of Sodium Hyaluronate and Tissue Adhesive in Penetrating Keratoplasty of Corneal Perforations. Ophthalmic Surg 155:55-57
14. Pouliquen Y, Petroutsos G, Goichot L (1983) Penetrating Keratoplasty in Corneal Perforations. J Fr Ophthalmol 11:145-148
15. Sanitato JJ, Kelley CG, Kaufman HE (1984) Surgical Management of Peripheral Fungal Keratitis (Keratomycosis). Arch Ophthalmol 102:1506-1509
16. van Rij G, Rinkel van Direl B, Beekhuis WH et al (1987) Conjunctival Transplantation. Doc Ophthalmol 47:145-150
17. Völcker HE, Naumann GOH (1984) Excentric Tectonic Mini-Keratoplasty in Corneal, Corneosceral and Scleral Processes. Klin Mbl Augenheilkd 185:158-166
18. Weidle EG, Thiel HJ (1984) Keratoplasty à chaud as a Therapeutic Measure in Acute Corneal Infections. Klin Mbl Augenheilkd 184:520-528

Triple Therapeutic Approach for Keratitis

Alexander A. Bialasiewicz, Ulrich Schönherr, Thomas Schmitt and Gottfried O.H. Naumann

Abstract. A new regimen to treat corneal ulcers more effectively was initiated in the University Eye Hospital Erlangen-Nürnberg in 1985 using a triple therapeutic approach. Since then, 223 eyes of 205 patients with severe keratitis have been treated, 163 eyes with a culture-established bacterial and 60 with a herpetic etiology. 169 different aerobic fast-growing bacterial strains were isolated (85% Gram positive, 15% Gram negative).

Therapeutic options included topical and systemic antibiotics (54), antibiotics with corticosteroids (84), and antibiotics, corticosteroids and early tectonic penetrating keratoplasty à chaud (25).- Hospital stay was shortest for the keratoplasty groups and visual rehabilitation was significantly better in the corticosteroid groups and best in the keratoplasty group.

Therapeutic alternatives for herpetic corneal lesions consisted of Acyclovir (11), Acyclovir and corticosteroids (40), and Acyclovir plus tectonic keratoplasty (6). Tectonic keratoplasty was only done with imminent or existent perforation.- Visual rehabilitation was best in the Acyclovir medical group, whereas the addition of corticosteroids did not result in a persistent increase of visual acuity or lesser morbidity.

Long-term secondary complications consisted of recurrences (18 in the bacterial =11%, 40 in the herpetic groups =40%), secondary glaucomas (6 in the bacterial, 16 in the herpetic groups =24.6%) and repeat keratoplasty (2 in the bacterial =10%, 4 in the herpetic groups =45%).

This study outlines the benefits of a triple therapeutic approach with effective antibiotics, corticosteroids and early tectonic penetrating keratoplasty for severe culture-established bacterial keratitis. Furthermore, these data suggest the application of corticosteroids in severe herpetic keratitis patients not to be beneficial.

Introduction

Eyes formerly doomed by severe bacterial infections have become treatable and curable in the recent past through better understanding of the immunology of infection and the advance of newer chemotherapeutic agents as well as surgical refinements in tectonic corneal grafting (28,31). Adequate management of eyes suffering from bacterial keratitis relies on a sound microbiological diagnosis (4,16).

Immediate broad-spectrum antibiotic therapy has been proven effective, particularly with a combination of systemic and topical/ local drug regimens (4). Decision-making in a second step may necessitate a change of antibiotic drug regimens according to susceptibility patterns and the introduction of intraocular pressure-lowering substances (4,13,18).

It is still felt by most corneal surgeons that tectonic keratoplasty should generally be performed only after the infiltrate has shown a tendency for scar formation in order to minimize the risk of recurrence of the disease and graft failure. A poor outcome of infected corneal ulcers and grafts in these patients can be associated with either a persistence of the live pathogens (attraction of Ia-expressing macrophages, directly destructive effects), or leuko-attractive cell wall fragments after effective anti-infective therapy (glycoconjugates provoking macrophage activation, polyclonal B-cell activation, adjuvans function in delayed type hypersensitivity).

It is generally accepted that corticosteroids are a valuable means to decrease the destructive phase of infection pathogenesis and therefore reduce morbidity and hospitalization (2,22,34). Furthermore, excision of an infective lesion seems the best way to get rid of infected tissue and may further contribute to the benefit of lesser morbidity (28).

The rationale for successfully coping with the destructive phase of infection pathogenesis must therefore include:

1. elimination of the pathogen with agent-specific anti-infective drugs,
2. anti-inflammatory/immunosuppressive medication and
3. excision of remaining infective keratitic stromal tissue after resolution of the hypopyon using technically advanced tectonic corneal grafting.

To our knowledge, there has as yet been no larger study comparing the results of mono antibiotic-therapy with a combined approach including antibiotics, corticosteroids and tectonic corneal grafting à chaud. We have evaluated 205 patients with 223 eyes (163 eyes of culture-established etiology, 60 eyes with herpetic lesions) over a period of 4 years (1985-1988). Patients were divided into three separate management groups:

1. antibiotics,
2. antibiotics and corticosteroids and
3. antibiotics, corticosteroids and early tectonic perforating keratoplasty.

Short-term and long-term visual rehabilitation and secondary complications were moni-tored for the separate trial groups and compared to patients with herpetic keratitis.

Patients

1. Eligibility Criteria

A selected population of 205 patients (223 eyes) with severe keratitis were studied from January 1985 until December 1988 at the University Eye Hospital Erlangen-Nürnberg.

Criteria for eligibility to enrollment in the study protocols of bacterial keratitis were: (1) a culture-established diagnosis and exclusion of other infectious eye diseases and (2) completely documented follow-ups (5-28 months, mean 10 months).

Criteria for eligibility to enrollment in the study protocols of herpetic keratitis were: (1) absent corneal sensitivity measured by esthesiometry, (2) virologic tests and cultures for bacteria in uncertain cases and (3) completely documented follow-ups (2-15 months, mean 8 months).

2. Clinical Diagnoses

2.a) bacterial

163 eyes presented with bacterial keratitis/ulcers. Clinical diagnoses included:

- severe keratitis and serpent ulcers (n=114),

- endophthalmitis (n=25),
- panophthalmitis (n=4),
- complicated penetrating injury (n=10),
- complicated intraocular foreign body (n=6) and
- complicated graft rejection (n=4).

2.b) herpetic

60 eyes with infectious keratitis were of clinically presumed or virologically established herpetic etiology. Clinical diagnoses included:

- (sub)epithelial keratitis with stromal involvement (n=9)
- corneal ulcers (n=10)
- keratouveitis with severe corneal involvement (n=39)
- severe (sub)epithelial keratitis and stromal involvement during Varicella zoster reactivation (n=2).

Materials and Methods

1. Bacteriological Work-Up

In each case, corneal smears were taken with MW 142 swabs (MAST Diagnostica, Hamburg, West Germany) directly from the ulcers including those of presumed herpetic etiology. The probes were directly applied to agar plates (blood, chocolate, Endo and Sabouraud), and the MW 142 swabs placed into a nutrient broth for enrichment and further culture. In selected cases, Gram and Giemsa stains were performed immediately. Agar plates were incubated at 37°C, 5% CO_2 and evaluated morphologically after 18-24 hours for the first time, and again after another 24 hours. Further identification and antibiotic susceptibility testings were done at the Institute for Clinical Microbiology (Chairman: Prof. M. Röllinghoff, M.D.). Anaerobic cultures were not done.

2. Herpes Virus Infections Work-Ups

Corneal ulcers of presumably herpetic origin were worked-up clinically by corneal esthesiometry. Verification with monoclonal antibody direct immunofluorescent assays was performed in selected cases. Agar plating to rule out bacterial or fungal coinfections was done in each single case.

3. Documentation of Therapeutic Trials

3.a) bacterial

In a partly prospective, partly retrospective study, each patient received topical aminoglycosides (preferably Tobramycin (10)) and a combination of systemic cephalosporins (Cefotiam, 2x2g/d) with aminoglycosides (Amikacin, 2x500mg/d for three days, then tapered according to drug monitoring) as a first-line therapy. Six to 12 hours after starting with antibiotics, 250 mg (or more) of methylprednisolone were given IV and tapered in a daily two-step-fashion. The following days, topical corticosteroids (Pred A) were applied under strict slit-lamp control. After the evaluation of antibiotic susceptibility data, antibiotics were changed or added respectively.

Treatment groups to be compared included:

- topical and systemic antibiotics (54),

- antibiotics with topical and systemic corticosteroids (84),
- antibiotics with corticosteroids combined with a tectonic keratoplasty (25).

In each case, tectonic keratoplasty à chaud was done only after resolution of the hypopyon when only the stromal keratitic lesion remained. Morbidity and visual rehabilitation of this patient group was compared to a patient group receiving a graft long time after medical therapy.

3.b) herpetic

Patients with herpetic infections were divided into four groups receiving:

- Trifluorthymidine (3),
- Acyclovir (11),
- Acyclovir and corticosteroids (40) or
- Acyclovir, corticosteroids and penetrating keratoplasty (6).

4. Statistical Evaluation

Data obtained retrospectively and prospectively were evaluated with the SPSS statistics program and the chart-graphics program (MICROSOFT) for statistical significance. Chi-square tests and t-tests were performed where indicated.

Results

1. Microbiology

1.a) Spectrum of Isolates (Tab.1)

Cultures of probes taken from corneal ulcers of presumed bacterial origin revealed 20 different bacteria with 169 different strains. Staphylococci represented the most frequently isolated pathogenic agents with S. aureus found in 27% of cases. 15% of isolates were traditionally pathogenic Gram-negative strains.

Coinfections were found in 6 cases of the older age groups (mean 72 yrs.) with Staphylococc aureus coinfecting coagulase-negative Staphylococci strains, Gram-positive cocci and aerobic sporulating agents, and pneumococci coinfecting Moraxella species, Corynebacteria and alpha-hemolysing Streptococci.

Isolates from patients with metastasising carcinomas included coagulase-negative (2x) and coagulase-positive (2x) Staphylococci.

In patients with Diabetes mellitus, coagulase-negative Staphylococci (9x), coagulase-positive Staphyloccoci (4x), Morganella mor-ganii (1x), P.aeruginosa (1x), L.monocytogenes (1x) and alpha-hemolysing Streptococci (1x) were found.

A high incidence of Gram-negative bacteria and each case of Moraxella could be correlated with the patient group consisting of (presumed) alcoholics.

The incidence of pathogenic bacteria peaked at age 30-40 with a substantial amount of Gram-negative bacteria (frequent sequelae after contaminated foreign body injuries) and increased with older age (>60 yrs.).

1.b) Antibiotic Susceptibility Testing

Gram-positive organisms were susceptible to Erythromycin, Ciprofloxacin, Norfloxacin, Imipenem, and Chloramphenicol at a rate of more than 90%. Gentamycin and Tobramycin were less effective vs. staphylococci (80%) in vitro. Tetracyclines, an often used topical antibiotic for external infectious eye diseases, had a less than satisfactory efficacy with an in vitro susceptibility rate of less than 40%. Erythromycin was effective in vitro of 85%.

Gram-negative rods and cocci (excluding H.influenzae) showed a very good overall sensitivity to Ciprofloxacin, Norfloxacin, Amikacin, Tobramycin, Gentamycin, Imipenem, Cefotaxime and Cefotiam. Less than satisfactory results were achieved with Tetracyclines, Cefazoline, and Chloramphenicol.

Topical/local antibiotics are known to achieve fastest and highest concentrations in the cornea. Immediate therapy for any possible pathogen can only be recommended on the basis of known susceptibility data including Gram-positive as well as Gram-negative bacteria. Topically applied Ciprofloxacin, Erythromycin, Chloramphenicol, Tobramycin and Tetracyclines were compared in that respect: Ciprofloxacin was effective in more than 90% of isolated strains from 163 culture-established bacterial corneal ulcers and ranged significantly before Chloramphenicol, Tobramycin and Tetracylines. Ciprofloxacin was only marginally statistically superior to Erythromycin resulting from the good susceptibility of the majority of Gram-positive organisms to Erythromycin.

Ciprofloxacin has yet not been approved for topical application in clinical settings in Germany, and has thus not been used in this study. In this study, treatment with topical antibiotics was started with Gentamicin or Tobramycin drops hourly, and was changed to Erythromycin, if the respective bacteria turned out to be Gram-positive.

2. Patient Risk Factors

2.a) Age, Gender, Laterality

The mean age of the patients with bacterial infections was 61 years, the range being 11-96. Older age groups were most frequently affected with the 7th, 8th and 9th decades taking a relative percentage of the total of 15.6%, 23.2% and 13.8% respectively.

No statistically significant differences existed for the correlations of gender ratios with bacterial keratitis (45.4% female, 54.6% male, $X^2=1.76$, $X_{Crit.}=3.84$: not significant) nor between the left or right eyes involved (48.5% L.E./51.5% R.E.; $X^2=0.18$, $X_{Crit.}=3.84$: not significant).

2.b) Compromising Diseases

Immunocompromising diseases associated with corneal ulcers were found in 41 patients, most frequently in the 60-80 yrs. age group (34 cases =84.3%). Diabetes (mean age 70 yrs.) and metastasizing carcinomas (mean age 72 yrs.) were found most frequently, followed by a variety of other acquired or drug-induced (alcoholics, IV-drug abusers, immunosuppressed) secondary immunodeficiencies.

2.c) Antibiotics/Corticosteroids Pretreatment

When this study was started, antibiotic pretreatment or combined pretreatment with corticosteroids was thought to be a risk factor particularly associated with a more servere course of bacterial disease. Antibiotic pretreatment and combination ointments with corticosteroids were documented in 52 corneal ulcer patients, 16 of whom were of presumed herpetic (=21%) and 36 of culture-established bacterial origin (=22.5%). The herpetic corneal ulcers had had no microbiologically relevant colony counts of pathogenic organisms, and treatment for a presumed bacterial cause had to be judged as a wrong indication.

Thus, less than a quarter of patients with proven bacterial corneal ulcers admitted to our hospital had been pretreated with antibiotics thereby resulting in less difficulties to interprete culture results.

2.d) Contact Lenses, Mascara

Contaminated contact lenses, dispensers and mascara were not predominant causes of corneal ulcers in this patient population.

3.Procedures and Risk Factors

3.a) Surgical

Twenty-five tectonic corneal grafts were performed à chaud. Most frequently, corneal grafting was done in the third, eighth, ninth and tenth decades correlating with clinical severity and high colony counts of microbial infections. In certain cases in the very old age groups (5.6% of the total study group), tectonic keratoplasty was performed with only low-dosage topical and no systemic corticosteroids for fear of recurrence of the primary disease. Tectonic penetrating keratoplasties were only done after resolution of the hypopyon, in order to excise the keratitic stromal lesion.

Most of the 17 enucleations (=10.4% of the total) were done in patients of the eighth (=20%) and ninth decades (=45%). The need for enucleations in intractable cases was significantly correlated with diabetes (and other compromising diseases) in the respective higher age groups and preexisting secondary angle closure glaucoma with neovascularization.

Conjunctival flaps had to be done in two patients of the "antibiotics only" protocol.

3.b) Medical

Medical antibiotic therapy combined with corticosteroids was applied most frequently in the third (85.7%), fourth and fifth (65.3% each) and seventh decades (64.7%). Antibiotic therapy without corticosteroids was most frequently given to young patients in the third and to the very old patients in the tenth decades.

4. Visual Rehabilitation

Most patients (90%) suffering from bacterial corneal ulcers experienced some degree of visual rehabilitation when the visual acuities (V.A.) at admission and at dismissal were compared.

Significant discrepancies with respect to the mode of therapy, the age groups, and the incidence of diabetes could be observed in the short-term protocols for bacterial ulcer trials (see 4.a, 4.b). Short-term results as expressed by the V.A. at dismissal depended on the length of hospitalization.

Hospitalization was significantly different with respect to each treatment group and was estimated at a mean of 23 days for the "anti-infective only" compared to 15 days for the "keratoplasty plus corticosteroids" protocols.

Short-term visual results were documented at dismissal, long-term visual results covered a period of 5-28 months, with a mean of 10 months after dismissal.

4.a) Short-Term Visual Results:

V.A. at admisssion ranged from LP to 0.9 (mean 0.3): The younger the age group, the better the V.A. at admission.

V.A. at dismissal ranged from LP to 1.2 (mean 0.4). Visual recovery was best in the 20-30 year age group, and the greatest changes betweeen V.A. at admission and at dismissal were noted in the 30-40 year age group.

54 patients enrolled in the "anti-infective only"-protocol had a significant mean increase in V.A. from 0.02-0.25 (t-test: $p<0.013$).

84 patients of the "anti-infective plus corticosteroids"-protocol experienced a mean increase in V.A. from 0.1-0.4 (t-test: $p<0.001$).

25 patients treated with antibiotics, corticosteroids and early tectonic penetrating keratoplasty in addition had a mean increase from 0.02-0.6 (t-test: $p<0.005$).(Fig.5).

4.b) Long-Term Visual Results

Long-term visual results ranged from 5-28 months after dismissal (mean = 10 months). Visual results showed a significant decrease in all age groups compared to the V.A. on the day of dismissal, most pronounced in the "antibiotics only"-protocol.

A decrease of V.A. was observed in each of the long-term results of all protocols:

- antibiotic therapy without corticosteroids was worst: 0.01,
- antibiotics with corticosteroids: 0.2,
- keratoplasty with antibiotics without systemic corticosteroids: 0.01 and
- keratoplasty with antibiotics and corticosteroids: 0.3. At the end of the "anti-infective only" protocol, conjunctival flaps had to be done twice, which contributed additionally to the bad visual results of this group of patients.

Statistical evaluation of these data (t-test) showed the V.A. of the "antibiotics only"-protocol to be significantly different from the "keratoplasty plus corticosteroids"-protocol ($p<0.001$). Differences between V.A. for the "antibiotics plus corticosteroids"-protocol and the "keratoplasty plus corticosteroids" group were marginally significant. All the other visual results were not statistically different from each other.

Therefore, satisfactory short-term and long-term visual rehabilitation had only been documented consistently and significantly for the "keratoplasty" and "corticosteroids" groups of patients.

5. Secondary Complications and Late Events

5.a) Secondary Glaucomas

Reversible intraocular pressure elevations during hospitalization occurred in 20 patients, particularly in the older age groups at a mean frequency of 30% (61-70:9 =45%, 71-80:5 =25%, 81-90:4 =20%).- In the other age groups, the incidence of a secondary rise of intraocular pressure was estimated at 0-5%.

Long-term visual impairment due to secondary glaucomas requiring therapy was noted in 6 patients of the older age groups (60-80 yrs.) suffering from diabetes.

5.b) Recurrences of Infections or Second Episodes

Eighteen patients (=11%) experienced a second episode of infectious disease. All of these recurrences or second episodes could be observed during check-ups after dismissal. Infectious agents isolated from these cases were: Coagulase-negative Staphylococci at high colony counts (15x), S.aureus (1x), Corynebacteria (2x), alpha-hemolysing Streptococci (1x), P. aeruginosa (1x), Moraxella sp. (1x). Phage-typing or plasmid analysis to differentiate recurrences from newly acquired infections were not done.

Two of these patients were of the "penetating keratoplasty"-protocol and needed repeat corneal grafting, which subsequently developed uneventful.

5.c) Antiinfective Pretreatment is no Risk Factor for Enucleation

Antibiotic pretreatment had been documented in 36 patients with bacterial corneal ulcers. This patient group was compared to the trial group not pretreated, and V.A. was observed to be 0.1/0.08 at admission vs. 0.2/0.2 at dismissal with the long-term results of 0.15/0.07 at an average of 4 months after dismissal. In each case, the responsible organisms could be isolated, and pretreatment had to be judged ineffective.

Enucleations occurred no more frequently in the patient group pretreated with antibiotics or corticosteroids combination ointments compared to the patients not pretreated when statistical correction was applied to the absolute numbers (X^2=0.28, $X_{Crit.}$=2.71: not significant).

5.d) Late Procedures

In the first group of patients with the "antibiotics only" protocol, 6 penetrating keratoplasties were performed much later for clarification of the scarred corneas. These patients were not included in the study.

6. Comparison With Herpetic Corneal Ulcers

6.a) Risk Factors

Risk factors for the control population of herpetic ulcers were corticosteroids and a combination therapy with antibiotics and corticosteroids due to a missed diagnosis

(=69.5% of cases with therapy-resistant severe keratitis).

The mean age of patients suffering from herpetic corneal ulcers was similar to those of bacterial etiology with a peak at the 30-40 yr. age group and an increase from 60 yrs. up (mean: 61.5yrs.). Systemic compromising diseases could not be documented.

6.b) Visual Results

Short-term visual results were monitored at dismissal,long-term results were obtained after an observation period of 3-16 months (mean of 8 months after dismissal).

Patients with herpetic corneal ulcers commonly presented with a better V.A. than patients with bacterial keratitis (0.1 vs. 0.07).

The historic Trifluorthymidine trial group (3 patients) was too small to be included for statistically significant results.

Patients receiving Acyclovir only had an increase in V.A. from 0.15 at admission to 0.25 at dismissal, which was significantly better than the increase of the mean V.A. of all bacterial keratitis trials ($p < 0.005$).

There was no statistical difference of increase in V.A. between the use of Acyclovir or a combination with corticosteroids ($X^2 = 1.67$, $X_{Crit.} = 2.0$: not significant).

There were no significant differences between an increase in V.A. after medical or combined medical and surgical therapy ($X^2 = 0.66$, $X_{Crit.} = 1.98$: not significant) in this study: This observation may be correlated with the sole indication for tectonic keratoplasty to cover perforations or descemetoceles in active herpetic lesions.

Long-term visual results were disappointing in the "Acyclovir only" trial (0.06 five months after dismissal). Additional therapy with corticosteroids did not help to achieve a significantly better V.A. (0.08).

6.c) Secondary Complications

- Recurrences

In general, morbidity was much higher in the herptic group compared to the bacterial ulcer group.

When relapses were compared, herpetic corneal ulcers recurred in 40 out of 60 patients (=40%), whereas a relapse of bacterial etiology was noted in only 18/163 (=11%) of cases. A repeat keratoplasty had to be performed in 4 patients (45%), a high rate when compared to the bacterial ulcer group (2 patients=10%).

Bacterial coinfections of clinical relevance were only observed after dismissal with simultaneous reactivation of the Herpes lesions. Coagulase-negative Staphylococci (10x), S.aureus (2x) and corynebacteria (2x) were isolated. Since the use of corticosteroids was limited to the period of hospitalization, corticosteroid treatment could not be correlated with the ensuing bacterial complications.

- Enucleations and Secondary Glaucomas

No enucleations were necessary in the observation period in contrast to the bacterial corneal ulcers.

Secondary glaucomas were the most common complications of herpetic corneal ulcers occurring in 16 patients (=24.6%) compared to only 6 (=3.7%) with ulcers of bacterial etiology. The long-term risk for the development of severe secondary glaucomas in the herpetic keratitis group was significantly higher than in the bacterial ulcer group ($p<0.001$).

Thus, significant differences between the prognosis of cure, visual rehabilitation, patient morbidity and long-term complications such as secondary glaucomas and relapses of the primary diseases could be observed.

Discussion

In this partly prospective, partly retrospective study of 205 selected patients with 223 eyes and 163 bacterial and 60 herpetic corneal ulcers, an attempt was made to define the role of topical/local and systemic corticosteroids and tectonic perforating keratoplasty for morbidity and visual outcome.

Compared to previous investigations carried out on the basis of a clinical diagnosis with a high percentage of negative culture results, this study of 163 bacterial corneal ulcers has included only patients with correctly culture-established microbiological diagnoses (4,13,27). Patients with fungal or parasitic infections have not been included in this study, and only patients with complete follow-ups have been evaluated.

Bacterial keratitis may be etiologically defined, if repeat cultures grow the same organism, or if traditionally pathogenic agents may be cultured from the respective lesions. For any first-line therapy to make sense, the spectrum of pathogens in the respective area of a referral center must be known (9,17,32,36). In this study, coagulase-negative and coagulase-positive staphylococci at high colony counts were most frequently isolated from corneal ulcers. 15% of isolates were Gram negative bacteria. This included 6 patients with coinfections. Moraxella was found with a relatively high incidence. Moraxella has been reported earlier to be significantly correlated with alcoholism, which may also hold true for these patients living either in neglected circumstances or being employed in the alcoholic beverage industry with an enormous daily consumption of beer (5,24). The spectrum and incidence of bacteria correlates well with earlier studies from 1972 (27) and 1985 (6) in our hospital as well as many previous reports on the spectrum of microbial keratitis in adults in the Northern parts of the USA (25). Attempts for isolation of anaerobic organisms have not been done in this study as they were thought not to play as great a role in acutely diseased infectious keratitis patients than aerobic organisms (12,15,30). This, however, may not be a correct assumption considering recent literature and anaerobes should - particularly in rural areas as ours - be looked for more closely in the future (1,7).

Diabetes and advanced age have been identified as risk factors in this population of corneal ulcer patients. Most of the tectonic keratoplasties and enucleations were performed in the higher age groups, partly due to the severity of the infection, partly because of in vivo intractibility despite in vitro antibiotic susceptibility. The male gender of the younger age groups seemed to be prone to develop infectious bacterial keratitis only with a history of previous foreign body lesions (1).

Pretreatment of patients with antibiotics or corticosteroids combination ointments did not represent a risk factor for a more complicated clinical course in this study, which is in accordance with previously controversial experimental and clinical works (2,11,19,23,33). Contaminated contact lenses or mascara play a significant role for corneal ulcers in this rural patient population.

Antibiotic susceptibility with respect to overall Gram-negative and Gram-positive strains was best for the topical ointments of Ciprofloxacin, followed by Erythromycin. This observation is in support of previously published findings for Norfloxacin of conjunctival probes (10,14,29). From the microbiological standpoint, topical Ciprofloxacin may therefore be recommended as a first-line therapy without knowledge of responsible agents in severe keratitis of presumed bacterial etiology.

The combination of systemic Cephalosporins with Aminoglycosides (Amikacin) for immediate therapy was effective in vitro as well as clinically in 85% of cases (26).

Therapeutic modalities were elaborated with topical and systemic corticosteroids and antibiotics and additional penetrating tectonic keratoplasty à chaud. All trials resulted in an increase of V.A. at the end of hospitalization.

Statistically significantly better V.A. was obtained with a regimen of corticosteroids during the acute phase of infection and with a "corticosteroids plus keratoplasty"-protocol. The rationale for using corticosteroids from the beginning of treatment was to reduce the inflammatory reaction, which might have been be elicited by live bacteria as well as cell wall fragments (Lipopolysaccharides etc.). From the point of infection immunology, this destructive phase involving a completely activated amplification system can only be overcome by topical/local and systemic corticosteroids (3,21). Superiority of endophthalmitis trials using high-dosage corticosteroids has been suggested recently (35).

Corneal grafting à chaud after the disappearance of a hypopyon was done to excise the infectious lesion and thereby achieve an enhanced cure with a shortened hospital stay (8,28). This latter management was chosen because antibiotics are known to only slowly if ever reach pathogenic organisms located in the stromal tissue of the cornea (36). Only twice, repeat keratoplasties had to be carried out for late secondary infections. This is a low incidence considering the severe clinical pictures at admission.

The fear of secondary angle closure glaucomas due to formation of anterior synechiae had led to a recommendation for "postponement of keratoplasty in the acutely inflamed and/or perforated cornea" (18) in the past. Thanks to advanced viscoelastic anterior segment surgery, this standpoint is no longer tenable.

Despite good experimental evidence against it, the utilization of corticosteroids in infectious inflammatory eye diseases had long been neglected by clinicians because of fear to enhance pathogen replication and produce a deleterious result. With the advent of newer and better antibiotics, well-controlled application of corticosteroids systemically and topically may now lend a broader support to the research results of infection immunologists in the late 1970s (2,34).

Long-term V.A. of patients treated for bacterial corneal ulcers showed best results with a combination therapy of antibiotics, corticosteroids and keratoplasty. Unsatisfactory results were seen with antibiotics only, because of frequent development of corneal scars in the visual axis.

When the treatment results of the 163 bacterial corneal ulcers were contrasted to the 60 herpetic keratitis patients, it was noted that hospitalization of herpetic keratitis patients was significantly shorter, however, morbidity due to recurrences and visual impairment because of secondary glaucomas and corneal scarring was much higher. In comparison to the bacterial corneal ulcers, patients with herpetic lesions experienced an increase in short-term and long-term V.A. only in the Acyclovir (medical treatment) group. Tectonic keratoplasties resulted in a decrease of V.A. in the long run, and 44% of patients had suffered episodes of recurrences with graft rejections at the time of check-ups. This high rejection rate of corneal grafts for herpetic corneal ulcers has been documented previously, and an increased expression of MHC II antigens during HSV reactivation has been proposed as a pathogenic mechanism (20).

In conclusion, recognition of pathogenic mechanisms of destructive bacterial ocular infections has resulted in a fair chance for conservation of the eye and restoration of useful V.A. as well as a decreased hospital stay through the application of a triple therapeutic approach with

- agent-specific topical/systemic anti-infective drugs,
- topical/systemic corticosteroids and
- excision of the infected area (=tectonic corneal grafting).

The rationale for this approach may be found in the knowledge that factors responsible for a poor outcome of corneal ulcers (and corneal grafts in corneal ulcer patients) are not primarily bacterial in nature, but onsist of the destructive host response mediated by bacterial glycoconjugates.

Clinical management of herpetic keratitis is different from bacterial keratitis, and the use of corticosteroids may not be helpful in this condition, particularly since the prevention of frequent recurrences is not possible.

Table 1. Spectrum And Incidence of Bacterial Pathogens From 163 Corneal Ulcers

Isolates	Incidence		%
Coagulase negative Staph	74		44%
S. aureus	44		26%
Streptococcus pneumoniae	8		5%
hemolysing Streptococci	7	Gram-positive= 85%	4%
Streptococcus faecalis	5		3%
Corynebacteria	5		3%
Moraxella sp.	5		3%
Pseudomonas aeruginosa	4		2%
Hemophilus influenzae	3		2%
Proteus mirabilis	3	Gram-negative = 15%	2%
Morganella morganii	2		1%
other Gram negative bacteria	9		5%
Total	169		100%

References

1. Affeldt JC, Flynn HW, Forster RK et al (1987) Microbial Endophthalmitis Resulting from Ocular Trauma. Ophthalmology 94:407-413
2. Aronson SB, Moore TE (1969) Corticosteroid Therapy in Central Stromal Keratitis. Am J Ophthalmol 67:873-896
3. Aronson SB, Elliot JH (1972) Ocular Inflammation. CV Mosby St.Louis pp.28-33
4. Baum JL (1979) Initial Therapy of Suspected Microbial Corneal Ulcers. I.Broad Antibiotic Therapy Based on Prevalence of Organisms. Surv Ophthalmol 24:97-105
5. Baum JL, Fedukowicz HB, Jorden A (1980) A Survey of Moraxella Corneal Ulcers in a Derelict Population. Am J Ophthalmol 90:476-480
6. Bialasiewicz AA, Radtke U, Maywald M (1987) Ätiologie von Hornhautulzera unter besonderer Berücksichtigung der bakteriellen Genese. Klin Mbl Augenheilkd 190:161-166
7. Boldt HC, Pulido JS, Blodi DF et al (1989) Rural Endophthalmitis. Ophthalmology 96:1722-1726
8. Boruchoff SA, Donshik PC (1975) Medical and Surgical Management of Corneal Thinnings and Perforations. Int Ophthalmol Clin 15(4):11-123
9. Byrne-Rhodes KA, Anicete GR (1988) Common Isolates and in vitro Antibiotic Susceptibility in Microbial Keratitis in Saudi Arabia Saudi Bull Ophthalmol 3:17-24
10. Chi NX, Neu HC (1984) Ciprofloxacin, a Quinolone Carboxylic Acid Compound Active Against Aerobic and Anaerobic Bacteria. Antimicrob Ag Chemother 25:319-326
11. Hyndiuk RA, Chin GN (1973) Corticosteroid Therapy in Corneal Diseases. Int Ophthalmol Clin 13:103
12. Hyndiuk RA, Nassif KF, Burd EM (1983) Bacterial Diseases.
13. In: Smolin G, Thoft RA (eds) The Cornea. Scientific Foundations and Clinical Practice. Little, Brown & Co., Boston pp. 147-167
14. Hyndiuk RA, Skorich DN, Burd EM (1986) Bacterial Keratitis. In: Tabbara KF, Hyndiuk RA (eds) Infections of the Eye. Little, Brown & Co., Boston pp.303-330
15. Jacobson JA, Call NB, Kasworm EM et al (1988) Safety and Efficiency of Topical Norfloxacin vs. Tobramycin in the Treatment of External Ocular Infections. Antimicrob Ag Chemother 32:1820-1824
16. Jones DB (1979) Initial Therapy of Suspected Microbial Corneal Ulcers. II. Specific Antibiotic Therapy Based on Corneal Smears. Surv Ophthalmol 24:97-116
17. Jones,DB (1981) Decision-Making in the Management of Microbial Keratitis. Ophthalmology 88:814-820
18. Jones RN (1985) Selection of Antimicrobial Agents for Susceptibility Testing. Coll American Pathol Summing Up 15(2):3
19. Kenyon KR (1982) Decision-Making in the Therapy of External Eye Disease: Noninfected Corneal Ulcers. Ophthalmology 89:44-51
20. Kleinert RW (1986) Corticosteroid Use in Ocular Infectious Disease. In: Tabbara KF, Hyndiuk RA (eds) Infections of the Eye. Little, Brown & Co, Boston pp.293-202
21. Langston RHS, Pavan-Langston D (1975) Penetrating Keratoplasty for Herpetic Keratitis: Decision Making and Management. Int Ophthalmol Clin 15(4):125-140
22. Leibowitz HM, Lass JH, Kupferman A (1974) Quantitation of Inflammation in the Cornea. Arch Ophthalmol 92:427-430
23. Leibowitz HM, Kupferman A (1975) Bioavailability and Therapeutic Effectiveness of Topically Administered Corticosteroids. Trans Am Acad Ophthalmol Otolarlyngol 79:78-88

24. Leibowitz HM, Kupferman A (1980) Topically Administered Corticosteroids: Effect on Antibiotic Treated Bacterial Keratitis. Arch Ophthalmol 98:1287-1290
25. Leibowitz HM, Ryan W, Kupferman A et al (1985) The Effect of Alcohol Intoxication on Inflammation of the Cornea. Arch Ophthalmol 103:723-725
26. Liesegang TJ, Forster RK (1980) Spectrum of Microbial Keratitis in South Florida. Am J Ophthalmol 90:38-47
27. McNamara BT, Meyer RD, Pasiecznik KA (1982) In vitro Susceptibility of Cephalotin-Resistant Enterobacteriaceae and Ps.aeruginosa to Amikacin and Selected New ß-Lactam Agents. Antimicrob Ag Chemother 21:753-575
28. Meythaler H, Schick A (1972) Klinische und statistische Untersuchungen über das Ulcus corneae serpens. Ber Dtsch Ophthalmol Ges 71:594-597
28. Naumann GOH, Sautter H (1988) Chirurgie der Kornea.In: Mackensen G, Neubauer H (eds) Augenärztliche Operationen I. Springer Verlag Heidelberg pp.492-555
29. O'Brien TP, Sawusch MR, Dick JD et al (1988) Topical Ciprofloxacin Treatment of Pseudomonas Keratitis in Rabbits. Arch Ophthalmol 106:1444-1446
30. Ormerod D, Murphree AL, Gomez DS (1986) Microbial Keratitis in Children. Ophthalmology 93:449-454
31. Proeller O (1903) Über die Verwendbarkeit der Hornhauttransplantationen bei schweren ulzerativen Prozessen der Kornea. Graefes Arch Ophthalmol 56:315-325
32. Richardson JF, Marples RR (1982) Changing Resistance to Antimicrobial Drugs and Resistance Typing in Clinically Significant Strains of Staph.epidermidis. Med Microbiol 15:475-484
33. Smolin G, Okumoto M, Leon-Sit L (1980) Combined Gentamicin-Tobramycin-Corticosteroid Treatment. II Effect on Gentamycin-Resistant Pseudomonas Keratitis. Arch Ophthalmol 98:473-474
34. Snip RC, Kenyon KR (1978) Acute Inflammatory Cells in Melting Human Corneas. Invest Ophthalmol Vis Sci 17(S):252
35. Stern DA, Engel HM, Driebe WT (1989) The Treatment of Postoperative Endophthalmitis: Results of Differing Approaches to Treatment. Ophthalmology 96:62-67
36. Wilhelmus KR (1984) Bacterial Corneal Ulcers. Int Ophthalmol Clin 24:1-16
37. Wilhelmus KR, Gilbert ML, Osato MS (1987) Tobramycin in Ophthalmology. Surv Ophthalmol 32:111-122.

Penetrating Keratoplasty for Acanthamoeba Keratitis

Linda Ficker and Colin Kirkness

Abstract. Eighteen penetrating keratoplasties were performed for Acanthamoeba keratitis (1985-1989) in 13 eyes. Diagnostic delay contributed to scarring (n=6), uncontrolled infection (n=7) and perforation (n=5). Five eyes achieved 6/9 vision and 50% of penetrating keratoplasties remained clear (mean follow-up 34 months). Graft rejection episodes were common (50%), but did not cause failure.

Risk factors for graft survival were recurrence, scleritis and glaucoma. Recurrence occurred in 50% of cases and was associated with the finding of trophozoites in excised corneal tissue. One bilateral case developed a temperature-sensitive mutant, resistant to Brolene, and required regrafting for recurrence. Scleritis was managed with periopera

tive intravenous corticosteroids in two perforated eyes. Although the scleritis was controlled, recurrence required regrafting and these penetrating keratoplasties failed. Eight eyes developed cataract and underwent cataract extraction. Three intumescent cataracts were associated with ocular hypertension and vision was lost due to uncontrolled glaucoma.
Keratoplasty in quiet eyes had a good prognosis, but inflamed eyes compared poorly with grafting for Herpes Simplex Virus or suppurative (bacterial/fungal) keratitis, the hazard ratios at 36 months being 9.4 and 5.9 respectively.

Introduction

Acanthamoeba sp. was first identified as pathogenic for microbial keratitis in 1974 (10). A patient sustained a corneal abrasion which was irrigated with tap water. He subsequently developed microbial keratitis which was treated with antibiotics and antivirals without microbiological investigation. Treatment was ineffective and a corneal scrape was subsequently performed. Giemsa staining of the smear revealed thick-walled cysts, and wave-like tracks were observed a few days later on the surface of the blood agar culture. A direct wet-mount of the agar revealed both cysts and trophozoites indicating the diagnosis of a free-living amoeba, indentified as Acanthamoeba sp. The infection was treated with an antiamoebic drug, Sulphadiazine, but was not controlled and the patient required excisional penetrating keratoplasty.

Diagnosis

An increasing number of case reports of Acanthamoeba keratitis followed, which described progressive keratitis and a poor prognosis. This usually followed delay in the identification of Acanthamoeba. The keratitis often masqueraded as herpetic keratitis at the time of presentation and was treated initially with antivirals. The epithelial defect frequently healed on such treatment, but an indolent course followed which was characterised by recurrent epithelial breakdown, progressive corneal infiltration and lysis. Corneal scrapes at this stage often gave a culture-negative result.

Special staining techniques were recommended to facilitate early diagnosis. These included specific immunofluorescent antibody staining in addition to non-specific stains, such as lectins and calcofluor white, which stain cyst walls. Special culture techniques were advocated as Acanthamoebae grow best on non-nutrient agar seeded with live Escherichia coli.

Deep stromal invasion and encystment occur with time and in association with keratocyte depletion. This is the likely reason why corneal scrapes are often microscopy and culture negative if the infection has been established for a few weeks. A biopsy is then required to obtain deeper tissue containing viable amoeba.

Treatment

Medical therapy has been based on in vitro sensitivity data and the first successful treatment with topical Neomycin and Brolene (Propamidine drops and Dibromopropamidine ointment) was reported in 1985 (20). A number of additional drugs have since been found to be effective in combination therapy for acanthamoebic keratitis including Paromomycin, Polyhexamethonium Biguanide, Ketoconazole and Clotrimazole. Brolene resistance has been reported (6) for a temperature-sensitive mutant which could only be cultured at 25°C. Clotrimazole has provided effective therapy for recurrence of infection post-penetrating keratoplasties (4).

Topical coricosteroids are often administered to control the limbitis which is often a feature of the disease. Crystalline keratopathy was first described in such patients. It is a low-grade mid-stromal keratitis due to non-virulent bacteria including Streptococcus viridans and causing corneal opacities resembling crystals (3).

The increasing incidence of Acanthamoeba keratitis was associated with contact lens wear including hard, gas permeable, Saturn, soft and disposable lenses (8,17). Contamination of homemade saline solutions was established as the most common etiological-factor in the United States and these solutions were withdrawn. Amoebae have also been found in domestic water supplies, which are used by lens wearers to rinse lenses.

Excisional Keratoplasty

There are a number of surgical principles, which have been advocated for microbial keratitis (12). Early surgery with reformation of the anterior chamber angle performed within 24 hours following perforation reduces the risk of peripheral anterior synechiae and secondary glaucoma ($p<0.001$). In the perforated eye, the cord length of the excised host disc is often greater than the trephine diameter used to mark the epithelium. The donor trephine must be selected on the basis of the host cord length to ensure an adequately sized donor disc. This avoids trabecular distortion and outflow obstruction caused by an undersized disc. Cataract extraction is avoided unless the lens is intumescent. Interrupted suturing permits removal of loose sutures without compromising wound stability.

Before the introduction of effective medical therapy in 1984, uncontrolled amoebic keratitis resulted in progressive stromal collagenolysis. It has been demonstrated that Acanthamoeba-conditioned culture medium produces collagenolysis in corneal tissue due to collagenase (21). Excisional keratoplasty was performed as a therapeutic procedure both to debulk infection and to avoid perforation.

Among early case reports there was often delay in establishing the diagnosis and penetrating keratoplasties were performed for uncontrolled keratitis or corneal perforation. In some cases the diagnosis was made by histopathological examination of the excised cornea. Penetrating keratoplasty was performed from 2-13 months after the onset of infection and graft diameter ranged from 7.5mm to 10mm (1,10,11,14,18,19). Recurrence, reported in about 57% of eyes, resulted in graft failure within a month of the surgery. The reports do not indicate whether there was a correlation between histopathological clearance of infected tissue and graft survival. It is difficult therefore to comment on the success of "excisional" penetrating keratoplasty without adjunctive topical therapy.

After 1984 antiamoebic drugs were used, but the regimes reported varied considerably. The diagnosis of Acanthamoeba keratitis continued to be made after significant delay. There was a lag between onset of keratitis and commencement of antiamoebic treatment which ranged from one to seven months (mean 3.1 months). Infection was therefore advanced before appropriate therapy was initiated and patients continued to require penetrating keratoplasty if the clinical disease failed to respond or if there was impending or actual perforation. Some patients were treated preoperatively with both Brolene and Neomycin, although for periods ranging from one week to 17 months (2,3,4,20). Graft survival without recurrence appeared better for patients pretreated for at least one month. Numbers were too small for statistical analysis; 6/7 penetrating keratoplasties survived in cases pretreated for a month or more while only 2/5 penetrating keratoplasties survived in cases pretreated for less than a month despite postoperative Brolene and Neomycin therapy. It is not known how long treatment must be continued without the risk of recurrence although it is likely to be in part dependent on the duration of infection. Neomycin and Brolene have cysticidal activity, but corneal tissue excised from patients often contains demonstrable cysts after several months of treatment. Antiamoebic therapy is generally administered for several months after penetrating keratoplasty, particularly in patients with a long history prior to surgery in whom amoeba may have invaded the peripheral cornea.

Stromal keratocytes are depleted in the superficial stroma from which amoeba have migrated and inflammatory cells migrate to these areas. Infiltrates may not necessarily be a focal sign of infection and resolution of stromal infiltration does not necessarily indicate control of the infection.

Acanthamoeba keratitis can cause anterior scleritis with the onset ranging from 1-8 months (10,15,17). Treatment with high dose systemic corticosteroids (80mg) is generally effective and penetrating keratoplasty may later be performed. Late scleritis is usually associated with extensive peripheral corneal infiltration and has been associated with recurrence of infection in the graft. This suggests that peripheral scleral invasion by amoebae has occurred in these eyes.

Complications

The sequelae of inflammation include trabecular outflow obstruction and raised intraocular pressure. The anterior chamber of the eye is often relatively quiet in Acanthamoeba keratitis, but there can be severe limbitis which accounts for the pressure rise. Since the keratitis may only subside over a period of several weeks, it is important to achieve medical control of the intraocular pressure in order to protect the optic disc. This requires both hypotensive and antiinflammatory therapy. Glaucoma may be difficult to control after penetrating keratoplasty and a number of eyes were treated with cyclocryotherapy (2,10,17). Only one penetrating keratoplasty remained clear following this cyclodestructive procedure and the eye became blind. A preferable management strategy is to perform trabeculectomy in the first instance, followed by tube drainage in the event of trabeculectomy failure (9).

Cataract is not an uncommon complication of Acanthamoeba keratitis, although combined penetrating keratoplasty and cataract extraction has only rarely been reported as a primary procedure (6). Cataract extraction has been performed subsequently, both extracapsular and intracapsular cataract extraction, at intervals ranging from 4-12 months post penetrating keratoplasty in eyes free from recurrent infection. Penetrating keratoplasty survival curves cannot be constructed from the data available in this report, but individual survival ranged from 6-36 months which was the duration of follow-up.

The incidence of transplant rejection episodes is about 50% which compares with the incidence for Herpes simplex grafts (7). It is therefore especially important in this group, comprising mostly young patients, to prevent the progression from minimal anterior chamber inflammation to destructive endothelial rejection with a Khodadoust line. Early rejection episodes manifesting anterior chamber cells and occasional penetrating keratoplasty precipitates should be aggressively treated with intensive topical corticosteroids to minimize endothelial cell loss.

Comment

Acanthamoeba keratitis is associated with contact lens wear. Increasing awareness of the clinical signs have led to earlier diagnosis and treatment. The role of penetrating keratoplasty in the management of Acanthamoeba infection is changing. Adequate pretreatment with antiamoebic therapy and aggressive corticosteroid therapy for rejection episodes appear especially important for graft survival.

References

1. Blackman HJ et al (1984) Acanthamoeba Keratitis Successfully Treated with Penetrating Keratoplasty. Cornea 3:125-130
2. Cohen EJ et al (1987) Medical and Surgical Treatment of Acanthamoeba Keratitis. Am J Ophthalmol 103:615-625
3. Davis RM (1987) Acanthamoeba Keratitis and Infectious Crystalline Keratopathy. Arch Ophthalmol 105:1524
4. Driebe WT et al (1988) Acanthamoeba Keratitis: Potential Role for Topical Clotrimazole in Combination Chemotherapy. Arch Ophthalmol 106:1196
5. Epstein RJ et al (1986) Rapid Diagnosis of Acanthamoeba Keratitis from Corneal Scrapings Using Indirect Fluorescent Antibody Staining. Arch Ophthalmol 104:1318
6. Ficker LA et al. Acanthamoeba Keratitis - the Challenge of Resistance to Medical Therapy.
7. Ficker LA et al (1989) The Changing Management and Improved Prognosis for Grafting in HSK. Ophthalmol 96:1587
8. Ficker LA et al (1989) Acanthamoeba Keratitis Occuring with Disposable Contact Lens Wear. Am J Ophthalmol 108:453
9. Gilvarry A et al (1989) The Management of Post-Keratoplasty Glaucoma by Trabeculectomy. Eye 96:1587
10. Jones DB et al (1975) Acanthamoeba Polyphaga Keratitis and Acanthamoeba Uveitis Associated with Fatal Meningoencephalitis. Trans Ophthalmol Soc UK 95:221
11. Key SN et al (1980) Keratitis Due to Acanthamoeba castellanii. Arch Ophthalmol 98:475
12. Kirkness CM et al (1991) Penetrating Keratoplasty in the Management of Perfo-

ration Complicating Microbial Keratitis. Eye 5:431
13. Lindquist TD et al (1988) Clinical Signs and Medical Therapy of Early Acanthamoeba Keratitis. Arch Ophthalmol 106:73
14. Lund OE et al (1978) Amoebic Keratitis: A Clinicopathological Case Report. Br J Ophthalmol 62:373
15. Mannis MJ et al (1986) Acanthamoeba Sclerokeratitis. Arch Ophthalmol 104: 1313 - 1317
16. Mathers W et al (1987) Immunopathology and Electron Microscopy of Acanthamoeba Keratitis. Am J Ophthalmol 103:626
17. Moore MB et al (1985) Acanthamoeba Keratitis Associated with Soft Contact Lenses. Am J Ophthalmol 100:396
18. Nagington J et al (1974) Amoebic Infection of the Eye. The Lancet 1537
19. Samples JR et al (1984) Acanthamoeba Keratitis Possibly Acquired from a Hot Tub. Arch Ophthalmol 102:707
20. Wright P et al (1985) Acanthamoeba Keratitis Successfully Treated Medically. Br J Ophthalmol 69:778
21. YuGuang HE et al (1990) In Vivo and In Vitro Collagenolytic Activity of Acanthamoeba castellanii. Invest Ophthalmol Vis Sci 31:2235

IV. NOSOCOMIAL INFECTIONS

- Basics, Surveillance Programs

Epidemiology of Nosocomial Infections

S. Lemmen und Franz Daschner

Abstract. Nosocomial infections in ophthalmology are rare, and severe events estimated at an incidence of approximately 0.05%.
Most infections are endogenous; very rarely are microorganisms transmitted from an exogenous source, e.g. hands, air, medications etc. The most common nosocomial pathogens are S.aureus, S.epidermidis, some Gramnegative organisms, as P.aeruginosa and viruses.
Diagnosis and therapy of nosocomial infections of the eye do not significantly differ from non-hospital-acquired infections.

Introduction

Nosocomial infections are defined by the fact that the disease has not manifested itself clinically at admission nor that it has been incubating. Infections, which have been acquired during the hospital stay and may become apparent only after dismissal are classified as nosocomial, such as epidemic keratoconjunctivitis, postoperative endophthalmitis or hepatitis B (4).

Infections becoming apparent during hospitalization but which may be seen in the context of another infection present at admission (as for example metastatic endophthalmitis may develop on the basis of infectious endocarditis) are not defined as nosocomial.

Infections of neonates acquired at birth (for example with chlamydiae) are usually characterized as nosocomial, however, transplacental infections diagnosed after birth (for example toxoplasmosis or listeriosis) are not accounted for nosocomial infections (4).

The incidence of nosocomial infections has until now only been evaluated systematically and nation-wide in the USA (Study on the Efficacy of Nosocomial Infection Control (SENIC (5). According to this study, 6% of all in-patients in the USA acquire nosocomial infections. Nosocomial infections prolong the length of hospitalization and increase mortality. Thus, 0.6% of all nosocomial infections in the USA in 1984 were fatal, and in 2.3% they represented a cofactor for the fatal outcome (7). As a matter of fact, nosocomial infections present a medical and economic as well as a social problem.

Incidence of Nosocomial Infections and Microbial Spectrum

We have monitored the incidence of nosocomial infections in the various departments of the Freiburg University Hospital in a prospective study for several years. High rates of nosocomial infections have occurred particularly in the Children's Hospital (16.3%) due to infections of preterm babies and neonates and in the Surgical Department (6.4%) because of an increased exposure to microbes during surgery. An increased risk of nosocomial infections is known for intensive care units due to invasive diagnostic and therapeutic regimens, e.g. intubation, urethral and venous catheters and in addition because of the often decreased defense mechanisms of the respective patients. In this study, the lowest incidence of nosocomial infections has been found in the Eye Hospital (0.03%).

The Study on the Efficacy of Nosocomial Infection Control in the USA has shown urethritis (45%) to be the most frequently occurring nosocomial infection (5). Postoperative wound infections are the second most frequent (30%) and septicemia the third most frequent (19%) reason for nosocomial infections. Various ocular nosocomial infections comprise postoperative endophthalmitis, dacryocystitis and episcleritis as well as hospital-acquired nonsurgically related blepharitis, conjunctivitis and keratitis.

The most frequent etiologic organisms in urethral infections are E.coli and S.faecalis; infections of the skin and mucous membranes are mainly caused by S.aureus and C.albicans. In hospital-acquired pneumonitis, P.aeruginosa can be isolated most frequently; in nosocomial septicemia, S.aureus is the most frequently found organism. Overall, S.aureus is the most frequent microbe causing nosocomial infections followed by miscellaneous Gram-negative bacteria (3,8). The most frequent organisms in nosocomial ocular infections are shown in Tab.2 (8):

- Coagulase negative Staphylococci (22%),
- S.aureus (19%) and
- P.aeruginosa (9%).

Epidemiology of Nosocomial Infections

In nosocomial infections endogenous and exogenous sources of pathogens can be identified. Infections caused by organisms originating from the bodily flora are defined as "endogenous" (e.g. wound infections due to microbes of the gut flora subsequent to gastrointestinal surgery). Two thirds of hospital-acquired infections are thought to be "endogenous". This is the reason why nosocomial infections may not necessarily be linked to a lack of hygiene in medical or nursing care. These infections are extremely difficult to prevent.

Transmission of exogenous pathogens occurs directly via the hands of the personnel and indirectly via contaminated instruments/devices and solutions.

Colonisation of the eye lids and conjunctiva with "physiologic" as well as pathogenic organisms may represent a risk factor for postoperative endophthalmitis in elective intraocular surgery. Hematogenous spread of pathogens from distant sites may involve the eye, e.g. in endocarditis, catheter septicemia or translocation of intestinal facultatively intracellular bacteria.

The most important exogenous source of pathogens are the hands of caring personnel; direct contact with infected mucous membranes is particularly frequently the cause for hand-borne transmission of epidemic keratoconjunctivitis and neonatal ophthalmitis. Epidemics of nosocomial infections may be caused by inadequate disinfection of instruments, e.g. tonometers, other diagnostic devices as well as contamination of eye drops or solutions. With regard to the surgical environment, contaminated gels and solutions, devices such as surgical microscopes, implants (e.g. intraocular lens) or transplants (e.g. corneal buttons) may give rise to nosocomial postoperative infections. Frequently isolated pathogens in this setting comprise coagulase negative staphylococci, enterobacteriaceae, streptococcal species and fungi.

During surgical interventions, the oropharyngeal and nasal cavities are of particular importance as a source of pathogens: with continued conversation, respiratory secretions and pathogens (e.g. S.aureus, coagulase negative Staphylococci and Streptococcus viridans) may sediment directly into the surgical area, since the surgical mask may only be of limited value for the prevention of air-borne transmission, particularly when it has been soaked. Vectors and modes of transmission have been characterized; air has not been shown to play any major role. Therefore, ocular surgery does not necessarily have to be performed in operating rooms separated from operating theaters used by other surgical disciplines.

Nosocomial Infection Risk Estimation by Invasive Procedures

Invasive diagnostic and therapeutic procedures increase the risk for directly and indirectly caused nosocomial infections. This may explain the relatively high infection rates in surgical and intensive care units. The risk of urethral infections caused by catheters increases day by day at a rate of 3-5%, and in peripheral/central vein catheters, the risk of septicemia increases at a rate of 0.1-1%. In aseptic surgery, the postoperative incidence of wound infections is estimated at 0.5-2%. In tracheal intubation for respiratory failure, the risk of pneumonitis is approximately 3-5% per day. Following an intubation under general anesthesia, 0.5-1% of patients develop pneumonitis.

Nosocomial Ocular Infections - Postoperative Ocular Infections Endophthalmitis

Postoperative endophthalmitis is a rare complication of elective intraocular interventions and is estimated at a rate of 0.05-0.5%. Endophthalmitis most frequently occurs subsequent to glaucoma surgery (3). Postoperative endophthalmitis manifests itself in the first 24-72 hours after surgery. This interval may be prolonged due to perioperative antibiotic prophylaxis or application of corticosteroids. If pathogens are slowly replicating bacteria or fungi, postoperative endophthalmitis may develop up to three or four weeks after the intervention. Most frequently isolated agents are Coagulase negative Staphylococci (42%), S.aureus (22%) and Streptococci (10%) (3). Previous reports have dealt with epidemics of endophthalmitis caused by instruments, intraocular solutions and lens implants contaminated with Gram-negative organisms or fungi (3).

Acute fulminant painful endophthalmitis with blurred vision and lid edema, conjunctival hyperemia and a hypopyon in the first days after surgery may be indicative for an infection by S.aureus or Gram-negative bacteria. The clinical diagnosis of subacute postoperative endophthalmitis is more often associated with agents such as Cagulase negative Staphylococci, P.acnes or fungi. Even with an invasive (intraocular) approach for sampling a negative microbiologic result is obtained in approximately 30% of cases (3).

Therapy for infections due to S.aureus may involve intraocular instillation of antibiotics and vitrectomy. Infections due to coagulase negative staphlyococci may often be successfully managed by topical, subconjunctival and/or systemic antibiotics. Lens implants do not necessarily have to be explanted in endophthalmitis following cataract extraction. Application of corticosteroids (topical and, in case of severe infections, intraocular or systemic) may result in a reduction of the inflammatory response and therefore faster cure (9).

Dacryocystitis

Postoperative dacryocystitis after dacryocystorhinostomy with a hydrophile implant is differentiated into an acute and chronic disease. Both entities are mainly caused by Pneumococci, Staphylococci or P.aeruginosa. H.influenzae may additionally cause an acute disease, whereas candida or atypical mycobacteria may play a role in the chronic course (8).

The incidence of postoperative dacryocystitis is not known. The diagnosis is established clinically with an increased mucopurulent lacrimal secretion, sometimes accompanied by pain and developing into a chronic disease. Therapy consists of the systemic administration of cephalosporins or of piperacillin when P.aeruginosa has been isolated. In addition, topical antibiotics may be instilled.

Episcleritis

The most frequently isolated causative agents in episcleritis are coagulase negative staphylococci, S.aureus and enterobacteriaceae (8). Episcleritis may develop some weeks after retinal detachment surgery in 0.24-4% of cases, particularly if an episcleral silicone device has been used. The clinical picture is characterized by ocular pain, conjunctival hyperemia and secretion, subconjunctival hematoma, blood-tinged tears and/or development of fistulas (8). The removal of the silicone device is the therapy of choice, and additional cephalosporins or flucloxacillin or vancomycin should be administered depending on the organism cultured.

Nosocomial Ocular Infections Not Related to Surgery

Endophthalmitis

Hematogenous spread during septicemia/viremia and local invasion are the most frequent causes of non-surgically related nosocomial endophthalmitis. Severely diseased or immunocompromised patients are particularly prone to these infections (8). The most important primary infection sites for septicemia/fungemia are endocarditis, contaminated venous catheters and gastrointestinal colonisation or central nervous system infections (8). The most important agents are Staphylococci, Streptococci, Gram-negative organisms (particularly Proteus and P.aeruginosa) as well as candida (8).

Candida endophthalmitis may represent the first and sometimes the only clinical manifestation of a disseminated fungal infection. This can be observed particularly in patients receiving long-lasting broad-spectrum antibiotics or intravenous hyperalimentation and suffer from immunodeficiency syndromes (8). Cytomegalovirus retinitis has been observed in patients suffering from the acquired immunodeficiency syndrome.

Blepharitis

Nosocomial blepharitis is often caused by hematogenous spread from distant sites of primary infection, e.g. bacteremia in osteomyelitis (3), or subsequently by an anatomically restricted lesion of the eye, e.g. in trauma. The clinical presentation is characterized by lid edema and erythema with crusts or a yellowish exudate at the lid margins. Eye burning, itching, persistent tearing and photophobia is often found as well.

No data are available concerning the incidence of nosocomial infections; it may be hypothesized, however, that this infection is not a rare event in a hospital setting. The most frequently found pathogens include Staphylococci and Gram-negative rods, e.g. P.aeruginosa; even viruses of the Herpes family like Herpes Simplex Virus and Varicella Zoster Virus may be causative for blepharitis.

Conjunctivitis

Conjunctivitis is the most frequent nosocomial ocular infection, which is not related to ophthalmic surgery (8). A viral etiology (Adenovirus) can often be determined, and the disease occurs in epidemic dimensions at times (10). Conjunctivitis is often accompanied by blepharitis and keratitis. Clinically, a red eye with chemosis and serous or purulent exudate can be observed; itching may be an additional sign.

The incidence of conjunctivitis in neonates ("neonatal ophthalmitis") is particularly high at approximately 0.2% (8). In developed countries, chlamydial infections range at about 14:1000 live births, a rate much higher than gonococcal infections ranging at 0.4:1000 live births. Staphylococci play the most important role for infections of the newborn.

Keratitis

Nosocomial keratitis may be induced by endogenous reactivation of latent Herpes Simplex Virus in the trigeminal ganglion. This reactivation commonly occurs in immunocompromised and fatally ill patients. The most frequent cause of nosocomial keratitis are bacterial pathogens (65-90%), e.g. S.aureus, Pneumococci, P.aeruginosa and B.catarrhalis. Fungi may be isolated in up to 20-35%. Aspergillus and Candida may be found particularly in immunocompromised patients (8).

Nosocomial Bacterial Ocular Infections in Intensive Care Units

With tracheal intubation in patients suffering from pneumonitis, repeat endotracheal lavage is demanding. A contamination of the eye by aerosolized tracheal secretions may result from a misplacement of the tracheal extubation tube during lavage of a patient. The same organisms were found in infected eyes and tracheal secretions when patients with tracheal intubations were studied (6). Therefore, it is recommended to cover the eyes of the mostly comatose patients and to eliminate the horizontally via the lower part of the patient's face.

New Quinolones in Ophthalmology

Recently, topical New Quinolones have been introduced into Ophthalmology, which have been recommended as an alternative to standard antibiotics, e.g. Polymyxin, Bacitracin, Neomycin, Gentamicin, and Tobramycin. With regard to the sensitivity patterns of S.aureus, Coagulase negative Staphylococci, Pneumococci and Streptococci, the New Quinolones show a reduction of in vitro activity compared to standard antibiotics. The in vitro sensitivity of Enterococci and P.aeruginosa may be even less.

Furthermore, increasing resistance vs. Staphylococci (S.aureus 4%) and P.aeruginosa (up to 20%) has been reported for the New Quinolones (11). Up to date there has been no convincing prospective randomized clinical study comparing the efficacy of New Quinolones with standard antibiotics, which have been applied successfully over so many years. We feel that New Quinolones should not be primarily applied in ocular infections, but should be prescribed in more severe infections involving multiresistant pathogens comparable to therapeutic standards in other medical therapeutic disciplines (2).

Table 1. Incidence of nosocomial infections in different hospital departments

Department	Patients	Nosocomial Infections (%)
Children's	2950	16.3 %
Obs-Gyn	3188	7.4 %
ENT	3123	0.5 %
Eye	3137	0.03%
Neurosurgery	2981	5.3 %
Surgery	8621	6.4 %
Medical	15802	1.8 %

Table 2. Most frequently isolated pathogens in nosocomial ocular infections

Organism	Isolation Frequency (%)
Coagulase negative Staphylococci	22%
S.aureus	19%
P.aeruginosa	9%

References

1. Daschner F (1981) Krankenhausinfektionen in einem Universitätsklinikum. Dtsch Med Wschr 106:101-105
2. Daschner F (1991) Gyrasehemmer in der Ophthalmologie - Werbung und Wirklichkeit. Z prakt Augenheilkd 12:362
3. Elston RA, Chattopadhyay B (1991) Postoperative Endophthalmitis. J Hosp Inf 17:243-253
4. Garner JS, Jarvis WR, Emori TG et al (1988) CDC Definitions for Nosocomial Infections, 1988. Am J Infect Control 16:128-140
5. Haley RW (1986) Managing Hospital Infection Control for Cost-Effectiveness. Am Hospital Publishing Inc Chicago,USA
6. Hilton E, Uliss A, Samuels S et al (1983) Nosocomial Bacterial Eye Infections in Intensive Care Units. Lancet 2:1318-1320
7. Horan TC, White JW, Jarvis WR et al (1986) Nosocomial Infection Surveillance. Morb Mort Weekly Rep 35:17-29
8. Peacock JE (1987) Uncommon Infections: Eye and Central Nervous System. In: Wenzel,RP (ed.) Prevention and Control of Nosocomial Infections. Williams & Wilkins, Baltimore pp.440-466
9. Shrader SK, Band JD, Lauter CB et al (1990) The Clinical Spectrum of Endophthalmitis: Incidence, Predisposing Factors, and Features Influencing Outcome. J Inf Dis 162:115-120
10. Warren D, Nelson KE, Farrar JA et al (1989) A Large Outbreak of Epidemic Keratoconjunctivitis: Problems in Controlling Nosocomial Spread. J Inf Dis 160:938-943
11. Wolfson JS (1989) Quinolone Antimicrobial Agents: Adverse Effects and Bacterial Resistance. Eur J Clin Microbiol Infect Dis 8:1080-1092

Principles of Hygiene and Prevention of Infections

Konrad Botzenhart and Peter Heeg

Abstract. Hospital acquired infections in ophthalmology may cause severe ocular disease or the loss of eyes, and may interrupt the operative or consultative practices of the ophthalmologist. Prevention of infections is of prime importance, because antibiotic therapy is frequently not effective.

Introduction

In the last century one of the most important discoveries concerned the recognition of hygienic measures decreasing the risk of interventions by physicians, namely by sterilisation of instruments and disinfection of hands. These discoveries have been associated primarily with the names of Wendell-Holmes, Semmelweis and Lister (7). From their work - performed without any knowledge of microorganisms as causative agents of infection -, the concept of asepsis and antisepsis evolved at the turn of the century: a concept that has determined hygienic measures in surgery until today.

According to existing law, the physician treating a patient in the hospital is responsible for the enforcement of hygienic measures. Therefore, the detection, treatment and prevention of nosocomial infections is the definite task of the physician and his responsibility cannot be annihilated and transferred to a third party. The responsibility of the physician is further established by the sequelae of an infection for the individual patient and the causal relationship of diagnostic and therapeutic measures as well as nursing care. In the scope of his responsibility, the physician should ensure that qualified personnel assists him in the task of detection, treatment and prevention of nosocomial infections.

Epidemiology of Nosocomial Infections

Infections after medical interventions and hospital treatment are still of great importance with approximately 5-6% of all treated patients being affected. Hospital acquired infections in Germany are estimated at a frequency of one million per year (6). This incidence at the respective localizations (see below) has also been found in large studies in the United States (5) and in previous studies in Germany (4). Ocular involvement only represents a small fraction of these infections, however, it is often very severe in the individual patient and may eventually lead to blindness.

The major part of nosocomial infections involves infections of the urinary tract (42%) followed by wound infections (22%) and infections of the respiratory tract (15%)(4).

Infections of the urinary tract occurring in hospitals are most frequently caused by permanent indwelling catheters, associated in part with transurethral interventions. Typically, these infections develop with the insertion or application of a foreign body as a leading device for bacteria ascending from the colonized distal part of the urethra into the physiologically sterile bladder. Although it may be possible to decrease the incidence of infection by application of careful hygienic regimens to tubing as well as maintenance of the catheter, however, the unphysiologic irritation of the urethra may suffice to acquire an infection.

A prerequisite for wound infections - representing the second most frequently occurring nosocomial infections - is provided by compromised normal skin or mucous membranes and other tissues usually representing a barrier to infectious agents. The more the tissue is qualitatively compromised (cf. hematoma, ischemia, necrosis), the easier infections may manifest themselves; e.g. the necessary numbers (infectious dose) and virulence of infecting organisms may be lower. Plastic implants are a particular risk factor because of microbial colonization, for example by Coagulase negative Staphylococci.

The third most frequent infections in the hospital are those of the respiratory tract, e.g. pneumonias and bronchopneumonia with often severe sequelae. In certain groups, for example infections with P.aeruginosa, fatality reaches 70%. Tracheal intubation of patients facilitates the infection and may be compared to catheterization of the urinary tract with respect to its abnormal irritation of the respiratory tract. As well, a significant etiopathologic factor consists of the compromised local defense mechanisms of the respiratory tract in unconscious and intubated patients without a cough reflex and with a reduced ciliary clearance.

This short survey of hospital acquired infections elucidates on the fact that most of these infections do not occur because of preventable negligence or omission of established hygienic measures but are closely linked to the immunocompetence of the patient and the underlying disease as well as the mode and duration of medical treatment.

Prevention

From this one may derive that the contemporary and future incidence of hospital acquired infections may not necessarily decrease. A reduction or minimizing of these infections may primarily be achieved in elective surgical interventions, e.g. for inguinal hernias or artificial joints. Success in some certain areas may, however, eventually be equalized by an increased infection rate due to the introduction of modern therapy (e.g. transplantation) or by up to now untreatable patients. In order to minimize infection rates in certain procedures, strict regulations and standards must be instituted. Only thus may regulations for medical and nursing personnel be established. Furthermore, quality standards of medical care can thus be ensured.

Prevention of infection cannot only be restricted to the elimination of negligence, but has to analyze the factors facilitating infection and the source of infectious agents. Since an endogenous infection uncontrolled by hygienic regimens may eventually become as important a cause for the failure of an intervention as an exogenous infection, a careful work-up of all aspects of medical care is demanding in the interest of the patient and for the success of any intervention.

Empirical and theoretical knowledge of infections subsequent to medical interventions is large and has been documented in a voluminous body of literature. The treating physician is responsible for infection prevention and must know the state of the art in his operational area either himself or must be advised by a specialist. Similar obligations exist for the nursing care, medical technical and hospital technical sectors. Professional hospital infection control by educated and knowledgeable staff is therefore demanding.

In ohthalmology, conditions are relatively well-defined and there are few sources of infection. Despite this fact, incidents have been documented in the literature when institutions, maintaining hospitals were organisationally incriminated with an insufficient, e.g. non-professional institution of basic hygienic prerequisites (1).

Professional establishment of hospital hygiene means the staffing of one infection control nurse per 300 beds in hospitals to monitor the incidence and clinical features of apparent infections and to care for necessary procedures in the nursing and, as far as feasible, in the medical areas.

One medically trained person should care for medical and scientific problems of hospital infection control in emergency care hospitals of more than 450 beds (2).

The specific areas of professional activity of these persons is given in Tables 1 and 2.

Furthermore, it may be advisable to know about and follow the constantly updated recommendations of the committees of hospital hygiene and infection prevention of higher public health authorities (such as the Bundesgesundheitsamt in Germany)(2). These comprise the multiple constructional, technical and organizational problems with regard to infection prevention. Since these cannot be explained in detail in this short survey, a simple scheme is used to demonstrate the basics of infection prevention (Fig.1). In this figure, the risk of infection is visualized depending on certain sources and modes of spread of infection, thereby resulting in a grading of significance and urgency of preventive measures.

The emergence of an infection is easiest if infected organs or tissues are operated on or if contaminated material is inserted, e.g. by contaminated corneal buttons or intraocular lens implants. Manifestation or aggravation of local infections and the spread and further distribution of infectious agents with subsequent complications may be possible in these conditions.

It may sometimes be difficult to decide whether an infection prevails or a colonization, not necessarily resulting in invasion of the organism exists. Decision may be made clinically (on the basis of inflammation symptoms) or microbiologically (by detection of agents in tissue). Absence of infection in the tissues to be operated on is certainly one of the most important prerequisites for a non-infected postoperative course.

All devices used during surgery or other medical or nursing measures touching disclosed, overt, possibly compromised tissues (hands or gloves of the surgeon, instruments, solutions, swabs, suture material etc.) range second in the risk of infection. Particular attention must be paid to thermolabile devices, which cannot be sterilized by steam. Chemical sterilization of those instruments requires specific know-how.

The risk of infection also depends on the care and preservation of tissue during surgery and smaller invasive interventions. Thus, the level of skill and education and the sufficient number of treating physicians and assistants is an important factor for achieving optimized results. This has been clearly shown in epidemiological studies in the USA and Canada (3). It is self-explaining that safe procedures of sterilization and effective disinfection of the skin of the patient and hands of the personnel are demanding.

The risk of infection is diminished when tissues or organs remain intact and not injured. Any abnormal irritation, however, results in a compromised local defense with subsequent risk of infection (see: urinary tract infections). In ophthalmology, this is applicable to tonometry and contact lens fitting.

Everything not brought in direct contact with the respective organ and with increasing distance may be seen as less important a source of infection. This applies to devices in surgical theaters distant from the patient or to treatment rooms (e.g. X-rays, monitors), cleanliness of floors, air quality etc. The surroundings of the room where medical interventions and other treatment regimens are performed are even more apart; and the spread of organisms to the patient via textiles, hands or the air may be imaginable, but may not be brought into a causal relationship with hospital acquired infections without an additional lack of hygiene, e.g. omission of hand disinfection. Cleanliness in these areas should not be omitted; however, it is certainly ineffective to intensify disinfection of the floor in the operating theater or on the wards in an attempt to compensate for faults during a medical procedure. Measures taken in the periphery of interventions endangered by the risk of infection may only prove beneficial when optimized conditions have previously been achieved in the central area.

Recommendations for Infection Prevention

In summary, the following statements can be made comprising the principles of hygiene and infection prevention:

- Medical science including ophthalmology may not be further advanced, if infections are accepted as non-preventable.
- Infection prevention requires an analysis of etiology and accompanying conditions and cannot be achieved by abolishing putative understood negligence in traditional procedures.
- Infection prevention at a high level can only be achieved with the help of professional medical and paramedical infection control personnel.
- An effective prevention of infections requires a high level of knowledge and strict discipline of all personnel involved irrespective of education or hierarchical position, as well as an increased volume of work and materials.
- Greatest care should be taken and the most intense attention should be given to those conditions or devices, which are most probably related to an infection, since they are closest to the infectious event.
- Peripheral measures cannot compensate for negligence in the immediate patient area. However, even away from the infectious event, hygienic and reproducibly meticulous work should be done concerning peripheral devices and functions.

Table 1. Tasks of the hospital epidemiologist (2)

1.	Recommendations for the personnel concerning hospital hygiene and infection prevention.
2.	Inspection of hospital areas on a regular basis.
3.	Establishment and enforcement of infection control policies for the individual areas of the hospital.
4.	Continuing education for the hospital personnel.
5.	Control of epidemiologically relevant technical devices and instruments.
6.	Evaluation of infectious events.
7.	Work-up and interpretation of infection statistics.
8.	Recommendations for the acquisition of devices, disinfectants, antiseptics.
9.	Recommendations for planning and instituting hospital constructions.
10.	Recommendations for environmental health in hospitals.
11.	Chairmanship in the infection control committee.

Table 2. Tasks of the infection control nurse (officer) (2)[1]

1.	Inspection of hospital areas on a regular basis and monitoring of functions.
2.	Providing help in establishing infection control policies.
3.	Collecting and work-up of data for the recognition of nosocomial infections.
4.	Recommendations for the prevention and abolishment of nosocomial infections.
5.	Education of and practicing preventive procedures with hospital staff.
6.	Providing help in the selection of hygienically relevant procedures and products.
7.	Providing help in the planning of hospital constructions and functional devices.
8.	Work in the infection control committee including preparations for the sessions.
9.	Cooperation with the educational institutions for paramedics.

[1] In accordance with the medical hospital hygiene personnel and the Chairman of the Department.

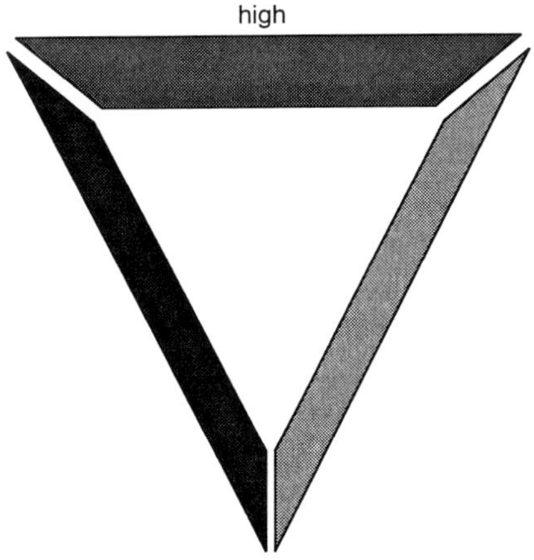

Fig.1. Risk of infection relating to various sources and modes of infection. SOURCE OF INFECTION
infected or contaminated organs, tissues, transplants, implants contaminated solutions and instruments in invasive interventions
contact with mucous membranes, droplet,
skin contact,
indirect contact with infected devices, dust.

References

1. Brandis H (1965) Infektionen im Krankenhaus. Med Mschr 19:57-61
2. Bundesgesundheitsamt (ed) (1991) Richtlinie für die Erkennung, Verhütung und Bekämpfung von Krankenhausinfektionen. Fischer Verlag Stuttgart
3. Cruse PJE, Foord R (1973) A Five Year Prospective Study of 23649 Surgical Wounds. Arch Surg 107:205-209
4. Daschner F (1981) Krankenhausinfektionen in einem Universitätsklinikum. Dtsch Med Wschr 106:101-105
5. Horan TC, White JW, Jarvis WR et al (1986) Nosocomial Infection Surveillance, 1984. Morb Mort Weekly Rep 35(1SS):17-29
6. Norden G (1989) Ermittlung und Analyse von Krankenhausinfektionen. Das Krankenhaus 81:420-424
7. Pulverer G, Schaal KP (1983) Geschichte der Krankenhausinfektionen. In: Thofern E, Botzenhart K (eds) Hygiene und Infektionen im Krankenhaus. G. Fischer Verlag Stuttgart

Perioperative Prophylaxis in Ophthalmology

Jörg Draeger, Jörn-Wolff Prüter, Manfred Förtsch

Abstract. The possible causes of intraocular infections after microsurgical interventions of the eye are reviewed. Extensive experiments were carried out to investigate infections caused by the patient himself, by the surgeon and by the surgical surroundings. In order to consider the different aspects involved in perioperative prophylaxis, we investigated the pre-, intra- and postoperative periods. Work-ups of conjunctival smears and antisepsis of the conjunctiva are important preoperative precautions to be taken. Microbiological investigations were carried out to check for the possibility of contamination of eye drops, the operating theater equipment and the micrsocopes. The sterilization of microsurgical instruments using different procedures was monitored in particular. During the intraoperative period, surgical clothing like face masks, gloves and gowns were examined. Patient drapings were monitored for sterility.

The results are evaluated with respect to their significance for perioperative prophylaxis and the practical consequences for optimized infection control measures.

Introduction

The body of evidence reported in the literature causing perioperative infections led us to study the issue of prophylaxis (6, 11,12). Most frequently, contamination of eye drops and ointment have been described.

An inquiry performed among West German surgical eye centers revealed that there were no standard preoperative procedures. 75% of the 58 surgical centers used topical/local antibiotics and 16% did not take any prophylactic measures at all to avoid postoperative infections.

Ophthalmic surgery is privileged with very few infections, because of the metabolic properties and the anatomy of the eye itself. However, despite comprehensive concepts of hygiene, postoperative sporadic infections do occur. Instituting preventive measures is what we would like to call "Perioperative Prophylaxis". We propose a three-step approach:

1. The preoperative work-up of the patient including a conjunctival smear and disinfection of the eye and its vicinity as well as the correct sterilization of the instruments to be used.
2. Intraoperative protection using textile covers and plastic films for the surgical area and protective clothing for the surgeon and personnel.
3. Postoperative antiinfective treatment.

These three steps are divided into three sections concerning the patient, surgeon and environmental factors.

Study

In the preoperative phase, conjunctival smears are taken from the patients. The main issue for the environmental factors consists of the sterilization of instruments. During this phase, there are only few risk factors, which deserve particular attention: Diabetics, immunosuppressed and one-eyed patients.

1. Conjunctival Smears and Disinfection: First of all, conjunctival swabs from patients undergoing surgery are taken, however, although this step may seem simple, there are many sources for mis-interpretations. Results are not reproducible, if smears are taken from certain parts of the cul de sac or the eye lids (13).- Surface antisepsis should be done with PVP-iodine (2), however, it might be argued that this agent is not sufficiently bactericidal for S.aureus, coliform bacteria and P.aeruginosa.

2. Sterilization: Sterilization of instruments is one of the most important measures to be taken for preoperative prophylaxis. Various procedures are currently available and their effects on micro-surgical instruments are highly variable (5). Sterilization itself generally poses no problem at all with respect to the microbiological results, but it may cause a problem if combinations of thermolabile and water absorbing materials are used. As a result, many different ways for sterilization have been proposed. This has led to a costly and highly time-consuming procedure. Hot air and hot steam sterilization methods are most popular for sterilization of thermostaabile materials. Frequent autoclaving may lead to corrosion in highly sensitive microsurgical instruments limiting their proper functions (4).

Thermolabile materials can be sterilized using ethylene oxide, but materials may be affected by color changes. There is a lot of breezing time involved and since the gas is carcinogenic, this procedure is potentially dangerous for the personnel involved. Complete sterilization of electric motors is impossible with this procedure.

A new technique for sterilization of sensitive materials has recently been introduced. It is called low temperature plasma sterilization (STERRAD), which may open new horizons (Fig.1). STERRAD utilizes hydrogen peroxide, which is transformed into plasma in a vacuum. Sterilization runs at a temperature of 37°C and takes only one hour to perform. At the end of the process, the product consists of water and oxygen. The remaining air has a maximal humidity of 5%. Advantages are the low temperature and no breezing time at the end of the sterilization with prompt availability of instruments right after the procedure. However, this method cannot be used for sterilization of cellulose, linen and cotton. These materials absorb hydrogen peroxide and prevent its diffusion (10).

We have tested the compatibility and microbiological reliability of this new method and found that all instruments tested were essentially sterile. A multi-center evaluation is currrently under way in several German institutes of hygiene. In our hands, sterilization appears to be highly efficient and, in addition, it seems not to act adversely on sensitive thermolabile and corroiable materials.

Plasma sterilization might be an alternative to gas sterilization and it seems most advantageous in the field of microsurgery, because it will be good for most surgical materials.

This provides completely new possibilities for the concept of pre-packaged surgery cassettes for elective surgery in that a risky adding of thermolabile instruments is not any longer required. This would significantly decrease the risk of secondary contamination. The development of special sets of cassettes for the use in ophthalmic microsurgical interventions is under way in our institution (Fig.2).

In the future, plasma sterilization may provide an ability to use completely novel materials. Theoretically, it will be possible to combine highly sensitive precision instruments including electric motors simultaneously with conventional instruments.

During surgery, there are many factors to be considered for infection control measures. The surgeon and surgical personnel have to put on conventional protective clothing, e.g. coat, mask, cap and gloves. This outfit works as a barrier for infections from the standpoints of the surgeon as well as the patient.

3. Covers: In the operating theater it is demanding to care for the safety of the patient. Two alternatives exist in order to cover the non-sterile body, e.g. reusable cotton or disposable (plastic) materials. Several comparative studies have come to the conclusion that the risk of infection is lower by a factor of 2-5.2 with the use of disposable sheets (1,7,8,9).

In ocular surgery, some other important implications have to be considered. A large amount of the sugical interventions is performed using local anesthetics, and the head should be covered. All materials should be air-permeable to a sufficient extent in order to prevent hypoxia. We have made an analysis of the breathing air under the patient cover and there had been no increase in CO_2 concentrations. No significant differences have been found comparing cotton or disposable covers.

4. Surgical Films: Despite adequate skin disinfection, pathogenic organisms may appear from the lower layers of the skin during surgery and may be a cause of contamination. Therefore, it is important to cover the immediate vicinity of the eye with sterile materials. Simple plastic films are not good enough for the eye, since they do not cover the eye lid completely.

We have therefore developed a new kind of surgical film. With the use of a lid opener, it automatically covers the margins of the eye lids.

During surgery, the surgeon's protective measures must be considered as well. Studies of the coats have resulted in similar findings as with the patient covers, because of identical materials used (Fig.3).

5. Surgical Masks: Since the surgeon's mouth and nasopharynx may come close to the operating sites (Fig.4), this part of the body should be protected. However, a surgical mask does not represent an absolute protection (13). Our studies have shown that masks worn for more than one hour exhibit an appreciable quantity of organisms on the outer surface. In fact, a high risk of contamination is possible with a free exit of exhaled air from the sides of the mask. We have used thermography to investigate this phenomenon and have compared inhaled to exhaled air fluxes (Fig.5). The pictures from the exhalation phase have demonstrated that most of the air escapes laterally and from the nasal areas. We were able to improve the perfomance of these masks by introducing a foam rubber segment along the top, which prevents the escape of the exhaled air into the nasal areas.

6. Gloves: Most ophthalmic microsurgeons use surgical gloves. There is no question as to the impairment of tactile and micromotor actions. 3.7% of gloves tested after surgery have been found punctured indicating the necessity for the disinfection of hands preoperatively.

7. Eye Drops and Ointment: As mentioned in the introduction, medications such as eye drops and ointment may become contaminated. Single-dosage ophthioles may be very useful for the prevention of this risk. They have been available in Germany since 1987, made according to the directions of the DAB 9.

Despite all these preventive measures, it is only possible to reduce the amount of pathogens, however, it is not possible to completely sterilize the surgical field.

Postoperative treatment is much simpler. Antibiotic dressings should be done with the same medications used for prophylaxis.

Discussion

Ten fundamental rules should be observed for proper perioperative prophylaxis, which cannot rule out infections completely, but may help to minimize the incidence of infections:

1. The sterile zone and the non-sterile zone should be strictly separated in the operating theater (3).
2. Conjunctival smears from the cul de sac should be properly taken in order to ensure a significant result.
3. For infection control, it is mandatory to reduce the amount of organisms in the eye preoperatively (by the use of antibiotics) and to prepare the patient with antiseptics/antibiotics.
4. With respect to sterilization, some materials of microsurgical instruments have been shown not to be compatible with the sterilization process. Specific prepacked cassettes, which may be opened only immediately before surgery should be used.
5. Topical medications should be applied from single-dosage ophthioles only.
6. The patient should be covered with disposable drapings, which must be sterile and comfortable.
7. The surgical film (as described by us) must cover the close vicinity of the eye and the eye lids.
8. The surgeon's coat should be a barrier of infections and comfortable to wear in addition.
9. Since all of these procedures still do not guarantee a complete eradication of infections, local and topical antibiotics should in addition be applied after the surgical interventions.
10. In case of postoperative infections, prophylactic and the rapeutic regimens should be analysed systematically step by step. It appears not to be warranted to change procedures before an overall prior assessment of risk factors involved in current measures has been done.

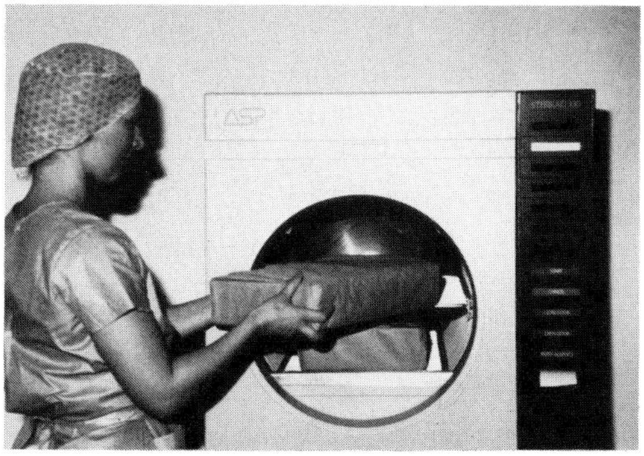

Fig. 1 Low temperature plasma sterilization (STERRAD)

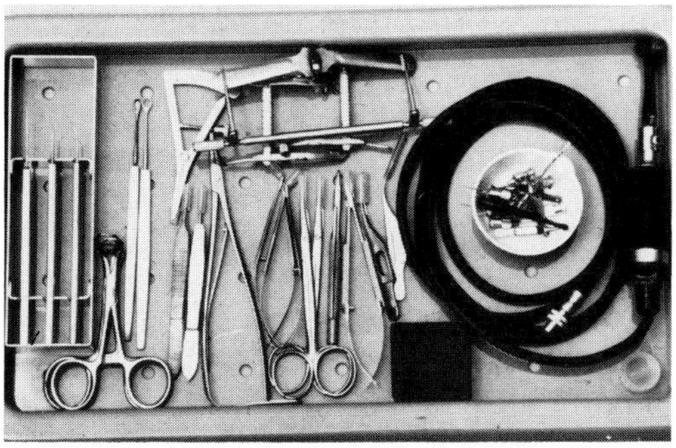

Fig. 2 Cassette for plasma sterilization

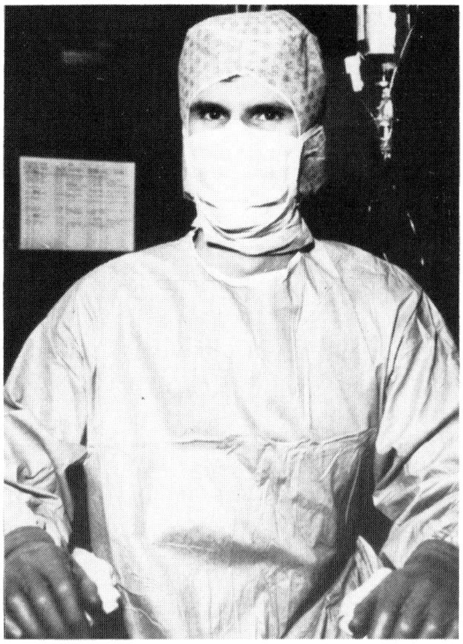

Fig.3 Single-use surgical coat

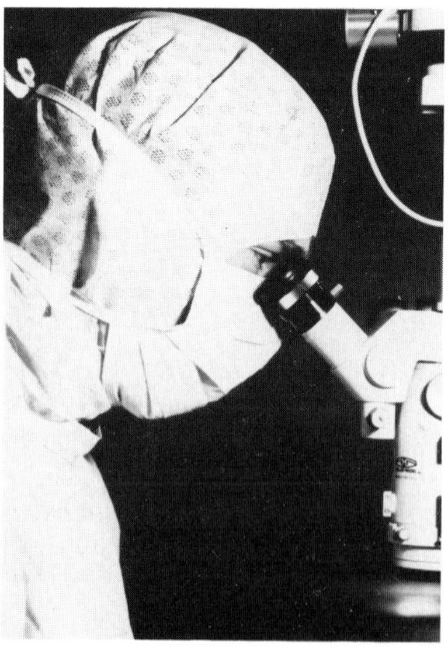

Fig. 4 Surgical mask

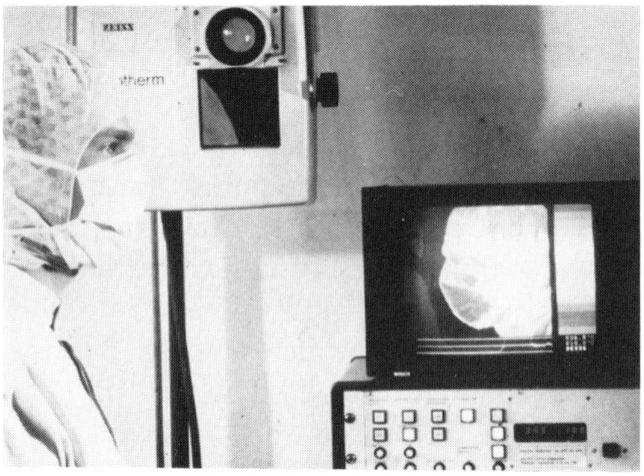

Fig. 5 Theomography

References

1. Baldwin BC, Fox IL, Russ C (1981) Effect of Disposable Draping on Wound Infection Rate. VA Med 108:477
2. Beck EG, Schmidt P (1988) Hygiene und Präventivmedizin. 3.Auflage, ENKE Verlag, Stuttgart
3. Draeger J, Kirchner M (1988) Technische Ausstattung und Organisation einer ophthalmologischen Operationseinheit.
   In: Mackensen G, Neubauer H (eds) Augenärztliche Operationen I.Springer Verlag, Heidelberg
4. Draeger J, Klein L (1987) Microsurgical Instruments.
5. In: Drager J (ed) Ophthalmic Microsurgery Instrumentation, Microscopes and Technique. S.Karger Verlag, Bern
6. Draeger J, Prüter JW (1990) Eignung verschiedener Verfahren zur Sterilisation von mikrochirurgischen Instrumenten. Klin Mbl Augenheilk 133-137

7. Hallermann W (1963) Infektionsprobleme der Augenheilkunde. Klin Mbl Augenheilk 142:414-418
8. Knippenberger H, Krauch H, Heinrich D (1988) Einweg-OP-Abdecksystem oder textiles Abdeckmaterial? Klinikarzt 17:234-241
9. Moylan A, Fitzpatrick KT, Davenport KE (1987) Reducing Wound Infections. Arch Surg 122:152-157
10. Moylan A, Kennedy BV (1981) Die Bedeutung von Kitteln und Tüchern als Schranke bei der Verhütung von Wundinfektionen. Krankenhaushygiene 3:46-52
11. Prüter JW, Förtsch M, Draeger J (to be published) Niedrigtemperatur-Plasmasterilisation (NTP), Neue Möglichkeiten in der Augenchirurgie. Fortschr Ophthalmol
12. Rauh W (1953) Sulfonamidpuder und Infektion nach der Staroperation. Klin Mbl Augenheilk 122:257
13. Rintelen F (1951) Infekte durch infizierte Argentumtanninoalbuminat Lösungen bei bulbuseröffnenden Operationen. Klin Mbl Augenheilk 119:94
14. Thofern E, Botzenhart K (1983) Hygiene und Infektionen im Krankenhaus. G Fischer Verlag,Stuttgart

Molecular Epidemiology of Adenovirus Strains

Koki Aoki and Morikazu Shinagawa

Abstract. Adenovirus has been found to cause epidemic keratoconjunctivitis and pharyngoconjunctival fever and these infections have been included in a nation-wide surveillance program in Japan.

DNA restriction endonuclease analysis for genome typing of Adenovirus DNA was performed on a total of 118 Adenovirus isolates including serotypes Adenovirus 3, Adenovirus 4, Adenovirus 7, Adenovirus 8, Adenovirus 11, Adenovirus 19 and Adenovirus 37 from patients with epidemic conjunctivitis obtained in Japan, Australia and the Philippines.

In Japan, 46 Adenovirus 3 isolates obtained from 1983 to 1986 were either Adenovirus 3f or Adenovirus 3g. Yearly alternations of predominance of both genome types was observed in the Northern part of Japan during this period.

The genome types in Australia were Adenovirus 3p and Adenovirus 3f, and those in the Philippines were Adenovirus 3p, respectively. Nine Adenovirus 8 isolates in Australia and in the Philippines were typed as Adenovirus 8p, but 11 Adenovirus 8 isolates in Japan were Adenovirus 8b. Thirteen Adenovirus 19 isolates were identified as Adenovirus 19a. All 3 isolates of Adenovirus 37 in Japan and three isolates in Australia before 1982 were typed as Adenovirus 37p, however, five isolates in Australia after 1983 were identified by genome type as Adenovirus 37d.

A total of 165 Adenovirus type 3 and 4 strains from epidemic keratoconjunctivitis at an eye clinic in Sapporo from 1983 to 1989 were classified into either genome types of Adenovirus 3f, 3g, and 4a. By the use of Hinf1 and Tap1, these were classified into 11, 3 and 12 subgenome types, respectively. During this period, four epidemics of Adenovirus 3 (1983 and 1986) and Adenovirus 4 (1985 and 1986) infections relating to epidemic keratoconjunctivitis occurred. The prevalent strains of Adenovirus 3g in 1983 belonged to a single subgenome type, but in the Adenovirus 3f epidemic in 1986, an alteration of the subgenome type was observed. In this year only a few Adenovirus 3 were isolated, such Adenovirus 3f strains were classified into many types, and seemed to be less stable than those of Adenovirus 3g in regard to the alteration of subgenome types.

All Adenovirus 4a strains in 1988 belonged to a single subgenome type except for one, but in 1985, three subgenome types became predominant in due order. With Adenovirus 4, the prevalent types tended to change within several years.

The method using enzymes recognizing four or five base pair sequences is a powerful tool for investigating the epidemiology of Adenovirus in local microenvironments.

Introduction

In Japan, Adenovirus 4 has been the most important agent of epidemic keratoconjunctivitis caused by Adenovirus strains and accounted for 42% of the cases; Adenovirus 3 was the second most prevalent (19%) from 1982 to 1988 according to our report of Sapporo in Japan. Recently, many genome types have been recognized in Adenovirus strains by using restriction endonuclease analysis, and this genome typing is an extremely useful tool in the field of epidemiology.

Epidemiological Study

In order to classify genome types in more detail to monitor the alteration of prevalent Adenovirus strains, we employed Hinf I and Taq I, which recognize 5- and 4-base pair sequences, respectively, and cleave virus DNA into many fragments. We investigated the alterations of prevalent Adenovirus 3f, Adenovirus 3g and Adenovirus 4a strains in epidemic keratoconjunctivitis from an epidemiological point of view (Tab.1).

In 1983, increases of Adenovirus 3g and in 1986, increased prevalence of Adenovirus 3f were observed. All Adenovirus 3g strains isolated in 1983 belonged to a single subgenome type. However, in Adenovirus 3f, one possible derivative of the subgenome type that dominated until the middle of the increase became predominant late in the increase. In 1984 only very few Adenovirus 3f strains were isolated and the subgenome types of these strains tended to be new.

All 49 Adenovirus 3 strains used in our study were isolated from patients in a single eye clinic from 1983 through 1986.

Among the 26 strains of Adenovirus 3f, nine enzyme restriction patterns were able to be identified with each of the enzymes, and the patterns were numbered from one to 9 in chronological order of isolation of the strains. Consequently, the 26 strains were classified into 11 subgenome types by the combination of both enzymes. Adenovirus 3fH1T1 was the dominant subgenome type in 46% of cases (Fig.1).

The 23 strains of Adenovirus 3g were classified into three subgenome types, and Adenovirus 3gH1T1 was the dominant type rendering 74% of cases (Tab.2).

Adenovirus 3fT1H1, which was isolated in 1983, could again be identified in 1986, and this subgenome type was dominant until August of 1986. Thereafter, this subgenome type was replaced by a new genome type,

Adenovirus 3fH9T8, derived from Adenovirus 3fH1T1.

The major strain in 1983 was Adenovirus 3g, and one single subgenome type, Adenovirus 3gH1T1, was predominant. In 1985, Adenovirus 3gH2T1 appeared and took the place of Adenovirus 3gH1T1, and in 1986, 11 strains were also of this type.

Chronological arrangement of the subgenome types indicated the slight alterations of Adenovirus DNA, even within the prevalent strains (Fig.2).

During the period from 1985 through 1989, 122 strains of Adenovirus 4 were isolated. Of these, 68 strains (56%) were obtained in 1985, 12 strains (10%) in 1986, 12 strains (10%) in 1987, 21 strains (17%) in 1988 and 9 strains (7%) in 1989. All of the 122 Adenovirus 4 strains were identified as Adenovirus 4a with BamHl, EcoRl, Hind III and Sma I, as reported by Guo and coworkers (1,2). In 1985 and 1988, epidemics of Adenovirus 4a were observed; the one in 1985 being of a rather large scale.

All Adenovirus 4 strains were isolated in same eye clinic during the period from 1985 through 1989.

Among the 122 strains of Adenovirus 4a, nine restriction patterns were observed and classified into 12 subgenome types with Adenovirus 4aH3T3 being the most frequently identified type (36%) (Tab.3).

All Adenovirus 4a strains were arranged according to the isolation dates, so that we were able to detect any chronological changes of the subgenome types. When Adenovirus 4a was prevalent in 1985, 68 strains were isolated and they were classified into four subgenome types. At first, Adenovirus 4aH1T1 was the predominant subgenome type followed by Adenovirus 4aH3T3 and finally Adenovirus 4aH4T1, possibly derived from Adenovirus 4aH1T1, was most frequent.

In 1987, two new subgenome types, Adenovirus 4aH7T7 and Adenovirus 4aH8T8 were detected.

In 1988, another increase in frequency of Adenovirus 4a was observed. Among 21 strains, two subgenome types, which were identical to those in the previous year, were obtained; one strain was Adenovirus 4aH7T7 and the remaining 20 were Adenovirus 4aH8T8.

In 1989, two subgenome types were identified. One of them was Adenovirus 4aH7T7, which had also been isolated in 1987 and 1988.

Adenovirus 4 infections had been rarely detected in Japan before 1978. However, since 1978 when the first strain was isolated from a patient with pharyngitis in the Aichi Prefecture, Adenovirus 4 infections have increased in various parts of the country. In the present study, Adenovirus 4 strains evaluated from 1985 through 1989 belonged to the single genome type of Adenovirus 4a.

Li and Wadell reported that genome types of Adenovirus 4a were highly conserved, and that they had been isolated during the past 19 years (5). However, the present study showed that prevalent strains of Adenovirus 4a tended to change within two years, except for Adenovirus 4aH7T7, at the level of subgenome type (Fig.2).

In the survey of 1985, the subgenome type Adenovirus 4aH3T3 was isolated from 43 cases of epidemic keratoconjunctivitis, eight of which were suspected of nosocomial infection. We found six genome types in 1986 and two in 1987 without epidemics. The Adenovirus with the genome type 4aH8T8, which occurred originally in the winter of 1987, gave rise to 20 cases, including four hospital acquired infections in the Summer of 1988. The genome type Adenovirus 4aH7T7, which originated in 1988, was the etiologic agent of seven cases in the Winter of 1989. From these findings, we could determine the index cases and reservoir of infections which could not have been traced before specific enzymes recognizing 6-bp sequences were.

Conclusion

We have studied the molecular epidemiology of conjunctivitis caused by Adenovirus in Asia (6).

The analysis of prevalent genome types of Adenovirus 3f, Adenovirus 3g and Adenovirus 4a with Taq I and Hinf I has indicated a variation of subgenome types with time (3,4).

This molecular epidemiologic approach gives us vital information for the surveillance of epidemic Adenovirus conjunctivitis not only in Japan but also in Asia (Tab.3).

Table 1. Annual Incidence of Ad conjunctivitis (Sapporo/Japan)

	1982	1983	1984	1985	1986	1987	1988	Total
Ad 3		42	3	11	31	24	11	122
Ad 4	59	8	30	80	9	21	57	264
Ad 8	6	33	19	4	27	4	20	113
Ad 19		8	15	5	3	1	7	39
Ad 37	4	33	14	3	29	2	5	90
Total	69	124	81	103	99	52	100	628

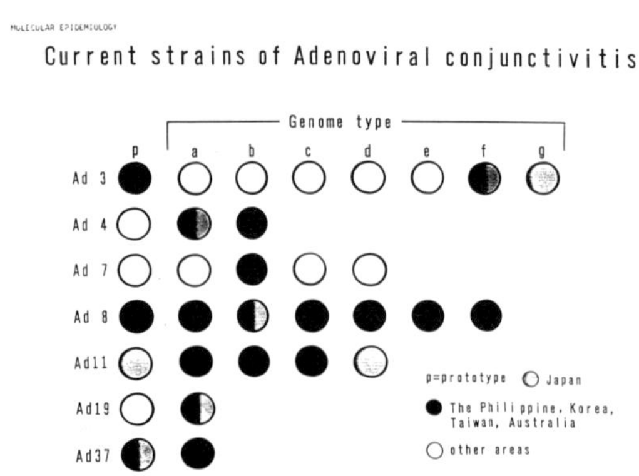

Table 2. Subgenome types of ad3 classified with hinf I and Taq I enzymes

Ad3f

Subgenome type	RE Profile HinfI	TaqI	No. of strains isolated (%)
Ad3fH1T1	1	1	12 (46.2%)
Ad3fH2T2	2	2	1 (3.8)
Ad3fH3T1	3	1	1 (3.8)
Ad3fH4T3	4	3	1 (3.8)
Ad3fH5T4	5	4	1 (3.8)
Ad3fH4T5	4	5	1 (3.8)
Ad3fH6T6	6	6	1 (3.8)
Ad3fH7T7	7	7	1 (3.8)
Ad3fH8T8	8	3	1 (3.8)
Ad3fH9T8	9	8	5 (19.2)
Ad3fH9T9	9	9	1 (3.8)

Ad3g

Subgenome type	RE Profile HinfI	TaqI	No. of strains isolated (%)
Ad3gH1T1	1	1	17 (73.9)
Ad3gH2T1	2	1	5 (21.7)
Ad3gH3T2	3	2	1 (4.3)

Table 3. Subgenome types of ad4a classified with hinf I and Taq I enzymes

Subgenome type	RE Profile HinfI	TaqI	No. of strains isolated (%)
Ad4aH1T1	1	1	14 (12.0)
Ad4aH2T2	2	2	1 (0.9)
Ad4aH3T3	3	3	42 (35.9)
Ad4aH4T1	4	1	12 (10.3)
Ad4aH3T4	3	4	1 (0.9)
Ad4aH5T1	5	1	1 (0.9)
Ad4aH6T5	6	5	2 (1.7)
Ad4aH6T1	6	1	2 (1.7)
Ad4aH5T6	5	6	1 (0.9)
Ad4aH7T7	7	7	16 (13.7)
Ad4aH8T8	8	8	23 (19.7)
Ad4aH9T9	9	9	2 (1.7)

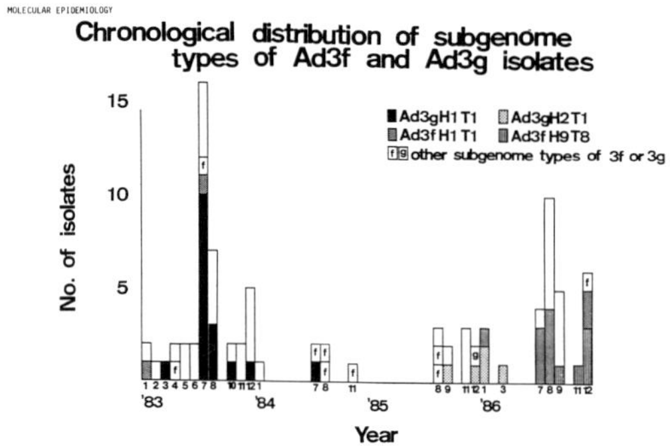

Fig.1. Chronologic distribution of subgenome types of Adenovirus 3f and Adenovirus 3g isolates.

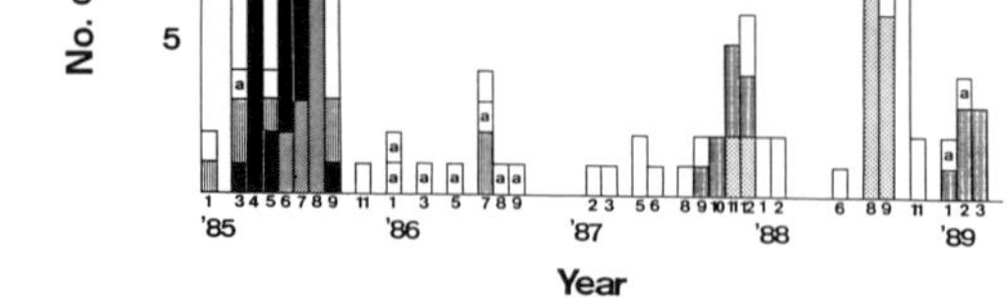

Fig.2. Chronologic distribution of subgenome types of Adenovirus 4a isolates.

References

1. Guo DF, Shibata R, Shinagawa M et al (1988) Genomic Comparison of Adenovirus Type 3 Isolates from Patients with Acute Conjunctivitis in Japan, Australia, and the Philippines. Microbiol Immunol 32:833-842
2. Guo DF, Shinagawa M, Aoki K et al (1988) Genome Typing of Adenovirus Strains Isolated from Conjunctivitis in Japan, Australia, and the Philippines. Microbiol Immunol 32:1107-1118
3. Itakura S, Aoki K, Sawada H et al (1990) Analysis with Restriction Endonucleases Recognizing 4- or 5-Base-Pair Sequences of Human Adenovirus Type 3 Isolated from Ocular Diseases in Sapporo, Japan. J Clin Microbiol 28:2365-2369
4. Itakura S, Aoki K, Sawada H et al (1990) Analysis with Restriction Endonucleases Recognizing 4- or 5-Base-Pair Sequences of Human Adenovirus Type 4 Isolated from Ocular Diseases in Sapporo, Japan. J Clin Microbiol 29:1740-1743
5. Li QG, Wadell G (1988) The Degree of Genetic Variability Among Adenovirus Type 4 Strains Isolated from Man and Chimpanzee. Arch Virol 101:65-77
6. Sawada H, Aoki K, Kawana R et al (1987) Molecular Epidemiology of Adenoviral Conjunctivitis in Sapporo, Japan, and Manila, Philippines. Jpn J Ophthalmol 31:546

Nationwide Surveillance Program of Epidemic Conjunctivitis in Japan

Koki Aoki, K. Isobe, and S. Ohno

Abstract. In Japan, the Infectious Diseases Surveillance Program started in July 1981 under the control of the Ministry of Health and Welfare. Approximately 250 ophthalmologists were designated as index stations and have reported a large number of pharyngoconjunctival fever, epidemic keratoconjunctivitis, and acute hemorrhagic conjunctivitis.
We reviewed the surveillance data from January 1986 to December 1989. A total of 136,814 cases in the reports included 35 577 (26%) cases of pharyngoconjunctival fever, 86 402 (63.2%) of epidemic keratoconjunctivitis, and 14 835 (10.8%) of hemorrhagic conjunctivitis. All three diseases, especially pharyngoconjunctival fever and hemorrhagic conjunctivitis, recently decreased in number. Pharyngoconjunctival fever and epidemic keratoconjunctivitis were more frequently seen in Summer (from the 34th to the 36th week of the year) than in other seasons in Japan. Acute hemorrhagic conjunctivitis used to have a similar epidemic tendency, but its incidence has averaged throughout the year in recent years. We have organized a Viral Conjunctivitis Study Group in Japan starting in July 1990 and consisting of 22 ophthalmologists.
Materials were collected from 588 patients with conjunctivitis in whom viral infections were suspected. The etiologic diagnosis could be established from appropriate specimens in 311 cases (53%). It was shown that Adenovirus infections were diagnosed in 297 cases, Herpes simplex virus in 12 cases, Enterovirus 71 and Coxsackievirus B2 in one case, respectively, and Chlamydia trachomatis in 9 cases. Evaluations of conjunctival smears revealed that Adenovirus type 8 was detected in 104 cases (33%) Adenovirus 3 in 37 cases (12%), Adenovirus 4 in 81 cases (26%), Adenovirus 37 in 21 cases (7%), Adenovirus 19 in 4 cases, and Adenovirus 11 in one case.
Conjunctivitis is caused by many kinds of viruses, however, Adenovirus 8 is currently most frequently isolated.

Introduction

Among viral conjunctivitis, epidemic keratoconjunctivitis and pharyngoconjunctival fever caused by Adenovirus, and acute hemorrhagic conjunctivitis caused by Enterovirus 70 or Coxsackie virus A24 are highly contagious. Even a small prevalence of these infections may evoke a large-scale epidemic and subsequently, a serious problem for the whole area in some instances.

Early and correct recognition of the prevalence is extremely important for the prevention of these diseases. We have reviewed the Annual Report of National Surveillance of Infectious Diseases, in order to get to know the epidemiological data including the seasonality of these diseases from 1982 to 1990 in Japan (5,6,8).

National Epidemiological Data

In Japan, the National Epidemiologic Surveillance of 21 infectious diseases had been started under the patronage of the Ministry of Health and Welfare in July 1981. The program selected three epidemic eye diseases such as epidemic keratoconjunctivitis, pharyngoconjunctival fever and acute hemorrhagic conjunctivitis for the infectious ocular diseases to be reported to the surveillance committee. A number of eye clinics and hospitals were appointed as index stations dependent of the population of certain areas. The number of stations amounted to 297 in 1991. They have reported patient and laboratory data of the monitored diseases, and the information has statistically been evaluated referring to etiology and seasonal prevalence. The program then has offered informational feedbacks to the respective areas (Fig.1).

In 1984, the total number of new patients approximated 70000. This number decreased in 1985. Epidemic keratoconjunctivitis was invariably the largest fraction for nine years. Pharyngoconjunctival fever was next followed by acute hemorrhagic conjunctivitis. This order remained almost the same every year. Epidemic keratoconjunctivitis occurred in approximately 23000 patients in 1984 and in 22000 in 1989 showing some decrease in incidence. The number of new cases decreased from 9966 in 1986 to 984 in 1989. It was reduced to one tenth in four years (Fig.2).

Analysis of the seasonal incidences of each disease by weekly evaluations has shown that each year from 1982 to 1990 epidemic keratoconjunctivitis was most frequently reported in Summer (1). The largest number of cases was reported in 1984. After 1984, the incidence decreased and remained unchanged for the next six years (Fig.3).

Data including 2659 reported cases of pharyngoconjunctival fever of all stations, showed a peak incidence in the period between the 29th and the 36th week, which belongs to the Summer season in Japan. In 1984 41% of all the outbreaks were reported during this period. On the other hand, the number of reported cases decreased in Winter. This tendency remained the same for nine years in all areas except for the Okinawa Island (Fig.4).

There was a large outbreak of acute hemorrhagic conjunctivitis due to Enterovirus 70 and Coxsackie virus A24 reported in the Summers of 1985 and 1986. 47% of all the patients of these two years were reported in a time period of four weeks (37th to 40th weeks) in the Okinawa Island (3). However, the reported numbers of acute hemorrhagic conjunctivitis have decreased since 1987. As the total number of new cases decreased, the seasonal incidences showed a less distinct peak, and only a small number of patients have been reported (Fig.5).

The reports from 1982 to 1990 showed large outbreaks of pharyngoconjunctival fever and epidemic keratoconjunctivitis in 1984, and one of acute hemorrhagic conjunctivitis in 1985. After those outbreaks, newly referred patients with one of these viral infections decreased gradually, and there was no remarkable seasonal prevalence of these diseases. By this method of reporting, information of the surveillance program is employed to distribute knowledge of the frequency of conjunctivitis patients and to prevent epidemics.

Epidemiological Study

A Viral Conjunctivitis Study Group in Japan has been organized starting in July 1990 and consisting of 22 ophthalmologists, who are located from Hokkaido to Kyushu, all over Japan. Samples have been collected from 698 patients with suspected viral conjunctivitis.

The conjunctival swabs collected at the first presentation were inoculated into the cultures of HeLa cell and of human embryonic kidney cells, and inoculated tubes were incubated at 35°C rotating. The cytopathogenic agents detected were identified by neutralization tests using antisera.

Since it may somtimes be difficult to differentiate between viral and chlamydial infections clinically, Chlamydia trachomatis antigen was tested for by an indirect enzyme immunoassay in some of the cases in addition to viral isolation procedures.

An etiologic diagnosis could be established in 367 out of 698 cases by virus isolation. The frequency of positive isolates was 53%. Adenovirus infections were diagnosed in 352 cases (96%), Herpes simplex virus in 13 cases (4%), and Enterovirus 71 and Coxsackie virus B2 in one case each, respectively. Enterovirus 70 could not be isolated in this study. Chlamydia trachomatis infections were diagnosed in nine cases.

Among 352 adenoviruses, type 8 was detected in 158 cases, type 4 in 104 cases, type 3 in 46 cases, type 11 in 4 cases, type 19 in 3 cases, type 37 in 7 cases, and type 19 or 37 in 30 cases. Adenovirus types 19 and 37 are very similar and it is sometimes difficult to differentiate these viruses by neutralization tests (2,7). In this study, without DNA analyses, types 19 and 37 could not be separated in some cases. However, we suspect that almost all of them might have been Adenovirus 37 (Tab.1).

Data after the onset of disease are shown in Tab.2. Most of the viruses were isolated 1-8 days after onset. Only once, Adenovirus 8 was isolated on day 30. Average duration of virus isolation was almost the same in each virus.

Viruses were isolated in 50% to 60% of the patients until eight days after the onset, and in less than 20% after day nine (Tab.2).

The clinical diagnosis and types of virus were correlated. 271 viruses were isolated from patients diagnosed as epidemic keratoconjunctivitis. Adenovirus 8 was the most frequent, followed by types 4, 19/37 and 3. Most of the causative viruses of pharyngoconjunctival fever were Adenovirus types 3 and 4. Seventy percent of the obtained viruses from patients with acute hemorrhagic conjunctivitis were Adenovirus 8.

Considering the causative viruses, half of Adenovirus 3 came from patients with pharyngoconjunctival fever, followed by those with epidemic keratoconjunctivitis. In Adenovirus 4, epidemic keratoconjunctivitis was more prevalent than pharyngoconjunctival fever. Although Adenovirus 8 was obtained most frequently from patients with epidemic keratoconjunctivitis, it was also isolated from the cases with acute hemorrhagic conjunctivitis and pharyngoconjunctival fever. Adenovirus 11 was rare and most of the isolates came from patients suffering from epidemic keratoconjunctivitis. It was thought that main clinical manifestation of Adenovirus 19/37 was epidemic keratoconjunctivitis (90%). In three patients, Herpes simplex virus type 1 was correlated with a clinical diagnosis of keratitis or dermatitis. The other cases were not suspected to be Herpes simplex virus type 1 infections. In these cases, 80% of the patients showed the clinical signs of epidemic keratoconjunctivitis. Herpes simplex virus type 1 may therefore be an important causative agent not only for keratitis but also for conjunctivitis together with Chlamydiae (4) (Tab.3).

Table 4 shows the annual incidence of etiological infectious agents in my hospital from 1980 to 1990. The most frequent agents were Adenovirus 8 in 1980, Enterovirus 70 in 1981, Adenovirus 4 in 1982, Adenovirus 3 in 1983, Enterovirus 70 in 1984, Adenovirus 4 in 1985, Adenovirus 3 in 1986 and 1987, Adenovirus 4 in 1988 and Adenovirus 8 in 1990 (Tab.4).

Conclusions

1) Epidemic keratoconjunctivitis was most frequent and there was a remarkable prevalence of epidemic keratoconjunctivitis and pharyngoconjunctival fever in the Summer of 1984.
2) A diagnosis of viral infection was established in 367 patients (=53%) out of 698 with acute conjunctivitis seen by 22 ophthalmologists in Japan.
3) Adenovirus infections were diagnosed in 352 cases (96%), Herpes simplex virus in 13 cases, Enterovirus 71 and Coxsackie virus B2 in one case each, respectively.
4) Evaluations of conjunctival smears revealed that Adenovirus 8 was detected in 158 cases (45% of adenoviruses), Adenovirus 4 in 104 cases (30%), Adenovirus 3 in 46 cases (13%), Adenovirus 19/37 in 40 cases (11%), and Adenovirus 11 in four cases.
5) Virus could be isolated in about 60% until eight days after onset, but less than 20% after day nine.
6) The annual incidence of etiologic agents showed a remarkable prevalence of one particular virus each year.

Table 1. Nationwide surveillance program of epidemic conjunctivitis in Japan. 367 positive isolates

Adenovirus	352	(95.9%)
Ad 3	46	(13.1%)
Ad 4	104	(29.6%)
Ad 8	158	(44.9%)
Ad11	4	(1.1%)
Ad19	3	(0.9%)
Ad37	7	(2.0%)
Ad19/37	30	(8.5%)
HSV-1	13	(3.5%)
EV71	1	(0.3%)
CB2	1	(0.3%)
Total	367/698	

Table 2. Rate of success of isolation as a function of the number of days after onset

Days after onset	1	2	3	4	5	6	7	8	9	10	11	12	13
Virus (+)	43	83	79	53	37	19	17	17	1	1	1	2	4
	----------- * 348 ------------								-------- **9 --------				
Virus (-)	29	83	53	42	18	12	12	14	4	2	5	2	27
	----------- 263 -------------								-------- 40 ---------				
%	60	50	60	56	67	61	59	55	20	33	17	50	13

*348 (57%)
611

**9 (18%)
49

Table 3. Virus isolation from patients as a function of clinical diagnosis

Virus	EKC	PCF	AHC	Conjunctivitis	HSV	Others	Total
Ad 3	15	27	0	2	0	2	46
Ad 4	71	28	2	2	0	1	104
Ad 8	139	4	8	5	0	2	158
Ad11	3	0	0	0	0	1	4
Ad19/37	35	0	2	1	0	2	40
HSV-1	8	0	0	2	3	0	13
EV71	0	1	0	0	0	0	1
CB2	0	0	0	1	0	0	1
Total	271	60	12	13	3	8	367

Table 4. Etiologic agents of conjunctivitis. 1980-1990 (Sapporo)

Virus Years	1980	´81	'82	'83	'84	'85	'86	'87	'88	'89	1990	Total
Ad *	19		7	11	7				3	86	9	142
Ad 1					3							3
Ad 3		7		42	3	11	31	24	11	9	1	139
Ad 4		3	59	8	30	80	9	21	57	10	5	282
Ad 8		76	6	33	19	4	27	4	20	2	23	214
Ad11						1			3		2	6
Ad19		7		8	15	5	3	1	7		5	51
Ad35					1							1
Ad37		2	4	33	14	3	29	2	5	2	13	107
EV70		61		23		37	14					135
HSV			6	6	9	18	10	14	13	5	10	91
VZV					3							3
Chlamydia				5	7	33	15	13	11	13	10	107
Total	114	61	105	146	148	169	124	82	127	127	78	1281

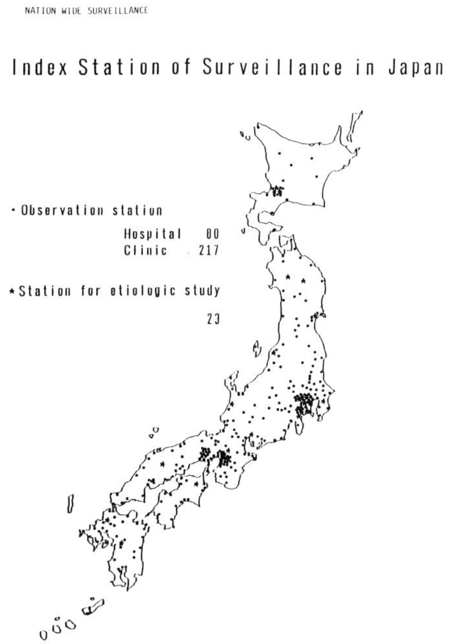

Fig.1. Index stations of surveillance program in Japan

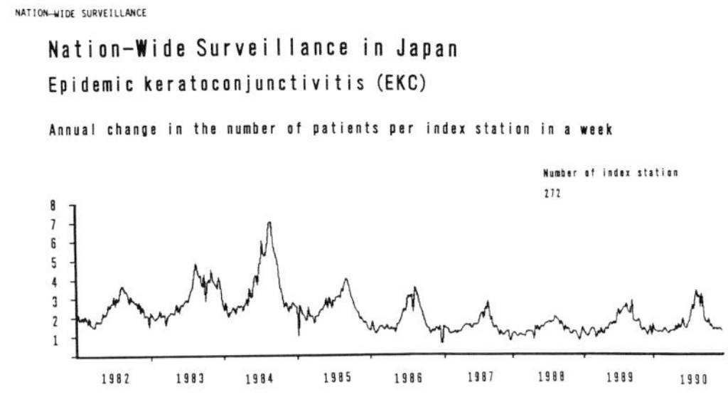

Fig.3. Nationwide Surveillance in Japan: Epidemic keratoconjunctivitis

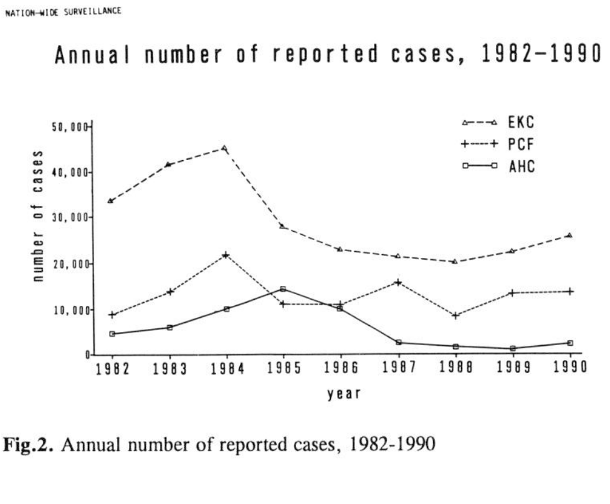

Fig.2. Annual number of reported cases, 1982-1990

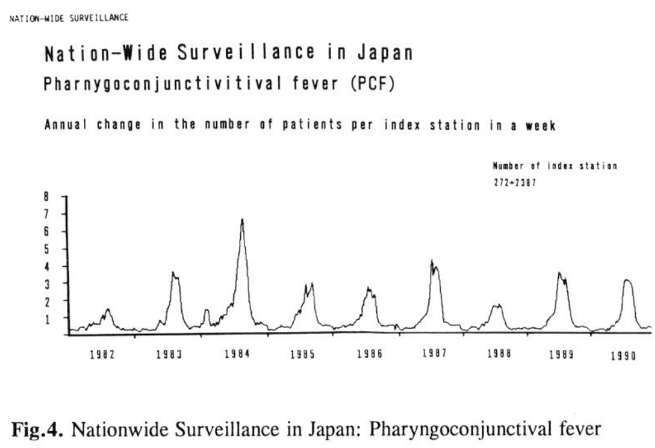

Fig.4. Nationwide Surveillance in Japan: Pharyngoconjunctival fever

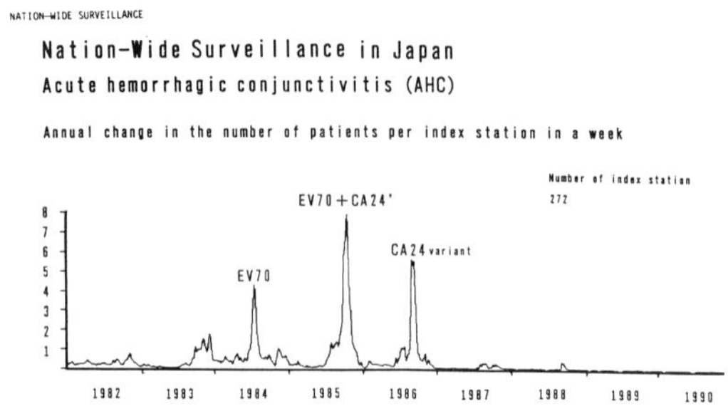

Fig.5. Nationwide Surveillance in Japan: Acute hemorrhagic conjunctivitis

References

1. Aoki K, Kato M, Ohtsuka K et al (1981) Clinical and Etiological Study of Viral Conjunctivitis During Six Years, 19741979, in Sapporo, Japan. Ber Dtsch Ophthalmol Ges 78:384-391.
2. Aoki K, Kawana R, Matsumoto I et al (1986) Viral Conjunctivitis with Special Reference to Adenovirus Type 37 and Enterovirus 70 Infection.
3. Aoki K, Sawada H, Ishikawa H et al (1988) An Outbreak of Acute Hemorrhagic Conjunctivitis Due to a Coxsackie Virus Type A24 Variant in Japan. Jpn J Ophthalmol 32:15
4. Aoki K, Sato C, Hashimoto N et al (1988) Clinical Conjunctivitis in Sapporo, Japan. Jpn J Ophthalmol 32:444-449'
5. Annual Report of the National Surveillance of Infectious Diseases, 1986-1989 (1990). Office of Infectious Diseases Control, Health Service Bureau, Ministry of Health and Welfare, Japan.
6. Hatano H, Tanaka N, Soda K (1988) Prevention of Acute Conjunctivitis: Epidemiological and Preventive Study in Japan. In: Friedlander MH (ed) Prevention of Eye Disease. Mary Ann Liebert, New York pp.41-46
7. Higushi M, Nakjazono N, Ishii K et al (1987) Antigenic and Restriction Endonuclease Analyses of New Adenovirus Types 19 and 37 Causing Acute Conjunctivitis. Jpn J Ophthalmol 31:547-557
8. Oya A (1989) Annual Report on Findings of Infectious Agents in Japan 1986-1988. Jpn J Med Science and Biology, 1987-1989, pp.40-42

Bacterial Endophthalmitis: The French Prospective Multicenter Study

Annie Salvanet-Bouccara, Francoise Forestier, Gabriel Coscas

Abstract. A prospective multicenter study about bacterial endophthalmitis (BE) in France, was carried out for one year long under the aegis of the GEEP (Groupement d'Etudes Epidémiologiques et Prophylactiques) with the contribution of 64 French hospital departments of ophthalmology.
During this survey, 143 cases of post surgical endophthalmitis (PSE) were recorded: 111 of them were secondary to preprogrammed surgery (PPS), 32 happened after penetrating eye injury (PEI).

Twenty four BE collected apart from surgery were named "medical" endophthalmitis. The frequency of Bacterial Endophthalmitis is 0.32% after PPS, and 2.8% after PEI. Intraocular samples were taken out in 61.5% of the PSE. From 50 PSE, 53 germs were isolated.

Bacterial etiology was established in 35% of these PSE. Bacteria isolated were Gram positive in 86.7% of these PSE (among which were 20 Staphylococcus epidermidis and 20 Streptococcus), and Gram-negative in 13.3%. From pseudophakic eyes, 20 bacteria were isolated, 10 of them were Staphylococcus epidermidis and 6 were Streptococcus. From 11 post PEI BE, 13 germs were isolated, among which 5 Staphylococcus epidermidis and 4 Streptococcus. BE visual prognosis depends on the bacterial nature: visual acuity is more than 1/10 in 68% of the Staphylococcus BE but only in 7% of the Streptococcus BE.

Intraocular injections of antibiotics both in the anterior chamber and in the vitreous, and vitrectomy also increase the quality of the visual result. Three months after PSE, 35% of those who received systemic and periocular antibiotics, added with intraocular antibiotics and with or without vitrectomy, recovered a visual acuity of 4/10 or more, instead of only 18% of which without any intraocular therapy.

Introduction

Under the auspices of the Groupement d'Etudes Epidémiologiques et Prophylactique (Group for Epidemiological and Prophylactic Studies), a prospective multicenter study on bacterial endophthalmitis was carried out in 64 French hospital departments (Fig.1) including all of the cases recorded during a follow-up period of one year (from February 1988 through January 1989).

The purpose of this prospective study was to determine the incidence of endophthalmitis and risk factors and to collect all available additional information using a standardized questionnaire for each case of endophthalmitis. This questionnaire was conceived in order to find out details on the incidence and clinical characteristics, the nature and incidence of microorganisms isolated from intraocular aspirates as well as the treatment, the prognosis and the outcome after three months.

Systemic antibiotic prophylaxis was not administered in any of the centers involved. Records of overall surgical activities (data concerning surgical procedures, penetrating injuries, and clinically diagnosed endophthalmitis cases) were kept by each hospital and reported monthly.

Results - Epidemiology

During the year of survey, 36241 surgical procedures have been recorded including 1148 cases of penetrating ocular injuries.

In this prospective study, 167 cases of endophthalmitis have been recorded including 143 cases of postoperative endophthalmitis with 32 cases of endophthalmitis having occurred after penetrating ocular trauma and 111 cases after elective intraocular surgery.

Twenty-four cases of endophthalmitis not related to surgical interventions were labelled "medical" endophthalmitis.

Among 111 postoperative endophthalmitis cases after elective procedures, 83 cases occurred after cataract surgery and 28 cases were reported after various different planned procedures (retinal detachment, glaucoma, keratoplasty, refractive surgery, and secondary intraocular lens implantation).

In this French survey, the incidence of endophthalmitis was 0.32% after planned surgery and 2.80% after penetrating ocular injury. Thus, the risk of endophthalmitis was almost 10 times greater in cases of ocular trauma.

Diabetes mellitus was found in 15 patients with post surgical endophthalmitis. The rate of diabetes mellitus (13.5%) was higher than in the general population. None of the patients with penetrating ocular injury were known to be diabetics.

Risk of Different Procedures

Among the 83 patients with endophthalmitis after cataract surgery, 23 patients had undergone intracapsular surgery and 60 extracapsular surgery. Among the 23 patients with endophthalmitis after intracapsular surgery, 12 had received an anterior chamber lens, and among the 60 patients with endophthalmitis after extracapsular surgery, 48 had received a posterior chamber lens, and 6 of them an anterior chamber lens.

Vitreous loss was reported in 6 cases of intracapsular surgery and in 5 cases of extracapsular surgery. An intraocular foreign body was detected in 8 of the 32 cases of posttraumatic endophthalmitis.

Clinical Characteristics

Two thirds of the cases of endophthalmitis after cataract surgery occurred between the second and the seventeenth day after surgery, regardless of the mode of extraction, the location of the intraocular lens or its presence or absence.

In our survey, cases of chronic endophthalmitis accounted for approximately 20% of endophthalmitis cases after surgery for cataract.

In other planned surgical procedures except from cataract surgery, the onset of endophthalmitis was:

- between the second and the fifth days: in 9/12 patients with retinal detachments,
- between the second and the fifth days: in the 3 secondary intraocular lens implantations reported,
- between the sixth and the sixtieth days: in 5/6 patients with keratoplasties,
- after the sixtieth day: in 2/4 patients with glaucoma filtering surgery.

Endophthalmitis occurred in the first 24 hours following trauma in 46.4% of the cases due to penetrating ocular injury. The rate was 75% when a foreign body had penetrated the eye.

Clinical Signs and Symptoms

Ocular pain was the usual sign in 90% of the acute cases and in 87% of the chronic cases of postoperative endophthalmitis. In contrast, pain occurred in only 62.5% of the subacute cases. Thus, it is demanding to examine the eye in the postoperative days.

In cases of postoperative endophthalmitis, Tyndall's phenomenon in the aqueous humor was present in 95.3%, Tyndall's phenomenon in the vitreous in 86.3%, and a hypopyon in 78.3%.

Intraocular Samples

Smears were performed in 70% to 76% of postoperative endophthalmitis and in 56.5% of "medical" endophthalmitis cases.

Anterior chamber taps and, more often, vitreous aspirates were taken and worked up in almost 50% of patients suffering from postoperative endophthalmitis after cataract surgery, in 46.4% postoperative endophthalmitis after various other planned surgical interventions, and in up to 36% of posttraumatic endophthalmitis.

Overall, intraocular specimens (aqueous humor and/or vitreous) from postoperative endophthalmitis were sampled in 61.5% of cases. The rate of bacterial growth from intraocular samples was 56.8%.

Bacterial Spectrum

All of the intraocular fluids were cultured. Fifty-three pathogenic organisms were isolated from intraocular taps of 50 cases of postoperative endophthalmitis. The distribution of these 53 strains isolated from intraocular taps in post-operative endophthalmitis was:

- 86.7% Gram-positive, with S.epidermidis: 37.7%, S.aureus: 7.5% and Streptococcus: 37.7%; and
- 13.3% Gram-negative organisms (Tab.2).

In 28 endophthalmitis cases after cataract surgery 29 strains could be isolated from intraocular taps:

- 86.2% were Gram-positive with S.epidermidis: 41.4%, S.aureus: 3.4% and Streptococcus: 38%, and
- 13.7% were Gram-negative (Tab.3).

In 20 pseudophakic endophthalmitis cases 20 strains were isolated from intraocular taps:

- 85% were Gram-positive with S.epidermidis:50%, S.aureus:5% and Streptococcus:30%) and
- 15% were Gram-negative (Tab.4).

In 11 endophthalmitis cases after "other" planned surgical interventions 11 strains were isolated from intraocular taps:

- 90.9% were Gram-positive and
- 9.1% were Gram-negative (Tab.5).

In 11 posttraumatic endophthalmitis cases 13 strains were isolated from intraocular taps:

- 84.6% were Gram-positive with S.epidermidis: 38.5%, S.aureus: 7.7% and Streptococcus: 30.7% and
- 15.4% were Gram-negative (Tab.6).

In 10 cases of "medical" endophthalmitis 12 bacterial were isolated from smears and intraocular samples:

- 58.3% were Gram positive,
- 33.3% were Gram negative with Pseudomonas accounting for 25% of cases (Tab.7).

Modes of Treatment

The modes of treatment were chosen independently by each department of ophthalmology. The most frequent systemic antibiotic combination were Fluoroquinolones

(76.9%) and Fosfomycin (30%); Ureido-Penicillins (17%) and Cefotaxime (7%).

Periocular antibiotics were applied in 70% of the patients by subconjunctivally or peribulbar. The most frequently used periocular antibiotics were Gentamicin and Chloramphenicol. Many different topical antibiotics were used.

Intraocular antibiotics were given in 50% of patients either in the anterior chamber or in the vitreous. The most frequently used antibiotic was Chloramphenicol (80%) in the anterior chamber and Aminoglycosides (70%) in the vitreous.

Vitrectomy was performed in 50% of postoperative endophthalmitis cases. In 50% of the cases, vitrectomy was carried out in the first two days after the onset of endophthalmitis, and in 85% of cases in the first week.

Topical, periocular and sometimes systemic corticosteroids were given additionally.

Results of Treatment

At a three-month follow-up visit, visual acuity was better than 20/50 in 35% of the postoperative endophthalmitis cases treated with systemic and periocular antibiotics combined with intraocular treatment, e.g. injection of antibiotics with or without vitrectomy.- In contrast, only 18% of the patients given systemic and periocular antibiotics without intraocular treatment had achieved comparable results of visual acuity.

At a three-month follow-up visit, visual acuity was better than 20/200 in 77% of the postoperative endophthalmitis cases after cataract that had been treated with intraocular antibiotics (anterior chamber and vitreous).- In contrast, only 52% of the patients treated with intraocular antibiotics in either the anterior chamber or the vitreous had achieved comparable results of visual acuity.

Enucleations were done in 11.4% of the endophthalmitis cases after planned surgery, and in 13.6% of the endophthalmitis cases after penetrating injury.

At a three-month follow-up the visual outcome was better than 20/200 in 68% of the patients infected with Staphylococcus and only in 7% of the patients infected with Streptococcus.

Discussion

The data of this French prospective study organized by the Groupement d'Etudes Epidémiologiques et Prophylactique have been collected by mail through a standardized endophthalmitis questionnaire enclosing 85 items. The answer rate obtained for this type of study was high at an average of 90% per item, compared to an usual answer rate of 75%.

The incidence of postoperative endophthalmitis in this prospective study was 0.32%. The frequency in previous retrospective studies had been approximately 0.50% (0.49% from 1957 to 1972 (3) and 0.53% from 1964 to 1974 (6)).

The incidence of posttraumatic endophthalmitis in our study was 2.8%. Similarly, the retrospective study of Haut and coworkers (8) had assessed a frequency of 2.0% for endophthalmitis after penetrating injuries. Modern surgical techniques and intraocular lens implantations do not seem to have increased the risk of endophthalmitis as shown by our study.

After extracapsular cataract extraction almost two thirds of endophthalmitis cases had occurred before the 17th day.

This survey has confirmed Deutsch's (4) findings about painless endophthalmitis induced by staphylococcal infections. In subacute post-cataract endophthalmitis we have found that the onset was painless in 37.5% of the cases. Thus, it is imperative to repeat examinations of the eye, especially for outpatients, in the first two weeks following surgery.

In this survey, the overall rate of evidence for growth of bacteria in postoperative endophthalmitis was 35%.- In chronic endophthalmitis, cultures of intraocular fluids failed (14): Evidence for growth of bacteria was seen in only 13% of these cases, even though in 73% intraocular taps had been taken.

In this study, when intraocular samples were available, bacteria could be isolated in 56.8%. In the study of Driebe and coworkers (5), bacterial isolation rate was given at 75%. In accordance with other studies, it is pointed out that vitreous cultures may be positive for bacterial growth despite negative aqueous cultures. Bacteria have more often been isolated from the vitreous than from the aqueous humor samples (7). Thus, in 39 cases in which one vitreous and one aqueous humor aspirations had been carried out at same time, 27 bacteria have been isolated from 25 vitreous samples and only 19 bacteria from 17 aqueous samples. The same organism was isolated from the vitreous and aqueous fluids in 14 cases of endophthalmitis.

This prospective study has confirmed the great diversity of isolated bacterial strains, which is similar to the distribution reported in the literature (1,5,10,12,13,16). Gram positive bacteria account for more than 80% of isolates. Our study has emphasized a higher rate of Streptococcus (33%) than previous studies and the absence of Bacillus.

Our study has confirmed that the visual outcome may be improved by intraocular antibiotics and vitrectomy (2,9,15). After the third month, visual acuity is better than 20/50 in 36% of the patients treated with intraocular treatment combined with systemic and periocular antibiotics for post-cataract endophthalmitis. This visual acuity was achieved in only 23% of the patients treated with systemic and periocular antibiotics alone. Similar to the report of Parrish and coworkers (11), the French study has confirmed the very aggressive characteristics of streptococcal endophthalmitis when compared with the prognosis of staphylococcal endophthalmitis.

Conclusions

The results of this prospective multicentric study are presented as information only. Our survey has confirmed the importance of intraocular samples as an aid to early diagnosis of endophthalmitis. This should be done for identification of microbes and for antibiotic susceptibility testing.

The modes of the best choice of treatment regimens for postoperative endophthalmitis are still controversial. Information obtained from this survey might initiate further controlled studies comparing different therapeutic regimens. Further studies as being performed in the USA right now are needed to define the role of vitrectomy.

Figure 1

Antibes	(Dr. De Laage)	Montelimar	(Dr. Quanquin)
Argenteuil	(Dr. Hart)	Montfermeil	(Dr. Bodard Rickelman)
Avignon	(Dr. Genevet)	Montpellier	(Dr. Boudet)
Belfort	(Dr. Rollin)	Montreuil	(Dr. Zenatti)
Besancon	(Pr. Montard)	Paris - C.N.O. des Quize-Vingts	(Dr. Haut)
Blois	(Dr. Francois)	Paris - C.N.O. des Quize-Vingts	(Pr. Limon)
Bobigny	(Dr. Chaine)	Paris - C.N.O. des Quize-Vingts	(Pr. Massin)
Bordeaux	(Pr. Verin)	Paris - C.N.O. des Quize-Vingts	(Dr. Ruellan)
Bourg-en-Bresse	(Dr. Roussille)	Paris - Foundation Rothschild	(Dr. Aron-Rosa)
Brest	(Pr. Colin)	Paris - Foundation Rothschild	(Pr. Ganem)
Briancon	(Dr. Decornez)	Paris - Foundation Rothschild	(Dr. Moraz)
Caen	(Pr. Lecoq)	Paris - Hospital Bichat	(Dr. Mondon)
Cannes	(Dr. Chagnon)	Paris - Hospital Cochin	(Dr. Pr. Hamard)
Clermont-Ferrand	(Pr. Rigal)	Paris - Hospital Lariboisière	(Pr. Campchini)
Corbeil	(Pr. Chaneac)	Paris - Hospital Saint-Antoine	(Pr. Saraux)
Creil	(Dr. Curan)	Paris - Hospital Saint-Joseph	(Dr. Demailly)
Creteil	(Pr. Coscas)	Paris - Hospital Saint-Michel	(Pr. Bouchat)
Dax	(Dr. Peyresblanques)	Poitiers	(Pr. Risse)
	(Dr. Rousse)	Reims	(Pr. Ducasse)
Evreux	(Dr. Onfray)	Rouen	(Pr. Brasseur)
Gonesse	(Dr. Cochet)	Saint-German-en-Laye	(Dr. Theron)
Gueret	(Dr. Slaouti)	Saint - Nazaire	(Dr. Guillaumat)
Lannion	(Dr. Coat)	Strasbourg	(Pr. Flament)
Les Mans	(Dr. Banchereau)	Suresnes	(Dr. Lebuisson)
Lille - C.H.R.	(Dr. Rouland)	Tarbes	(Dr. Poletti)
Lille - Hop. Huriez	(Pr.Constantinides)	Valenciennes	(Dr. Fallas)
Limoges	(Pr. Adenis)	Vandoeuvre-Les-Nancy	(Pr. George)
Lyon	(Pr. Bonnet)	Vannes	(Dr. Perchereu)
Marseille	(Pr. Metge)	Poissy	(Dr. Bonsch)
Meaux	(Dr. Salès)	Pontivy	(Dr. Langlois)
Metz	(Dr. Lévy)	Vichy	(Dr. Pataa)
Mont-de-Marsan	(Dr. Dahan)	Villeneuve-St.-Georges	(Dr. Salvanet-Bouccara)

Figure 2: Isolated Bacteria Post Surgical Endophthalmitis

GRAM +	S. epidermidis	20	24	37,7%	45,2%	86,7%
	S.aureus	4		7,5%		
	Streptococcus NG	9	20	16,9%	37,7%	
	Streptococcus A	1		1,9%		
	Streptococcus C	1		1,9%		
	Streptococcus D	4		7,6%		
	Pneumococcus	5		9,4%		
	Micrococcus	1	2	1,9%	3,8%	
	Corynebacterium	1		1,9%		
GRAM -	E.Coli	1	7	1,9%	13,3%	13,3%
	P.aeruginosa	3		5,7%		
	P. Mirabilis	1		1,9%		
	Citrobacter	2		3,8%		
	Total bacteria	53				(ACA+VA)
	Cases with Numerous bacteria	3				

Figure 3: Isolated Bacteria in Post Cataract Endophthalmitis

GRAM +	S. epidermidis	12	13	41,4%	44,8%	86,2%
	S. aureus	1		3,4%		
	Streptococcus NG	6	11	20,8%	38%	
	Streptococcos A	1		3,4%		
	Streptococcus D	2		6,9%		
	Pneumococcus	2		6,9%		
	Micrococcus	1		3,4%	3,4%	
GRAM -	E. coli	1	4	3,4%	13,7%	13,7%
	P. awruginosa	2		6,9%		
	P. mirabilis	1		3,4%		
	Total bacteria	29				
	Caeses with Numerous bacteria	1				(ACA+VA)

Figure 4: Isolated Bacteria in Pseudophakic Endophthalmitis

GRAM +	S. epidermidis	10	17	50%	55%	85%
	S.aureus	1		5%		
	Streptococcus NG	3		15%	25%	
	Streptucuccus A	1		5%		
	Streptococcus D	1		5%		
	Pneumococcus	1		5%	5%	
GRAM -	P. mirabilis	1	3	5%	15%	15%
	P. aeruginosa	2		10%		
	Total Bacteria	20				(ACA+VA)

Figure 5: Isolated Bacteria After Other Regular Procedures

GRAM +	S. epidermidis	3	10	27,3%	45,5%	91%
	S. aureus	2		18,2%		
	Streptococcus NG	1		9,1%	45,5%	
	Streptococcus C	1		9,1%		
	Streptococcus D	1		9,1%		
	Pneumococcus	2		18,2%		
GRAM -	Citrobacter	1	1	9,1%	9,1%	9,1%
	Total Bacteria	11				
	Caeses with Numerous bacteria	0				(ACA+PA)

Figure 6: Isolated Bacteria Post-Traumatic Endophthalmitis

GRAM +	S. epidermidis	5	11	38,5%	46,2%	84,6%
	S. aureus	1		7,7%		
	Streptococcus NG	2		15,3%	30,7%	
	Streptocuccos D	1		7,7%		
	Pneumococcus	1		7,7%		
	Corynebacterium	1		7,7%	7,7%	
GRAM -	P. aeruginosa	1	2	7,7%	15,4%	15,4%
	Citrobacter	0		7,7%	.	
	Total bacteria	13				
	Cases with Numerous bacteria	2				

(ACA-VA)

Figure 7: Isolated Bacteria in "Medical" Endophthalmitis (Smears + Intraocular Samples)

GRAM +	S. epidermidis	3	7	25%	50%	58,3%
	S. aureus	3		25%		
	Pneumococcus	1		8,3%	8,3%	
GRAM -	Pseudomonas	3	4	25%	33,3%	33,3%
	Proteus	1		8,3%	8,§%	8,3%
Fungi	Candida	1	1	8,3%	8,3%	8,3%
	Total bacteria	12				
	Cases with numerous bacteria	2				

Acknowledgement. This study has been partly supported by a grant from Groupement d'Etudes Epidemiologiques et Prophylactiques (Lafaix Ch, Fisch A).

References

1. Bohigian GM, Olk RJ (1986) Factors Associated with Poor Visual Results in Endophthalmitis. Am J Ophthalmol 101:332-334
2. Carney M, Peyman GA (1987) Vitrectomy in Endophthalmitis. Int Ophthalmol Clin 27:127-134
3. Christy NE, Lall P (1973) Postoperative Endophthalmitis Following Cataract Surgery. Effects of Subconjunctival Antibiotics and Other Factors. Arch Ophthalmol 90:361-366
4. Deutsch TA, Goldberg MF (1984) Painless Endophthalmitis After Cataract Surgery. Ophthalmic Surg 15:837-840
5. Driebe N, Mandelbaum S, Forster R et al (1986) Pseudophakic Endophthalmitis: Diagnosis and Management. Ophthalmology 93:442-447
6. Fahmy JA (1975) Endophthalmitis Following Cataract Extraction: A Study of 24 Cases in 4498 Operations. Acta Ophthalmol 53:522-536
7. Forster RK, Abbott RL, Gelender H (1980) Management of Infectious Endophthalmitis. Ophthalmology 87:313-319
8. Haut J, Liotet S, Chermet H (1980) Inutilite et danger des frottis avec culture pre-operatoire. Bull Soc Ophthalmol Fr 80:33-40
9. Mandelbaum S, Forster RK (1987) Postoperative Endophthalmitis. Int Ophthalmol Clin 27:95-106
10. Olson JC, Flynn HW Jr, Forster RW (1983) Results in the Treatment of Postoperative Endophthalmitis. Ophthalmology 90:692-699
11. Parrisch CM, O'Day DM (1987) Traumatic Endophthalmitis. Int Ophthalmol Clin 27:112-119
12. Puliafito CA, Baker AS, Haat J et al (1982) Infectious Endophthalmitis, Review of 36 Cases. Ophthalmology 89:1055-1066
13. Rowsey JJ, Newson DL, Sexton DJ et al (1982) Endophthalmitis. Current Approaches. Ophthalmology 89:1055-1066
14. Salvanet-Bouccara A, Cherifi M, Serrhini A et al (1990) Endophtalmies torpides chez le pseudophake. J Fr Ophthalmol 13:333-338
15. Salvanet-Bouccara A, Dubayle Ph, Forestier F et al (1986) Vers une strategie raisonnee du traitement des endophtalmies bacteriennes post-operatoires. J Fr Ophthalmol 9:523-532
16. Weber DJ, Hoffmann KL, Thoft RA et al (1986) Endophthalmitis Following Intraocular Lens Implantation. Report of 30 Cases and Review of the Literature. Rev Infect Dis 8:12-20

- Postoperative Infections

Management of Acute Endophthalmitis: The European Standpoint

Anselm Kampik and Hans-Peter Heidenkummer

Abstract. Endophthalmitis after any type of ocular trauma remains one of the most sight-threatening complications. Whereas twenty years ago an eye suffering from endophthalmitis was essentially lost, today's possibility to save the eye is up to 85%. This improvement in management of acute endophthalmitis is due to three major therapeutic steps:

- Immediate evaluation of vitreous aspirate.
- Early diagnostic and therapeutic vitrectomy.

- Intraocular application of antiinflammatory and antibacterial drugs.

The essential components of this approach to the management of acute endophthalmitis are demonstrated.

The efficacy of the present mode of therapy has been evaluated in a retrospective study of a consecutive series of 27 cases of acute endophthalmitis. Applying this mode of management to acute endophthalmitis, 85% of eyes could be saved. The most important prognostic criterium in this series of similarly treated cases was the interval between the onset of symptoms and the time of vitrectomy. This interval was 2.4 days in average in cases with functional improvement, and was 4.1 days in average in cases without improvement.

Thus, immediate diagnostic and therapeutic vitrectomy appears to be the most effective mode of treatment of acute endophthalmitis.

Introduction

Acute endophthalmitis caused by infectious organisms remains to be one of the most sight-threatening complications of accidental or surgical trauma to the eye. Despite modern antibiotic treatment, vision in endophthalmitis may only be restored with a very early and effective management of the intraocular infection.

Although acute infectious endophthalmitis has to be differentiated from other non-infectious severe intraocular inflammations (e.g. toxic, phakogenic or sterile) it is usually feasible to obtain a diagnosis of endophthalmitis very early. This early diagnosis is particularly important, because many of the mostly fulminant cases of endophthalmitis may be treated successfully only during the first 24 to 48 hours after onset of the infection. Only about 10 years ago the diagnosis of an acute and massive endophthalmitis most likely implicated loss of visual function and eventually loss of the globe. During the last 10 years intravitreal application of antibiotics combined with pars plana vitrectomy has been advocated and has led to a better prognosis of this very severe disease (3,5,10,14,17-20,28-31). However, the management of these severe forms of intraocular inflammations or infections is still discussed controversially. This dispute has led to an ongoing multicenter randomised clinical trial (6). For the time being, clinical management particularly with regard to severe endophthalmitis remains to be a matter of clinical evidence and personal experience, which has been pointed out by various authors over the last ten years (3,8,10-12,14,17-20,24-26,28-31).

This survey describes our choice of therapy for acute and severe endophthalmitis, which has evolved from clinical experience and experimental research during the past 10 years, and is supported by our own results.

Incidence and Grading of Severe Endophthalmitis

The reported incidence of endophthalmitis varies greatly, since "endophthalmitis" is a clinical, comprehensive term for a disease with a wide range of severity. After intraocular surgical procedures, the incidence has been reported to range from 0.05% to 0.5% (1,2,4,15,27,32). For further details on the incidence of postsurgical endophthalmitis see Pflugfelder and coworkers (pp. 342-352) in this volume.

The diagnosis of endophthalmitis usually is made by the presence of the following signs and symptoms, which may not always be observed in full, thus possibly obscuring a very early diagnosis:

- Pain usually is present, but may be attributed to preceding trauma or surgery and therefore not be reported.
- Conjunctival chemosis and injection vary greatly depending on the current medication.
- One of the most important signs of a beginning endophthalmitis is the status of the anterior chamber with cells, flare, hypopyon, and fibrinous exudate.
- The time course of these findings in the anterior chamber frequently is correlated to the development of inflammatory signs of the vitreous body.
- Corneal haze or edema is a worrying event and immediate ultrasonography of the eye is demanding to rule out vitreous involvement as soon as fundus details or fundus red reflex may no longer be observed.

Cellular and fibrinous involvement of the anterior chamber and the vitreous may hinder visualization of the retina to a variable degree. Endophthalmitis is considered "mild" or "severe" according to the visibility of the fundus and visual acuity. Endophthalmitis is usually considered to be "mild" as long as the visual acuity is better than hand motions and details of the fundus are visible. Endophthalmitis is considered to be "severe" as soon as ophthalmoscopic details of the fundus are no longer visible.

Between these corner stones of an arbitrary grading of endophthalmitis varying degrees of severity may be found, which may frequently and sometimes suddenly change in the time course of a developing acute endophthalmitis. Therefore, decision-making in the management of acute endophthalmitis primarily relies on the time course and the specific individual pattern of the development of infection.

Goal and Rationale of Management

The reasons for the loss of visual acuity in acute endophthalmitis are

- destruction of intraocular tissue due to direct action of the infectious agent,
- release of toxins and enzymes from bacteria,
- destruction caused by the local inflammatory response to the infectious agent.

In the very early stages of infectious endophthalmitis, the inflammatory process is predominantly located in the retina, the retinal vessels and at the vitreous base (14). Even in the early stages of an acute endophthalmitis the vitreous base may be infiltrated densely by polymorphonuclear leucocytes. Subsequently, necrosis of the ciliary body and the retina may result in a destruction of intraocular tissues. Inflammation may be enhanced by a phacogenic factor in cases where nuclear or cortical remnants of the lens have remained in the eye after cataract extraction. This latter combination of an infectious and phacogenic inflammation carries a worse prognosis (14).

The goal in the management of acute endophthalmitis is the elimination of the intraocular infectious agents including toxins, proteolytic enzymes, and inflammatory products to prevent secondary tissue destruction and to restore visual function. In order to achieve this goal drugs such as antibiotics, corticosteroids or antimycotics have to be applied sufficiently high in concentration in order to achieve a therapeutic level.

Topical or systemic application of these drugs is limited by the anatomical barriers such as the cornea or the blood-retinal barrier. Therefore, intravitreal application of drugs should be considered to guarantee significant therapeutic intraocular levels of antibiotics.

The rationale to perform a pars plana vitrectomy together with i.o. application of antibiotics at the same time and very early in the disaease is twofold:

- By performing a vitrectomy sufficient material is obtained to perform smears, histopathology, and culture techniques. The value of a vitreous biopsy alone is limited by the rather low percentage of positive findings at these biopsies (8,11,15).

Although no statistical data are available so far, the combined information from smears, histopathologic examination, and culture tests from vitrectomy material appears to be superior to a fine needle vitreous biopsy.

- Vitrectomy results in an immediate reduction of the intravitreal amount of pathogens and therefore to an increased ratio of antibiotics against bacteria. The vitreous seen as a "nutrient broth" is also removed by the procedure (22). Additionally, bacterial enzymes, toxins and possible diffusion barriers for intravitreal drugs are removed.

With regard to these two statements, the reasons for vitrectomy in endophthalmitis are simultaneously diagnostic as well as therapeutic.

Management by Vitrectomy and Intravitreal Drug Application

As soon as an acute endophthalmitis reaches a stage with no fundus details visible, the decision for an immediate pars plana vitrectomy even as an emergency procedure should be made. Fibrin and pus must be removed from the anterior chamber before performing the complete vitrectomy. We recommend to remove the natural lens if present, but to leave a previously implanted artificial lens in place. However, the posterior lens capsule is always torn in order to improve diffusion of intravitreal drugs, and to drain possible lens remnants from the capsular bag.

Vitrectomy usually is performed according to the following scheme: Vitreous material is removed for smears and sufficient material for bacterial cultures after opening the pars plana with sclerotomies. A fast preliminary diagnosis is made by staining the smears and decide whether bacteria or fungi are present. In addition, Gram-positive bacteria can usually be differentiated from Gram-negative bacteria.

It is our goal to remove the vitreous as completely as possible especially to clean the vitreous base and the area over the ciliary body being almost always infiltrated by leucocytes and/or covered with fibrin. Membraneous structures on the surface of the retina may be removed carefully. This procedure, however, needs very careful manipulations, since the inflammatory changes of the retina may easily lead to iatrogenic lesions. Performing such a vitrectomy in endophthalmitis therefore needs a fully trained vitreous surgeon.

After vitrectomy intravitreal drugs are applied, and anibiotics may be given according to the recommendations of Pflugfelder and coworkers (this volume). We feel that antibiotics in the irrigation fluid should not be recommended, since there is great variation in the amounts of irrigation fluid needed for each individual case. Therefore, the calculation of retinal toxicity for a certain antibiotic is rather unpredictable.

Lately it has also been suggested to instill corticosteroids into the vitreous cavity. It has been shown experimentally that corticosteroids may have beneficial effects on the course of bacterial endophthalmitis (13). Other studies have found a stabilisation of the blood-ocular barriers by corticosteroids (26). Three further experimental studies have confirmed the beneficial effects of corticosteroids in the treatment of bacterial endophthalmitis in conjunction with an antibiotic therapy (21,23,25). Therefore, there is good reason to instill up to 1mg of Dexamethasone additionally to the chosen intraocular antibiotic into the vitreous cavity after vitrectomy.

Results of Combined Diagnostic and Therapeutic Vitrectomy

We have treated 27 cases of endophthalmitis over three years from 1988 to 1990 at the Eye Hospital of the University of Würzburg. Fourteen eyes had had a previous extracapsular cataract surgery, four patients a pars plana vitrectomy, 6 patients a penetrating injury, three patients had a metastatic endophthalmitis. All patients had visual acuity of light perception before vitrectomy. Although in all cases the diagnosis could be made on histopathological grounds only 13 out of 27 cases (48%) disclosed a culture-positive bacterial etiology. The following bacteria were found: S.epidermidis, S.aureus, Streptococci, and P.aeruginoasa.

The visual outcome after this mode of treatment demonstrated that 14 out of these 27 eyes obtained a useful vision (VA >1/35). Twelve achieved a visual acuity above 0.1. Four very severely damaged eyes had to be enucleated. Those eyes are remarkable for their rather long history of endophthalmitis, before a vitrectomy was performed. These figures imply that

- 85% of the eyes with severe acute endophthalmitis could be saved,
- 52% regained ambulatory vision, and even
- 44% achieved useful visual acuity.

In analyzing the data of this cohort of patients it was of note, that - from a retrospective point of view - the most important prognostic criterium in this series of similarly treated cases was the average intervall between the onset of symptoms and the time of vitrectomy. This average intervall was 2.7 days in cases which retained useful vision, and was 4.4 days in cases with remaining light perception and was 13 days in cases where an enucleation had to be performed.

Proposed Guidelines for Management of Acute Endophthalmitis

Although there is some dispute on the best mode of treatment of acute endophthalmitis, there is enough evidence for a very early and rather aggressive approach in the treatment of acute and severe endophthalmitis as described above. By summarizing the discussed rationale for treatment of acute endophthalmitis the following guidelines might be proposed:

- Immediate vitreoretinal surgery should be performed as an emergency procedure as soon as fundus details are obscurred and ultrasound demonstrates vitreous infiltrates.
- A vitreous aspiration at the beginning of surgery has to be performed for diagnostic processing of intraocular tissue during the time of surgery.
- The anterior chamber has to be cleaned from fibrin and other cellular debris.
- Vitrectomy should be performed as complete as possible with a special emphasis on cleaning the vitreous base.
- The natural lens or lens remnants should be removed at the time of surgery.
- In our experience, the artificial lens should be left in place in order to avoid additional surgical tissue damage.
- Finally, intravitreally antibiotics and corticosteroids at appropriate non-toxic concentration should be instilled into the vitreous cavity.

Following these guidelines is a matter of clinical experience and - so far - a matter of uncontrolled personal experiences of various groups of researchers. With regard to the data obtained until now, this mode of treatment is probably most effective to treat fulminant endophthalmitis. Most importantly, treatment should not be delayed and be performed as soon as endophthalmitis becomes severe. Delaying this mode of treatment in the very aggressive cases of endophthalmitis may lead to a worsened prognosis of the disease in an individual patient.

However, more controlled studies are needed in order to achieve consensus on the best management of acute endophthalmitis.

References

1. Allen HF, Mangiaracine AB (1964) Bacterial Endophthalmitis after Cataract Extraction: A Study of 22 Infections in 20000 Operations. Arch Ophthalmol 72:454
2. Cameron ME, Forster TDC (1978) Endophthalmitis Occurring During Hospitalization Following Cataract Surgery. Ophthalmol Surg 9(5):52
3. Chen CJ (1983) Management of Infectious Endophthalmitis by Combined Vitrectomy and Intraocular Injection. Ann Ophthalmol 15:968
4. Christy NE, Lall P (1973) Postoperative Endophthalmitis Following Cataract Surgery. Arch Ophthalmol 90:361
5. Davidson SI (1985) Post-Operative Bacterial Endophthalmitis. Trans Ophthalmol Soc UK 104:278
6. Doft BH (1991) Endophthalmitis Vitrectomy Study. Arch Ophthalmol 109:487
7. Doft BH, Weiskopf J, Nilsson-Ehle I et al (1985) Amphotericin Clearance in Vitrectomized versus Nonvitrectomized Eyes. Ophthalmology 92:1601
8. Driebe WT Jr,, Mandelbaum S, Forster RK et al (1986) Pseudophakic Endophthalmitis. Diagnosis and Management. Ophthalmology 93:442
9. Ficker LA, Peacock J (1986) Infectious Endophthalmitis. Trans Ophthalmol Soc UK 105:319
10. Ficker LA, Meredith TA, Wilson LA et al (1988) Role of Vitrectomy in Staphylococcus Epidermidis Endophthalmitis. Br J Ophthalmol 72:386
11. Forster RK, Abbott RL, Gelender H (1980) Management of Endophthalmitis. Ophthalmology 87:813
12. Forster RK, Abbott RL, Gelender H (1980) Management of Infectious Endophthalmitis. Ophthalmology 87:313
13. Graham RO, Peyman GA (1974) Intravitreal Injection of Dexamethasone.

Treatment of Experimentally Induced Endophthalmitis. Arch Ophthalmol 92: 149
14. Kampik A, Dabov B (1986) Akute Endophthalmitis. In: Lund OE, Waubke TN (eds) Akute Augenerkrankungen - Akute Symptome. Bücherei des Augenarztes, Ferd.Enke Verlag Stuttgart 109: 177-193
15. Kattan HM, Pflugfelder SC (1989) Complications of Intraocular Microbial Agents. Int Ophthalmol Clin 29:188
16. Kattan HM, Flynn HB, Pflugfelder SC (1991) Nosocomial Endophthalmitis Survey. Current Incidence of Infection after Intraocular Surgery. Ophthalmology 98: 227
17. Kroll P, Busse H (1981) Ergebnisse der Vitrektomie bei akuter und chronischer Endophthalmitis. Klin Mbl Augenhlkd 179: 514
18. Laatikainen L, Tarkkanen A (1987) Early Vitrectomy in the Treatment of Post-Operative Purulent Endophthalmitis. Acta Ophthalmol 65:455
19. Lund OE, Kampik A (1983) Vitrektomie bei Endophthalmitis. Klin Mbl Augenhlkd 182:30
20. Majerovics A, Tanenbaum HL (1984) Endophthalmitis and Pars Plana Vitrectomy. Can J Ophthalmol 19:25
21. Maxwell DP, Brent BD, Diamond JD et al (1991) Effect of Intravitreal Dexamethasone on Ocular Histopathology in a Rabbit Model of Endophthalmitis. Ophthalmology 98:1370
22. Maylath FR, Leopold FH (1955) Study of Experimental Intraocular Infection. Am J Ophthalmol 40:86
23. Meredith TA, Aguilar HE, Miller MJ et al (1990) Comparative Treatment of Experimental Staphylococcus epidermidis Endophthalmitis. Arch Ophthalmol 108: 857
24. Peyman GA, Herbst R (1974) Bacterial Endophthalmitis. Arch Ophthalmol 91:416
25. Peyman GA (1977) Antibiotic Administration in the Treatment of Bacterial Endophthalmitis. II Intravitreal Injections. Surv Ophthalmol 21:332
26. Raichand M, Peyman GA, Schwartz H et al (1982) Antiinflammatory Action of Dexamethasone in Vitrectomy Infusion Fluid. Ophthalmic Surg.13:493
27. Stark WJ, Worthen DM, Holladay JT et al (1983) The FDA Report on Intraocular Lenses. Ophthalmology 90:311
28. Talley AR, D'Amico DJ, Talamo JH et al (1987) The Role of Vitrectomy in the Treatment of Postoperative Bacterial Endophthalmitis. Arch Ophthalmol 105:1699
29. Vastine DW, Peyman GA, Guth SB (1979) Visual Prognosis in Bacterial Endophthalmitis Treated with Intravitreal Antibiotics. Ophthalmic Surg.10:76
30. Verbraeken H, Geeroms B, Karemera A (1988) Treatment of Endophthalmitis by Pars Plana Vitrectomy. Ophthalmologica, Basel 197:19
31. Verbraeken H, van Leathem,J (1985) Treatment of Endophthalmitis with and without Pars Plana Vitrectomy. Ophthalmologica, Basel 191:1
32. Wilson LA (1986) Acute Bacterial Infection of the Eye: Bacterial Keratitis and Endophthalmitis. Trans Ophthalmol Soc UK 105:43

Diagnosis and Management of Acute Postoperative Endophthalmitis: The American Standpoint

Stephen C. Pflugfelder, Harry W. Flynn Jr., William W. Culbertson

Abstract. Infectious endophthalmitis continues to be a rare sight-threatening complication following intraocular surgery and trauma.

We recently reviewed the incidence of postoperative endophthalmitis after extracapsular cataract extraction with intraocular lens implantation in a modern eye hospital and found it to be 0.072%. This was not significantly different than the incidence following intracapsular cataract extraction with or without intraocular lens implantation performed at the same eye hospital from 1976 to 1982. A statistically significant increase in the incidence of endophthalmitis was found in diabetic patients, and patients undergoing secondary intraocular lens implantation.

Coagulase-negative Staphylococci are the most common causative organisms for acute postoperative endophthalmitis, followed by Staphylococcus aureus, Gram-negative bacteria, Streptococcus species and fungi. Microbiologic studies indicate that the majority of cases of postoperative endophthalmitis are caused by external ocular microflora.

This suggests that prophylactic therapy to decrease or eliminate ocular surface microflora immediately prior to surgery may decrease the incidence of endophthalmitis.

Bacillus species are the most common isolates from posttraumatic endophthalmitis, and they are frequently associated with retained intraocular foreign bodies and soil-related injuries. Other Gram-positive bacteria and fungi are less common causes of posttraumatic endophthalmitis.

Currently recommended management of acute endophthalmitis includes microsurgical biopsy of intraocular fluids for microbiologic analysis followed by intraocular administration of antibiotics and corticosteroids. Topical, periocular and systemic antimicrobial and anti-inflammatory therapy are also recommended. Clinical features and management of typical and atypical cases of postoperative and posttraumatic endophthalmitis are discussed.

Introduction

Acute inflammation following intraocular surgery may be infectious, requiring prompt identification of the infecting organism and initiation of appropriate antibiotic therapy, or sterile and responsive to anti-inflammatory therapy. In some cases, differentiating sterile postoperative inflammation from acute infectious endophthalmitis may be difficult. Certain clinical features and appropriate microbiologic laboratory studies are helpful in determining the cause of acute postoperative inflammation.

Differentiating Postoperative Sterile Inflammation from Infectious Endophthalmitis

Signs and symptoms typically observed in patients with acute postoperative sterile and infectious inflammation are compared in Table 1. Patients with acute postoperative infectious endophthalmitis tend to have significantly more inflammatory signs and symptoms than patients with sterile inflammation. Certain conditions may masquerade as infectious endophthalmitis in the early postoperative period (Table 2). In most cases, sterile postoperative inflammation can be easily distinguished from infectious endophthalmitis; however, in a small percentage of cases, early mild acute postoperative infectious endophthalmitis may be indistinguishable from sterile inflammation. In these mild cases,it is reasonable to treat the eye with topical corticosteroids, and closely monitor the condition over the next 24 hours. Cases of infectious endophthalmitis will usually worsen over this time period, whereas sterile postoperative inflammation generally improves with anti-inflammatory therapy. When doubt exists whether significant acute postoperative inflammation is sterile or infectious, diagnostic procedures are recommended to obtain intraocular fluid for microbiologic studies.

Epidemiology of Infectious Postoperative Endophthalmitis

Kattan and coworkers recently reported the incidence of acute postoperative endophthalmitis following 22791 cases of extracapsular cataract extraction with intraocularlens implantation performed at the Bascom Palmer Eye Institute during a five and one-half year period during the late 1980's was 0.070% (15).

This was statistically significantly lower than the incidence of acute postoperative endophthalmitis in 2978 cases of intracapsular cataract extraction with intraocular lens implantation (0.20%) performed at the same institution during a six year period in the late 1970's and early 1980's. In the study reported by Kattan and coworkers (15), a significantly greater incidence of acute postoperative endophthalmitis was also noted in patients undergoing secondary intraocular lens implantation and in diabetic patients.

A recent study by Javitt and associates analysed the likelihood of rehospitalization for endophthalmitis in 338141 Medicare beneficiaries over age 65 who were previously admitted to United States hospitals for cataract extraction in 1984 (12). The risk of developing endophthalmitis in this cohort was 0.17% for intracapsular cataract extraction compared with 0.12% for extracapsular cataract extraction or phacoemulsification ($p<0.002$).

Based on these two studies, it appears that the incidence of acute endophthalmitis in patients undergoing extracapsular cataract extraction with intraocular lens implantation in a modern surgical facility is between 0.07% and 0.12%. The significantly lower incidence of acute endophthalmitis in extracapsular procedures compared to intracapsular cataract extraction suggests that preservation of the posterior lens capsule may offer some protection against postoperative infectious endophthalmitis.

For years, ocular surface microflora have been postulated to be the causative agents of acute postoperative endophthalmitis. This theory is supported by a previous report from our institution that the majority (60%) of the cases of acute postoperative infectious endophthalmitis are caused by Staphylococcus species (7), the most common microbial inhabitants of the lids and ocular surface. Several recent studies have confirmed that endophthalmitis is most often caused by ocular surface microorganisms. Kattan and coworkers have found identical antibiograms between the intra- and extraocular isolates from patients with acute postoperative endophthalmitis (15).

Using DNA probes, Speaker and coworkers have found genetic identity between bacteria cultured from intraocular fluid and the ocular surface and/or nasal cavity of patients with acute postoperative endophthalmitis (18).

Since bacteria can be cultured from the ocular surface of almost all individuals, it appears that certain risk factors may make patients more susceptible to infection by ocular surface microflora. Several risk factors for development of acute postoperative endophthalmitis have been identified, and include

- chronic bacterial blepharitis,
- silent dacryocystitis,
- tear drainage obstruction,
- contaminated eye drops,
- preoperative contact lens wear,
- prosthesis in the fellow eye, and
- active nonocular infections.

These conditions may lead to an abnormally elevated population of ocular surface microbes, or colonization of the ocular surface by atypical organisms with greater virulence than the normal microflora. Intraocular entry of ocular surface microflora following intraocular surgery may be facilitated by mechanical wound problems.

Driebe and coworkers have reported that 22% of patients treated for pseudophakic endophthalmitis had wound leaks or vitreous wicks (6).

Host factors, which lower resistance to infection such as chronic immunosuppressive therapy and diabetes mellitus (15) have also been found to be significant risk factors for acute postoperative endophthalmitis.

Diagnosis of Infectious Postoperative Endophthalmitis

Successful treatment of endophthalmitis often depends on early recognition of ocular infection and prompt institution of appropriate antimicrobial therapy. Cultures of aqueous and vitreous humor obtained from diagnostic anterior chamber and vitreous biopsies are recommended to confirm clinical suspicion of infection and to guide therapy. Both diagnostic anterior chamber and vitreous biopsies are performed because organisms are often recovered in only one of these fluids when both are sampled. In cases where it is possible to obtain only one intraocular fluid for culture, we recommend obtaining vitreous, since microorganisms are cultured from the vitreous more frequently than from the aqueous (Table 3).

Intraocular fluid specimens for culture are obtained using the operating microscope. Diagnostic anterior chamber tap is performed by passing a 25 gauge needle attached to a tuberculin syringe through the limbus into the anterior chamber. Approximately 0.1ml of aqueous is aspirated and placed directly on the appropriate microbiologic culture media.

There are several options for obtaining a vitreous o.k. The simplest technique is to aspirate vitreous humor using a 25 or 23 gauge needle attached to a tuberculin syringe. If a peripheral iridectomy is present, the needle can be passed through the limbal incision and peripheral iridectomy into the anterior vitreous cavity. Alternatively, the needle can be placed through the pars plana into the anterior vitreous cavity. The optimal technique for vitreous biopsy is the use of an automated vitrectomy instrument placed into the vitreous cavity through a pars plana sclerotomy. Approximately 0.1ml of vitreous is cut and aspirated into a syringe attached to the aspiration line (a 3-way stopcock can be attached to the aspiration line of the Micro Vit^{R} instrument several centimeters behind the handpiece). Since only a small amount of vitreous is removed by this technique, an infusion line is not required.

After obtaining the diagnostic specimen, appropriate microbiologic culture media are immediately inoculated with the intraocular fluid specimens (13). Typically, the specimens are directly inoculated onto sheep blood and chocolate agar and thioglycollate broth and placed in a 37°C incubator. To enhance recovery of fungi, sheep blood and Sabouraud's agars are inoculated and incubated at 25°C. In order to maximize the chance of a positive culture result, a membrane filter system has been recommended to concentrate dilute vitrectomy specimens, prior to inoculation of culture media (13).

Despite adherence to these diagnostic microbiological protocols, positive cultures were obtained in only 58% of cases of clinically suspected infectious postoperative endophthalmitis in a 1980 study performed at our institition (8). Possible explanations for this low recovery rate include:

1) the low concentration of organisms present in intraocular fluids,
2) delay in transporting and processing specimens,
3) the fact that diagnostic procedures on patients with suspected postoperative endophthalmitis were frequently performed on nights and weekends when specimens were processed by the treating physicians without assistance from the microbiology staff.

Realizing that many treating physicians do not have access to microbiology laboratories with experience in culturing intraocular fluid, Joondeph and coworkers have evaluated the use of blood culture bottles for culturing intraocular fluid specimens (14). They found that blood culture bottles were as effective as both direct media inoculation and membrane filter systems for culturing both reference strains of bacteria and clinical specimens obtained from patients with endophthalmitis. Blood culture bottles provide a simple and effective culture technique for ophthalmologists who do not have access to microbiology laboratories with personnel experienced in processing ocular specimens. Even at institutions with ocular microbiology laboratories, blood culture bottles are useful for culturing specimens obtained on nights and weekends.

Because 24 to 48 hours are often required to culture organisms from intraocular fluid specimens, and Gram stained smears of intraocular fluid specimens are often falsely negative, the selection of intraocular antibiotics is usually made empirically before culture results are available. Rapid and specific microbiologic diagnostic tests for intraocular fluid specimens would assist in the management of endophthalmitis in several ways. First, they would allow rapid distinction between sterile and infectious causes of postoperative endophthalmitis. Sterile postoperative inflammation could be treated aggressively with anti-inflammatory medications and these patients could be spared the risk of toxicity associated with intraocular antibiotic administration. Second, specific rather the empiric antibiotic therapy could be administered in cases where rapid microbiologic identification of the infecting organism has been made.

Over the past few years, several nonculture antigen and DNA detection techniques have become available for rapid detection of microbial infections. Antigen techniques rely to the ability of specific antibodies to react with antigens produced by microorganisms. There are several different methods for detecting the reaction between an antibody and its target antigen, including agglutination, formation of a precipitate line, and a colormetric reaction. Several agglutination assays are currently available for detecting antigens produced by several common bacterial species causing endophthalmitis, including Staphylococcus, Streptococcus and Hemophilus species in intraocular fluid specimens in as little as 15 minutes. Although these tests have not been evaluated for diagnosis of endophthalmitis, they have been found to have a greater sensitivity than Gram stains for diagnosis of experimental keratitis.

All living organisms possess a unique complement of genetic material (DNA) that encodes the amino acid sequences for their structural proteins and enzymes. DNA detection tests rely on this genetic uniqueness by the use of complementary DNA probes. A recently described molecular biology technique, the polymerase chain reaction, appears to be ideally suited for detecting microbial DNA in intraocular fluid specimens. Microbial DNA sequences in microliter specimen volumes can be specifically amplified over a million times within several hours. This amplified DNA can then be easily detected with complementary DNA probes.

Using the polymerase chain reaction, we recently found 100% sensitivity in detecting Cytomegalovirus genomes in aqueous humor aspirates obtained from enucleated eyes of patients with the acquired immunodeficiency syndrome and Cytomegalovirus retinitis (9). Application of the polymerase chain reaction for diagnosing intraocular bacterial or fungal infections has not been reported; however, this technique appears to be most promising for diagnosis of fastidious or slow-growing organism such as anaerobic and mycobacterial species which may take several weeks to grow in culture. The polymerase chain reaction may also prove to be useful for diagnosis of partially treated infections in which cultures are negative, but DNA from dead organisms is still present in intraocular fluid specimens.

Therapeutic Recommendations for Acute Infectious Postoperative Endophthalmitis

Our therapeutic approach for acute postoperative endophthalmitis, presented in Table 4, varies depending on the severity of infection.

In order to achieve therapeutic concentrations of recommended antibiotics in intraocular fluids as rapidly as possible, we currently treat all cases of acute postoperative endophthalmitis with intravitreal antibiotics (7). After intraocular fluid specimens have been obtained, a combination of intraocular antibiotics consisting of Vancomycin and an aminoglycoside or ceftazidine (table 5) is injected into the anterior vitreous cavity in a drop-by-drop fashion with the bevel of the needle facing anteriorly. Removal of the needle used for antibiotic injection from the eye is delayed for several seconds to allow diffusion of the antibiotic away from the injection site and limit the amount of antibiotic leaking out of the eye through the needle tract. In 1986, we substituted Vancomycin for Cefazolin because of an increase in cephalosporin resistance exhibited by the most common bacterial isolates in acute postoperative endophthalmitis (Staphylococcus and Streptococcus species) (4).

In addition to intraocular antibiotic administration, we routinely treat acute postoperative endophthalmitis with periocular and topical antibiotics (Table 5).

We generally treat only severe cases of postoperative endophthalmitis with intravenous antibiotics. Since negligible or subtherapeutic aqueous and vitreous humor concentrations are achieved following intravenous administration of most antibiotics (10), the potential systemic side-effects of systemic antibiotics outweigh the minimal therapeutic benefit. We currently treat postoperative endophthalmitis caused by Coagulase negative Staphylococcus with oral Ciprofloxacin, since aqueous and vitreous humor concentrations approaching the minimal inhibitory concentration for this organism have been detected in human eyes following one 750mg oral dose (17). Intravenous Ceftazidime, a third generation cephalosporin antibiotic, is currently used to treat severe postoperative endophthalmitis caused by Gram-negative bacteria, since therapeutic vitreous humor concentrations of this antibiotic have been measured following intravenous administration (1).

We generally recommend intravitreal Dexamethasone administration in eyes with moderate to severe endophthalmitis (Table 5). In severe cases of endophthalmitis, there is intense infiltration of the anterior chamber and vitreous cavity by polymorphonuclear neutrophils. These white blood cells are capable of destroying tissue by liberating oxygen metabolites such as superoxide and hydrogen peroxide as well as proteolytic enzymes (elastase, collagenase, gelatinase). It is likely that the intense neutrophil response in eyes with endophthalmitis may contribute to the retinal damage frequently seen in these eyes. In experimental pseudomonal endophthalmitis in rabbits, combined intravitreal Dexamethasone and Gentamicin administration has been found to decrease anterior chamber and vitreous cellular infiltration and retinal necrosis when compared to cases treated with intravitreal Gentamicin administration alone (11). In addition to standard intravitreal antibiotics, intravitreal injections of 1200μg of Dexamethasone was found to have no adverse affects in the treatment of 20 consecutive cases of endophthalmitis (3). Intravitreal Dexamethasone appears to be well tolerated by the retina. Graham and Peyman have found no retinal toxicity after intravitreal injection of 400μg of commercially available Dexamethasone

(11). We have found no histologic or electroretinographic evidence of retinal toxicity with up to 4mg of intravitreal Dexamethasone (16).

These preliminary clinical and laboratory studies indicate that intraocular corticosteroid therapy is well tolerated and may improve the visual outcome of endophthalmitis treatment by decreasing media opacity and inflammatory-mediated retinal damage. Although concern has been expressed about the possibility of potentiating or prolonging intraocular infection by use of intraocular steroid, no adverse effects attributable to intraocular Dexamethasone administration have been observed in the treatment of over 60 consecutive cases of acute postoperative endophthalmitis in the last two years at the University of Miami.

Vitrectomy is usually performed in severe cases of acute postoperative endophthalmitis where no red reflex is noted, and a significant abscess in the vitreous cavity is noted echographically. The rationale for performing vitrectomy in cases of postoperative endophthalmitis include the following:

1) obtaining an adequate specimen for microbiologic studies;
2) improving the distribution of intraocular antibiotics;
3) removing infectious material (draining the abscess);
4) clearing opaque debris from the visual axis.

The specific vitrectomy approach selected depends on the media clarity and the experience of the individual surgeon (pars plana vs.limbal approach). We generally avoid three-part posterior vitrectomy in severely inflamed endophthalmitis eyes because of the risk of creating iatrogenic retinal tears. In very severe cases with intense intraocular inflammation, we perform open-sky vitrectomy to remove the intraocular lens and opaque anterior vitreous.

Rarely the intraocular infection progresses following the initial therapy, and repeat intraocular injections of the most appropriate antibiotic based on sensitivity testing are given. The selection of systemic antibiotic(s) may also be modified based on sensitivity testing. In addition, pars plana vitrectomy can be performed, if this procedure was not performed initially.

The diagnostic and therapeutic protocol presented herein may improve the visual prognosis for patients with acute infectious postoperative endophthalmitis. In our most recent report of "in house" cases managed between 1984 and 1989, 15 of 24 (62.5%) of culture-proven cases have achieved 20/200 or better visual acuity.

Table 1. Clinical features differentiating sterile postoperative inflammation from infectious endophthalmitis

Signs/symptoms	sterile	infectious
Pain	none or minimal	moderate to severe
Conjunctival Injection	minimal	moderate to severe
Chemosis	none or minimal	moderate to severe
Corneal Edema	none or minimal	moderate to severe
Hypopyon	rare	common
Fibrin in Anterior Chamber	occasionally	common
Vitritis	none	common

Table 2. Conditions masquerading as acute infectious postoperative endophthalmitis

1. Anterior and vitreous hemorrhage
2. Excessive postoperative inflammation resulting from:
   - retained lens cortical material
   - intraocular medication toxicity
   - corneal edema
   - vitreous loss
   - chronic preoperative miotic therapy
   - surgical iris trauma
3. Wound and suture abscesses

Table 3. Value of vitreous biopsy for culture diagnosis of postoperative endophthalmitis

Study/year (ref.)	% positive vitreous/negative aqueous cultures
Forster 1980 (7)	35%
Driebe 1986 (5)	52%
Kattan 1991 (1)	28%

Table 4. Recommended initial therapy of acute postoperative endophthalmitis

Therapy	mild cases*	severe cases*
intraocular AB	+	+
topical & periocular AB	+	+
intravenous AB	optional	+
intraocular ST	optional	+
vitrectomy	optional	generally +**

AB = Antibiotics
ST = Corticosteroids
*+ = recommended
mild= visual acuity better than hand motions, minimal anterior segment inflammation, ophthalmoscopic view of optic nerve head or retinal vasculature or good red reflex
severe = visual acuity better or worse of hand motions, advanced anterior segment inflammation, no ophthalmoscopic view of fundus details (poor or no red reflex)

** value of vitrectomy for endophthalmitis is currently being studied in a prospective, randomized multicenter study ("Endophthalmitis Vitrectomy Study")(5,2)

Table 5. Recommended initial antibiotic and corticosteroid therapy for infectious acute postoperative endophthalmitis

1. Intraocular
- Gentamicin 0.1mg/0.1ml* (or Amikacin 0.4mg/0.1ml) or
- Ceftazidim 2.25 mg and Vancomycin 1mg/0.1ml
- Dexamethasone 400μg/0.1ml (optional)
2. Periocular
- Gentamicin 20mg (or Ceftazidime 50mg) and Vancomycin 25mg
- Dexamethasone 4-12mg
3. Topical (start on first postoperative day)
- Gentamicin 9.0mg/ml q 1 hour and Vancomycin 50mg/ml q 1 hour
- Prednisolone acetate 1% q 1 hour
4. Systemic
- Coagulase Negative Staphylococci: Ciprofloxacin 750mg p.o. q 12 hours
- Gram-negative bacteria: Ciprofloxacin 750mg p.o. q 12 hours and Ceftazidime 1-2mg i.v. q 12 hours

References

1. Boisjoly HM, Jotterand VH, Bazin R et al (1987) Metastatic Pseudomonas Endophthalmitis Following Bronchoscopy. Can J Ophthalmol 22:378-380
2. Caskey PJ, Folk JC (1987) Accurate Gentamicin Solution for Intravitreal Injection. Arch Ophthalmol 105:454
3. Cole HP, Stallmann J, Diamond J et al (1989) High-Dose Intravitreal Dexamethasone for Infectious Endophthalmitis. Invest Ophthalmol Vis Sci 30(suppl):509
4. Davis JL, Koidu-Tsiligianni A, Pflugfelder SC et al (1988) Coagulase Negative Staphylococcal Endophthalmitis: Increase in Antibiotic Resistance. Ophthalmology 95:1404-1410
5. Doft BH (1989) Endophthalmitis Vitrectomy Study. Arch Ophthalmol 109: 487-489
6. Driebe WT Jr, Mandelbaum S, Forster RK et al (1986) seudophakic Endophthalmitis: Diagnosis and Management. Ophthalmology 93:442-448
7. Flynn HW, Pflugfelder SC, Culbertson WW et al (1989) Recognition, Treatment, and Prevention of Endophthalmitis. Sem in Ophthalmol 4:69-83
8. Forster RK, Abbott RL, Gelender H (1980) Management of Infectious Endophthalmitis. Ophthalmology 87:313-319
9. Fox GM, Crouse CA, Chuang E et al (1991) Detection of Herpesvirus DNA in Vitreous and Aqueous Specimens by the Polymerase Chain Reaction. Arch Ophthalmol 109:226-271
10. Glasser DB, Hyndiuk RA (1986) Antibacterial Agents. In: Tabbara KF, Hyndiuk RA (eds) Infections of the Eye. Little Brown Co, Boston
11. Graham RO, Peyman GA (1974) Intravitreal Injection of Dexamethasone: Treatment of Experimentally Induced Endophthalmitis. Arch Ophthalmol 92: 149-154
12. Javitt JC, Vitale A, Canner JK et al (1991) National Outcomes of Cataract Extraction. Endophthalmitis Following In-Patient Surgery. Arch Ophthalmol 109:1085-1089
13. Jones DB, Liesegang TJ, Robinson NM (1981) Laboratory Diagnosis of Ocular Infections. In: Washington, JA (ed) Cumulative Techniques and Procedures in Clinical

Microbiology. American Society for Microbiology, Washington
14. Joondeph BC, Flynn HW, Miller D et al (1989) A New Culture Method for Infectious Endophthalmitis. Arch Ophthalmol 107:1334-1337
15. Kattan HM, Flynn HW, Pflugfelder SC et al (1991) Nosocomial Endophthalmitis Survey. Current Incidence of Infection After Intraocular Surgery. Ophthalmology 98:227-238
16. Kattan HM, Flynn HW, Pflugfelder SC et al (1990) Retinal Toxicity of Intravitreal Dexamethasone in the Pigmented Rabbit Eye. Invest Ophthalmol Vis Sci 31 (suppl):308
17. Keren G, Ahalel E et al (1991) The Intravitreal Penetration of Orally Administered Ciprofloxacin in Humans. Invest Ophthalmol Vis Sci 32:2388-2392
18. Speaker MG, Milch FA, Shah MK et al (1991) Role of External Bacterial Flora in the Pathogenesis of Acute Postoperative Endophthalmitis. Ophthalmology 89:639-650

Localized Endophthalmitis

Manfred R. Tetz, David J. Apple

Abstract. Following extracapsular cataract extraction and implanation of posterior chamber intraocular lenses, 0.07 to 0.6% of patients may develop an endophthalmitis. Clinically, such cases were and often are referred to as toxic lens syndrome. With increasing knowledge about the difference etiologies of post implantation inflammation, one has to differentiate various conditions. Import etiologies for such inflammations include 1) true toxic lense syndrome, 2) intraoperative intraocular lens contamination with non-infectious agents such as glove powder, 3) phacoanaphylactic endophthalmitis, 4) and inoculation of bacteria leading to either the less frequently occuring fulminant general postoperative endophthalmitis or a condition termed localized endophthalitis. The latter condition was described by Apple and coworkers 1986 and has gained more importance in the differential diagnosis of post-implantation inflammation ever since. Its clinical course, causative organismus, pathogenesis, therapy and differential diagnosis are elaborated upon.

Introduction

Historic review and differentiation from the "toxic lens syndrome": Currently, extracapsular cataract extraction (ECCE) with implantation of a posterior chamber intraocular lens (IOL) is the cataract operation most commonly performed in the western hemisphere. Fortunatelly, few patients show an intense or prolonged postoperative intraocular inflammation (4) and only about 0.07% to 0.6% develop an endophthalmitis (28,33,34,36,48,56).

Clinically, such cases were and often still are referred to as toxic lens syndrome. The spectrum of inflammation may vary from recurrent anterior chamber cell and flare, keratic precipitates with or without a hypopyon, to a severe endophthalmitis involving the vitreous cavity (46,58,75). According to its original meaning, a toxic lens syndrome by definition implicates the IOL itself as the cause for a sterile inflammation. IOL materials most commonly used include polymethylmethacrylate and polypropylene, both of which have been proven safe and effective. Therefore the term toxic lens syndrome did not actually refer to the IOL biomaterial but rather to poor manufacturing quality.

For many years, many IOLs had poorly polished optic surfaces and loop-optic junctions. These mechanically irritated the uveal tissues leading to a prolonged breakdown of the blood-aqueous barrier or postoperative uveitis (4,39). In severe cases, such manufacturing defects were the cause of the so called uveitis-glaucoma-hyphema (UGH) syndrome - a term coined by Ellingson (19) - though it had been well-known to physicians since the introduction of IOLs. A very high incidence of this condition occured in the 1980s, when the frequency of implantation of IOLs increased (4).

The term toxic lens syndrome was established in the ophthalmic literature just around the same time, in the late 70s, early 80s, when several series of postimplantation inflammation differing from the UGH syndrome were observed. In some instances there was a contamination of the implant by polishing substances (47,86). Another etiologic factor included defective sterilisation processes. Certain wet pack as well as ethylene-oxide sterilisation methods lead to several occurences of toxic lens syndrome (71,72). At present, with improved manufacturing and sterilization processes, as well as much better quality control standards, these IOL production-related problems have largely been solved by most manufacturers (4).

However, there are still sporadic instances when a severe post-implantation inflammation occurs. Recent reports have undoubtedly shown that in many of these instances the term toxic lens syndrome is a misnomer. The offending substance in these patients is neither the IOL nor a contamination that occured during the manufacturing process, but rather 1) the exposition of crystalline lens proteins to the body's immune system or 2) the inoculation of substances like surgical glove powder (5) or 3) infection by organisms during surgery (4, 23, 25, 41, 42, 58, 75, 76, 77).

Whereas the first two conditions still represent a sterile inflammation with an inflammatory stimulus similar to that with polishing compounds, the third denotes an only recently identified special form of a true infectious inflammation, a localized endophthalmitis (3,58,75). This term was coined in 1986 by D.Apple and coworkers at the 1. Meeting of the DGII in Gießen, Germany and published in the proceedings of this meeting (3).

Clinical Course of Localized Endophthalmitis

There is a variation in clinical presentation of localized endophthalmitis, but there are some clinical hallmarks commonly present that provide a clear differentiation from a fulminant general postoperative endophthalmitis. The latter has an acute onset, pain and rapid loss of vision; it is commonly caused by organisms of high virulence.

With localized endophthalmitis, one usually finds a delayed or late onset of inflammation occuring over a range of several days to months and even years after the primary surgery (3,4,6,22,46,65,75, 76,77,78,79).

Thus, when referring to the clinical course, or, when a histological examination of intraocular tissues, i.e. the capsular bag, is lacking, some authors prefer the terms late or delayed-onset endophthalmitis, chronic postoperative endophthalmitis, and pseudophakic endophthalmitis (8, 11, 20, 21, 22, 24, 25, 27, 57, 62). Despite the use of different terms, depending on different clinical or pathological presentations, they often may describe the same entity.

The severity of the inflammation may vary. Quite often at some point a hypopyon is present. Typical clinical features are illustrated in Figs. 1 and 2. Recurrences are common and a waxing and waning of the inflammation - especially when treated with topical antibiotics and steroids - may be seen (4, 53, 74, 75, 76, 77).

Posterior capsule opacification and whitish precipitates within the capsular bag do occur and sometimes a Nd:YAG posterior capsulotomy may be required (9,46,52,76). Even an in-the-bag hypopyon has been observed (73).

Causative Organisms of Cases of Localized or Delayed Onset Endophthalmitis

Many types of organisms have been isolated by positive cultures or histological examination of intraocular tissues. The microorganisms found include Propionibacterium species (22), Propionibacterium acnes (1, 3, 11, 45, 46, 61, 62, 66, 74, 75, 76, 77, 87), Coryneform bacteria (22, 43, 44), Bacteroides fragilis (35), Coagulase negative Staphylococci (63,85), Staphylococcus epidermidis (3, 6, 22, 74, 75, 76, 77, 78, 84), Staphylococcus aureus (69), Enterococci (63), Group D Streptococci (74), Group G Streptococci (59), Proteus mirabilis (74), Proteus aeruginosa (74), Fungi (14), Alternaria alternata (63,64), Candida parapsilosis (22), Actinomyces species (62), Paecilomyces lilacinus (38), and others.

There is a predominance for organisms of low virulence, especially S. epidermidis and P.acnes. Mixed infections with these two organisms have been observed (53). Coagulase negative Staphylococci, like S.epidermidis, are the predominant causative organisms in infections associated with vascular catheters and implanted foreign bodies (16,17,28). The nature of these organisms and findings by several authors suggest that these organisms probably originate from the patient's cul de sac, periorbital skin, lid or lid lashes, rather than from a contaminated non-sterile IOL or endogenous infection via the blood stream (12,16).

Means of Intraocular Invasion and Sequestration from the Host's Immune System

Most evidence indicates that organisms enter the patients eye at the time of surgery. Dickey et al (16) found culture-positive anterior chamber aspirates in 43% of 30 patients at the end of surgery (ECCE or phacoemulsification). Sherwood et al (67) reported intraocular bacteria in 29 of 101 patients, with a total of 90% positive cultures of the conjunctival sac in the same patients. The intraocular lens is probably the most important vehicle of intraocular invasion. Bacterial adhesions on the IOL surface have been demonstrated experimentally and clinically (15,26,32,68). Other potential means of inoculation include contamination of irrigation solutions, surgical instruments or viscoelastic substances (4,67). In most cases frank intrusion of organisms does not necessarily lead to a subsequent infection. None of the 13 patients of Dickey's et al. (16) series with culture-proven presence of intraocular organisms developed an endophthalmitis. Organisms seem to cause intraocular infections only sporadically and under certain conditions. How do the inoculated organisms avoid or overcome the host's immune response?

Sequestration of organisms within the closed compartment of the capsular bag or between IOL optic and intact posterior lens capsule may play an important role (58, 66, 75, 76), see Fig 3 and 4. P.acnes seems to enjoy nearly perfect anaerobic growth conditions in this environment. Most authors found no difference of the incidence of localized endophthalmitis depending on the IOL fixation site. Treumer (78,79) has suggested that there may be a higher risk for this type of infection with capsular bag fixation.

Other potential physical refuges from marauding leukocytes may be provided by early postoperative fibrin reactions (16). In the case of S.epidermidis such refuge may be rendered by the potential of this bacterium to produce a protective glycocalyx or extracellular slime matrix following initial polymer surface adhesion and reproduction (15, 16, 28). This protection works twofold: 1. against the host's immune response protecting the bacteria from opsonophagocytosis and 2. against antibacterial drugs physically preventing them to penetrate the matrix (26,28).

Pathomechanism of Inflammation

There may be other mechanisms contributing to the smoldering low grade uveitis in addition to commonly observed inflammatory responses with the body's unspecific and specific defense system against microorganisms. The slime protection of S.epidermidis may provoke a subacute inflammation that only partially responds to therapy since access of therapeutic drugs is limited.

In cases of infection with P.acnes lipolytic enzymes produced by the organism may support an inflammatory response as seen with the same bacterium in acne vulgaris.

The inflammation may become manifest following certain therapeutic measures. Tetz et al (76) were the first to describe a Nd:YAG laser induced exacerbation of a previously "quiet infection" with P.acnes sequestered within the confines of the lens capsular sac, see Fig 3. Following this report other case reports have confirmed these findings (9,61).

Further research will be necessary to evaluate whether a synergistic effect that has been experimentally proven with mycobacterial protein and crystalline lens material in the sense of the Freund's adjuvant theory truly plays a role in the human eye (Literature reviewed in 58, see also differential diagnosis).

Diagnosis

The diagnosis of the disease often has to be based on the clinical course. Diagnostic anterior chamber or vitreous taps are often falsely negative (46,58). In case of positive culture results from different ocular tissues and fluids proof of a clone identity of the isolated strain by molecular typing methods is helpful to rule out a secondary contamination of the asservates (28). Sometimes, direct proof of bacteria in removed parts of the capsular sac is possible by culture and histologically (58,66,75), see Figure 4.

Differential Diagnosis

The differential diagnosis of localized endophthalmitis comprises such entities as true toxic lens syndrome, sympathetic ophthalmia, chronic iris chafing, posterior iris tuck, recurrent anterior chamber microhyphema and others (4,60). A very important condition in the differential diagnosis includes the so-called phacoanaphylactic reaction. This condition consists of a granulomatous inflammation associated with residual crystalline lens protein. Histologically, this disease has also been found in eyes following ECCE with posterior chamber IOL implantation (2,51). Commonly, with phacoanaphylactic endophthalmitis there is a time lag between the cataract procedure and the onset of the inflammation ranging from days to several weeks. In certain instances, there may be a very late onset of this type of inflammation (30). Meisler and coauthors (45) have suggested that in some eyes a synergistic action of both bacteria and lens protein may be involved in the pathogenesis of this specific inflammation. This relates to the Freund's adjuvant theory of mycobacterial protein and crystalline lens material. In this context, Apple et al (4) have called attention to a statement of Verhoeff and Lemoine (82) that has gained new importance. These authors noted the following, when reviewing the histopathology of their cases: "In connection with the Gram stain it may be well to state here that the cataractous lens, after fixation, often in places appears to have undergone transformation into fine granules, some of which are basophilic and stain deeply by the Gram method. Such granules sometimes appear in pus cells, possibly due to precipitation of lens material within the latter, and often closely resemble large cocci." Apple et al suggested that perhaps they were unknowingly seeing organisms, and they therefore have actually introduced the concept of synergism in their original work 70 years ago.

Therapy

Whereas there is consensus that in cases of generalized endophthalmitis early vitrectomy is an important measure to eradicate the organisms and improve the patient's chances not to suffer from severe visual loss (37), therapy of localized endophthalmitis remains somewhat controversial. Due to the relative low incidence of the disease most published data on therapeutic regimens is based on case reports. Thus in the absence of a prospective, randomized clinical therapeutic trial, very different means of prevention (7, 20, 31, 40), conservative treatment (8, 10, 22, 24, 28, 46, 48, 50, 54, 55, 78, 87), and surgical treatment (8, 10, 24, 29, 46, 48, 50, 54, 56, 80, 81, 87) have been suggested.

In light of the fact that it is always better to prevent a disease than to have to treat it later, preventing the infection an obvious first objective. Sterile operative conditions, draping of the patient's eye, desinfection of the lids and lashes are some commonly used prophylactic techniques. It is still somewhat unclear as to what effect the use of perioperative topical antibiotics has and which substances and which type of regimen of application seem optimal (28,40).

From experimental animal test results there is evidence that additional use of dexamethasone eye drops has no negative effects and does not increase the risk of infection (83). On the other hand, patients with diabetes mellitus seem to be at a higher risk for developing a postoperative endophthalmitis (34). However, as to whether a specific prophylaxis in such patients is advantageous remains speculative.

Various conservative treatments with antibiotics with or without steroids have been suggested using topical, systemical and/or intraocular applications (8, 10, 22, 24, 28, 46, 48, 50, 54, 55, 78, 87). Recommendations for surgical therapy include anterior chamber lavage, vitrectomy, posterior capsulotomy with in the bag application of antibiotics, removal of the implant, removal of the capsular sac and combinations thereof (8, 10, 18, 24, 46, 48, 49, 50, 54, 56, 80, 81, 87). Some authors recommend early vitrectomy (48) as in generalized endophthalmitis.

Interestingly, Seymour and Ramsey (70) found that in the meantime localized endophthalmitis is among the three most common reasons for IOL removal.

Conclusion

Localized endophthalmitis has been established as an important and quite common source of delayed or late onset post-IOL implantation inflammation. The future will have to show whether new sources for the latter condition will be identified, especially with rapidly evolving IOL technology, as new biomaterials and surface modifications. A clinical awareness of this condition is necessary for prevention and/or early diagnosis and treatment. This is the only means of reducing the need for undesirable clinical sequelae of IOL explantation.

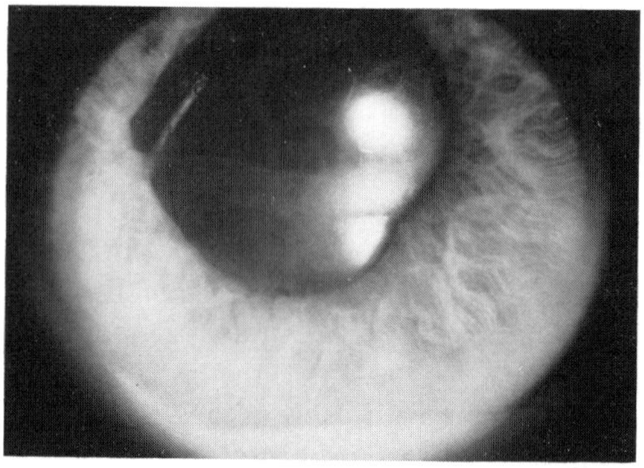

Fig. 1: Second occurence of an inflammation in the left eye of a 75 year old female patient 4 months after ECCE with a 3-piece posterior chamber IOL implantation. Two months postoperatively, an inflammation had been successfully treated with topical and systemic antibiotics. Note the presence of fibrinous exsudates surrounding the IOL.

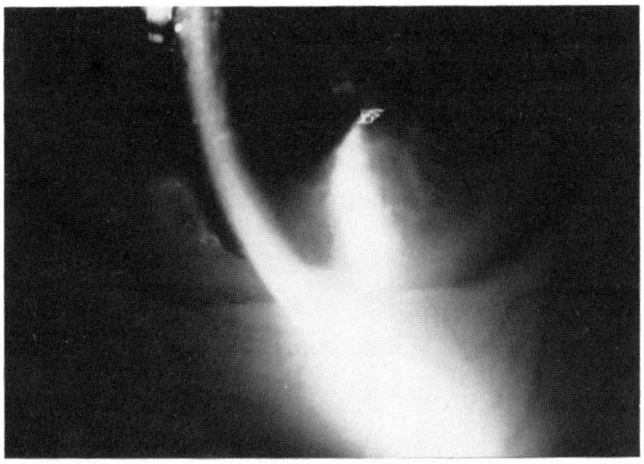

Fig. 2: Slit lamp photograph of the same eye as illustrated in Fig 1. Note the presence of a hypopyon without any ciliary injection. With such relatively "quiet" eyes one may assume a sterile inflammation rather than a true infection. The patient suffered from a total of 4 inflammatory episodes, that could be successfully treated with antibiotics.

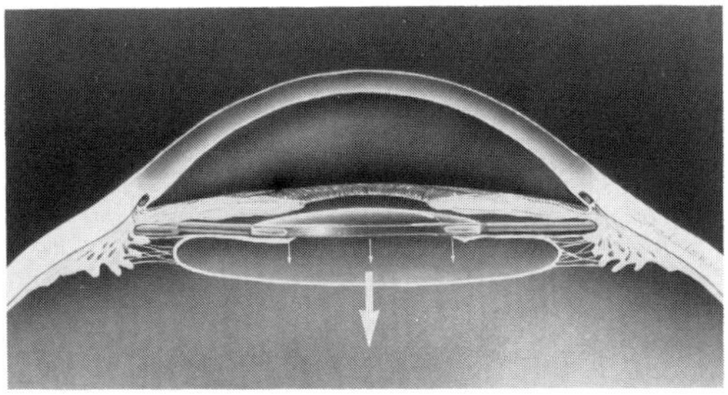

Fig. 3: Schematic illustration demonstrating the concept of organisms sequestered within the lens capsular sac between IOL optic and posterior lens capsule (small arrows). They may often present as whitish plaques or opacification of the posterior capsule and Nd:YAG laser treatment may liberate the bacteria into the vitreous cavity causing an endophthalmitis (large arrow).

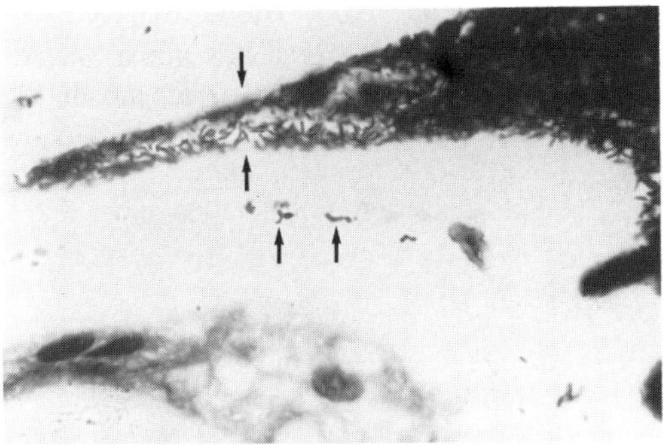

Fig. 4: Higher power photomicrograph of a part of a lens capsular sac. The IOL and lens capsular sac were removed due to a localized endophthalmitis. Histologically, the presence of Gram-positive pleomorphic bacilli (arrows) could be shown.

References

1. Abrahams IW (1989) Propionibacterium acnes Endophthalmitis: An Unusual Manner of Presentation. J Cataract Refract Surg 15:698-701
2. Apple DJ, Mamalis N, Steinmetz RL et al (1984) Phacoanaphylactic Endophthalmitis Associated With Extracapsular Cataract Extraction and Posterior Chamber Intraocular Lens. Arch Ophthalmol 102: 1528-32
3. Apple DJ, Tetz MR, Hunold W: (1988) Lokalisierte Endophthalmitis: Eine bisher nicht beschriebene Komplikation der extrakapsulären Kataraktextraktion. In: Jacobi KW, Schott K, Gloor B (eds) 1. Kongress der Deutschen Gesellschaft für Intraokularlinsen Implantation. Springer-Verlag, Berlin Heidelberg New York pp.6 - 14

4. Apple DJ, Mamalis N, Olson RJ et al (1989) Intraocular Lenses. Evolution, Designs, Complications and Pathology. Williams and Wilkins, Baltimore
5. Bene C, Kranias G (1986) Possible Intraocular Lens Contamination by Surgical Glove Powder. Ophthalmic Surg 17:290-291
6. Bialasiewicz AA, Koniszewski G, Naumann GOH (1988) Pseudo-"Toxic lens"-Syndrom über vier Jahre durch Staphylokokkus epidermidis Endophthalmitis. Klin Mbl Augenheilk 193:142-145
7. Böke W (1987) Intraokulare Entzündungsreaktionen nach Implantation einer retropupillaren Linse. Klin Mbl Augenheilk 190:393-402
8. Brady SE, Cohen EJ, Fischer DH (1988) Diagnosis and Treatment of Chronic Postoperative Bacterial Endophthalmitis. Ophthalmic Surg 19:580-584
9. Carlson AN, Koch DD (1988) Endophthalmitis Following Nd: YAG Laser Posterior Capsulotomy. Ophthalmic Surg 19:168-170
10. Carlson AN, Tetz MR, Apple DJ (1989) Infectious Complications of Modern Cataract Surgery and Intraocular Lens Implantation. Infect Dis Clin North Am 3: 339-55
11. Cohen G, Colin J, Anguil MY, Le-Gouil JY (1988) Endophthalmie chronique au Propionibacterium acnes chez un pseudophake. J Fr Ophthalmol 11:521-522
12. Comte P, Verin P, Gauthier L (1988) Endophthalmie chez un porteur d'implant: metastase septique ou inoculation locale. Bull Soc Ophthalmol Fr 88:261-262
13. Cotticelli L, Russo S, Costagliola C et al (1991) Moraxella laconata Endophthalmitis After Intraocular Lens Implantation. Europ J Implant Ref Surg 3:152-155
14. Cusumano A, Busin M, Spitznas M (1991) Mycotic infection of the capsular bag in postoperative endophthalmitis. J Cataract Refract Surg 17: 503-505
15. Cusumano A, Busin M, Spitznas M (1991) Rasterelektronenmikroskopische Untersuchungen an explantierten Intraokularlinsen. In: Schott K, Jacobi KW, Freyler H (eds) 4. Kongress der Deutschen Gesellschaft für Intraokularlinsen Implantation. Springer-Verlag, Berlin Heidelberg New York pp. 184-189
16. Dickey JB, Thompson KD, Jay WM (1991) Anterior Chamber Aspirate Cultures After Uncomplicated Cataract Surgery. Am J Ophthalmol 112:278-82
17. Dougherty SH, Simmons RL (1989) Endogenous Factors Contributing to Prosthetic Device Infections. Infect Dis Clin North Am 3:199-209
18. Durquety MC, Guetari MC, Le-Rebeller MJ (1990) Indications d'explantation. Bull Soc Ophthalmol Fr 90:329-333
19. Ellingson FT (1978) The Uveitis-Glaucoma-Hyphema Syndrome Associated With the Mark VIII Anterior Chamber Lens Implant. J Am Intraocul Implant Soc 4:50-53
20. Elliott RD, Katz HR (1987) Inhibition of Pseudophakic Endophthalmitis in a Rabbit Model. Ophthalmic Surg 18:538-541
21. Ficker L, Meredith TA, Wilson LA et al (1987) Chronic Bacterial Endophthalmitis. Am J Ophthalmol 103:745-748
22. Fox GM, Joondeph BC, Flynn HW Jr et al (1991) Delayed-onset Pseudophakic Endophthalmitis. Am J Ophthalmol 111: 163-73.
23. Garner A (1989) Complications of Prosthetic Intraocular Lens Implantation: A Histopathological Study. Br J Ophthalmol 73:940-945
24. Gloor B (1990) Behandlung der akuten und chronischen Endophthalmitis nach Hinterkammerlinsen-Implantation. Klin Mbl Augenheilk 196:325-328
25. Gloor B, Messmer E, v. Ziegler C (1991) Akute und chronische Endophthalmitis nach Hinterkammerlinsenimplantation. In: Schott K, Jacobi KW, Freyler H (eds)

26. Kongress der Deutschen Gesellschaft für Intraokularlinsen Implantation. Springer-Verlag, Berlin Heidelberg New York pp. 162-169
27. Griffiths PG, Elliot TS, McTaggart L (1989) Adherence of Staphylococcus epidermidis to Intraocular Lenses. Br J Ophthalmol 73:402-406
28. Haimann MH, Weiss H, Miller JA (1991) Delayed-onset Pseudophakic Endophthalmitis (letter). Am J Ophthalmol 111:656-657
29. Hartmann C, Jansen B, Schumacher-Perdreau F et al (1991) Bakterielle Spätendophthalmitis nach Kunstlinsenimplantation: Eine chronische, IOL-assozierte "Plastikinfektion". In: Schott K, Jacobi KW, Freyler H (eds) 4. Kongress der Deutschen Gesellschaft für Intraokularlinsen Implantation. Springer-Verlag, Berlin Heidelberg New York pp. 170-178
30. Heimann K, Lemmen KD, Hartmann C (1991) Die Therapie der postoperativen Endophthalmitis. In: Wenzel W, Reim M, Freyler H, Hartmann C (eds) 5. Kongress der Deutschen Gesellschaft für Intraokularlinsen Implantation. Springer-Verlag, Berlin Heidelberg New York pp.629-640
31. Holz FG, Tetz M, Völcker HE (1991) Extrakapsuläre Kataraktextraktion mit Hinterkammerlinsenimplantation bei umschriebener Endophthalmitis phacoanaphylactica. In: Wenzel W, Reim M, Freyler H, Hartmann C (eds) 5. Kongress der Deutschen Gesellschaft für Intraokularlinsen Implantation Springer-Verlag, Berlin Heidelberg New York pp. 570-574
32. Imbert P, Comte P, Lagoutte F et al (1990) Implantation et endophtalmie: Moyens de prevention. Bull Soc Ophtalmol Fr 90(3):323-324.
33. Jansen B, Hartmann C, Schumacher-Perdreau F et al (1991) Late Onset Endophthalmitis Associated With Intraocular Lens: A Case of Molecularly Proved S.epidermidis Aetiology. Br J Ophthalmol 75:440-441
34. Javitt JC, Vitale S, Canner JK et al (1991) National Outcomes of Cataract Extraction. Endophthalmitis Following Inpatient Surgery. Arch Ophthalmol 190:1085-1089
35. Kattan HM, Flynn HW Jr, Pflugfelder SC et al (1991) Nosocomial Endophthalmitis Survey. Current Incidence of Infection After Intraocular Surgery. Ophthalmology 98:227-38
36. Kelly LD, Gaynon M (1990) Bacteroides fragilis Endophthalmitis: A Case Report. Can J Ophthalmol 25:208-209
37. Koul S, Philipson A, Philipson BT Incidence of Endophthalmitis in Sweden. Acta Ophthalmol Copenh 6:499-503
38. Laatikainen L, Tarkkanen A (1987) Early Vitrectomy in the Treatment of Post-Operative Purulent Endophthalmitis. Acta Ophthalmol Copenh 65:455-460
39. Levin PS, Beebe WE, Abbott RL (1987) Successful Treatment of Paecilomyces lilacinus Endophthalmitis Following Cataract Extraction with Intraocular Lens Implantation. Ophthalmic Surg 18:217-219
40. Liesegang TJ, Bourne WM, Brubaker RF (1984) The Effect of Cataract Surgery on the Blood Aqueous Barrier. Ophthalmology 91:32-39
41. Lommatzsch PK, Lössner A, Kohlmann et al (1991) Ist eine antibiotische Vorbehandlung von Intraokularlinsen zur Vermeidung der polymerassoziierten Endophthalmitis sinnvoll? In: Schott K, Jacobi KW, Freyler H (eds). 4. Kongress der Deutschen Gesellschaft für Intraokularlinsen Implantation. Springer-Verlag, Berlin Heidelberg New York pp. 179-183
42. Magnocavallo M, Cassina T, Lo-Votrico A et al (1988) Endophtalmite et pseudophaquie. Klin Mbl Augenheilk 192:440-443
43. McClellan K, Coster DJ, Badenoch PR et al (1987) Endophthalmitis Following Cata-

ract Extraction. Aust N Z J Ophthalmol 15:19-23
44. McManaway JW, Weinberg RS, Coudron PE (1990) Coryneform Endophthalmitis. Two Case Reports. Arch Ophthalmol 108: 942-944
45. McManaway JW, Weinberg RS, Coudron PE (1991) Coryneform Group A-4 Endophthalmitis. An Experimental Animal Model. Invest Ophthalmol Vis Sci 32: 2696-2699
46. Meisler DM, Palestine AG, Vastine DW et al (1986) Chronic Propionibacterium Endophthalmitis After Extracapsular Cataract Extraction and Intraocular Lens Implantation. Am J Ophthalmol 102:733-739
47. Meisler DM, Mandelbaum S (1989) Propionibacterium-associated Endophthalmitis After Extracapsular Cataract Extraction. Review of Reported Cases. Ophthalmology 96:54-61
48. Meltzer DW (1980) Sterile Hypopyon Following Intraocular Lens Surgery. Arch Ophthalmol 98:100-104
49. Metge P, Cohen H, Cadiou D et al (1990) Endophthalmies du pseudophake. Bull Soc Ophthalmol Fr 90:531-535
50. Metge P, Cohen H, Cadiou D et al (1990) Indications d'explantation. Bull Soc Ophthalmol Fr 90:329-333.
51. Momose A (1987) Management of Post operative Inflammation in Lens Implant Surgery. Indian J Ophthalmol 35:72-74
52. Necker HP, Weidle EG, Steuhl KP (1989) Endophthalmitis phakoanaphylactica mit Uveitis anterior am Partnerauge. Klin Mbl Augenheilk 195:248-253
53. Neuteboom GH, de-Vries-Knoppert WA (1988) Endophthalmitis After Nd:YAG Laser Capsulotomy. Doc Ophthalmol 70: 175-178
54. Nishi K, Nishi O, Apple DJ et al (1988) A Case of Localized Endophthalmitis Due to Propionibacterium acnes and Staphylococcus Epidermidis Following Extracapsular Cataract Extraction. Jpn J Clin Ophthalmol 42:931-935
55. Okl RJ, Bohigian GM (1987) The Management of Endophthalmitis: Diagnostic and Therapeutic Guidelines Including the Use of Vitrectomy. Ophthalmic Surg 18:262-267
56. Pflugfelder SC, Hernandez E, Fliesler SJ et al (1987) Intravitreal Vancomycin. Retinal Toxicity, Clearance, and Interaction With Gentamicin. Arch Ophthalmol 105:831-837
57. Pham-Duy T, Wollensak J, Schnitzkewitz G (1988) Endophthalmitis und Toxic lens-Syndrom. Differentialdiagnose und Therapie. Klin Mbl Augenheilk 193:243-248
58. Pichto-de-Chamfleury A (1987) Endophthalmies du pseudophake. Bull Soc Ophthalmol Fr 90:531-53
59. Piest KL, Kincaid MC, Tetz MR et al (1987) Localized Endophthalmitis: A Newly Described Cause of the So-Called Toxic Lens Syndrome. J Cataract Refract Surg 13:498-510
60. Posenauer B, Funk J (1991) Streptokokken der Gruppe G als Erreger einer postoperativen Endophthalmitis. Klin Mbl Augenheilk 199:45-47
61. Rochels R (1991) Klassifikation, Ätiologie, Pathogenese, Klinik und Differentialdiagnose der intraokularen Entzündungsreaktionen nach Kataraktextraktion mit Kunstlinsenimplantation. In: Schott K, Jacobi KW, Freyler H (eds) 4. Kongress der Deutschen Gesellschaft für Intraokularlinsen Implantation. Springer-Verlag, Berlin Heidelberg New York pp. 153-161
62. Roussel TJ, Culbertson WW, Jaffe NS (1987) Chronic Postoperative Endophthalmitis Associated With Propionibacterium acnes. Arch Ophthalmol 105:1199-1201
63. Roussel TJ, Olson ER, Rice T et al (1991) Chronic Postoperative Endophthalmitis Associated With Actinomyces Species. Arch Ophthalmol 109:60-62

64. Rummelt V, Ruprecht KW, Bialasiewicz AA (1990) "Toxic-lens-Syndrom" In: Freyler H, Skorpik C, Grasl M (eds) 3. Kongress der Deutschen Gesellschaft für Intraokularlinsen Implantation. Springer-Verlag, Berlin Heidelberg New York pp. 269-271
65. Rummelt V, Ruprecht KW, Boltze HJ et al (1991) Chronic Alternaria alternata Endophthalmitis Following Intraocular Lens Implantation (letter). Arch Ophthalmol 109:178
66. Salvanet-Bouccara A, Cherifi M, Serrhini A et al (1990) Endophthalmies torpides chez le pseudophake: Difficultes diagnostiques et therapeutiques. A propos de 4 cas. J Fr Ophthalmol 13:333-338
67. Sawusch MR, Michels RG, Stark WJ et al (1989) Endophthalmitis Due to Propionibacterium acnes Sequestered Between IOL Optic and Posterior Capsule. Ophthalmic Surg 20:90-92
68. Sherwood DR, Rich WJ, Jacob JS et al (1989) Bacterial Contamination of Intraocular and Extraocular Fluids During Extracapsular Cataract Extraction. Eye 3:308-312
69. Schemann JF (1987) Scanning Electron Microscopic Study of an Anterior Chamber Intraocular Lens: Latent Endophthalmitis. Ophthalmologica 195:7-12
70. Seedor JA, Koplin RS, Shah M et al (1990) Chronic Postoperative Endophthalmitis from Staphylococcus aureus. J Cataract Refract Surg 16:512-513
71. Seymour RG, Ramsey MS (1989) Cause of Intraocular Lens Removal. Can J Ophthalmol 24:152-154
72. Stark WJ (1978) Wet-pack vs. Dry Pack Lenses. (letter to the editor) J Am Intraocul Soc 4:213
73. Stark WJ, Rosenblum P, Maumenee AE et al (1980) Postoperative Inflammatory Reactions to Intraocular Lenses Sterilized With Ethylene-Oxide. Ophthalmology 87:385-389
74. Stefansson E, Cobo LM, Carlson AN et al (1990) Endocapsular Hypopyon: A Clinical Sign of Localized Endophthalmitis. Ophthalmic Surg 21:221-222
75. Stern GA, Engel HM, Driebe WT Jr (1990) Recurrent Postoperative Endophthalmitis. Cornea 9:102-107
76. Tetz MR, Apple DJ, Hansen SO et al (1987) "Localised Endophthalmitis": A Complication of Extracapsular Cataract Extraction. Implants in Ophthalmology 1:93-97
77. Tetz MR, Apple DJ, Price FW et al (1987) A Newly Described Complication of Neodymium-YAG Laser Capsulotomy: Exacerbation of an Intraocular Infection. Arch Ophthalmol 105:1324-1325
78. Tetz MR (1990) "Toxic Lens Syndrom" im Wandel? Editorial. Ophthalmochirurgie 2:1
79. Treumer H, Böke W (1989) Zur mikrobiell induzierten Entzündungsreaktion nach Implantation endokapsulärer sulkusfixierter Intraokularlinsen. In: Lang GK, Ruprecht KW, Jacobi,KW, Schott,K (eds.): 2. Kongress der Deutschen Gesellschaft für Intraokularlinsen Implantation. Enke Verlag, Stuttgart pp. 221-226
80. Treumer H (1990) Akute und chronische Entzündungsreaktionen nach Implantation künstlicher Linsen. Fortschr Ophthalmol 87 Suppl:33-40
81. Treumer H (1990) Zur chirurgischen Therapie der bakteriellen Entzündung nach Intraokularlinsenimplantation. In: Freyler H, Skorpik C, Grasl M (eds) 3. Kongress der Deutschen Gesellschaft für Intraokularlinsen Implantation. Springer-Verlag, Berlin Heidelberg New York pp.403-409
82. Verbraeken H, Geeroms B, Karemera A (1988) Treatment of Endophthalmitis by Pars plana Vitrectomy. Ophthalmologica 197:19-25
83. Verhoeff FH, Lemoine AN (1922) Endophthalmitis Phacoanaphylactica. Am J Ophthalmol 5:737-744

84. Wahl JC, Elliott RD, Katz HR (1991) The Effect of Dexamethasone on the Inhibition of Pseudophakic Bacterial Endophthalmitis. Ophthalmic Surg 22:348-349
85. Wenzel M, Reim M (1988) Eine Klassifizierung intraokularer bakteriologischer Befunde nach Linsenimplantation. Klin Mbl Augenheilk 193:589-593
86. Wenzel M, Reim M (1989) Bakterielle intraokulare Entzündungen nach Linsenimplantation. In: Lang GK, Ruprecht KW, Jacobi KW, Schott K (eds) 2. Kongress der Deutschen Gesellschaft für Intraokularlinsen Implantation. Enke Verlag, Stuttgart pp. 227-229
87. Wilbrandt HR (1982) Presumed Polishing Compound Remnants on Surfaces on Intraocular Lenses. J Am Intraocul Implant Soc 8:251-253
88. Zambrano W, Flynn HW Jr, Pflugfelder SC et al (1989) Management Options for Propionibacterium acnes Endophthalmitis. Ophthalmology 96:1100-1105

- Metastatic Infections

Metastatic Bacterial and Fungal Endophthalmitis: Microbial Aspects

Alexander von Graevenitz

Abstract. Metastatic endophthalmitis has become rare in the antibiotic era. Its microbial spectrum has also changed. Formerly, Neisseria meningitidis, Streptococcus pneumoniae, streptococci and Staphylococcus aureus were the main agents; today, Candida albicans, Bacillus cereus, Enterobacteriaceae, S.aureus and Haemophilus sp. lead the list.
Important host factors are diabetes, hyperalimentation, recent surgery, cardiac abnormalities, intravenous lines, drug abuse, previous antimicrobial therapy and immunosuppression. The main foci are the meninges, endocardium, urinary, gastro-intestinal, and wound sites. Diagnosis is made by culture of intraocular fluid, blood, and/or suspected other sources (e.g. CSF, urine). Conjunctival cultures do not correlate with vitreal ones. Inoculation of solid and liquid media as well as most stains should be done in the operating room. Therapeutically, systemic and perhaps intravitreal broad-spectrum antibiotics should be administered although no controlled studies exist reagarding choice of antibiotics and route of administration. Prevention of loss of the eye includes periodic ophthalmoscopy in patients with candidemia

(of whom 25-40% show ocular involvement), early aspiration, and immediate antibiotic administration.

Introduction

Metastatic endophthalmitis is defined as an inflammatory process of the internal ocular spaces secondary to an infective focus elsewhere. It is a rare disease today. There have been two reviews of bacterial metastatic endophthalmitis, one from 1977 covering 102 cases reported between 1935-1975 (15); and the other from 1986 which has added 6 cases to the first series and has covered 72 new ones reported between 1976 and 1985 (8). This paper will review the present situation regarding bacterial and fungal infections. It will, however, not discuss localization, clinical signs and symptoms, and surgery since they do not belong to the domain of the microbiologist.

Pathogenesis, Risk, and Etiology

Metastatic endophthalmitis is characterized by hematogenous spread of microorganisms from a focus to the ocular blood vessels, followed by their crossing of the "blood-ocular barriers", their deposition and subsequent multiplication in the ocular tissues, and the host's inflammatory response. Most diseases or factors predisposing to septicemia could, then, predispose to metastatic endophthalmitis as well. In bacteremia, however, the risk seems extremely small and associated with the site of the focus (e.g., meninges) (4) although no figures exist for particular constellations. In contrast, fungemia with Candida albicans carries a significant risk of endophthalmitis (4%-39% in 5 series; with a mean of 27%) (6,10). Figures are considerably lower for fungemia with non-albicans Candida spp. (C.tropicalis, C.parapsilosis, C.glabrata) (4-20% with a mean of 9.5%) (10).

Metastatic endophthalmitis may occur at any age and with equal frequency in both sexes, is bilateral in approximately 25% of cases, but affects the right eye about twice as often as the left one (8). Prior to the antibiotic era, the majority of patients with metastatic endophthalmitis had shown no risk factors predisposing to septicemia; rather, metastatic endophthalmitis occurred in sydromes such as meningitis.

Nowadays, antibiotic treatment, diabetes mellitus, intravenous drug abuse, recent surgery, intravenous catheters, cardiac anormalies, and corticosteroid therapy are found in a majority of those patients; only about one quarter is free of these predisposing factors (8) (Tab.1). Surprisingly, however, neutropenia is not among the factors predisposing to recognizable metastatic endophthalmitis although it predisposes to septicemia.

The prevalence of foci has also changed over time (Tab. 1). The percentage of bacterial metastatic endophthalmitis with a meningeal focus has decreased from 56% (1935-1975) (15) to 26% (1976-1985) (8) while cases related to intravenous drug abuse now constitute a plurality, the "focus" either being unknown or found in the paraphernalia, drugs, or the skin flora (16). Such cases are difficult to identify in earlier series because of the low incidence of drug abuse, failure to inquire or to recognize this factor as predisposing, and use of insufficient techniques for the culture of fungi.

No significant difference over time is evident with regard to other foci (endocardium, urinary tract, abscesses, wounds, and respiratory tract; 7-14% each). Puerperal foci have by now disappeared altogether. Usually, a septic focus becomes evident before metastatic endophthalmitis appears.

The infecting microorganisms have also shown a change in ranking over time (Tab.1). From 1935-1975, Neisseria meningitidis and Streptococcus pneumoniae accounted for two-thirds of the causative agents, with the meninges being the main focus (8). From 1976 on, these agents together had dropped to 14% but the spectrum had enlarged, reflecting intravenous drug abuse but also nosocomial septicemia with gram-negative rods. Table 1 also lists localization, prognosis, and special factors associated with each bacterial species. Only the more common agents are mentioned; for the unusual agents the reader will have to consult individual case reports since a quotation of that literature would go beyond the framework of this review.

Three bacteria, however, deserve special mention. Coagulase-negative staphylococci have only recently been reported in metastatic endophthalmitis, in contrast to postoperative endophthalmitis where they have always been the most frequently observed agents (7,17). Mycobacterium tuberculosis has also been observed as an agent of metastatic endophthalmitis (8,15); in one recent series, one of 109 patients with miliary tuberculosis showed choroidal tubercles (13). Treponema pallidum causes a systemic disease in the later stages; thus, one may question the appropriateness of the word "metastatic" for these cases involving the choroid, retina, and iris.

Since fungal endocarditis is not covered in either of the two reviews mentioned a few remarks are indicated. Candida albicans is now the most frequently reported agent of metastatic endophthalmitis. This is due to the increase in predisposing factors for C.albicans fungemia such as intravenous cannulation and hyperalimentation, intravenous drug abuse, diabetes, corticosteroid treatment, surgery, multiple antibiotic therapy, etc. The high incidence of metastatic endophthalmitis has been mentioned earlier but, unfortunately, none of the predisposing factors is predictive for its development, and neither is the number of positive blood cultures or of isolations from sources other than blood (3,14). Interestingly, while C.albicans causes fungemia in drug addicts much more rarely than the non-albicans species, it is the only species in this subpopulation that causes metastatic endophthalmitis (3,6,10,14). Usually, the intraocular lesions are located posteriorly and appear between 3 and 20 days after the onset of the septicemia and may cause no subjective symptoms at all (6,14). In drug addicts, the disease tends to be unilateral; bilaterality is seen in patients with other predisposing factors (6,14). In a large majority of patients, the organism can be isolated from other sites, notably cutaneous ones (6,14), although it should be stressed that only approximately 50% of the cases of disseminated candidiasis recognized post mortem are diagnosed intravitam (10). The source of the organism remains mostly unknown (6). Determinations of antibody titers are not helpful but progressive antigenemia may be detected over time (14). With appropriate treatment, the course is favorable although some visual defects are likely to remain.

Metastatic endophthalmitis with non-albicans Candida spp. has been reported a few times and was only observed in patients on hyperalimentation, multiple antibiotic treatment, and previous surgery (10).

Metastatic endophthalmitis due to Aspergillus may remain localized to the eye, as in drug abusers, or it may occur in the course of disseminated aspergillosis, e.g. in patients with endocarditis or in those with neutropenia or under immunosuppression (5). The former type carries a good, the latter a poor prognosis. Since cultures of the vitreous have been done rarely, the diagnosis had to rely on culture from other sites or on histological evidence, blood cultures being rarely positive in aspergillosis.

Diagnosis

The diagnosis of metastatic endophthalmitis may be made by examining ocular and/or systemic samples.

Most reliable are, of course, ocular samples obtained by anterior chamber taps in cases of anterior localization, and of the vitreous (taken either by aspiration or by vitrectomy) in cases of posterior localization. It should be emphasized that a microbiology technician or, better yet, a clinical microbiologist ought to be present when the sample is taken because of its unique value, the necessity for an immediate diagnosis (and, perhaps, intraocular therapy), and the danger of the specimen drying up in transport. An aspirate, not a swab, should be used, because too much of the sample may be lost in a swab. From the fluid (0.1-0.2ml of aqueous or 0.5-2.0ml of vitreous augmented by saline) the microbiologist should perform smears and cultures. Microscopic preparations done in the operating room are generally limited to Gram stains and potassium hydroxide preparations while acid-fast, PAS, or other fungal stains should be performed in the laboratory. Analysis of the leucocytic reaction, is, of course, important not only for the assessment of inflammatory changes but also because microorganisms tend to concentrate in areas with polymorphonuclear leucocytes. Needless to say: the area of the drop should be marked on the slide.

It may also be a good idea to obtain cultures from both conjunctivae since they may be of help in differentiating contaminants from true pathogens present in the ocular fluid (which are not found on the conjunctiva) (8,9). Media to be inoculated in the operating room include at least chocolate agar and brain heart infusion broth, but supplemented thioglycollate (anaerobes generally being found in exogenous endophthalmitis only), sheep blood agar, and Sabouraud dextrose agar are also recommended. The use of an alcohol lamp for sterilizing the needle or loop should be discussed with the anesthesiologist and the operating surgeon. The fluid should be distributed over the surface of the plate, but not on the edges, and broth should be inoculated with 1 or 2 drops. If the volume is too large, sterile filtration is recommended (9).

Recently, the technique of fine-needle retinal biopsy has been developed (11) for cases in which empiric therapy yields no improvement. In such instances it may be advisable to use media for the culture of mycobacteria as well.

Cultures of the suspected focus (urine, CSF) or of the blood are very helpful, although they lack the specificity of intraocular cultures. In 16 of the 72 cases (22%) reported between 1976 and 1985, identical bacterial species were identified in ocular and extraocular samples (8). Eye samples were positive in 29 of 44 (66%), blood in 42 of 59 (71%), and blood or nonocular fluids in 52 of 65 (80%) (8) ($p>0.05$ for all comparisons).- The role of Candida serology has been mentioned before.

Antibiotic Treatment and Prevention

The basis for antibiotic treatment of ocular infections has recently been summarized by Barza (2). Elimination routes (anterior/posterior) are also discussed by this author. Briefly, the barriers to the penetration of antimicrobials are:

a) the retinal capillaries, which are non-fenestrated. As a consequence, non-lipid-soluble drugs pass poorly into the vitreous in the normal as well as in the inflamed state;

b) the retinal pigment epithelium with its tight intercellular junctions, which inhibit the passage of periocularly injected drugs into the vitreous;

c) the lens-iris apparatus which inhibits drug passage between anterior and posterior chamber;

d) the flow of aqueous humor from the posterior chamber to the anterior chamber which inhibits anterior-posterior drug flow.

For example, intravenous administration of ß-lactam antibiotics (2g of oxacillin, cephalothin, cefotaxime, cefamandole) results in vitreous levels of 0.3-2mg/l; 1.6mg/kg of intramuscular gentamicin yields levels of <0.2mg/l (2). Such levels (measured in the uninflamed eye) would be insufficient for an effective treatment of metastatic endophthalmitis.

Peak vitreal concentrations of 40-80mg/l gentamicin or 400mg/l cefazolin can be reached, however, by intravitreal injection in rabbit eyes of 200-400μg and 2000μg, respectively, if a 3-day dosage interval is maintained. For vancomycin, 1000-2000μg every 6 days led to 200-400mg/l peak levels(2).

Therefore, most ophthalmologists will today use intravitreal antibiotics (often a combination of vancomycin and amikacin; in Bacillus cereus infection, clindamycin) although it should be stressed no that controlled studies exist comparing the efficacy of intravenous with intravitreal antibiotics. Greenwald et al (8) believe that the outcome is equally good in anterior and focal (anterior or posterior) metastatic endophthalmitis with either mode of application, and that posterior diffuse metastatic endophthalmitis carries a poor prognosis for vision even when intravitreal antibiotics are given.

The benefit of periocular injection continues to be discussed (2,8) as does the benefit of corticosteroid therapy, which, however, is contraindicated in fungal metastatic endophthalmitis.

Greenwald et al have also reviewed the outcome of metastatic endophthalmitis in their 1976-1985 series. Forty-one percent of the affected eyes retained useful vision (finger counting or better), 30% became blind and 29% had to be enucleated (8).

The management of nocardial and fungal metastatic endophthalmitis is even more difficult. In metastatic nocardial endophthalmitis, antibiotic therapy with sulfonamides has had no influence on the poor visual prognosis; only one patient has been cured with intravenous trimethoprim-sulfamethoxazole (11). Metastatic fungal endophthalmitis has been treated with intravenous amphotericin B (at least 3mg/kg total dose) sometimes combined with 5-fluorocytosine, with oral ketoconazole alone, and with ketaconazole plus amphotericin B or 5-fluorocytosine (6,10).

In view of its extremely low incidence, I do not see how bacterial metastatic endophthalmitis can be prevented effectively. It is, however, well known that periodic ophthalmoscopy in patients with candidemia helps in pinpointing ocular lesions, which - as any case of metastatic endophthalmitis - call for immediate aspiration and treatment in order to achieve a favorable outcome (8). A 24-hour delay in the onset of treatment rendered imipenem, gentamycin, and ciprofloxacin unable to reduce bacterial counts in the rabbit eye (2).

References

1. Auerbach SB, Leach CT, Bateman BJ et al (1989) Meningococcal Endophthalmitis Without Concomitant Septicemia or Meningitis. Pediatr Infect Dis J 8:411-413
2. Barza M (1989) Antibacterial Agents in the Treatment of Ocular Infections. Infect Dis Clin North Am 3:533-551
3. Brooks RG (1989) Prospective Study of Candida Endophthalmitis in Hospitalized Patients with Candidemia. Arch Intern Med 149:2226-2228
4. Cheesbrough JS, Williams CL, Rustom R et al (1990) Metastatic Pneumococcal Endophthalmitis: Report of Two Cases and Review of Literature. J Infect 20:231-236
5. Demicco DD, Reichman RC, Violette EJ et al (1984) Disseminated Aspergillosis Presenting with Endophthalmitis: a Case Report and a Review of the Literature. Cancer 53:1995-2001
6. Dupont B, Drouhet E (1985) Cutaneous, Ocular, and Osteoarticular Candidiasis in Heroin Addicts: New Clinical and Therapeutic Aspects in 38 Patients. J Infect Dis 152:577-591
7. Fisch A, Salvanet A, Prazuck T et al (1991) Epidemiology of Infective Endophthalmitis in France. Lancet 338:1373-1376
8. Greenwald MJ, Wohl LG, Sell CH (1986) Metastatic Bacterial Endophthalmitis: A Contemporary Reappraisal. Surv Ophthalmol 31:81-101
9. Jones DB, Liesegang TJ, Robinson NM (1981) Cumitech 13, Laboratory Diagnosis of Ocular Infections. Washington II,JA (coordinating ed) Am Soc Microbiol, Washington DC, pp. 16-17
10. Joshi N, Hamory BH (1991) Endophthalmitis Caused by Non-Albicans Species of Candida. Rev Infect Dis 13:281-287
11. Knouse MC, Lorber B (1990) Early Diagnosis of Nocardia Asteroides Endophthalmitis by Retinal Biopsy: Case Report and Review. Rev Infect Dis 12:393-398

Table 1: Bacterial Agents of Metastatic Endophalmitis

Organism	Ref.	Numbers of cases 1973-75	1976-85	Localization a)	Prognosis re. vision	Predisposing Factors	Foci
Gram-Positve:							
Streptococcus pneumoniae	4,8,15	14	2	P/A,B/U	mixed	asplenia, M.Hodgkin	meninges, lung
Other streptococci	8,15	9	10	P/A	mixed	newborn age (grp. B), malignancies (other groups)	meninges, skin
Staphylococcus epidermidis	7,17	0	0	b)	b)	b)	b)
Staphylococcus aureus	8,15	11	7	P	mixed	diabetes, renal failure	skin
Bacillus cereus	8,15	1	11	P,U	poor	i.v. drugs	skin
Listeria monocytogenes	8	1	3	A	good	may be none	b)
Nocardia asteroides	8,11	6	3	P	poor	immunosuppression	lung
Gram-Negative:							
Neisseria mening-	1,8,15	56	8	A,B	good	may be none	meninges
Haemophilus influenzae	8	-	7	A,U	good	may be none (<3 yrs.)	meninges
Actinobacillus actinomycetemcomitans	8	-	2	P	good	valvular defect	endocardium
Enterobacteriaceae	8,12,15	7	16	P, U/B	poor	diabetes	urinary, intestinal tract
Pseudomonas aeruginosa	8,15	2	2	P/A	mixed	divers	divers

a) A, anterior; B, bilateral; P, posterior; U, unilateral
b) data not available

12. Liu YC, Cheng DL, Lin CL (1986) Klebsiella Pneumoniae Liver Abscess Associated with Septic Endophthalmitis. Arch Intern Med 146:1913-1916
13. Maartens G, Willcox PA, Benatar SR (1990) Miliary Tuberculosis: Rapid Diagnosis, Hematologic Abnormalities, and Outcome in 109 Treated Adults. Am J Med 89:291-296
14. Parke II DW, Jones DB, Gentry LO (1982) Endogenous Endophthalmitis Among Patients with Candidemia. Ophthalmology
15. Shammas HF (1977) Endogenous E.coli Endophthalmitis. Surv Ophthalmol 21:429-435
16. Shamsuddin D, Tuazon CU, Levy C et al (1982) Bacillus Cereus Panophthalmitis: Source of the Organism. Rev Infect Dis 4:97-103
17. Shrader SK, Band JD, Lauter CB (1990) The Clinical Spectrum of Endophthalmitis: Incidence, Predisposing Factors and Features Influencing Outcome. J Infect Dis 162:115-120
18. Wyler DJ, Glickman MG, Brewin A (1975) Persistent Serratia Bacteremia Associated with Drug Abuse. West J Med 122:70-73

Candida Endophthalmitis: Late Septic-Metastatic Complication of a Systemic Infection

Karl-Heinz Emmerich and W.Fegeler

Abstract. Septic metastatic Candida endophthalmitis is a late complication of Candida septicemia. With the appearance of the first signs and symptoms of a suspected Candida endophthalmitis, a combined diagnostic and therapeutic approach involving ophthalmologists, internists and bacteriologists is mandatory. This cooperative approach is elucidated.

Introduction

Mycotic diseasies that may affect man have been classified by Vanbreuseghen into four different entities:

- Acute intoxication by fungi, e.g. has been named mycetism.
- Mycotoxicosis is defined as clinical manifestations provoked by certain metabolites of toxic fungi, examples being Aflatoxin produced by moulds that may result in liver cancer or ergotaminic substances produced by Claviceps that had been of particular importance in the Middle Ages.
- Mycoallergic reactions are diseases ascribed to allergy and to sequelae of the presence of transient growth of fungi, which have been suggested in the pathogenesis of nail mycosis.
- Mycoses are the clinical manifestations of the disease caused by fungi in living tissues.

From the standpoint of biology, fungi are undifferentiated primitive plants with a habitat of soil and air. They are saprophytic on non-viable organic substances as well as parasitic in live tissues.

Fungi may be described according to Rieth and be classified as

- dermatophytes (e.g. Trichophyton and Microsporium),
- yeasts (e.g. Candida, Torulopsis and Cryptococcus) and
- moulds (e.g. Aspergillus and Penicillium).

Fungal Infections in Ophthalmology

In ophthalmology, exogenous as well as endogenous mycoses are clinically important.

Exogenous infections may occur in an otherwise healthy organ, e.g. due to a traumatic corneal lesion. Around the eye brows, blastomycosis or sporotrichosis caused by dermatophytes may be seen. Conjunctivitis may be caused by yeasts in predisposed persons. Mycotic corneal ulcers may be caused by infections with moulds or yeasts, e.g. Fusarium, Aspergillus, Cephalosporium and Candida.

Endogenous infections of the eye or its adnexae may be observed during fungal septicemia or asymptomatic fungemia with an otherwise visibly preserved integrity of tissues. Thus, aspergillomas of the orbit may occur during a pulmonary aspergillosis. Fungal endophthalmitis, therefore, is a classical organ manifestation of fungal septicemia or asymptomatic fungemia.

Over the last decades, the frequency of fungal diseases of the eye has increased a lot. This is thought to be due to the introduction of antibiotics and corticosteroids into medical treatment regimens. The elimination of bacteria by antibiotics may leave saprophytic fungi without competitive partners for nutrients. Fungal infections occur more frequently and extensively when the cellular immune system has been suppressed with the application of corticosteroids or cytotoxic agents. Decisive advances in intensive care, oncology and antimicrobial chemotherapy have resulted in an enlarging patient population at risk for these infections.

Diagnosis of Fungal Endophthalmitis

Candida albicans has been recognized to be the most frequent pathogen of fungal endophthalmitis. Aspergillus fumigatus, Fusarium or Cryptococcus neoformans are less frequently associated with endophthalmitis. Due to the rise in frequency of patients seroconverted for the Human Immunodeficiency Virus, cryptococcal infections will probably be observed more often in the next couple of years. Single case reports have been published on fungal endophthalmitis due to infections with Coccidioides immitis, Blastomyces dermatitidis and Sporothrix schenckii.

Immunocompromised patients treated for

- gastro-intestinal diseases,
- tumors,
- immunodeficiency diseases or
- bacterial infections and
- long-term i.v. catheterized patients in intensive care units are at high risk for fungal infections. One or more of these factors can always be found in the history of patients suffering from fungal endophthalmitis. The threat of fungal endophthalmitis rises as more risk factors can be substantiated.

Treatment

In ophthalmology, septic-metastatic Candida endophthalmitis represents the most feared complication of a septicemia or an asymptomatic fungemia with yeasts in patients at risk (3,7,8,10,12,15). Since penetration of antimycotics into the vitreous may not be sufficient to achieve therapeutic levels in many cases, systemic antimycotic regimens alone may render treatment unsuccessful (5,6). Pars plana vitrectomy accompanied by intravitreal application of Amphotericin B resulted in a reportedly better outcome (1,2,11,13,15,18).

The beneficial effects of intravitreal instillation of Amphotericin B has been controversially discussed as this substance at higher concentrations may damage the retina in addition to the preexistent inflammatory changes (16). Therefore, studies have been published reporting on pars plana vitrectomy without the use of intravitreal antimycotics avoiding the known local toxicity (9).

Clinical Features and Practical Approach

Patients at risk for a Candida endophthalmitis may complain of a progressive slow reduction of visual acuity and sometimes the appearance of a red eye. Biomicroscopically, a moderate iridocyclitis is accompanied by vitreous clouding, snow balls and focal or multifocal whitish lesions localized intraretinal or at the borderline of the inner retina and posterior vitreous layers (preretinal).

In patients with a suspected Candida endophthalmitis mycologic evaluations should be initiated and an internist's diagnosis should be sought (14). Mycologic basic tests should include Candida hemagglutination titers and Candida immunofluorescent tests. Oral and anal smears as well as urine samples should be obtained and evaluated for growth of Candida albicans or other pathogens in order to support positive serologic findings. A differential should be done and ultrasonography of the abdomen and chest X-rays are demanding. Renal functions should also be controlled, if antimycotic treatment with Flucytosin and Amphotericin B is instituted. Up to now, the therapy of choice for Candida endophthalmitis consists of a combination of Amphotericin B at 0.3mg/kg/day and Flucytosin at 150mg/kg/day for at least 14 days. During treatment, at least weekly clinical laboratory and mycologic-serologic parameters must be monitored to control for side-effects and ensure therapeutic success (4). The goals of treatment should be an elimination of viable organisms from the eye and prevention of relapsing fungemia.

Depending on the clinical condition, a pars plana vitrectomy may be considered either with a worsening of the ophthalmoscopic appaearance or after successful systemic treatment with a reduction in antibody titers. If lesions have completely healed during systemic antimycotic treatment, a pars plana vitrectomy may not be indicated. In some cases, retinal lesions in eyes with clear optical media may be coagulated by Argon laser.

The cessation of antimycotic treatment or the change of therapy involving oral antimycotics only can only be decided along the lines of ophthalmologic evaluations supported by mycologic and internist data.

References

1. Barrie T (1987) The Place of Elective Vitrectomy in the Management of Patients with Candida Endophthalmitis. Graefe's Arch Clin Exp Ophthalmol 225:107-113

2. Cantrill HL, Rodman WP, Ramsay RC et al (1980) Postpartum Candida Endophthalmitis. J Am Med Ass 243:1163
3. Griffin JR, Pettit TH, Fishman LS et al (1973) Bloodborne Candida Endophthalmitis. Arch Ophthalmol 89:450
4. Heidemann HT (1987) Verminderung der Nephrotoxozität von Amphotericin B durch NaCl-Beladung. Pilzdialog 2:23-24
5. Hinzpeter EN, Eisert S, Naumann GOH et al (1976) Zur Klinik der metastatischen mykotischen Endophthalmitis. Klin Mbl Augenheilk 168:303
6. Hoffmann DH (1965) Pilzinfektionen des Auges. Systematik, Klinik, Erkennung und Behandlung. In: Streiff EB (ed), Fortschr Augenheilk, Karger, Basel-New York
7. Jeker J, Leuenberger AE (1980) Zum klinischen Bild und zur Therapie der metastatischen Candida-Endophthalmitis. Klin Mbl Augenheilk 176:153
8. Jones BR (1975) Principles in the Management of Oculomycosis. Am J Ophthalmol 79:719
9. Kroll P, Emmerich KH, Fegeler W (1976) Candida albicans-Endopthalmitis: Ergebnisse der Pars plana-Vitrektomie ohne intraokulare antimykotische Therapie. Klin Mbl Augenheilk 168:137
10. Martenet AC, Wildberger H (1976) Die Soorendophthalmitis und ihre Behandlung. Klin Mbl Augenheilk 168:137
11. McCuen BW, Pakalnis A (1981) Endophthalmitis Management. In: Duke-Elder (ed) Advanced Vitreous Surgery Course, Durham, NC 10.Oct.
12. Michelson JB, Freedman SD, Boyden DG (1982) Aspergillus Endophthalmitis in a Drug Abuser. Ann Ophthalmol 14:1051
13. Peyman GA, Vastine DW, Diamond JG (1975) Vitrectomy in Exogenous Candida Endophthalmitis. Graefe's Arch Ophthalmol 197:55
14. Schmidt H, Fischedick AR, Peters PE et al (1986) Candida-Abzesse in Leber und Milz. Dtsch Med Wchschr 111:816-820
15. Snip RC, Michels RG (1976) Pars Plana Vitrectomy in the Management of Endogenous Candida Endophthalmitis. Am J Ophthalmol 82:699
16. Souri EN, Green WR (1974) Intravitreal Amphotericin B Toxicity. Am J Ophthalmol 78:89-92
17. Stern GA, Fetkenhour CL, O'Grady RB (1977) Intravitreal Amphotericin B Treatment of Candida Endophthalmitis. Arch Ophthalmol 95:89-92
18. Tavakolian U, Paulmann H, Heimann K et al (1981) Die pars plana-Vitrektomie in der Behandlung der bakteriellen und mykotischen Endophthalmitis. Ber. DOG. 253-257

V. SELECTED INTRAOCULAR INFECTIONS

- Zoonosis: Survey

Zoonoses and Ocular Infections

Harald L.J. Knorr and Albert Weber

Abstract. Diseases naturally transmitted from animals to man are defined as zoonoses (syn. anthropozoonoses). More than 200 zoonoses caused by virus, bacteria, chlamydia, rickettsia, fungi and parasites have been recognized and described.
A short survey is given on the epidemiology of the agents of some zoonoses that may involve the eye: Brucellosis, leptospirosis, Lyme disease, Newcastle disease, psittacosis/ornithosis, rabies, S.suis infection, visceral larva migrans, toxoplasmosis and tularemia.

Introduction

In the year of 1855, the well-known pathologist Rudolf Virchow affixed the subtitle "zoonoses" to the chapter "Infektionen durch contagiöse Thiergifte" written by himself in the "Handbuch der speziellen Pathologie und Therapie". Eight years later the word "zoonoses" received a twofold definition in the "Ethymologisches Wörterbuch der Veterinärmedizin und ihrer Hilfswissenschaften" plublished by W.Probstmayer: "Firstly, zoonoses are initial animal diseases and secondly they are diseases of man transmitted to the latter by a contagium from the animal".

In the year of 1958, an Expert Committee of the World Health Organization has defined "diseases and infections, which are naturally transmitted between vertebrates and man as zoonoses". This definition is still valid today (8). However, many attempts have been made to define the word "zoonoses" further. In order to reveal the way of the contagious agent, the expressions "zooanthroponoses" and "anthropozoonoses" were suggested. Hereby all those diseases (greek: nosos) which are transmitted from animal (greek: zoon) to man (greek: anthropos) were to be assigned to the "zooanthroponoses" whereas those diseases, which are transmitted from man to animal were to be assigned to the "anthropozoonoses". Due to a misunderstanding in the translation of these expressions they were unfortunately adopted to the Anglo-American literature in the inverse sense (17). Thus, the expression "zoonoses" is used in the further explanations instead of "anthropozoonoses".

According to the World Health Organization, approximately 200 zoonoses are known, caused by a multitude of viruses, chlamydia, rickettsia, bacteria, fungi, protozoa, helminths or arthropodes (8).

In the following review, the epidemiology of some zoonoses, which may also involve the eye of man and are relevant to Europe, are briefly described.

Zoonoses caused by virus

Rabies

This is the most significant, although fortunately not the most frequent zoonoses. Still, it has not at all lost its horror as it is lethal for man if it is not treated in time (8). Rabies occurs world-wide. Merely the Australian continent and countries with insular position (in Europe: Greece, Great Britain, Northern Ireland and Iceland) or with other favorable geographical conditions (in Europe: Norway and Sweden) presently lack cases of rabies. Northern America and most European countries have to deal with the so-called silvatic rabies. The most important reservoirs for the rabies virus are represented by skunks in the USA, and by the red fox in Europe (8).

In 1990, 21044 animal cases of rabies were diagnosed in Europe; 12833 (61%) were foxes, 2014 (9.6%) were cattle, 1282 (6.1%) were dogs, 1182 (5.6%) were cats, 864 (4.1%) were sheep or goats, 430 (2%) were roe deer and 278 (1.3%) were badgers among others. Furthermore, it is of epidemiological significance that in Europe the occurrence of rabies in bats, particularly in the species Epitesicus serotinus has been increasingly observed for the last couple of years (11).

Proceeding from the prevailing natural focus (fox), other game (predominantly roe deer and mustelides), domestic animals (predominantly cattle, sheep, goats, dogs and cats) and occasionally, man becomes infected directly by infected and/or diseased domestic animals (predominantly dogs and cats), whereas, according to existing knowledge, rodents (mice, rats) hardly play a role in the epidemiology of rabies (8).

According to the WHO, 108 cases of human rabies were officially registered between 1977 and 1990 in 14 European countries. In reality, however, figures are estimated to be much higher, because in Turkey there are said to be 30-60 cases annually and because reports from the GUS are still not reliable (11). In approximately 16% of the cases of human rabies noted in Europe, the subjects were infected during a stay in a non-European country - mostly in India, Pakistan and Africa. In Germany, a total of three persons with rabies was registered between 1980 and 1990, one of which could be linked to a dog attack in India (11).

The transmission of the rabies virus normally results from the bite of an infected animal of which the saliva contains virulent organisms (8). In this context, dogs play the most important role as vector in Europe, followed by cats, fox, cattle and bats. For the ophthalmologist it is probably of great significance that in one case in the USA and in two cases each in France and Thailand rabies was transmitted between humans by corneal transplantation (14).

Lymphocytic Choriomeningitis

The natural pathogen reservoir for the Lymphocytic Choriomeningitis Virus is the house mouse. Here the transmission of the virus occurs vertically. Mice, which have been infected intrauterine or directly after the birth are immunologically tolerant, e.g. hey do not produce any antibodies against the pathogen, but maintain a carrier and excretor status throughout their life (8). The elimination of the virus occurs through nasal mucus, saliva, urine or feces. Infections of other animals (mostly the golden hamster) and man is possible by contamination as well as by air-borne transmission (dust) (8).

In contrast to the mouse, the golden hamster is carrier and excretor of the Lymphocytic Choriomeningitis Virus for only 4-6 weeks. For this reason, man is only at risk of becoming infected by these animals within a short time period (8). Possibly, only those golden hamsters, which have recently been purchased in a pet shop or from a breeder where they had been infected via the feces of infected mice or other golden hamsters, may be infectious for man. Golden hamsters that have been in a family for more than three months will hardly be in quest for a source of infection. Latent infections with the Lymphocytic Choriomeningitis Virus have also been found in dogs, monkeys and guinea pigs. According to common knowledge these animals are of no significance for infections to man (8).

In connection with Lymphocytic Choriomeningitis Virus, prenatal infections occur and may cause internal hydrocephalus, uveitis and chorioretinitis in newborn (5).

Newcastle Disease

This virus disease, also known as atypical fowl plague occurs worldwide, mostly on fowl. Wild birds and waterbirds as well as parrots from Asia, Africa and Southern America must be reckoned with as an additional reservoir of virus. It is of further epidemiological significance that the pathogenic agent persists for weeks while the birds do not exhibit any clinically overt manifestations of the disease (8).

The human infection is acquired by air-borne transmission or by contamination and direct contact with the infected fowl, particularly chicken. In most cases, the infection leads to a unilateral follicular conjunctivitis, which may also be hemorrhagic (Fig.1,2). Occasionally, both eyes may become involved. Swelling of the preauricular lymph nodes and pain often go along with conjunctivitis. In general, this clinical manifestation persists for 3-4 days and is self-limited without any sequelae (8).

It is of epidemiological significance that veterinarians and poultry farmers can also be infected by the vaccine strain of Newcastle Disease virus which is apathogenic for the fowl, but has retained its pathogenicity for man. Infection is possible after disintegration of the lyophilized inoculum or by use of spray-vaccines (8).

Zoonoses caused by chlamydia

Psittacosis in man due to Chlamydia (C.).psittaci is caused by contact with psittacides, whereas the expression "ornithosis" is used for diseases transmitted from other bird species also caused by C. psittaci. The expression "ornithosis" is also used as a synonym for avian chlamydial diseases (8).

C.psittaci infections occur world-wide. The epidemiological relevance of C.psittaci infections of man, which have been proven in 130 birds for psittacosis (or ornithosis) has been known for a long time. Under present conditions, parrots and parakeets are the greatest sources of danger for man (8). Strains of C.psittaci can also cause infections in various species of vertebrates - so far, more than 22 are known. Therefore, it is not surprising that dogs and particularly cats are increasingly found to be responsible for C.psittaci infections in man. This is a fact which still draws too little attention not only in human medicine but also in veterinary medicine (19). The transmission of C.psittaci to man occurs primarily by inhalation of contaminated dust, further by direct contact with ocular and nasal secretions of infected animals. Acute follicular kerato conjunctivitis caused by C.psittaci (Fig. 3,4,5,) has been observed in man (19) after direct contamination with infected cats.

Zoonoses caused by bacteria

Brucellosis

The occurrence of this bacterial zoonosis of man is closely linked with the occurrence and distribution of brucellosis in animals, particularly in cattle, sheep, goat and pig (8). In Europe, brucellosis in animals is still frequent and most prevalent in Western European and Mediterranean countries like France, Portugal, Spain, Malta, Greece, and Turkey. Due to successful infection control, brucellosis in farm animals has been completely eradicated in Germany (8). In Africa, Asia, Latin America, particularly in Brazil and Mexico, some countries remain where brucellosis occurs frequently in farm animals (13). In countries harboring animal brucellosis, not only veterinarians, farmers, animal attendants, milkers, shepherds, abattoir staff and knackers, but also tourists are in danger to acquire this infectious disease (8).

Infection of man is caused either by direct contact with secretions of infected cattle, sheep, goats, pigs or dogs, by conjunctival or by minute skin lesions (8). Infections are possible by consumption of raw milk and its products like sheep and goat cheese. Brucella sp. is able to remain infectious for up to half a year. Pathogens may be transmitted by air, e.g. by infectious aerosoles, which occur in abattoirs (20).

Corresponding to the manifold general clinical manifestations, Brucella infections can be observed in all parts of the eye and its adnexa. In man, various ophthalmological findings have been reported including non-specific catarrhal conjunctivitis and tenonitis, motility pain, phlyctenular keratoconjunctivitis, dacryoadenitis, scleritis, nummular keratitis, corneal ulcers, iridocyclitis, retinitis, papillitis, and optic nerve atrophy (20).

Leptospirosis

Mainly rodents, particularly rats, mice and farm animals (pigs, cattle and domestic animals) are notable world-wide as carriers and excretors of leptospires (different serovars of Leptospira interrogans). Infections with leptospires can also be found world-wide in numerous game, particularly wild boars, foxes, hares and hedgehogs (latent infection). Infected animals often shed great amounts of leptospires in the urine (8).

Infection of man occurs primarily via minute skin lesions inflicted during professional work, bathing or walking on barefoot. Apart from this mode of transmission, cases have been reported after bites of mice, rats or hamsters. In these case reports, urine secreted by the animals at the same time had probably been the actual source of infection (8). Leptospires can also invade via compromised mucous membranes of mouth, nose or eyes, e.g. after a plunge into a canal or sewage water, or while diving or swimming in ditch water (3).

Nowadays, a change in the epidemiology of human leptospirosis can be noticed. Previously, miners or canal workers who had to deal with sewage water in any form most frequently fell ill on this disease (8). Due to improved working and hygienic conditions as well as adequate precautionary measures (protective clothes) the risk of infection could be drastically reduced for these persons.

Apart from rural workers (farmers, crop workers), abattoir workers, butchers and veterinarians, who belong to the classical high-risk groups even today, swimmers and kajakers, acquiring smaller or larger skin lesions in lakes, ponds or slow-moving rivers while practising their hobbies, are increasingly frequent at risk (3).

With all leptospiral infections a largely similar clinical picture develops, which is characterized by a biphasic course of illness (8). For the ophthalmologist it is important that in the first phase beginning abruptly with a high fever (39°C and above), shivering fit, violent muscle pain and headaches, conjunctivitis, episcleritis and photophobia are always observed (13). After a short interval of 5-7 days without fever, the second phase of organ manifestations follows. Infections with L.icterohaemorrhagiae (Morbus Weill) are characterized by icteric discoloration of the sclera. After one or two months, sometimes only after 6 months to one year, iridocyclitis and uveitis being the most important and most frequent late manifestations of leptospirosis may appear. Severe complications have hardly ever been reported due to the frequently bilateral iridocyclitis. Nevertheless, uveitis is usually very persistent and may often relapse (13). Furthermore, chorioretinitis with retinal exudates, retinal detachments and papillitis are not rare (13).

Lyme Borreliosis

Only recently, Lyme borreliosis, a previously little-known infectious disease caused by the spirochete Borrelia (B.) burgdorferi has been increasingly observed in humans and animals in Europe. The number of persons latently infected with B.burgdorferi is estimated at 30000 to 60000 per year (4). In Europe, the tick species Ixodes ricinus and in the USA, the tick species Ixodes dammini and Ixodes pacificus play the greatest roles as reservoirs and vectors of Lyme borreliosis. Epidemiological investigations recently performed in West Germany have demonstrated infected ticks in up to 20% in the area of Munich, up to 23% in Berlin (West) and up to 30% in the vicinity of Freiburg. In Austria and Switzerland similar rates of 34% to 40% were found (6). Further investigations revealed that not only game, but also domestic animals like horses, cattle, sheep and dogs are frequently latent carriers of B.burgdorferi (4). For this reason, ticks can acquire the infection from B.burgdorferi infected animals, the latter therefore forming a source of infection not only for the ticks, but indirectly for man, too.

Transmission of the pathogenic agent of Lyme borreliosis is not only possible by ticks but also by Stomoxyinae like Stomoxys calcitrans (4).

Human Lyme borreliosis shows a variety of clinical manifestations. Inflammatory lesions can be verified in all parts of the eye, such as conjunctivitis, keratitis, iridocyclitis, choroiditis, retinal pigment epithelitis, optic neuropathy, panophthalmitis, ocular muscle paresis or arcuate neuroretinitis (15).

Streptococcus suis infection

The occurrence of Streptococcus (S.) suis type 2 infections in man is closely linked with the occurrence of the pathogenic agent in pigs. According to current knowledge, these animals represent the main reservoir for S. suis type 2. This bacterial species has also been proven in wild boars (10). Pigs at the age of 4 - 12 weeks become ill with clinical symptoms of meningitis. Additionally, pigs which are clinically healthy can harbour S.suis type 2 for weeks and months in their tonsils (10).

Although the ways of transmission have still not been completely elucidated, the contamination of man seems to occur primarily by direct contact with infected pigs and pork via the conjunctiva or via minute skin lesions. Corresponding to the modes of infection, people processing pork and cooks are exposed to an increased risk of infection (10).

After an incubation period of several hours to two days, infections most frequently present with meningitis and impairment of the eighth cranial nerve including loss of hearing and balance. Numerous cases have reported uveitis, endophthalmitis or nystagmus with S.suis type 2 infections in man (10).

Tularemia

The occurrence of Tularemia in man corresponds with the geographical distribution of the zoonosis in animals. Up to now, the pathogen Franciscella (F.) tularensis has been proven in more than 125 different animal species (16). Particularly the hare (Lepus europaeus) is considered to be the main reservoir for the pathogenic agent.

European endemic areas are presently known in Sweden, Czechoslovakia, Hungary, Austria, Switzerland, and Germany (predominantly the Northern sea coast of Schleswig-Holstein and Mainfranken) (8). F.tularensis is transmitted by direct contact of secretions, blood, organs of infected animals, through minor or minute skin lesions or via the conjunctiva (8). Infections of man can also be caused by blood-sucking anthropodes and via airborne transmission by contaminated dust (16).

The human clinical manifestations are dependent on the entry of the pathogen. Four to 6% of all F.tularensis infections occur in an oculoglandular form, which is characterized by the Parinaud conjunctivitis, synonymous with conjunctivo-oculo-glandular syndrome (12).

Zoonoses caused by parasites

Toxocariasis

Toxocara (T.) canis, an ascarid worm of dogs is considered to be the most important pathogen of this zoonosis. In numerous reports it has been recorded that this nematode species may exist world-wide in dogs in varying frequency; isolation rates in dog feces can reach up to 80% (9). The environmental contamination by dog feces containing eggs of Toxocara is of particular epidemiologic significance. Three to 5% of the samples collected from streets and public places of six European metropolitan areas contain eggs of Toxocara (9). According to statistical evaluations of epidemiological studies on dogs in the USA, specific locations evidentially carry an increased risk of Toxocara infestations (2). The large infective potential for man can be derived from data on seroprevalence. Seroepidemiological investigations performed in Switzerland show antibodies against Toxocara in 2.3% of 1016 blood donors, while regional differences account for a range of zero to 8.9% (2). In Germany, a seroprevalence of 2.53% has been reported. Compared to the seroprevalence the number of clinically manifest human cases may obviously seem to be very small, but it may also be possible that many cases have simply been overlooked. In the USA, approximately 10000 new diseases of visceral Toxocariasis, and about 700 cases of ocular larva migrans are diagnosed yearly (2). According to surveys made among ophthalmologists in the state of Alabama (USA), at least one case of ocular larva migrans per 1000 patients is diagnosed (2).

Regarding ocular larva migrans, it is not only T.canis, but also nematodes of racoons, which are of importance (7). Similar diseases in man have been increasingly identified in the USA in the last years (7).

In Germany, Knorr and coworkers were the first to describe an infection due to Baylisascaris (B.) procyonis associated with the Diffuse Unilateral Subacute Neuroretinitis (DUSN) syndrome in a 48-year old woman, who kept a racoon at home. The DUSN syndrome is characterized by disseminated greyish-white retinal foci, intraocular inflammation, degeneration of pigment epithelium, optic atrophy and visual impairment (Fig.6-9).

The amount of embryonal eggs of T.canis of B.procyonis resp. determines the clinical manifestations in man. In many cases, toxocariasis lacks any clinical symptoms and is therefore not recognized (7,8). Ocular involvement is characterized by edema of the lids, chemosis, keratitis, granulomatous iridocyclitis, chorioretinitis and chronic endophthalmitis (13).

Toxoplasmosis

The domestic cat is the most important and in many regions the only final host for the world-wide distribution of Toxoplasma. Other felides like the wild cat (Felis silvestris), puma (F.concolor), ozelot (F.pardalis), lynx (Lynx rufus) and tiger (F.bengalis) can take over this function and shed infectious oocysts of T.gondii (1). In the cat populations of European countries the percentage of cats shedding oocysts of Toxoplasma gondii via the feces is estimated at 0.4 and 2.0%, and is rarely higher (2). Particularly young cats play an important role as excretors. The elimination of oocysts lasts for up to 20 days, and great amounts of about 100000 oocysts per gramm feces may be shed (1). After reinfection, diminished amounts of oocysts or none at all are shed with the feces of cats due to developing immunity (1).

Cats shedding oocysts may be seronegative or seropositive. Therefore, the results of serologic tests of cats do not permit any conclusions about whether or not the animal has been a shedder of oocysts at the time the test has been done and thus has been a risk of infection for man (1). The epidemiological role of the cat as a direct or indirect source of infection for man is undoubtable, although the percentage of man infected with oocysts of cat feces cannot be stated exactly (1).

With respect to food-borne infections, the consumption of raw pork products such as raw minced meat is of greatest epidemiological importance, because up to 97% of slaughtered pigs may be infected with cysts of T.gondii (18). Sheep may also be infected by T.gondii in up to 80%. As far as the population of Western Europe and Germany is concerned, the risk of an oral infection by eating sheep meat is almost negligible, because raw sheep meat is hardly ever being eaten in these countries. In addition, cysts of T.gondii have been certainly inactivated after deep-freeze storage (at least 11 days at -20°C) (18). The rate of cattle infected with T.gondii is between 6 and 21%. Only beef, which has not been done, and raw calf's liver are a possible source of infection for man (18).

Human toxoplasmosis may either be an acute, chronic or predominantly symptom-free latent infection (8). Congenital toxoplasmosis, which belongs to the most important protozoan infectious diseases of pregnancy, may cause internal hydrocephalus, retinochoroiditis and intracranial calcifications (1). Acquired toxoplasmosis (of adolescence or as an adult) may present with acute conjunctivitis and lid edema, retinochoroiditis, iridocyclitis and others (13).

Conclusions

Further pathogenic agents of zoonoses, which have not been mentioned, but may as well be important for an ophthalmologist in Europe are listed as Salmonella, Yersinia enterocolitica, Yersinia pseudotuberculosis, Listeria monocytogenes, Pasteurella multocida, Bacillus anthracis, Taenia solium and Trichinella spiralis (8,13).

This survey may have shown that occasionally, a causal relationship of zoonoses with ocular signs and symptoms may be detected by careful history-taking and inquiring for close contacts with animals.

With a more intense cooperation between human and veterinary physicians, it may be possible to identify some diseases as zoonoses and specific therapy may be instituted faster.

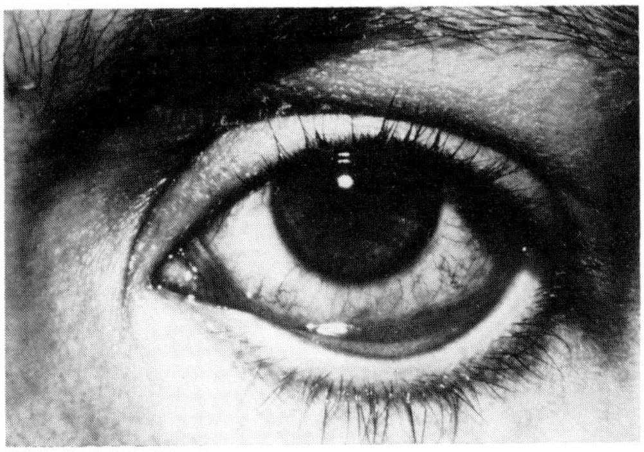

Fig.1. Serous follicular and hemorrhagic conjunctivitis by Newcastle Disease Virus

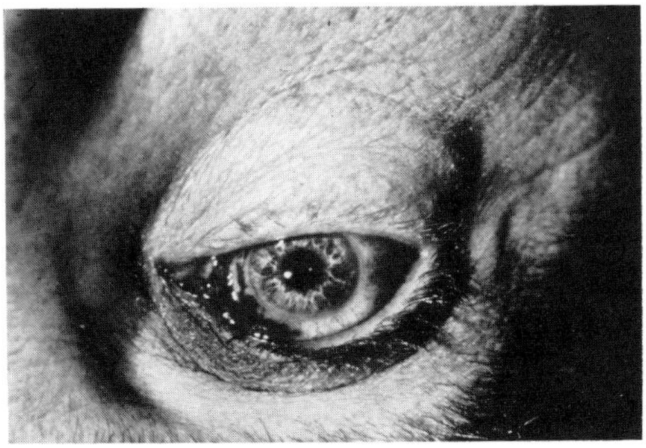

Fig.2. Hemorrhagic conjunctivitis by Newcastle Disease Virus

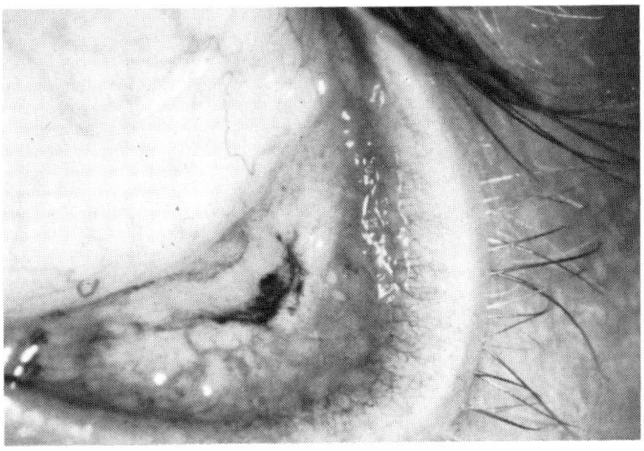

Fig.3. Acute follicular conjunctivitis by Chlamydia psittaci transmitted from domestic cat

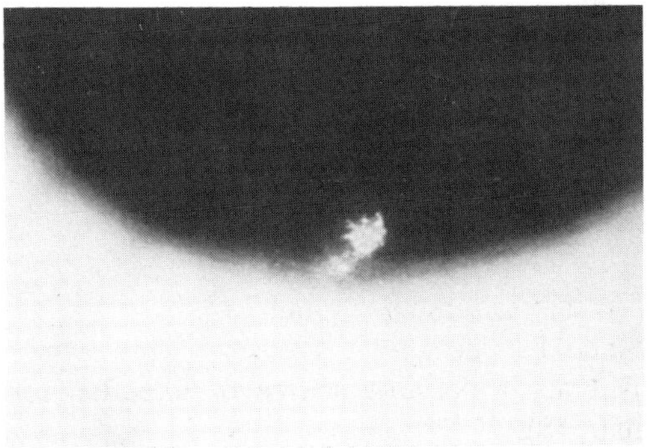

Fig.4. Superficial keratopathy with epithelial and subepithelial corneal infiltrates following an infection with Chlamydia psittaci

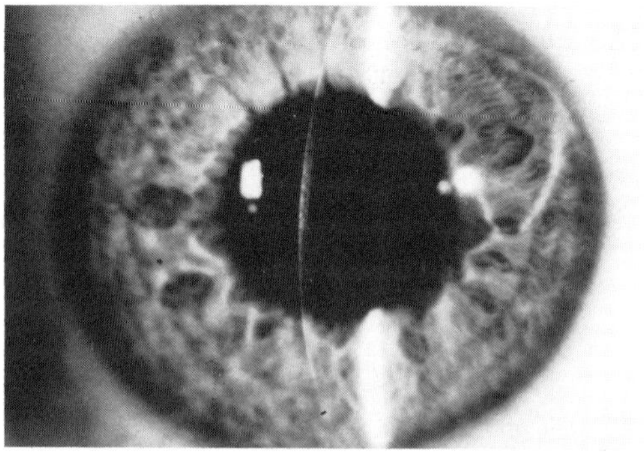

Fig 5. Slit lamp photograph showing the epithelial and subepithelial localisations of the corneal infiltrates, VA cc 0.6.

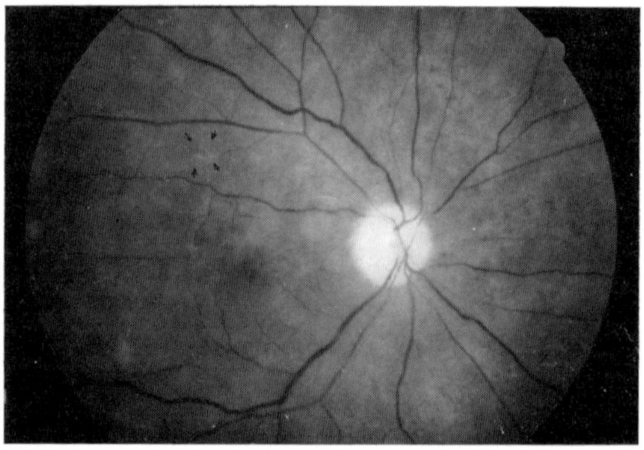

Fig. 6. Right eye showing unilateral disseminated intraretinal and subretinal, greyish-white lesions, and focal hypertrophy of the retinal pigment epithelium caused by the white shaped larvae of racoon roundworm, Baylisascaris procyonis (arrows).

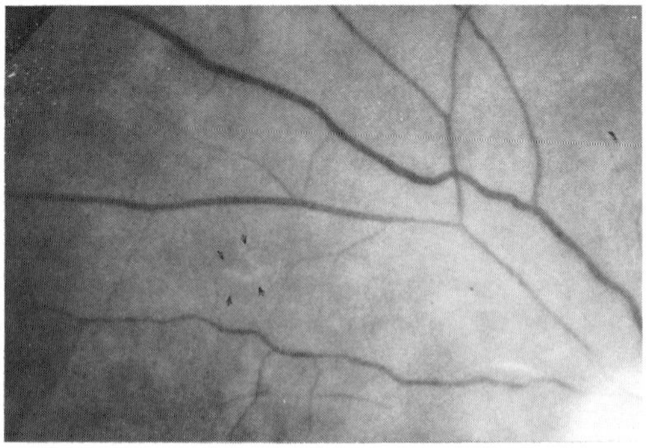

Fig.7. Higher magnification of the 1530μm larvae of the racoon roundworm, Baylisascaris procyonis (arrows)

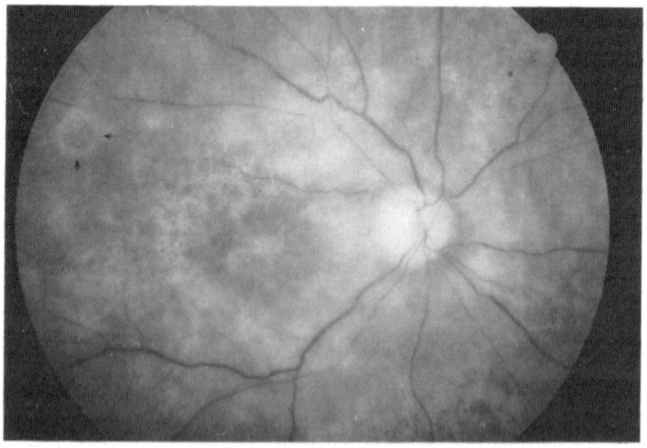

Fig. 8. Diffuse, unilateral, subacute neuroretinitis syndrome with atrophy of the retinal pigment epithelium and optic atrophy. Note the area of the larvae of the racoon roundworm after laser treatment (arrows).

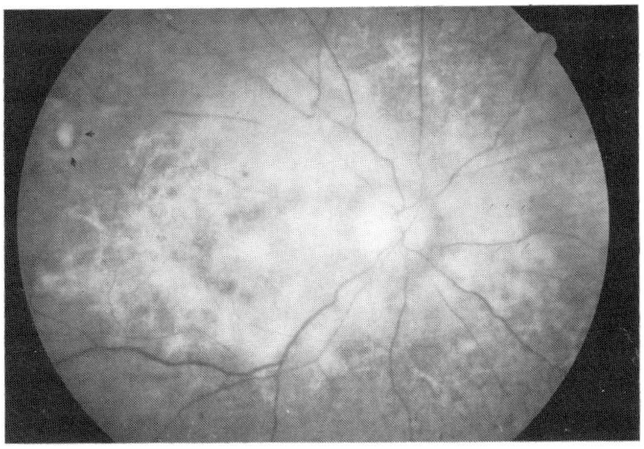

Fig. 9. Right fundus with progressive lesions and a serous detachment of the parapapillary retina one month after laser treatment.

References

1. Dubey JP (1986) Toxoplasmosis. JAVMA 189:165-169
2. Eckert J (1988) Zur Bedeutung von Hunden und Katzen in den Infektketten parasitärer Zoonosen in Europa. Wien Tierärztl Mschr 75:457-465
3. Ellis WA (1986) Leptospirosis. J Small Anim Pract 27:683-92
4. Herzer P (1989) Lyme Borreliose. Steinkopff, Darmstadt
5. Hochgesand P, Turss R, Ackermann R (1975) Goldhamster als Überträger einer pränatalen Chorioretinitis. Klin. Mbl. Augenheilk. 196:190-195
6. Käsbohrer A, Schönberg A (1990) Serologische Untersuchungen zum Vorkommen von Borrelia burgdorferi bei Haustieren in Berlin (West). Berl Münch Tierärztl Wchschr 103:374-378
7. Kazacos KR, Bayce WM (1989) Baylisascaris larva migrans. JAVMA 195:894-903
8. Krauss H, Weber A (1989) Zoonosen. Dtsch Ärzteverlag, Köln
9. Lamina J (1986) Ist die Toxocariasis auch bei uns eine bedeutsame Zoonose? Tierärztl Umschau 41:872-878
10. Lütticken R, Temme N, Hahn G et al (1986) Meningitis caused by Streptococcus suis: case report and review of the literature. Infection 14:181-185
11. Müller WW (1991) Review of reported rabies case data in Europe to the WHO Collaborating Centre Tübingen from 1977 to 1990. Rabies Bull 14(4):10-12
12. Ohara Y, Sato T, Fujita H et al (1991) Clinical manifestations of tularemia in Japan - Analysis of 1355 cases observed between 1924 - 1987. Infection 19:14-17
13. Sachsenweger M (1991) Taschenbuch der Augenheilkunde in den Tropen. Gustav Fischer Verlag. Stuttgart, New York
14. Schneider LG, Jackson C, Hohnsbeen KP (1981) Rabies transmission via corneal transplant. Rabies Bull.5(4):13
15. Schönherr U, Lang GE, Meythaler FH (1991) Bilaterale Lebersche Neuroretinitis stellata bei Borrelia burgdorferi Serokonversion. Klin Mbl Augenheilk 198:44-47
16. Selbitz HJ (1988) Die Tularämie - eine Zoonose mit Naturherdcharakter. Mh Vet Med 43:239-240
17. Stoll L (1969) Der Mensch als Infektionsquelle für Tiere. Blaue Hefte 41:24-31
18. Weber A (1988) Lebensmittelinfektionen und -intoxikationen durch Zoonosen. VET 3(7/8):32-39
19. Werth D (1989) Vorkommen und Bedeutung von Chlamydia psittaci und Coxiella burnetii bei Hund und Katze. Eine Literaturstudie. Berl Münch Tierärztl Wchschr 102:156-161
20. Young EJ (1983) Human Brucellosis. Rev Inf Dis 5:821-842

- Bacterial: Lyme Borreliosis

Serological Survey for Lyme Borreliosis in Ophthalmologic Patients

Andreas E. A. Hofmann, Thomas A. Berninger, Vera Preac-Mursic and Bettina Wilske

Abstract. In 4.6% of 517 patients evaluated for B.burgdorferi antibodies from 1988 until 03/91 significantly elevated IgG titers were found in comparison with a healthy control population (cut off 98-99%). IgM antibodies were not demonstrated.

There is no predilection of specific age groups or diagnoses in seroreactive patients in this study. As well, no characteristic clinicial criteria for the diagnosis of ocular Lyme borreliosis have been found. In four patients, the ocular disorder could be explained by other causes than borrelial infection. In two patients with iritis, suspicion of ocular Lyme borreliosis could be confirmed on the basis of cultural proof or erythema migrans in the history respectively; in one more patient (13 yrs.) suffering from VI nerve palsy and papilledema seroconversion to a titer of 1:64 leaded to the diagnosis of Lyme borreliosis. In the other patients Lyme borreliosis could not be substantiated further despite markedly elevated IgG antibody titers (up to 1:2048) since no other indications were present to support this diagnosis. Diagnostic criteria are suggested which may differentiate a highly suspicious from a presumed diagnosis of ocular Lyme borreliosis. To allow a clinical definition of ocular Lyme borreliosis application of stringent criteria seems to be mandatory.

Introduction

Lyme borreliosis is the most frequent tick-borne infectious disease in men in Europe and the USA and caused by the spirochete B.burgdorferi. Apart from the classical manifestations of Erythema migrans, meningo-polyradiculitis Bannwarth, acrodermatitis chronica atrophicans and Lyme arthritis, less frequently manifestations in other organs including the eye have been reported. In addition to the panophthalmitis caused by Borrelia observed by Steere and coworkers in 1985 (11), affections involving all segments of the eye including the optic nerve have been described (1-3,5,6,8,9,10,12,15,16).

As unequivocal clinical criteria for the diagnosis of ocular Lyme borreliosis have not yet been defined, diagnosis mostly is based only on serological findings. Characteristic history or evidence by culture cannot be obtained in most cases.

The aim of the present study was to evaluate the clinical findings of the ophthalmologic patients found to be seroreactive during the investigation period.

Patients and Methods

517 patients seen at the University Eye Hospital of Munich between 1988 and March 1991 have been tested for antibodies against B.burgdorferi. Antibody titers have been determined by indirect immunofluorescent tests after prior absorption with T.phagedenis. Antibody titers ≥ 1:64 were considered significantly elevated corresponding with a 98%-99% percentile of a healthy control population (13,14); i.e. among 100 healthy persons one or two will exhibit a titer of ≥ 1:64. Titers of ≥ 1:256 could not be found in the control population.

For seroreactive patients follow-up examinations were performed, either in the eye hospital or by the ophthalmologist. Included were detailed interviews, clinical examination and determination of antibodies against B.burgdorferi in parallel assay with previous sera.

One female patient with iritis was included in the study although no evidence had been shown for antibodies against B.burgdorferi. B.burgdorferi, however, had been cultured from a skin biopsy during a previously experienced erythema migrans.

Results

Twenty-four out of 517 examined patients showed significantly elevated IgG antibody titers; in 11 of these patients titers had been elevated two or more steps above the cut-off point (≥ 1:256, Tab.1). IgM antibodies could not be demonstrated. The age distribution of seroreactive patients is given in Fig.1.

IgG antibodies against T.gondii were found in 6 patients; however, there was no serologic evidence for an active infection. Neither was any clinical indication for a possible ocular toxoplasmosis to be found, except in patient 1.

In one other patient antibodies to Yersinia could be demonstrated; neither was there any serologic evidence for an active Yersinia infection.

None of the examined patients was seroreactive for syphilis (Treponema pallidum hemagglutination assay).

The ophthalmological diagnoses of 24 seroreactive patients are given in Table 2; antibody titers correlated with diagnostic groups are given in Fig.2.

16 patients were seen at the follow-up; Table 3 shows the clinical course in the respective diagnostic groups. At the time of the ocular disease none of the patients received specific therapy except for patients 1 and 4. Thus, in 7 patients amelioration of the clinical condition took place without therapy. At the time of the follow-up elevated antibody titers against B.burgdorferi could be confirmed in all patients; only in two patients we could demonstrate a significant change of titers (two or more titer steps) in parallel assay.

Case Reports of Selected Patients

Patient 1 (female, 59 yrs.) experienced an erythema migrans in April 1989 after a tick bite; at that time Doxycyclin was given (2x100mg/d for 10 days). In August 1989, severe iridocyclitis was diagnosed persisting for more than 4 weeks despite enforced medication with corticosteroids and Ceftriaxon; in this patient, the immunofluorescent antibody test for B.burgdorferi was non-reactive.

Patient 2 (male, 13 yrs.) had a papilledema and VI nerve palsy in November 1986; at this time serology was non-reactive for B.burgdorferi; however, in February 1987 seroconversion (IgG 1:64) could be demonstrated. In the cerebrospinal fluid, no specific antibody could be determined. Further data on this patient could not be obtained.

Patient 3 (male, 72 yrs.) experienced an erythema migrans in June 1990. He was treated with Doxycyclin (2x100mg/d for 20 days) and Isocillin (3x1200000 IU for another 20 days). In February 1991 an iritis was noted responsive to treatment with corticosteroids. The B.burgdorferi IgG antibody titer was 1:128.

Patient 4 (female, 47 yrs.) was diagnosed to have a recurrent chorioretinitis due to ocular toxoplasmosis. In 1987, Pyrimethamin and Sulfamethoxazole were administered. When another recurrence was noted in 1988, serology for B.burgdorferi showed an IgG titer of 1:256. Therefore treatment with Ceftriaxone (total dose of 21g over 14 days) followed. In February 1991, another relapse of chorioretinitis occurred; antibody titer control revealed a significant decrease of anti-Borrelia IgG to 1:64. Toxoplasma IgG antibody titer was constant 1:128, toxoplasma complement binding reaction <1:5.

Patient 5 (male, 51 yrs.) had a iuxtapapillar chorioretinitis in November 1989; antibody titers to B.burgdorferi were extremely elevated (1:2048). In June 1988, multiple oval-shaped erythematous skin lesions had occurred and been diagnosed clinically and histologically as Brocq's disease. No treatment was instituted and relapses did not occur. Toxoplasmosis IgG antibody titers were constantly at 1:1024, Toxoplasma complement binding reaction at <1:5.

Patient 6 (female, 87 yrs.) presented with a papilledema of vascular origin of her right eye and optic atrophy on her left (visual acuity R 2/5, L 1/50). Assuming a vascular opticopathy due to vasculitis systemic corticosteroids were administered. Serum IgG antibody titer against B.burgdorferi was constant at 1:512; in the cerebrospinal fluid no specific antibodies against B.burgdorferi were detected. At the follow-up the visual acuity on the right eye was 0.2 in the retinometer along with cataracta provecta. IgG antibody titers for toxoplasma remained unchanged at 107 IU/ml, the complement binding reaction was <1:5.

Patient 7 (male, 69 yrs.) on both eyes showed a progressive visual field loss suspicious for low-tension glaucoma. The IgG antibody titer to B.burgdorferi was found to be markedly elevated at 1:512. In the cerebrospinal fluid no specific antibody could be found.

Three more patients presented with papilledema and elevated B.burgdorferi IgG antibody titers (1:128-1:256). Up to now, they got no antibiotic therapy. In one of these patients, IgG antibody to toxoplasma (68 IU/ml) and complement binding reaction titers of 1:5 were found.

Discussion

The prevalence of elevated antibody titers among the examined patients has been found to range significantly above estimates for a healthy control population (13,14); therefore, it is tempting to suggest that at least part of the seroreactive patients actually suffered from Lyme borreliosis. A significant predilection of certain age groups as compared to the overall increased age of patients attending an ophthalmic care center was not found. The distribution of antibody titers over the diagnostic groups was even.

With regard to the etiology of ocular disease in our patients several statements may be made:

- In four of these patients other etiologies could be verified to explain the ophthalmologic disorder.
- Three patients (patients 1-3) were highly suspicious of suffering from a borrelia-caused eye disease.
- In patient 1 ocular Lyme borreliosis can be assumed because of the preceeding cultural proof of B.burgdorferi out of an erythema migrans skin biopsy. It is an interesting fact that no serum antibodies to B.burgdorferi could be identified; this may have been due to the early antibiotic treatment.
- In patient 2, a significant rise of antibody titer up to 1:64 had occurred; this seroconversion in association with the clinical finding of a VI nerve palsy suggests a clinical manifestation of Lyme borreliosis. In children B.burgdorferi is known to be the most frequent cause of facial palsies (4,7).
- In patient 3, clinical suspicion could be confirmed by the history of a preceding erythema migrans.
- In the other 18 seroreactive patients, Lyme borreliosis cannot be excluded; a definite etiology, however, could not be established on the basis of the present data.

The records of seven patients out of the last group are presented above. In patient 4, after anti-toxoplasmotic treatment another relapse of chorioretinitis occurred. Because of the elevated borrelia antibody titer, a short-term treatment with Cephalosporins was instituted in 1989. Although borrelia antibody titers decreased significantly within two years, further relapses occurred. The decrease of antibody titers could be due to the treatment as well as it could be the result of a normal course of the immune response. In the literature, relapses after antibiotic treatment have been reported in patients suspicious of ocular Lyme borreliosis. Because of the lack of further clinical or anamnestic data a possible causative relationship between the elevated Borrelia antibody titer and the relapsing chorioretinitis cannot be substantiated.

In patients 5, 6 and 7, B.burgdorferi antibody titers were found to be markedly elevated (≥1:256); in healthy control groups, IgG antibody titers of more than 1:128 have not been found (13,14). The height of the titers may just reflect seroprevalence titers after repeated earlier exposures to the infectious agent as well as a clinically manifest Lyme borreliosis. There were no historical or clinical indications to further endorse the suspicion of a borrelia-caused disorder. In these patients - quite as well as in the last three of the patients described above - no conclusions for a definite establishment of the diagnosis of ocular Lyme borreliosis may be drawn with sufficient certainty. In these cases ocular Lyme borreliosis represents only one of various possible differential diagnoses.

Conclusions

Our study could not bring forth unequivocal diagnostic criteria for ocular Lyme borreliosis. Since elevated antibody titers after exposure to the infectious agent are frequent in the healthy population (seroprevalence titer) a significantly elevated IgG antibody titer may not be an indicator of a clinically manifest Lyme borreliosis; on the other hand, lacking evidence of antibody titers against B.burgdorferi cannot definitely exclude Lyme borreliosis.

Therefore, the diagnosis of ocular Lyme borreliosis should only be established when stringent criteria have been fulfilled. The criteria applied to patients in this study are summarized in Table 4.

By a specifically directed history-taking in any ocular disease of undetermined etiology previous or present manifestations of Lyme borreliosis should always be asked for or ruled out respectively. Even if there is no evidence of Borrelia antibodies the etiology may be highly suspicious for Lyme borreliosis. If elevated antibody titers to B.burgdorferi are found, dermatologic, medical and neurologic examinations should be done to exclude other manifestations of Lyme borreliosis. If data do not provide enough information to ensure the diagnosis of Lyme borreliosis, antibiotic treatment should only be instituted after a thorough search for other possible causes. Treatment regimens been recommended by Winward and coworkers 1989 (15).

Application of stringent criteria for the diagnosis of ocular Lyme borreliosis is imperative, if future studies shall not be hampered by the inability to differentiate Lyme borreliosis from other clinical entities.

References

1. Aaberg TM (1989) The Expanding Ophthalmologic Spectrum of Lyme Disease. Am J Ophthalmol 107:77-80
2. Bialasiewicz AA, Huk W, Druschky KF et al (1989) Borrelia burgdorferi-Infektion mit beidseitiger Neuritis nervi optici und intracerebralen Demyelinisierungsherden. Klin Mbl Augenheilk 195:91-94
3. Bialasiewicz AA, Schönherr U (1990) Choriokapillaritis (sog. Pigmentepitheliitis) bei Borrelia burgdorferi-Serokonversion. Klin Mbl Augenheilk 196:481-483
4. Christen H-J, Bartlau N, Hanefeld F et al (1989) Lyme-Borreliose - häufigste Ursache der akuten peripheren Fazialisparese im Kindesalter. Monatsschr Kinderheilk 137:151-157
5. Kauffmann DJH, Wormser GP (1990) Ocular Lyme Disease: Case Report and Review of the Literature. Brit J Ophthalmol 74:325-327
6. Kehl F, Aust W (1990) Augenbefunde bei Zecken-Borreliose. Klin Mbl Augenheilk 193:66-68
7. Olsson I, Engervall K, Asbrink E et al (1988) Tick-Borne Borreliosis and Facial Palsy. Acta Otolaryngol, (Stockh.) 105:100-107
8. Schönherr U, Wilk CM, Lang GE et al (1990) Intraocular Manifestations of Lyme-Borreliosis. IV. International Conference on Lyme-Borreliosis, Stockholm, Sweden June 18-21,
9. Schönherr U, Lang GE, Meythaler FH (1991) Bilaterale Lebersche Neuroretinitis stellata bei Borrelia burgdorferi-Serokonversion. Klin Mbl Augenheilk 198:44-47
10. Seidenberg KB, Leib ML (1990) Orbital Myositis with Lyme Disease. Am J Ophthalmol 109:13-16
11. Steere AC, Duray PH, Kaufman G et al (1985) Unilateral Blindness Caused by Infection with the Lyme Disease Spirochete,

Fig. 1: Antibody Titer vs. Age group

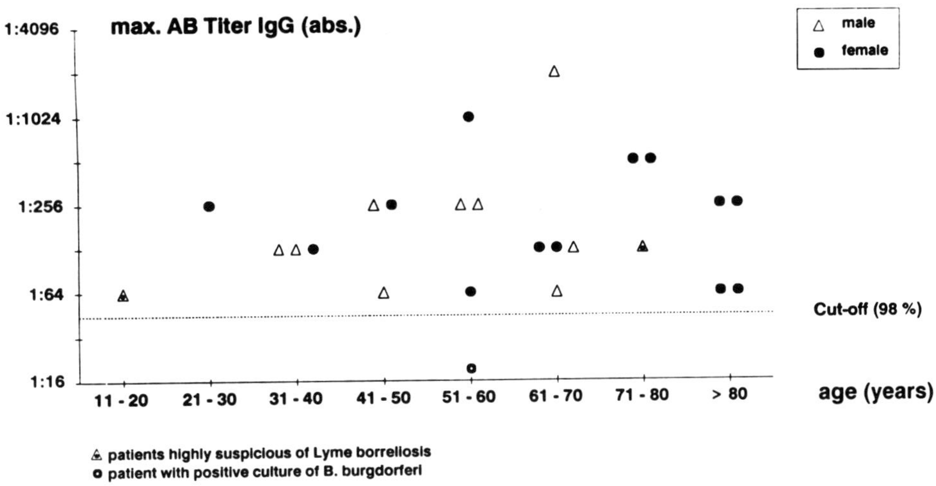

Fig. 2: Antibody Titers vs. Diagnostic Groups

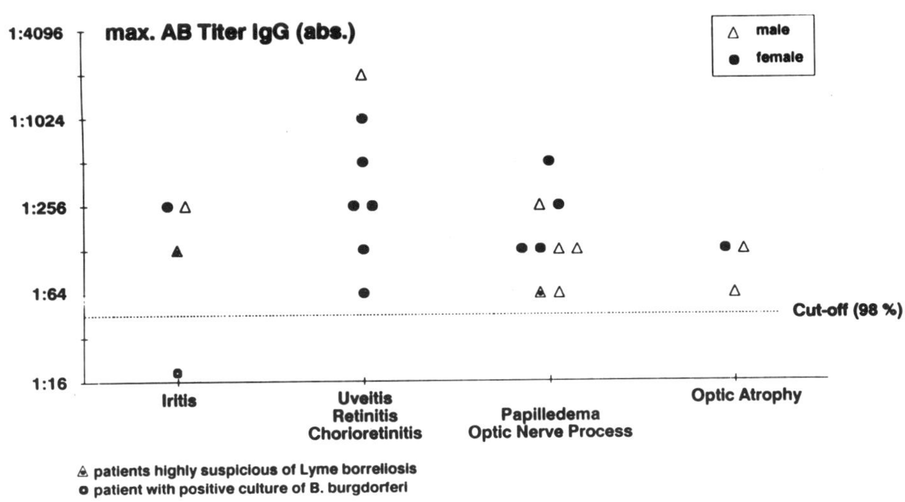

Tab. 1: Evidence Of Antibodies To Borrelia burgdorferi in Ophthalmologic Patients (1988 - 03/1991)

		1988	1989	1990	- 03/1991	total n	total %
total patients examined		71	184*	210	52	517	100
IgG#	borderline (1:32)	3	3	2	1	9	1,7
	elevated (≥ 1:64)	4	10	7	3	24	4,6
	from above: (≥ 1:256)	1	7	3	0	11	2,1

indirect immunofluorescent antibody test with prior absorption of sera with T. phagedenis

* One patient (female) with preceeding Erythema migrans lacking significantly elevated titers; cultural proof of Borrelia burgdorferi from skin biopsy by Dr. V. Preac-Mursic

Tab. 2: Ophthalmologic Diagnoses In Patients With Significantly Elevated Antibody Titers To Borrelia burgdorferi

Diagnosis	No. of Patients
Iritis	4 *
Uveitis	3
Retinitis	1
Chorioretinitis	4
Papilledema	10
Optic atrophy	5

* additionally 1 patient with cultural proof of B. burgdorferi

Tab. 3: Clinical Course Of Patients With Significantly Elevated Antibody Titers To Borrelia burgdorferi

Diagnosis	total no. of patients examined in follow-up	clinical findings ameliorated	unchanged	worsened
Iritis	4	3	1	-
Uveitis/Retinitis/ Chorioretinitis	5	1	2	2
Papilledema	6	4	1	1
Optic atrophy	1	-	-	1
total	16	8	4	4

Tab. 4: Criteria For The Diagnosis Of Ocular Lyme Borreliosis

strong suspicion of ocular Lyme borreliosis	- cultural proof in close relation to symptomatology - clinically unequivocal manifestations of Lyme borreliosis in history (Erythema migrans, Bannwarth's syndrome, ACA) - significant rise in IgG antibody titer (parallel assay) - demonstration of IgM antibody
B. burgdorferi as etiologic agent not ruled out	- significantly elevated IgG antibody titer; possibly additional: parallel occurrence of other, borrelia associated clinical manifestations

Borrelia burgdorferi. Ann Intern Med 103:382-384
12. Wilk CM, Bialasiewicz AA, Ruprecht KW et al (1989) Bilaterale akute konfluierende Chorioiditis disseminata bei Borrelia burgdorferi-Infektion. Klin Mbl Augenheilk 194:88-96
13. Wilske B, Münchhoff P, Schierz G et al (1985) Zur Epidemiologie der Borrelia burgdorferi Infektion: Nachweis von Antikörpern gegen Schildzeckenspirochäten bei Waldarbeitern aus Oberbayern. Münch Med Wochenschr 127:171-172
14. Wilske B, Steinhuber R, Bergmeister H et al (1987) Lyme-Borreliose in Süddeutschland. Dtsch Med Wochenschr 112:1730-1736
15. Winward KE, Smith JL, Culbertson WW et al (1989) Ocular Lyme Borreliosis. Am J Ophthalmol 108:651-657
16. Zaidman GW (1990) Episcleritis and Symblepharon with Lyme Keratitis. Am J Ophthalmol 109:487-488

Ocular Manifestations in Lyme Borreliosis

Ulrich Schönherr and Gottfried O.H. Naumann

Abstract. Lyme borreliosis plays an increasing role in Ophthalmology. While ocular symptoms due to conjunctivitis or paresis of cranial nerves are frequent, intraocular inflammations caused by B.burgdorferi seem to be rare and a main problem is the laboratory evidence for the establishment of the diagnosis. Mimicry of other diseases involving all of the ocular structures is typical for spirochetal infections. From 1985 until 1991, we have seen 17 patients with intraocular inflammations and evidence of active Lyme borreliosis, five with neuroretinitis, five with focal or disseminated choroiditis, three with diffuse choroiditis and serous retinal detachments, three with retinal vasculitis and one with iridocyclitis. Main diagnostic criteria were the presence of elevated IgM antibody titers or the new development of IgG titers against B.burgdorferi or simultaneous pathognomonic extraocular features. Ten patients remembered a tick bite, three had a proven erythema chronicum migrans, ten had extraocular manifestations such as arthritis, meningitis, meningopolyneuritis, demyelinating encephalitis and cardiac involvement.
Early-initiated systemic antibiotic therapy was rather effective in our patient population.

Introduction

Lyme borreliosis is a spirochetal infection mainly transmitted by ticks. In its multisystem involvement, its wide variability of manifestations and mimicry of other diseases, it is closely related to syphilis (65). Three different stages have been defined, but unlike syphilis later stages frequently occur without evidence of the previous stage. The eye may be involved primarily by inflammation of ocular tissues or secondarily by involvement of ocular adnexa. Ocular manifestations may be the first or even the only obvious manifestations of Lyme borreliosis (51,53).

History of Lyme Borreliosis

In Europe, the typical skin manifestations of erythema chronicum migrans (3), lymphadenosis cutis benigna (6) and acrodermatitis chronica atrophicans (18,25) as well as the typical neurological manifestations (7,21) have been well known since the beginning of this century. An association with tick bites was noted (22,41) and the infectious etiology was shown by transmission of acrodermatitis chronica atrophicans (22,23), erythema chronicum migrans (15) and lymphadenosis cutis benigna (43,44) using skin transplants. Even in acrodermatitis chronica atrophicans penicillin treatment was found to be beneficial (26,43). Although a spirochetal origin was assumed by several authors (35,67) the etiologic organism was not found.

The second part of the story began in North America in 1977 with the description of an epidemic oligoarthritis in Lyme, Connecticut by Allen C. Steere and coworkers.

It soon became apparent that the so-called "Lyme disease" was a multisystem infection, which most likely was transmitted by ticks and was associated with an ever since enlarging spectrum of skin, nervous system, heart, and joint manifestations (59,61).

In 1982, Willy Burgdorfer found an unknown spirochete in ticks which was shown to be the etiologic agent of Lyme disease (17). This spirochete was named Borrelia burgdorferi (28). Serologic tests were developed and Borrelia burgdorferi was isolated and cultured from erythema chronicum migrans, lymphadenosis cutis benigna, acrodermatitis chronica atrophicans, synovial fluid in Lyme arthritis and cerebrospinal fluid in neurologic manifestations (1, 4, 10, 46, 63, 69). The disease is now called "Lyme borreliosis" (65).

Course of Lyme Borreliosis and Staging

At the Fourth International Conference on Lyme Borreliosis in Stockholm in June 1990 an attempt was made to standardize the previous different classifications in agreement with the most active clinical researchers of Europe and North America (5).

The clinical pictures can be divided into acute and usually self-limiting signs or symptoms beginning several weeks to some months after inoculation with Borrelia burgdorferi or the slowly progressive form of late chronic manifestations appearing months to years after inoculation with Borrelia burgdorferi. Early Lyme borreliosis is further divided into a localized infection around the entry site of inoculation (for example around the tick bite) and an early disseminated infection. As the course in individual patients does not imply a uniform sequence with development of all three stages and as the infection may not become manifest until the second or third stage, a staging system without numbers has been preferred to avoid misunderstanding (Tab.1)(5).

Whether the late chronic manifestations may be due to a post-infection mechanism triggered by Borrelia burgdorferi or may be due to a persistence of the organism is still unknown. In several cases Borrelia burgdorferi has been cultured from patients months to years after a clinically successful antibiotic treatment (47). Probably both mechanisms are important (68).

Diagnosis of Lyme Borreliosis

In 1985, Steere and coworkers described the first isolation of spirochetes from a vitreous specimen obtained during vitrectomy in a patient with severe panophthalmitis in Lyme borreliosis (29,64). In experimentally infected animals Borrelia burgdorferi can usually be isolated from the eye (19,27).

Since direct visualization and cultivation of Borrelia burgdorferi from human eyes is rarely achieved, the main problem in ocular borreliosis is the establishment of the diagnosis. In cases of ocular inflammations in an endemic area it is demanding to evaluate for simultaneous evidence of extraocular active Lyme borreliosis.

Serology is the main aid in the diagnosis, but due to the lack of standardized tests for specific IgG and IgM antibodies against Borrelia burgdorferi the results of immunofluorescent antibody assays or enzyme-linked immunosorbent assays are not comparable with regard to different laboratories. To avoid false-positive results different methods of absorption with apathogenic Treponema are used leading to different titrations.

Thus, for the clinician it is necessary to be informed about the sensitivity and specificity of the immunofluorescent antibody assay or enzyme-linked immunosorbent assay results for interpretation. Positive IgG or IgM antibody titers may be confirmed by Western blots in selected cases (66). The persistence of positive IgG antibody titers may be the only sign of active borreliosis, but may also be due to a previous subclinical infection thus leading to substantial overdiagnosis of the disease. A single positive IgG antibody titer result must be interpreted with caution, since about 10-30% of a clinically healthy high-risk population, e.g. forest workers, have been found to be seropositive in screening tests in endemic areas (37,71).

The finding of specific IgM antibodies against Borrelia burgdorferi or the significant elevation of the IgG-titers during the course of the disease are important signs for active Lyme borreliosis (50). On the other hand,

- in early stage of localized infection only 20-50%,
- in early disseminated infection 70-90% and in the
- late chronic stage 90-100% of patients are seropositive.

In neuroborreliosis the detection of intrathecal antibody production (elevated cerebrospinal fluid/serum index for Borrelia-specific antibodies) is an important diagnostic marker (72).

Evaluation of the cellular immune response is a useful help in questionable cases, especially when the humoral antibodies are within the negative limits and borreliosis is suspected, a situation occurring after inadequate antibiotic treatment (31,32).

The diagnosis of Lyme borreliosis can be confirmed by the presence of pathognomonic clinical manifestations like

- Garin-Bujadoux-Bannwarth-syndrome,
- lymphadenosis cutis benigna (Fig.1),
- acrodermatitis chronica atrophicans (Fig.2) or
- a previous tick bite followed by an erythema migrans (Fig.3) in the absence of serologic test results (66).

Minor diagnostic criteria are a previous tick bite without erythema and the good response to antibiotic treatment.

Diagnosis of Ocular Lyme Borreliosis

In fact, only visualization and cultivation of Borrelia burgdorferi from the inflamed eye can lead to the diagnosis of proven ocular Lyme borreliosis. But ocular biopsies from cases of intraocular inflammations are generally not available. Therefore, diagnostic evidence has to be based on indirect criteria. In Tab.2 the diagnostic criteria for ocular Lyme borreliosis are listed and evaluated for clinical purposes. A probable ocular manifestation of Lyme borreliosis may be stated in cases of intraocular inflammations with at least one major criterion present and when other causes have been excluded. The microbiological and extraocular findings in 17 patients with intraocular inflammations and evidence of active Lyme borreliosis with one or more major criteria combined with one or more minor criteria seen in our institution from 1985 until 1991 are listed in Tab.3 and Tab.4.

Still many patients suffering from ocular inflammations with one or more minor diagnostic criteria and the suspicion of Lyme borreliosis may remain in whom an antibiotic treatment trial should be considered.

Clinical Spectrum of Ocular Lyme Borreliosis

Ocular biomicroscopy allows an exact localization of the inflammatory process due to the existence of boundary structures, which modify or limit the extension of intraocular inflammation (38). Lyme borreliosis like syphilis shows a wide variability of different inflammatory manifestations and seems to be a great imitator of ocular diseases (53).

Conjunctivitis

With a frequency of 11%, conjunctivitis is reported to be the most common ocular manifestation in early Lyme borreliosis in North America (62). However, there are regional differences. In South German patients, Weber and coworkers have found an incidence of only 1% while in 425 Slavonian patients with erythema migrans the rate of conjunctivitis was 5.4%. The frequency of conjunctivitis depends on the localization and amount of erythema migrans lesions (Tab.5) (53).

Iridocyclitis

Granulomatous iridocyclitis with posterior synechiae and cellular infiltrates may occur in the early disseminated stage and shows a good response to antibiotic treatment (53,73). One single case of Posner-Schlossmann syndrome with acute elevation of intraocular pressure and prompt response to antibiotic therapy has been observed in a patient with recurrence of lymphadenosis cutis benigna (54).

Retinal Vasculitis

Retinal vasculitis in Lyme borreliosis can manifest itself as the acute occlusive type leading to preretinal neovascularisation with recurrent vitreous hemorrhages requiring retinal laser treatment (34)(Fig.4) or as the chronic exudative type, leading to severe cystoid macular edema (50,55,58).

Choroiditis

Choroiditis in Lyme borreliosis may be the first sign of dissemination, which may be localized or multifocal (Fig.5) - sometimes resulting in subretinal neovascularisation - or diffuse with serous retinal detachment and lymphocytic meningitis imitating the Vogt-Koyanagi-Harada syndrome (Fig.6) (12, 14, 32, 53, 70).

Involvement of the Optic Nerve

Involvement of the optic nerve with distinctly different disease patterns in Lyme borreliosis may be encountered (39), such as optic disc edema due to an increased spinal fluid pressure in cases of encephalitis or pseudotumor cerebri (48).

Some cases of ischemic anterior optic neuropathy in patients with Lyme borreliosis have been reported (45,49).

Papillitis, a non-demyelinating inflammatory process of the optic disc with sudden loss of vision may occur in the early disseminating stage and may lead to severe optic atrophy (Fig.9) (13,16,20).

In neuroretinitis, inflammation of the optic disc may be associated with a vasculitis of the disc capillaries and the peripapillary vessels, leading to a macular star figure caused by lipids within Henle's layer (Fig.8). Neuroretinitis may be a sign of early disseminated borreliosis (13,33,52).

Ackermann (2) reported on 4 patients with retrobulbar neuritis in a group of 44 patients with late borrelial encephalomyelitis.

Keratitis

Keratitis may occur several years after infection with Borrelia burgdorferi with multiple and recurrent infiltration in all levels of the corneal stroma with changing locations. A good response to topical corticosteroids has been reported (9) as well as progression to vascularisation and scarring (8, 11, 30, 40, 53). This kind of stromal keratitis resembles interstitial keratitis with ghost vessels due to syphilis.

Involvement of the Eye Due to Extraocular Manifestations of Lyme Borreliosis

In Garin-Bujadoux-Bannwarth syndrome facial palsy is the most frequent cranial nerve involvement followed by palsies of the nerves of the oculomotoric system (III, IV, VI) (Fig.9).

Myositis is a common feature in Lyme borreliosis, a single case of orbital myositis has been reported in a child with active Lyme borreliosis (56).

Homonymous visual field defects may occur in cases of stroke due to cerebral vasculitis in Lyme borreliosis (24,36).

Therapy of Ocular Lyme Borreliosis

Before the etiology of Lyme borreliosis had become apparent, the benefit of penicillin in treating the dermatologic manifestations had been shown (26,43). Today, there is no consensus about the most effective antibiotic. It is difficult to evaluate the sensitivity of Borrelia burgdorferi to particular antibiotics in man because of the self-limiting character of the early manifestations.

Penicillin G, tetracyclines, doxycycline and cefotaxime seem to be effective but penetration into the cerebrospinal fluid is poor, if the meninges are not inflamed (44). Intravenous ceftriaxone is effective and seems to penetrate better into the cerebrospinal fluid as well as into the vitreous (44,57).

Knowing that there is no consensus about the best treatment we use intravenous ceftriaxone 2g daily for at least 2 weeks in cases of intraocular inflammation and one or more diagnostic criteria for ocular Lyme borreliosis (Tab.2). In cases of intraocular inflammation and possible Lyme borreliosis with minor diagnostic criteria we consider an oral doxycycline treatment of 200-400mg daily for at least two weeks.

However, Borrelia burgdorferi can persist despite antibiotic treatment (47). We have seen a patient in whom Borrelia burgdorferi was cultured from a joint after clinically successful treatment of two episodes of choroiditis with Doxycycline 200mg for two weeks and Ceftriaxone 2g for three weeks respectively.

Conclusions

The clinical spectrum of intraocular inflammations associated with Lyme borreliosis is not pathognomonic, however, presents the typical spectrum of an ocular spirochetosis especially with regard to its well-known variability. Intraocular inflammations may be the first or even the only overt clinical manifestation in Lyme borreliosis. Therefore, in cases of ocular inflammations exhibiting the known spectrum of spirochetal infections it is demanding to initiate a serologic work-up for Lyme borreliosis and a multisystem examination for extraocular manifestations including the skin, joints, nervous system and heart. Due to the multisystem and potentially chronic character of the disease, antibiotic treatment should be considered even in doubtful cases.

Systemic monotherapy with corticosteroids should not be initiated in cases of optic neuritis, unless spirochetal infection is ruled out.

Acknowlegdement. We thank Prof. G. Burmester, Dr. A. Krause, and T. Häubl from the Inst. of Clinical Immunology and Rheumatology, Dpt. of Med.III, University of Erlangen-Nürnberg for valuable discussing regarding the immunological and rheumatological aspects and for performing the T-cell proliferation assay and Dr.K.Weber, München, for valuable discussion regarding the dermatologic aspects.

Table 1. Stages of Lyme Borreliosis

EARLY LYME BORRELIOSIS		LATE LYME BORRELIOSIS
Localized infection:	Early disseminated infection:	Chronic infection:
Erythema migrans and borrelial lymphocytoma without signs or symptoms of disseminated infection. (Regional lymphadenopathy and /or minor constitutional symptoms may be present.)	Multiple erythema chronicum migrans-like lesions. Early manifestations of neuroborreliosis, arthritis, carditis or other organ involvement.	Acrodermatitis chronica atrophicans, neurologic, rheumatic or other organ or other organ manifestations-persistent or remitting for at least 12 (or 6) months.

from (5)

Table 2. Diagnostic Criteria for Ocular Lyme Borreliosis

Major diagnostic criteria
- Cultivation or visualization of Borrelia burgdorferi
- Previous erythema migrans
- Simultaneous extraocular active Lyme borreliosis,
- Elevated specific IgM antibody titer against Borrelia burgdorferi,
- Significant rising of IgG antibody titer against Borrelia burgdorferi
Minor diagnostic criteria
- Previous tick bite
- Response to antibiotic treatment
- Constantly elevated IgG antibody titer against Borrelia burgdorferi
- Positive T-lymphocyte proliferation assay[1]

[1] minor because method has not yet been established

Table 3. Seventeen Patients with Intraocular Inflammation in Active Lyme Borreliosis

Papillitis/Neuroretinitis	5 patients
Retinal vasculitis	3 patients
Choroiditis focal	2 patients
Choroiditis multifocal 3 patients	
Choroiditis diffuse	3 patients
Iridocyclitis	1 patient

Department of Ophthalmology, University Erlangen-Nürnberg, Germany. 1985-1991.

Table 4. Microbiological and Extraocular Findings in 17 Patients with Ocular Inflammation in Lyme Borreliosis

Culture of B.burgdorferi	1 of 17
Elevated specific IgG-titer	17 of 17
Elevated specific IgM-titer	6 of 17
Tick bite	11 of 17
Erythema migrans or lymphadenosis cutis benigna	4 of 17
Neurological manifestations	7 of 17
Oligoarthritis	5 of 17
Cardiac involvement	2 of 17
Without typical extraocular involvement	2 of 17

Table 5. Prevalence of Conjunctivitis in 425 Slavonian Patients with Erythema Migrans (Strle 1990)

	Total number of patients	Conjunctivitis patients	%	p value
Localization of erythema migrans:				
head	22	3	13.6	not
other	403	20	4.9	significant
Number of erythema migrans lesions				
more than one	38	6	15.8	significant
one	387	17	4.4	p < 0,01
Systemic symptoms				
present	195	15	7.7	not
absent	230	8	3.5	significant
Total	425	23	5.4	

from (53)

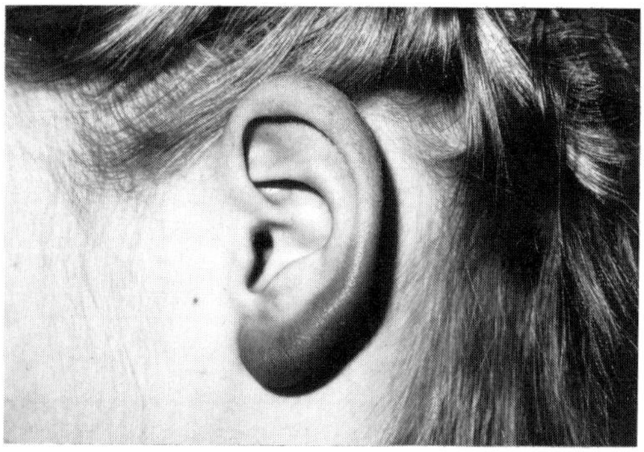

Fig.1. Lymphadenoma cutis benigna (permission of Dr.K.Weber,Munich)

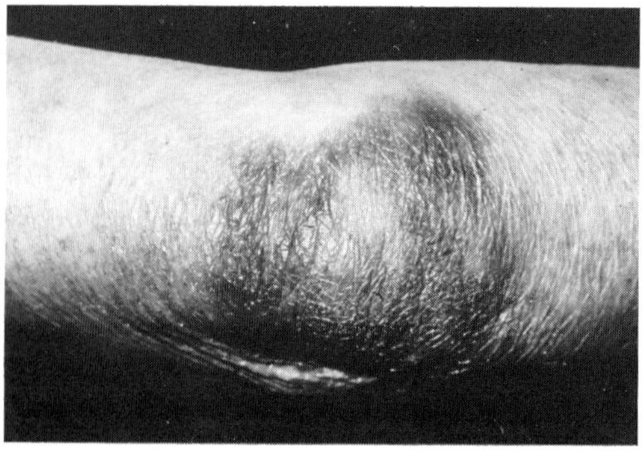

Fig.2. Acrodermatitis chronica atrophicans (permission of Dr.K.Weber, Munich

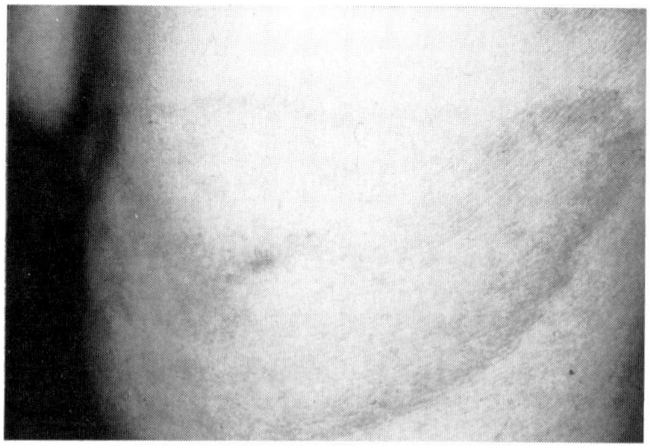

Fig.3. Erythema migrans (permission of Dr.K.Weber,Munich)

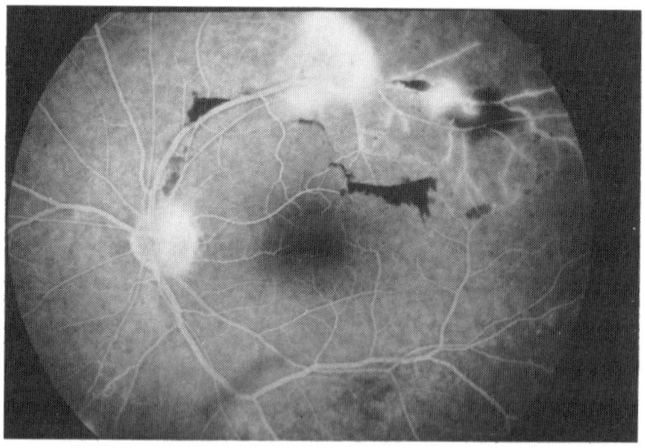

Fig.4. Retinal vasculitis in Lyme borreliosis (permision of Lang, Schönherr et al(31))

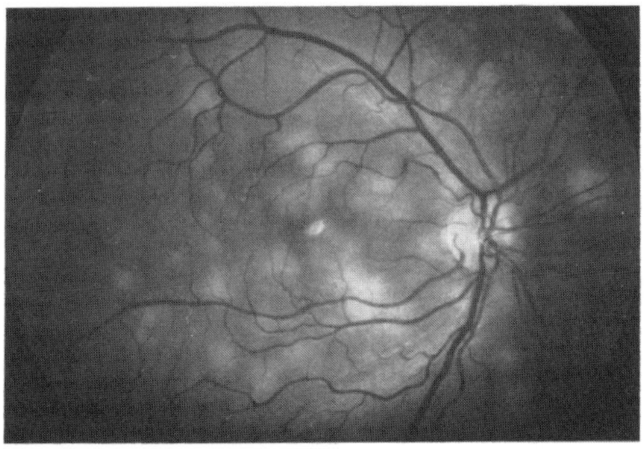

Fig.5. Multifocal choroiditis in Lyme borreliosis (permission of Schönherr et al (43))

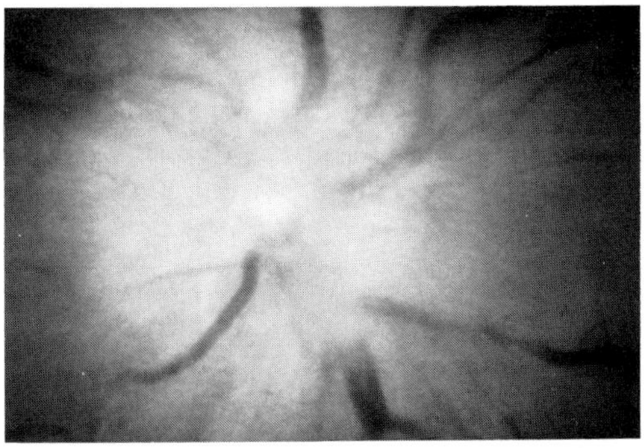

Fig.7. Papillitis in Lyme borreliosis (permission of Bialasiewicz et al (14))

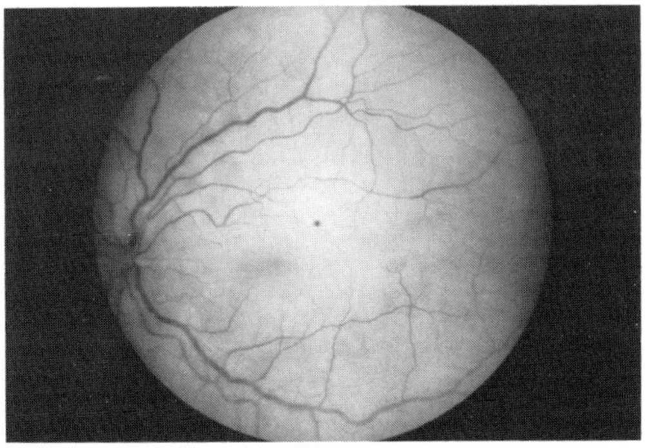

Fig.6. Diffuse choroiditis in Lyme borreliosis (permission of Wilk et al (61))

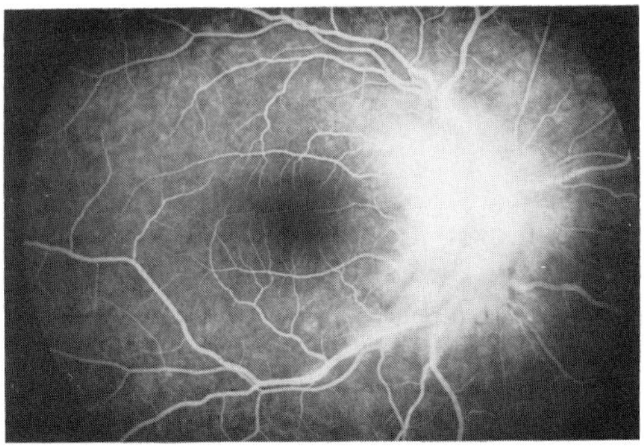

Fig.8. Neuroretinitis in Lyme borreliosis (permission of Schönherr et al(44))

References

1. Ackermann R, Kabatzki J, Boisten HP et al (1984) Spirochäten-Ätiologie der Erythema-chronicum-migrans-Krankheit. Dtsch Med Wochenschr 109:92-97
2. Ackermann R, Rehse-Küper B, Gollmer E et al (1988) Chronic Neurologic Manifestations of Erythema Migrans Borreliosis.Ann N Y Acad Sci 539:16-23
3. Afzelius A (1910) Verhandlungen der Dermatologischen Gesellschaft zu Stockholm. Sitzung vom 28. Oktober 1909. Arch Derm Syph (Berlin) 101:404
4. Asbrink E, Hovmark A (1985) Successful Cultivation of Spirochetes from Skin Lesions of Patients with Erythema Chronicum Migrans Afzelius and Acrodermatitis Chronica Atrophicans. Acta Pathol Microbiol Immunol Scand 93:161-163
5. Asbrink E, Hovmark A (1991) Comments on the Course and Classification of Lyme Borreliosis. Scand J Infect Dis Suppl 77:41-43
6. Bäfverstedt B (1943) Über Lymphadenosis cutis benigna. Eine klinische und pathologisch-anatomische Studie. PA Norstedt. Stockholm
7. Bannwarth A (1941) Chronische lymphocytäre Meningitis, entzündliche Polyneuritis und "Rheumatismus". Arch Psychiat Nervenkr 113:284-376
8. Baum J, Barza M, Weinstein P et al (1988) Bilateral Keratitis as a Manifestation of Lyme Disease. Am J Ophthal 105:75-77
9. Baum J, Barza M (1989) The Expanding Ophthalmologic Spectrum of Lyme Disease. Am J Ophthal 107:684-685
10. Benach JL, Bosler EM, Hanrahan JP et al (1983) Spirochetes Isolated from the Blood of Two Patients with Lyme Disease.N Engl J Med 308:740-742
11. Bertuch AW, Rocco E, Schwartz EG (1988) Lyme Disease: Ocular Manifestations. Ann Ophthalmol 20:376-378
12. Bialasiewicz AA, Ruprecht KW, Naumann GOH et al (1988) Bilateral Diffuse Choroiditis and Exudative Retinal Detachments with Evidence of Lyme Disease. Am J Ophthal 105:419-420
13. Bialasiewicz AA, Huk W, Druschky KF et al (1989) Borrelia burgdorferi-Infektion mit beidseitiger Neuritis nervi optici und intrazerebralen Demyelinisierungsherden. Klin Mbl Augenheilk 195:91-94
14. Bialasiewicz AA, Schönherr U (1990) Choriokapillaritis (sog. Pigmentepitheliitis) bei Borrelia burgdorferi-Serokonversion. Klin Mbl Augenheilk 196:481-483
15. Binder E, Doepfner R, Hornstein O (1955) Experimentelle Übertragung des Erythema chronicum migrans von Mensch zu Mensch. Hautarzt 6:494-496
16. Boutros A, Rahn E, Nauheim R (1990) Iritis and Papillitis as a Primary Presentation of Lyme Disease. Ann Ophthalmol 22:24-25
17. Burgdorfer W, Barbour AG, Hayes SF (1982) Lyme Disease - a Tick-Borne Spirochetosis? Science 216:1317-1319
18. Buchwald A (1883) Ein Fall von diffuser idiopathischer Haut-Atrophie. Arch Derm Syph (Berlin) 15:553-556
19. Duray PH, Johnson RC (1986) The Histopathology of Experimentally Infected Hamsters with the Lyme Disease Spirochete Borrelia Burgdorferi. Proc Soc Exp Biol Med 181:263-269
20. Farris BK, Webb RM (1988) Lyme Disease and Optic Neuritis. J Clin Neuro-Ophthalmol 8:73-78
21. Garin LH, Bujadoux C (1922) Paralysie par les tiques. J Med Lyon 71:765-767
22. Götz H (1954) Die Acrodermatitis chronica atrophicans Herxheimer als Infektionskrankheit. Hautarzt 5:491.504
23. Götz H (1955) Die Acrodermatitis chronica atrophicans Herxheimer als Infektionskrankheit. Ergänzung zur I. Mitteilung. Hautarzt 6:249-252

24. Hänny PE, Häuselmann HJ (1987) Die Lyme-Krankheit aus der Sicht des Neurologen. Schweiz Med Wochenschr 117:901-915
25. Herxheimer K, Hartmann K (1902) Über Acrodermatitis chronica atrophicans. Arch Dermatol Syph 61:57-76, 255-300
26. Hollström E (1951) Successful Treatment of Erythema Migrans Afzelius. Acta Derm Venereol (Stockholm) 31:235-243
27. Johnson RC, Marek N, Kodner C (1984) Infection of Syrian Hamsters with Lyme Disease Spirochetes. J Clin Microbiol 20:1099-1101
28. Johnson RC, Schmid GP, Hyde FW et al (1984) Borrelia Burgdorferi sp. Nov.: Etiologic Agent of Lyme Disease. Int J Syst Bacteriol 34:496-497
29. Kauffmann DJH, Wormser GP (1990) Ocular Lyme Disease: Case Report and Review of the Literature. Br J Ophthalmol 74:325-327
30. Kornmehl EW, Lesser RL, Jaros P et al (1989) Bilateral Keratitis in Lyme-Disease. Ophthalmology 96:1194-1197
31. Krause A, Brade V, Schörner C et al (1991) Cell Proliferation Induced by Borrelia Burgdorferi in Patients with Lyme Borreliosis - Autologous Serum Required for Optimum Stimulation. Arthritis Rheum T34:393-402
32. Krause A, Schönherr U, Schörner C et al (1991) Gonarthritis, Lymphadenopathie und disseminierte Chorioiditis als primäre Manifestation einer Lyme-Borreliose. Kasuistik und Diskussion der diagnostischen Möglichkeiten bei der Lyme-Borreliose. Z Rheumatol 50:10-15
33. Küchle M, Naumann GOH, Schönherr U (1990) Corneal Disorders, Infections, and Glaucoma in Pediatric Ophthalmology. Current Opinion in Ophthalmol 1:592-601
34. Lang GE, Schönherr U, Naumann GOH (1991) Retinal Vasculitis with Proliferative Retinopathy in a Patient with Evidence of Borrelia Burgdorferi Infection. Am J Ophthalmol 111:243-244
35. Lennhoff C (1948) Spirochaetes in Aetiologically Obscure Diseases. Acta Derm Venerol (Stockholm) 28:295-324
36. May EF, Jabbari B (1990) Stroke in Neuroborreliosis. Stroke 21:1232-1235
37. Münchhoff P, Wilske B, Preac-Music V et al (1986) Antibodies Against Borrelia Burgdorferi in Bavarian Forrest Workers. Zbl Bakt Hyg A 263:412-419
38. Naumann GOH, Naumann LR (1986) Intraocular Inflammation. In: Naumann GOH, Apple DJ (eds) Pathology of the Eye. Springer, New York Berlin Heidelberg Tokyo pp.99-184
39. Naumann GOH, Apple DJ (1986) Optic Nerve. In: Naumann GOH, Apple DJ (eds) Pathology of the Eye. Springer, New York Berlin Heidelberg Tokyo pp.723-770
40. Orlin SE, Lauffer JL (1989) Lyme Disease Keratitis. Am J Ophthalmol 107:678-680
41. Paschoud JM (1954) Lymphozytom nach Zeckenbiß. Dermatologica 108:435-437.
42. Paschoud JM (1958) Die Lymphadenosis cutis benigna (L.a.c.b.) als übertragbare Infektionskrankheit. II. Mitteilung. Übertragung in die Körperhaut. Hautarzt 9:153-165
43. Paschoud JM (1958) Die Lymphadenosis cutis benigna als übertragbare Infektionskrankheit. IV. Mitteilung. Besprechung der Untersuchungsresultate. Teil B: Penicillinbehandlung - Lymphadenosis cutis benigna und Erythema chronicum migrans: Zusammenhänge und Ätiologie - Zusammenfassung. Hautarzt 9:311-315
44. Philipson A (1991) Antibiotic Treatment in Lyme Borreliosis. Scand J Infect Dis Suppl 77:145-150
45. Pizzarello LD, MacDonald AB, Semlear R et al (1989) Temporal arteritis associated with Borrelia infection. A case report. J Clin Neuro Ophthalmol 9:3
46. Preac-Mursic V, Wilske B, Schierz G et al (1984) Repeated Isolation of Spirochetes

from the Cerebrospinal Fluid of a Patient with Meningoradiculitis Bannwarth. Eur J Clin Microbiol 3:564-565

47. Preac-Mursic V, Weber K, Pfister HW et al (1989) Survival of Borrelia Burgdorferi in Antibiotically Treated Patients with Lyme Borreliosis. Infection 17:355-359
48. Reik L, Burgdorfer W, Donaldson JO (1986) Neurologic Abnormalities of Lyme Disease without Erythema Chronicum Migrans. Am J Med 81:73-78
49. Schlechter SL (1986) Lyme Disease Associated with Optic Neuropathy. Am J Med 81:143-145
50. Schönherr U, Wilk CM, Lang GE et al (1990) IgM Borrelia Burgdorferi Antibody Titers in Patients with Ocular Manifestations of Lyme Borreliosis. Invest Ophthalmol Vis Sci 31/4:2804
51. Schönherr U, Wilk CM, Lang GE et al (1990) Augenbefunde bei Lyme-Borreliose. In: Burmester GR, Brade V (eds) Klinik und Diagnostik der Lyme-Borreliose. Bericht über das interdisziplinäre Lyme-Borreliose-Symposium in Erlangen am 18.11.89. Editiones Roche pp.65-74
52. Schönherr U, Lang GE, Meythaler FH (1991) Bilaterale Leber'sche Neuroretinitis stellata bei Borrelia burgdorferi-Serokonversion. Klin Mbl Augenheilk 198:44-47
53. Schönherr U, Strle F (1991) Ocular manifestations. In: Weber,K, Burgdorfer,W (eds) Lyme Borreliosis in Europe. Springer Verlag, Berlin, Heidelberg, New York, London, Paris, Tokyo. Chapter 28
54. Schönherr U (tp be published) Posner-Schlossmann-Syndrom ("Trabekulitis") und rezidivierendes Lymphadenoma cutis benigna Bäfverstedt bei Borrelia burgdorferi-Infektion.
55. Schönherr U, Leys AM, Lang GE et al (to be published) Retinal Vasculitis in Lyme Borreliosis.
56. Seidenberg KB, Leib ML (1990) Orbital Myositis with Lyme Disease. Am J Ophthalmol 109:13-16
57. Sharir M, Triester G, Kneer J et al (1989) The Intravitreal Penetration of Ceftriaxone in Man Following Systemic Administration. Invest Ophthalmol Vic Sci 30:2179-2183
58. Smith LJ, Winward KE, Nicholson DF et al (1991) Retinal Vasculitis in Lyme Borreliosis. J Clin Neuro Ophthalmol 11:7-15
59. Steere AC, Malawista SE, Hardin JA et al (1977) Erythema Chronicum Migrans and Lyme Arthritis: The Enlarging Clinical Spectrum. Ann Intern Med 86:685-698
60. Steere AC, Malawista SE, Snydman DR et al (1977) Lyme Arthritis: An Epidemic of Oligoarticular Arthritis in Children and Adults in Three Connecticut Communities. Arthr Rheum 20:7-17
61. Steere AC, Broderick TF, Malawista SE (1978) Erythema Migrans and Lyme Arthritis: Epidemiologic Evidence for Tick Vector. Am J Epidemiol 108:312-321
62. Steere AC, Bartenhagen NH, Craft JE et al (1983) The Early Clinical Manifestations of Lyme Disease. Ann Intern Med 99:76-82
63. Steere AC, Grodzicki RL, Kornblatt AN et al (1983) The Spirochetal Etiology of Lyme Disease. N Engl J Med 308:733-740
64. Steere AC, Duray PH, Kauffmann DJH et al (1985) Unilateral Blindness Caused by Infection with the Lyme Disease Spirochete Borrelia burgdorferi. Ann Intern Med 103:382-384
65. Steere AC (1989) Lyme Disease. N Engl J Med 321:586-596
66. Stiernstedt G, Dattwyler R, Duray PH et al (1991) Diagnostic Tests in Lyme Borreliosis. Scand J Infect Dis Suppl 77:136-142
67. Weber K (1974) Erythema-chronicum-migrans-Meningitis - eine bakterielle Infektionskrankheit? Münch Med Wschr 116: 1993-1998.
68. Weber K (1981) Treatment of Lyme Disease. Ann Intern Med 94:137

69. Weber K, Neubert U (1985) Das Lymphozytom - eine Borreliose? Z Hautkr 60:1585-1598
70. Wilk CM, Bialasiewicz AA, Ruprecht KW et al (1989) Bilaterale akute konfluierende Chorioiditis disseminata bei Borrelia burgdorferi-Infektion. Klin Mbl Augenheilk 194:88-96
71. Wilske B, Steinhuber R, Bergmeister H et al (1987) Lyme-Borreliose in Süddeutschland. Dtsch Med Wschr 112:1730-1736
72. Wilske B (1991) Epidemiologie und Diagnostik der Lyme-Borreliose (Borrelia-burgdorferi-Infektion). Med Welt 42:377-384
73. Winward KE, Smith LJ, Culbertson WW et al (1989) Ocular Lyme Borreliosis. Am J Ophthalmol 108:651-657

Recurrent Uveitis, Cystoid Macular Edema and Pericarditis in Lyme Borreliosis

Yan Guex-Crosier and Carl P. Herbort

Abstract. Lyme disease has been associated with many systemic and ocular. complications. We report on a 31-year-old man who suffered from recurrent pars planitis with two episodes of acute pericarditis. Extensive medical investigations were negative except for a highly positive Western Blot for B.burgdorferi.

Introduction

Lyme disease, first described by Steere and coworkers (7) in 1977 is now a well-known disease entity caused by B.burgdorferi affecting most organ systems, and which has been reviewed in detail by Asbrink (2).

Ocular complications are relatively rare, except for conjunctivitis, which is seen in about 11% of cases. Isolated cases of periorbital edema, oculomotor palsies, uveitis, papilledema from meningeal involvement, papillitis, interstitial keratitis and others have been reported (5,1).

Case Report

A 31-year-old man coming from a highly endemic area for B.burgdorferi was referred in January 1989. His medical history was characterized by an episode of bilateral intermediate uveitis in 1982 and an episode of pericarditis in 1988 that had responded to combined antibiotic (Amoxicillin and Clavulanic Acid 3x625mg for ten days) and acetyl salicylic acid treatment. Visual acuity was 0.6 OU. Bilateral uveitis associated with bilateral papillitis and cystoid macular edema was found. Inferior snowbanks and snowballs were present along the pars plana. Fluorescein angiography revealed diffuse leakage from the large and middle-sized vessels and confirmed the presence of cystoid macular edema as well as a massive leakage along the inferior vascular arcade temporally in the right eye

(Fig.1). Therapy including systemic Acetazolamide 500mg/d, Diclofenac eye drops, a potent non-steroidal antiinflammatory drug and Prednisolone Acetate 0.5% suspension was initiated. Because of persistent cystoid macular edema and inflammation, the patient was given three sub-Tenon's injections of corticosteroids (Triamcinolone,40mg) and his visual acuity improved to 1.0 OU. During this treatment, a new episode of pericarditis developed, which was successfully treated with systemic Indomethacin.

An extensive laboratory work-up was unremarkable. In particular, antinuclear antibodies were repeatedly negative, rheumatoid factor and HLA-B27 antigen were negative. A Tuberculin skin test was positive. Serological screening for syphilis, human immunodeficiency virus, Herpes simplex virus and toxoplasmosis remained negative except for a 1:128 positive indirect immunofluorescent antibody test for B.burgdorferi and a Western Blot highly positive for B.burgdorferi with 10 bands isolated.

No cardiac and valvular anbormalities were found. Cerebrospinal fluid analysis was unremarkable. A new course of antibiotic treatment by intravenous injections of Ceftriaxone 2g/d for 14 days followed by Doxycyline 200mg/d for another two weeks was initiated. No relapse of uveitis or pericarditis was seen during a follow-up period of nine months.

Discussion

The association of pericarditis and uveitis is unusual, although both manifestations have been described in systemic diseases like sarcoidosis, syphilis, tuberculosis, juvenile chronic rheumatoid arthritis, rheumatoid arthritis, systemic lupus erythematosus, psoriasis, human immunodeficiency virus seroconversion, Behcet's and Crohn's diseases. Very few cases of pericarditis have been reported in Behcet's disease (3). In most cases, no ocular involvement was described. The patient reported by us did not exhibit systemic sign suggesting Behcet's disease. He was HLA-B27 negative and had no evidence of collagenosis. Sarcoidosis was excluded by the absence of radiographically demonstrable changes in the lungs and the absence of cutaneous anergy (positive Tuberculin test following BCG). Cardiac involvement is seen in about 4-8% of patients with Lyme borreliosis, but an association of pericarditis and uveitis has not yet been described in this context. The most common clinical finding consists of a variable degree of atrioventricular block (first degree, Wenckebach or complete atrial ventricular block), but some patients suffer from (myo)pericarditis or minimal pericardial effusion.

Lyme disease is difficult to recognize when the hallmark of erythema chronicum migrans is missing during the first stage of infection. The presence of ocular inflammatory disease like keratitis, atypical pars planitis or ocular neuropathy shoud prompt a search for Lyme disease. The presence of antibodies to B.burgdorferi may be detected either by indirect fluorescent antibody staining or by enzyme linked immunosorbent assay or by immunoblotting, which is significantly more sensitive and specific (6).

The patient reported by us had a highly positive Western Blot for B.burgdorferi. However, even if an infection by B.burgdorferi had been most likely in this case, it did not prove B.burgdorferi to be the causative agent for the uveitis. A good response to systemic antibiotics in the first episode of pericarditis, however, suggested the presence of an infectious organism. Antibiotic treatment at that time had probably been insufficient, since only a prolonged treatment with high doses of Penicillin may be effective against B.burgdorferi. Amoxicillin, a second choice antibiotic, should be applied at a dosage of 500mg/tid with Probenicid 500mg/tid added for 10-30 days (8).

We think that our patient presented with a late-stage Lyme borreliosis including cardiac and ocular manifestations. The excellent effect of corticosteroids on the ocular inflammation suggests that the ocular involvement is mainly immunological in nature. Antibiotic treatment is less effective in more advanced stages. As demonstrated by Dattwyler and coworkers, Ceftriaxone may be effective for the treatment of patients with late-stage Lyme disease when Penicillin has failed (4). Although a good clinical effect had been seen, which might have been ascribed to the local corticosteroid therapy, we chose a long-term antibiotic therapy in order to avoid relapses of uveitis and, more important, to avoid further cardiac problems.

References

1. Aaberg TM (1989) The Expanding Ophthalmologic Spectrum of Lyme Disease. Am J Ophthalmol 107:77-80
2. Asbrink E, Hovmark A (1988) Early and Late Cutaneous Manifestations in Ixodes-Borne Borreliosis (Erythema Migrans Borreliosis, Lyme Borreliosis). Ann NY Acad Sci 539:4-15
3. Binak K, Ucak D, Yalcin B et al (1980) Left Ventricular Aneurysm and Acute Pericarditis in a Case of Behcet's Disease. J Rheumatol 7:578-580
4. Dattwyler RJ, Volkman DJ, Halperin JJ et al (1988) Treatment of Late Lyme Borreliosis - Randomized Comparison of Ceftriaxone and Penicillin. Lancet i:1191-1194
5. Flach AJ, Lavoie PE (1990) Episcleritis, Conjunctivitis and Keratitis As Ocular Manifestations of Lyme Disease. Ophthalmology 97:973-975
6. Grodzicki RL, Steere AC (1988) Comparison of Immunoblotting and Indirect Enzyme-Linked Immunosorbent Assay Using Different Antigen Preparations for Diagnosing Early Lyme Disease. J Infect Dis 157:790-797
7. Steere AC, Malawista SE, Hardin JA et al (1977) Erythema Chronicum Migrans and Lyme Arthritis: The Enlarging Clinical Spectrum. Ann Intern Med 86:685-698
8. Steere AC, Hutchinson GJ, Rahn DW (1983) Treatment of the Early Manifestations of Lyme Disease. Ann Intern Med 99:22-26

- Other Bacterical

T-Cell-Mediated Immune Response in Murine Brucellosis and Listeriosis: A Comparison

M.E.A. Mielke, H. Hahn

Introduction

The causative agent of M.Bang and Malta fever, members of the bacterial genus Brucella, belongs to the group of facultative intracellular bacteria. This group of pathogens, able to reside even in professional phagocytes, causes a wide variety of infectious diseases, including most anthropozoonoses, which range from acute illnesses such as listeriosis to chronic infections (Tab.1).

Despite its importance as a pathogen in cattle, sheep, and humans, studies on the immune response to Brucella are sparse. There have been some investigative activities focussing on the macrophage in the 1960s and 1970s shifting to the role of antibodies in the 1980s. Thus, much of our knowledge about immune mechanisms active in these infections stems from models other than brucellosis. However, each infection, despite similarities in the immune response, shows marked differences with respect to the susceptibility of the causative agent to the spectrum of effector mechanisms triggered by the host response. It therefore appeared worthwhile to study the mechanisms underlying immunity in Brucella infected animals. In doing so, we could include extensive studies on immunity to L.monocytogenes, this way being able to compare these two infections with respect to the immune response.

This brief overview summarizes our previous work on L. monocytogenes, and our results on Brucella infection will be discussed in the view of these data.

Immunity to Listeria monocytogenes

Murine Infection by Listeria monocytogenes

Murine infection by Listeria monocytogenes as a model was first introduced by Mackaness in 1962 (25, for review 16, 21, 37). The specific cellular immune response to this facultative intracellular bacterium results in inflammatory and protective phenomena, the most prominent ones being:

- delayed-type immune raction, granuloma formation, and splenomegaly which in turn are timely correlated with
- eradication of bacteria from infected organs.

In each case of infection with facultative intracellular bacteria, it has been found that macrophages of infected animals show greatly enhanced microbicidal properties (24,25,43). This enhanced bactericidal capacity is nonspecific, as evidenced by resistance to superinfection with unrelated bacteria (3,26), and is lost soon after the infection is terminated. However, it can be regenerated in an accelerated fashion by challenging the host with the homologous organism (36). The terms "cellular resistance" (nonspecific) and "cellular immunity" (specific) are used to define these two juxtaposed phenomena (1).

Mackaness (27) showed that macrophage activation is induced by specific lymphocytes. His conclusions were based on the results of adoptive transfer experiments in which viable spleen cells from immune animals could transfer specific cell-mediated immunity to non-immune recipients. The role of lymphocytes was substantiated further by the use of antilymphcyte globulin which suppressed immunity to Listeria (28). After the discovery that the lymphocyte surface antigen Thy-1 is a marker for thymus-dependent T cells, and antisera to this antigen had become available (39), it was shown that lymphocytes from Listeria-immune donor mice which transfer not only protection to Listeria (4,22,35), but also confer delayed-type hypersensitivity (DTH) (47), are T-cells. Experiments in T-cell-deficient nude mice further substantiated the assumed distinction between the mechanisms of non-specific resistance and the nature of specific cellular immunity. Thus, these animals are able to restrict replication of viable bacteria during the early phase of infection, but are incapable of forming granulomas and developing DTH and finally succumb to chronic infection (7,13). The most characteristic function of sensitized T-cells then seemed to be the attraction and accumulation of monocytes at foci of infections. The need for macrophages to cooperate with T-cells in the expression of immunity was also emphasized by adoptive immunization studies, which revealed that adoptive immunity cannot be expressed in recipients that have been treated with agents known to suppress the recipient's production and function of monocytes and macrophages (14,15,29).

T-Cell Subpopulation in Immunity to Listeria monocytogenes.

Experiments by Cantor and Boyse (5,6) provided evidence that T-cells form a heterogenous population. This and extending discoveries (46) prompted a new series of analysis asking in what way and to what extent, different T-cell subsets contribute to protective immunity and DTH. This analysis was facilitated by the development of a monoclonal antibody (mAb), GK1.5, with specificity to L3T4$^+$ (12) because of the expression of L3T4$^+$ (CD4) and Lyt-2$^+$ (CD8) cell surface molecules separates murine T-cells into two non-overlapping subsets. Four major experimental approaches were chosen:

- immunohistology,
- selective depletion of T-cell subsets in adoptive transfer systems,
- analysis of T-cell lines and clones, and
- in vivo depletion of T-cell subsets.

Immunohistology

The involvement of both, the L3T4$^+$ and Lyt-2$^+$, T-cell subsets in Listeria-induced immunity has been demonstrated by immunohistologic analysis of their distribution in granulomatous lesions in livers of infected mice (33). However, whereas the fraction of cells in granulomas bearing the L3T4$^+$ marker increased from 60 to 96 hours after adoptive transfer of immune T-lymphocytes, the relative amount of Lyt-2$^+$ cells remained constant, an observation that points to different mechanisms of activation.

Adoptive Transfer Experiments

Using subset-specific monoclonal antibodies, Kaufmann and coworkers (19) showed that the capacity of peritoneal exudate T-lymphocyte-enriched cells to adoptively mediate protection against Listeria monocytogenes and DTH to listerial antigens was markedly reduced by pretreatment of cells with either anti-L3T4$^+$ or anti-Lyt-2$^+$ antibodies plus complement, but that it could be restored by the addition of the two selected T-cell subsets. Therefore, a coopertion between specific L3T4$^+$ and Lyt-2$^+$ cells in mediating protection and DTH was assumed. Further evidence for a crucial role of Lyt-2$^+$ cells in antilisterial protection was obtained by transferring spleen cells from immune donors treated only by in vitro incubation with the appropriate monoclonal antibody. In these experiments (30), we were able to show that the strong protective capacity of splenic equivalents can be abrogated by anti-Thy-1 or anti Lyt-2$^+$ monoclonal antibody treatment., whereas there was only a slight inhibition after anti-L3T4$^+$ treatment. Similar results (23) were recently reported from other laboratories.

Based on the observation, that Lyt-2$^+$ cells are involved in protection and that these cells exert cytolytic activity against Listeria monocytogenes infected target cells, Kaufmann proposed a hypothesis according to which Lyt-2$^+$ cytolytic cells would establish direct contact with infected target cells, lyse them, and in this way release intracellular bacteria. The latter would subsequently be taken up by invading monocytes better equipped to kill the bacteria than the cells originally infected. Most recently (20), it has been reported that cloned L3T4$^+$ cells could also specifically lyse Listeria-infected Ia-positive bone-marrow macrophages in vitro. Thus, with the exception of the target cell spectrum, at the clonal level, there seems at present to be no clear-cut distinction between phenotype and function of the T-cell subsets involved in immunity against Listeria infection.

In Vivo Serotherapy with Monoclonal Antibodies Specific for T-cell and Monocyte Surface Structures:
As described here, the current view of immunoregulation is based mainly on studies of lymphcyte subsets either in vitro or by adoptive transfer to naive recipients. Recently, it has been shown (11) that unmodified monoclonal antibodies of the IgG2b type can be extremely effective in depleting cells in vivo and therefore can be used for the selective manipulation of the immune response. We, therefore, treated mice with three different monoclonal antibodies specific for Thy-1, L3T4$^+$, and Lyt-2$^+$, respectively, in order to assess the relative contribution of T-cell subsets to DTH, protection, and granuloma formation in murine listeriosis (30,31). Irrespective of whether monoclonal anitbodies were administered during the induction or the effector phase of DTH, the latter was affected by the application of anti-Thy-1 or anti-L3T4$^+$ monoclonal antibody only. The interrelatedness of DTH and protection against facultative intracellular bacteria has long been a subject of considerable controversy. The fact that animals can be desenitized without loss of resistance or, conversely, can be rendered hyper-

sensitive without causing a corresponding increase in resistance argued against the widely accepted view that both phenomena depend on the same mechanism. The possiblity of ablating DTH reaction by the administration of anti-L3T4+, but not by anti-Lyt-2+, monoclonal antibody in vivo offered the opportunity to investigate whether DTH and protection are indeed mediated by different T-cell subsets, as was assumed by the studies of Chen-Woan and coworkers (9,10) in the rat model. Therefore, the effect of monoclonal antibodies, administered during primary and secondary infection, on DTH, protection and granuloma formation was determined. Our data (30,31) demonstrate that in primary infection, bacterial clearance is inhibited by anti-Thy-1.2+ monoclonal antibody treatment and, to a lesser extent, by anti-Lyt-2+ monoclonal antibody treatment. Surprisingly, anti-L3T4+ monoclonal antibody treatment, although preventing expression of DTH, had no significant effect on the resolution of infection. Treatment with monoclonal antibodies shortly before secondary infection of animals which had been strongly immunized four weeks previously, yielded a comparable pattern. However, the effect of the anti-Lyt-2+ monoclonal antibody treatment was more pronounced. Anti-Thy-1.2 monoclonal antibody treatment abolished, and anti-Lyt-2+ monoclonal antibody treatment markedly reduced, established protective immunity, whereas anti-L3T4+ monoclonal antibody treatment had a negligible effect. On the bases of observations in nude (34) and SCID (2) mice that, despite macrophage activation, adequate protection can not be achieved in the absence of granuloma formation, we investigated (31) the effects of monoclonal antibody treatment on this essential feature of the host response. The examination of liver sections from immune animals 48 hours after reinfection showed complete absence of mononuclear foci in anti-Thy-1.2-treated animals. The typical Listeria-induced lesions in such treated animals were polymorphonuclear infiltrations similar to those that can be observed in the very early phase of primary infection. Most surprising was the fact that livers of anti-L3T4+-treated (CD8-sufficient) animals were free of any granulomatous lesions in the presence of protection. On the contrary, anti-Lyt-2+-treated (CD4-sufficient) animals were able to form granulomas.

The rapidly expressed CD8+ T-cell-mediated protection that can be observed in a secondary infection in the absence of granuloma formation, therefore, was argued to be the result of a rapid interaction with resident macrophages, shown to be activated by their elevated expression of MHC class II products in the absence of CD4+ T-cells (Mielke and Niedobitek, unpublished results). In order to prove this assumption, we employed the monoclonal antibody 5C6 (40,41,42), which has been shown to inhibit the recruitment of myelomonocytic cells into inflammatory foci and to exacerbate a primary Listeria infection by locking complement receptor type 3 (CR3, Mac-1, CD11b), a member of the leukocyte integrin family. If Listeria-primed CD8+ T-cells act independently of invading monocytes by rapidly activating resident macrophages for efficient listericidal activity, this antibody would have minimal effects on the outcome of a secondary infection in actively immunized mice. Our recent study (32), however, demonstrates that the inhibition of CR3-dependent

migration of phagocytes dramatically increased the susceptibility to Listeria monocytogenes, not only in primary but also in secondary infection, where potent, granuloma independent antibacterial mechanisms are expressed by $CD8^+$ T-cells. However, two elements of T-cell mediated immunity could be demonstrated even in the face of 5C6-treatment and therefore seem to be CR3/CD11b-independent, i.e. a) acquired immunity against low doses of viable Listeriae and
b) granuloma formation elicited in immune mice by heat killed bacteria.

In conclusion, the results of studies performed using the Listeria model and presented in this review may be summarized as follows:

1) Listeria-primed $CD8^+$ T-cells mediate protection by mechanisms dependent on a rapid interaction with phagocytes invading infected tissues within the first 24 hours after reinfection in a CR3/CD11b-dependent, but $CD4^+$ T-cell-independent manner. This $CD8^+$ T-cell-monocyte-interaction does not result in granuloma formation, DTH or splenomegaly.

2) Listeria-specific $CD4^+$ T cells act via
   a) a less protective early and
   b) a delayed but longlasting interaction with monocytes which results in DTH and granuloma formation and which is CR3/CD11b-independent.

It is well established that the aforementioned T-cell-dependent functions are mediated in vivo by cytokines. Based on the ability to dissociate protective from inflammatory effector mechanisms on the basis of T-cell subsets in the Listeria model, it should be possible to indentify the $CD4^+$ T-cell-derived granuloma inducing factor. We therefore analysed the patterns of cytokines secreted by spleen cells from naive and Listeria-primed T-cell-subset-depleted mice. Naive and immunized mice were challenged with a high, normally lethal dose ($1x10^6$/animal) of viable bacteria and sacrificed 6 hours later, a time at which antibacterial mechanisms begin to be expressed in immune mice. Spleens were removed and unfractionated, erythrocyte-depleted single cell suspensions were preincubated for 3 hours in Penicillin and Streptomycin containing tissue culture medium in order to prevent bacterial overgrowth in the following in vivo culture in the absence of antibodies (=viable antigen). Three other aliquots of cells were subsequently incubated in the presence of antibiotics and the presence or absence of any additional listerial antigen. Two different non-viable antigen preparations were used: heat killed bacteria ($1x10^7$/ml) and a culture filtrate (CF, 1:100) of Listeria monocytogenes (=soluble antigen, sAg). Spleen cell cultures ($1x10^8$ cells / 5ml = 1spleen equivalent) were set up in tissue culture flasks in an upright position and were incubated in the presence of Mercaptoethanol ($5x10^{-5}$ mol/l) and Indomethacin ($1x10^{-6}$ mol/l).

Depletion of T-Cell subsets was checked by cytofluorography at the midst of the incubation period. After 48 hours of incubation, a time which corresponds to a 10^{-4} reduction of the bacterial inoculum in the spleens and established granuloma formation in immune mice, supernatants were collected, filter sterilized and stored at -70°C until they were assayed for their content of several cytokines.

Interleukin-1 was only produced by spleen cells when stimulated in vitro by viable bac-

Interleukin-1 was only produced by spleen cells when stimulated in vitro by viable bacteria, regardless whether spleens were obtained from naive or immune mice. Interleukin-6 secretion could be induced in culture by all antigen preparations used. Spleen cells from immune mice produced more Interleukin-6 than those from primarily infected mice which, moreover, did not respond to soluble listerial antigen. A similar pattern of cytokine response could be shown for CSFs with the exception that the amount of colony stimulating activity in the supernatants of primarily or secondarily challenged mice was not significantly different when viable or heat killed bacteria were used for stimulation.

Most interesting was the analysis of inner necrosis factor TNF and interferon IFN-gamma production for which an important role in the eradication of Listeria is documented (17,18,44). TFN could be induced in spleen cells from primarily as well as T-cell-depleted secondarily infected mice when whole heat killed bacteria (=particulate antigen) were used for stimulation. However, the amount of TNF produced by spleen cells from previously immunized mice was very much increased. As shown for Interleukin-6 and colony stimulating factors CSFs, soluble antigen was able to selectively stimulate spleen cells from immune mice. The cells activated by soluble antigen were T-cells as was most clearly demonstrated by their sensitivity to anti-Thy-1.2 monoclonal antibody treatment. Neither anti-L3T4^{+} monoclonal antibody nor anti-Lyt-2^{+} monoclonal antibody treatment abolished soluble antigen-induced TNF secretion which points to the ability of both subsets to the secrete or, at least, induce the production of this important cytokine. The cytotoxic action of all supernatants tested was blocked or markedly inhibited by coincubation with anti-TNFalpha antibodies.

Interferon-gamma was the only cytokine tested that was produced by spleen cells from Listeria-challenged immune mice without the need for any additional stimulation in vitro. This rapidly induced IFN-gamma production was CD4^{+} T-cell-dependent. As shown for TNF, IFN-gamma production was induced in immune as well as non-immune spleen cells when heat killed bacteria were used for in vitro stimulation whereas soluble listerial antigen selectively stimulated T-cells of both the CD4^{+} and the CD8^{+} subset to produce IFN-gamma.

Interleukin-4 could not be detected in any of the supernatants tested.

In summary, the analysis of cytokines secreted in vitro by the spleens of mice infected with a high dose of Listeria monocytogenes revealed that Interleukin-1, Interleukin-6, CSFs, TNF and IFN-gamma can all be induced in both, naive as well as previously immunized animals. TNF and IFN-gamma, known to play a decisive role in protection against Listeria (2,17,18,44), are specifically produced by both, the CD4^{+} and the CD8^{+} T-cell subsets. Whereas Interleukin-1 could only be induced by viable bacteria present during in vitro vulture, Interleukin-6, CSFs, TNF, and IFN-gamma in addition were elicited from spleeen cells when cocultured with heat killed bacteria. The Listeria culture filtrate used as a soluble antigen preparation selectively stimulated T-cells from immune mice. Interleukin-4 could not be detected in either of the supernatants tested, which points to a preferentially Th_1-type cellular immune response.

The question remains whether the state of immunity and the differences in the histopathological appearance merely depend on differences in the kinetics, the amount, or the location of TNF and IFN-gamma production, or whether there are as yet non-identified T-cell-derived cytokines necessarily involved in protection and especially in granuloma formation?

The Brucellosis Model

General Features of Brucella Infection

Brucella abortus, a lipopolysaccharide LPS containing, Gram-negative rod, does not produce exotoxins but can inhibit the oxidative burst associated with phagocytosis as well as phagosome-lysosome fusion in macrophages. The course of Brucella infection in genetically resistant mice, which is highly reproducible (Fig.1.) On the basis of bacterial numbers in spleens, murine brucellosis can be divided into four phases:

1. an increase in bacterial numbers from day to day 6,
2. a steady state of bacterial multiplication during day 7 and 14,
3. the decline of bacterial load from day 15 to about day 36, and
4. subsequent bacterial persistance lasting for at least 10 weeks after infection.

Whereas in the Listeria-model T-cell-dependent functions can best be studied during secondary infection, immunity to reinfection in murine brucellosis is mediated in part by specific antibodies (38), making the recovery from a primary infection a more suitable experimental approach. Like in the Listeria-model the eradication of bacteria (phase 2-3 in brucellosis) is timely correlated to the expression of DTH to soluble antigen as tested by skin reaction.

T-Cell Depletion Studies

However, in spite of the aformentioned co-expression of DTH and the elimination of bacteria, the depletion of L3T4^{+} T-cells, although resulting in the failure to express DTH, allows normal recovery from infection. In the contrary, the depletion of Lyt-2^{+} T-cells prohibited the eradication of bacteria as did treatment with anti-Thy-1.2^{+} monoclonal antibodies, but did not influence the expression of DTH (Fig.1). Even on the histological level, the effects of a T-cell-subset-depletion in murine brucellosis resembled that in listeriosis. No focal accumulation of Thy-1.2^{+}, Lyt-2^{+}, or Mac1^{+} cells occurs in the liver of L3T4^{+} T-cell-depleted Brucella-infected mice. Resident F4/80+ macrophages as well as Ia+ cells are evenly distributed in the tissue. On the other hand, Lyt-2^{+} T-cell-depleted mice express a marked granulomatous inflammation constituted of L3T4^{+} T-cells and Mac1+ monocytes/macrophages.

Most impressive were the effects of a T-cell-subset depletion on splenomegaly, a leading symptom of many infections by facultative intracellular bacteria. The development of splenome galy, due to an increase in marginal zone macrophages, was shown to be totally dependent on L3T4^{+} T-cells and could even be enhanced by the depletion of Lyt-2^{+} T-cells. As could be shown by anti-Thy-1.2^{+} monoclonal antibody treatment, spleen weight, i.e. cellularity, was not correlated with bacterial load

1.2^+ monoclonal antibody treated mice contained high number of Brucella (unpublished data, manuscript in preparation).

Cytokines in Brucellosis

With the exception of studies about colony stimulating activity in the serum of Brucella infected mice, no data about the cytikine response to B. abortus are available. In the aforementioned study (8), Cheers and Young have shown that the level of CSFs in the serum was elevated transiently at the time of peak infection, 2-3 weeks after injection of the bacteria. The level of colony stimulating activity in serum correlated with an increase in the proportion of colony forming cells (CFC) in the spleens of infected animals, which in turn paralleled the degree of splenomegaly. However, neither the levels of colony forming cells in serum nor the colony forming cells response can explain differences in the ability of various mouse strains to control bacterial numbers. In a recent publication by Mosmann and coworkers (45), it was found that immunization with fixed B. abortus favors a Th1-type of T-cell response like it was demonstrated by us in the Listeria-model.

Conclusions

In conclusion, as shown in two different murine models using an acute and a more chronic infection, $CD4^+$ bacteria-induced T-cells mediate the inflammatory phenomena accompanying infections by facultative intracellular bacteria, i.e. DTH, splenomegaly, and granulomatous inflammation. In both systems, $CD8^+$ T-cells seem to be able to mediate protective mechanisms in the absence of any granulomatous monocyte accumulation. However, in spite of these similarities, differences in the ultimately protective mechanisms are most impressively demonstrated by distinct susceptibilities of infected animals to CR3-blocking antibodies (40). Whereas mice infected with Listeria monocytogenes are highly susceptible to monoclonal antibody 5C6 (32,41), there is no effect of such treatment on brucellosis (Mielke, Rosen, unpublished data) or BCG infection (Rosen, unpublished data).

Table 1. Facultative intracellular bacteria, grouped according to the duration of the natural course of infection in experimental animals

Listeria
- Yersinia
- Mycoplasma
- Legionella
- Rickettsia
- Salmonella typhi/paratyphi
- Bartonella
- Chlamydia
- Francisella tularensis
- Brucella
- Borrelia
- Treponema
- Nocardia
- Mycobacterium tuberculosis, leprae
- Mycobacterium avium-intracellulare

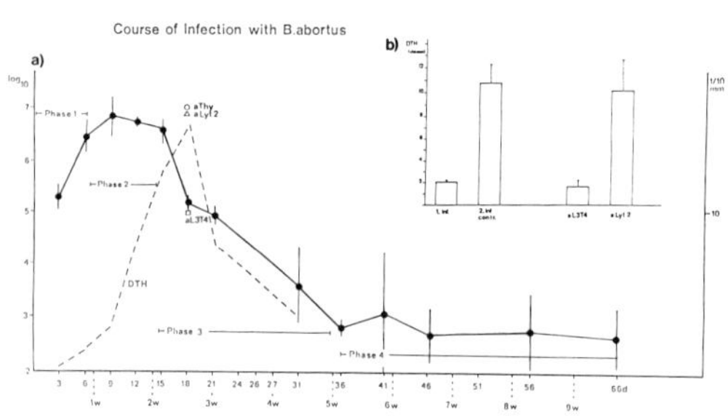

Fig.1. Course of Brucella abortus infection in mice. a) Male BALB/e mice were infected i.v. by 1×10^6 B. abortus, strain 19 and numbers of bacteria per spleen ($\log_{10}$) were determined at various intervals after infection. In parallel mice were challenged for DTH reactivity. Fifty μl of an appropriate antigen dilution was injected into the footpads of mice sacrified for the enumeration of bacteria/spleen 24h later. Skin reactivity was measured as specific footpad swelling (in 1/10mm). Three additional groups of five mice each were infected in parallel but treated with 500 μg of anti-Thy 1.2^+, anti-$Lyt2^+$, or anti-$L3T4^+$ monoclonal antibody respectively on day -3 and +10 of infection. On day 18 after infection, which represents the maximum of DTH reactivity and splenomegaly, these mice were sacrified and the numbers of B. abortus per spleen as well as DTH reactivity and efficiancy of T-cell-subset-depletion were determined. Whereas mice depleted from $L3T4^+$ T-cells (squares) were able to eradicate the bacteria as well as the controls, mice treated with anti-Thy 1.2^+ (circles) or anti-$Lyt2^+$ (triangles) monoclonal antibodies did not progress to phase 3 of an infetion in normal mice. DTH reactivity was suppressed by anti-$L3T4^+$ monoclonal antibody treatment in a primary as well as in a secondary response whereas the depletion of $Lyt2^+$ T-cells did not influence skin reactivity (b).

References

1. Armstrong AS, Sword C (1964) Cellular Resistance in Listeriosis.J Infect Dis 114:258
2. Bancroft GJ, Sheehan KCF, Schreiber RD et al (1989) Tumor Necrosis Factor is Involved in the T Cell-Independent Pathway of Macrophage Activation in SCID Mice. J Immunol 143:127
3. Blanden RV, Mackaness GB, Collins FM (1966) Mechanisms of Acquired Resistance in Mouse Typhoid. J Exp Med 124:585
4. Blanden RV, Langman RE (1972) Cell-Mediated Immunity to Bacterila Infection in the Mouse. Thymus-Derived Cells as Effectors of Acquired Resistance to Listeria monocyto genes. Scand J Immunol 1:379
5. Cantor H, Boyse EA (1975a) Functional Subclasses of T Lymphocytes Bearing Different Ly Antigens. I. The Generation of Functionally Distinct T-Cell Subclasses is a Differentiative Process Indipendent of Antigen. J Exp Med 141:1376
6. Cantor H, Boyse EA (1975b) Functional Subclasses of T Lymphocytes Bearing Different Ly Antigens. II. Cooperation Between Subclasses of Lyt Cells in the Generation of Killer Activity. J Exp Med 141:1390
7. Cheers C, Waller R (1975) Activated Macrophages in congenitally Athymic Nude Mice and Lethally-Irradiated Mice. J Immunol 115:844
8. Cheers C, Young AM (1987) Serum Colony Stimulating Activity and Colony Forming Cells in Murine Brucellosis: Relationship to Immunopathology. Microb Pathogen 3:185
9. Chen-Woan M, Sajewski DH, McGregor DD (1985) T-Cell Cooperation in the Medation of Acquired Resistance to Listeria monocytogenes. Immunology 56:33
10. Chen-Woan M, McGregor DD, Noonan SK (1986) Isolation and Characterization

of Protective T Cells Induced by Listeria monocytogenes. Infect Immun 52:401
11. Cobbold SP, Jayasuriya A, Nash A et al (1984) Therapy with Monoclonal antibodies by Elemination of T Cells Subsets in Vivo. Nature 312:548
12. Dialynas DP, Wilde DB, Marrack P et al (1983) Characterization of the Murine Antigenic Determinant, Designated L3T4a, Recognized by Monoclonal Antibody GK1.5: Expression of L3T4a by Functional T-Cell Clones Appears to Correlate Primarily with Class II MHC Antigen-Reactivity. Immunol Rev 74:29
13. Emmerling P, Finger H, Bockemühl J (1975) Listeria monocytogenes Infection in Nude Mice. Infect Immun 12:437
14. Hahn H (1974) Effects of Dextran Sulfate 500 on Cell-Mediated Resistance to Infection with Listeria monocytogenes in Mice. Infect Immun 10:1105
15. Hahn H (1975) Requirements for a Bone Marrow-Derived Component in the Expression of Cell-Mediated Antibacterial Immunity. Infect Immun 11:949
16. Hahn H, Kaufman SHE (1981) The Role of Cell-Mediated Immunity in Bacterial Infections. Rev Inf Dis 3:1221
17. Havel EA (1987) Production of Tumor Necrosis Factor During Murine Listeriosis. J Immunol 139:4225
18. Havel EA (1989) Evidence that Tumor Necrosis Factor has an Important Role in Antibacterial Resistance. J Immunol 143:2894
19. Kaufmann SHE, Hug E, Väth U et al (1985) Effective Protection Against Listeria monocytogenes and Delayed-Type Hypersenitivity to Listerial Antigens Depend on Cooperation Between Specific $L3T4^+$ und $Lyt2^+$ T Cells. Infect Immun 48:263
20. Kaufmann SHE, Hug E, Väth U et al (1987) Specific Lysis of Listeria monocytogenes-Infected Macrophages by Class II-Restricted $L3T4^+$ T Cells. Eur J Immunol 17:237
21. Kaufman SHE (1988) Immunity Against Intracellular Bacteria: Biological Effector Functions and Antigen Specificity of T-Lymphocytes. Curr Top Microbiol Immunol 138:141
22. Lane FC, Unanue ER (1972) J Exp Med 135:1104
23. Lukacs K, Kurlander R( )$Lyt\text{-}2^+$ T-Cell-Mediated Protection Against Listeriosis. Protection Correlates with Phagocyte Depletion but not with IFN-gamma Production.
24. Lurie MB (1942) Studies on the Mechanisms of Immunity in Tuberculosis: The Fate of Tubercle Bacilli Ingested by Mononuclear Phagocytes Derived from Normal and Immunized Animals. J Exp Med 130:247
25. Mackaness GB (1962) Cellular Resistance to Infection. J Exp Med 116:381
26. Mackaness GB (1964) The Immunological Basis of Acquired Cellular Resistance. J Exp Med 120:105
27. Mackaness GB (1969) The Influence of Immunologically Committed Lymphoid Cells on Macrophage Activity in Vivo. J Exp Med 129:973
28. Mackaness GB, Hill WC (1969) The Effect of Anti-Lymphocyte Globulin on Cell-Mediated Resistance to Infection. J Exp Med 129:993
29. McGregor DD, Koster FT (1971) The Mediator of Cellular Immunity. IV. Cooperation Between Lymphocytes and Mononuclear Phagocytes. Cell Immunol 2:317
30. Mielke MEA, Ehlers S, Hahn H (1988) T-Cell Subsets in Delayed-Type Hypersensitivity, Protection, and Granuloma Formation in Primary and Secondary Listeria Infection in Mice; superior Role of $Lyt2^+$ Cells in Acquired Immunity. Immun 56:1920

31. Mielke MEA, Niedobitek G, Stein H et al (1989) Acquired Resistance to Listeria monocytogenes is Mediated by Lyt2$^+$ T-Cells Independently of the Influx of Monocytes into Granulomatous Lesions. J Exp Med 170:589
32. Mielke MEA, Rosen H, Broche S et al (to be published) Listeria-Induced T-Cell-Monocyte Interactions in Protective Immunity and Granuloma Formation Depend on Two Distinct but TNF-and Gamma-IFN-Mediated Mechanisms. Dissociation on the Basis of CD11b-Dependency.
33. Näher H, Sperling U, Takacs L et al (1985) Dynamics of T-Cells of L3T4 and Lyt2 Phenotype within Granulomas in Murine Listeriose. Clin Exp Immunol 60:559
34. Newberg MF, North RJ (1980) On the Mechanisms of T-Cell-Independent Anti-Listeria Resistance in Nude Mice. J Immunol 124:571
35. North RJ (1973) Importance of Thymus-Derived Lymphocytes in Cell-Mediated Immunity to Infection. Cell Immunol 7:166
36. North RJ, Deissler JF (1975) Nature of Memory in T Cell-Mediated Immunity: Cellular Parameters that Distinguish Between the Active Immune Response and a State of Memory. Infect Immun 12:761-
37. North RJ (1981) Immunity of Listeria Monocytogenes. In: Nahmias AJ, O'Reilly RJ (ed) Immunology of Human Infection, Part 1, p.201. Plenum. New York
38. Plommet M, Plommet AM (1983) Immune Serum-Mediated Effects on Brucellosis Evolution in Mice. Infect Immun 41:97
39. Raff MC (1969) Theta Isoantigens as a Marker of Thymus-Derived Lymphocytes in Mice. Nature 224:378
40. Rosen H, Gordon S (1987) Monoclonal Antibody to the Murine Type 3 Complement Receptor Inhibits Adhesion of Myelomonocytic Cells and Inflammatory Cell Recruitment in Vivo. J Exp Med 166:1685
41. Rosen H, Gordon S, North RJ (1989) Exaverbation of Murine Listeriosis by a Monoclonal Antibody Specific for the Type 3 Complement Receptor of Myelomonocytic Cells. J Exp Med 170:27
42. Rosen G, Milon G, Gordon S (1989) Antibody to the Murine Type 3 Complement Receptor Inhibits T-Lymphocyte-Dependent Recruitment of Myelomonocytic Cells in Vivo. J Exp Med 169:535
43. Ruskin J, McIntosh H, Remington JS (1969) Studies on the Mechanisms of Resistance to Phylogenetically Diverse Intracellular Organisms. Immunol 103:252
44. Schreiber RD (1988) Validation of a Role for Endogenously Produced IFNg in Resolution of Listeria monocytogenes In fection in Mice. Adv Exp Med Biol 239:185
45. Street NE, Schumacher JH, Fong TA et al (1990) Heterogeneity of Mouse Helper T-Cells: Evidence from Bulk Cultures and Limiting Dilution Cloning for Precursors of Th1 and Th2-Cells. J Immunol 144:1629
46. Swain S (1983) T-Cells Subsets and the Recognition of MHC Class. Immunol Rev 74:129
47. Youdim S, Stutman O, Good RA (1973) Thymus Dependency of Cells Involved in Transfer of Delayed Hypersensitivity to Listeria monocytogenes in Mice. Cell Immunol 8:395

Ocular Brucellosis

Khalid F. Tabbara

Abstract. Brucellosis is a zoonotic disease caused by Brucella melitensis or Brucella abortus.
Three patients presented with clinical evidence of uveitis. Patients were referred by other ophthalmologists and had previously been treated with systemic corticosteroids. The patients were a 25 year old male, a 30 year old female and a 17 year old female.
Ocular findings consisted of anterior granulomatous uveitis in two patients and panuveitis in one patient. One patient had evidence of scleritis and peripheral corneal infiltrate.
Laboratory evaluation revealed serum titers for Brucella 1:320 in all three patients. Vitreous specimens were obtained from each of two patients and showed a high antibody titer for Brucella. In the 30 year old female patient, Brucella melitensis was recovered from a paravertebral abscess while in the 17 year old female patient, culture of the vitreous specimen revealed a heavy growth of Brucella melitensis.
All three patients were treated with systemic antibiotics and experienced complete recovery without the need for steroid therapy. Brucellosis, therefore, should be considered in the differential diagnosis of uveitis in the endemic areas.

Introduction

Brucellosis is a zoonotic systemic infection caused by the genus Brucella. The organism was first isolated by Colonel David Bruce (later Sir David) from the spleen of a soldier who died of Malta fever in 1887 in Malta (2). The agent of Malta fever (undulent fever) was later named Brucella honoring Sir David Bruce.

The disease had a major economic impact on meat and milk production throughout the world. Legislative measures in many countries have brought the disease of man and animals under control. Brucellosis continues to be a health problem in many regions of the world.

There are several species of Brucella and each species has one or more principal hosts. The principal hosts of
- Brucella melitensis are sheep, goats, and camels,
- Brucella abortus is cattle,
- Brucella suis is swine,
- Brucella canis is canine, and
- Brucella ovis is sheep (3).

The major causes of disease in man are B.melitensis, B.abortus, and B.suis.

Brucella melitensis infections have been reported in Kuwait and Saudi Arabia (6). With air travel, the geographic barriers of Brucellosis have been surpassed. Travellers to endemic areas may acquire the disease during their short visits by consumption of contaminated milk or milk products e.g.cheese. In addition, there has recently been an increasing intercontinental export by meat, milk products and animals.

In cows, Brucella abortus has a unique predilection to the lymphatics of the uterus. Infection of the placenta in cows is common and frequently leads to abortion. Organisms from infected placental tissue cause massive contamination of the environment and may cause infection in man. Cows may stay infected throughout their lives and successful deliveries are followed by excretion of the organisms in the milk.

Similarly, goats, camels and sheep may get infected with Brucella melitensis and may be the cause of contaminated milk. Cheese prepared from inadequate pasteurization of milk may contain viable Brucella organisms.

Transmission of the Disease

The disease is transmitted from animals to man by

- drinking raw or inadequately pasteurized milk, infected cheese, and meat (9). In addition, man may be infected by
- air-borne dissemination of the organism (5),
- person-to-person transmission and by
- rubbing the skin with infected cow's placental extracts (4).

Brucella are gram-negative intracellular coccobacilli that have the ability to persist in milk for several days and may remain viable in cheese for weeks. Also, the organism has been reported to survive in dust for several weeks (3).

The organism is killed when the milk turns sour because of its unique susceptibility to acidity. Similarly, the organism is killed by gastric acidity. The ingestion of milk, however, helps the organism to survive in the stomach. The consumption of antacids may also increase the susceptibility of the organism (7). Brucellae are killed by heating to 60°C for 10 minutes.

Systemic Manifestations

The systemic manifestations of brucellosis can be devided into two phases:
1) acute brucellosis and
2) chronic brucellosis.

The acute clinical manifestation of brucellosis includes fever, fatigue, malaise, anorexia, abdominal pain, night sweats, headache, and arthralgias. Children may display weight loss, malaise, arthralgia, hepatosplenomegaly, lymphocytosis, and elevation in liver enzymes (9).

The chronic phase of the illness occurs when the disease is left untreated or the diagnosis is missed. Skeletal and neurologic complications may occur in the chronic form of the disease. Patients may develop arthritis of the knees or ankles. Sacroileitis is also common. The disease may be confused with other autoimmune rheumatic disorders. Spondylitis, osteomyelitis and paravertebral abscess may occur. Skin rash may occur. Neurologic manifestations include meningitis, encephalitis, and peripheral nerve involvement e.g. sciatica. Other chronic manifestations include bronchopneumonia, pleuritis, endocarditis, orchitis and placentitis.

The eye may be involved in both phases of the disease.

Ocular Manifestations

Ocular brucellosis is uncommon in systemic brucellosis. We have studied the incidence of ocular brucellosis among patients with clinically manifest systemic brucellosis and found the incidence to be at 3%. Ocular findings are variable. They can be mild or severe leading to visual loss (1).

The ocular disease is usually unilateral. In the acute phase of the illness patients may develop unilateral endogenous endophthalmitis. I have seen one patient who developed endophthalmitis 17 days after the onset of systemic symptoms of fever, malaise, fatigue, night sweats and arthralgias. The only clinical finding was the presence of unilateral endophthalmitis with hypopyon. Blood IgG and IgM for Brucella melitensis were elevated and the organism was isolated from the vitreous.

Patients with brucellosis may develop scleritis. Scleritis is usually diffuse but may be nodular.

The intraocular inflammation presents as an anterior uveitis, choroiditis, or panuveitis with vitreous exudate. The anterior uveitis can be granulomatous or non-granulomatous (8). Posterior synechiae are common and secondary cataract may occur. Mutton fat keratic precipitates may be found. Patients treated with topical corticosteroids show an anterior nongranulomatous uveitis. Ocular brucellosis may lead to unilateral geographic choroiditis. Choroiditis may involve the retina and progress into a localized necrotic granuloma (8). Vitreous exudates and cells are common. In late forms of the disease, vitreous fibrotic bands may occur resulting in traction retinal detachment.

Retinal vasculitis may occur. The clinical ocular findings of ocular brucellosis are summarized in Table 1.

Furthermore, optic neuritis has been described by Abd Elrazak (1) in a 13-year-old female with systemic brucellosis. The patient presented with unilateral loss of vision of four days duration. The findings may suggest involvement of the optic nerve sheaths by the inflammatory process and may represent an extension of meningeal infection.

Another 20-year-old female presented to her neurologist with a headache and bilateral papilledema. The diagnosis of a pseudotumor cerebri was made. Further laboratory work-up revealed evidence of neurobrucellosis and meningeal involvement.

Laboratory Findings

Several serologic testing methods for Brucella are available. IgG and IgM antibodies can be detected with agglutination test, complement fixation or Enzyme-Linked Immunosorbent Assay. By far the Enzyme-Linked Immunosorbent Assay is superior to other methods. IgM antibodies are elevated in the acute phase of the disease.

The definitive diagnosis is made by isolation of the organism. The use of trypticase soy broth is valuable for the recovery of the organism. Brucella may be isolated from the vitreous in patients with endophthalmitis or with severe uveitis and vitreal exudates. Culture medium should be observed for three weeks.

Treatment

The treatment of choice for brucellosis, systemic or ocular, consists of the simultaneous administration of Doxycycline 100mg orally twice daily and Rifamycin 300mg orally twice daily. For ocular brucellosis, therapy consists of subconjunctival injections of Tobramycin 20mg every other day for a total of five doses. In patients with acute systemic brucellosis, treatment is given for three to four weeks but in chronic systemic disease, it should be given for a period of three months.

Conclusions

In conclusion, brucellosis is a curable and preventable cause of uveitis and ocular morbidity. The disease should be discovered early and treated promptly and adequately to prevent damage of the ocular structures. With air travel, geographic barriers are overcome and the disease may be seen in any country.

The disease may present with vague and nonspecific symptoms. History of ingestion of raw milk or milk products in an endemic area should give a high index of suspicion. Patients with ocular brucellosis may present with uveitis that can be confused with tuberculosis or other rheumatic causes of uveitis. The predominant ocular manifestations include:
- scleritis,
- granulomatous uveitis,
- posterior choroiditis,
- vitreous bands,
- traction retinal detachment.

Early treatment with specific antibiotics can induce complete recovery of the ocular disease without major sequelae. Subconjunctival Tobramycin should be combined with oral Doxycycline and Rifamycin for an adequate therapy of the intraocular disease.

Table 1. Ocular Manifestations of Brucellosis

Findings:	Scleritis	Retinitis
	Granulomatous uveitis	Retinal vasculitis
	Nongranulomatous uveitis	Retinal vasculitis
	Vitritis	Optic neuritis
	Choroiditi	Papilledema (Pseudotumor cerebri)
Sequelae:	Posterior synechiae	
	Glaucoma	
	Cataract	
	Vitreous fibrosis	
	Traction retinal detachment	

References

1. Abd Elrazak M (1991) Brucella Optic Neuritis. Arch Int Med 151:776-778
2. Bruce D (1887) Note on the Discovery of Microorganism in Malta Fever. Practitioner 39:161
3. Christie AB (1987) Brucellosis. In: Infectious Disease; Epidemiology and Clinical Practice, 4th ed. Edinburgh: Churchill Livingstone pp 1130-1158
4. Grave W, Sturm AW (1983) Brucellosis Associated with a Beauty Parlour. Lancet 1:1326-1327
5. Kaufman AF, Fox MD, Anderson DC et al (1980) Airborne Spread of Brucellosis. Ann NY Acad Sci 353:105
6. Madkour MM, Mohamed AE, Talukder MAS et al (1985) Brucellosis in Saudi Arabia. Saudi Med J 6:324-332
7. Steffen R (1977) Antacids a Risk Factor in Travellers. Scand J Infect Dis 9:311

8. Tabarra KF, Al Kassimi H (1990) Ocular Brucellosis. Br J Ophthalmol 74:249-250
9. Young EJ (1983) Human Brucellosis. Rev Infect Dis 5(5):821-842

Uveitis and Leptospirosis

Irene Castagna, R. Piparo, S. Dolci, R. De Natale

Abstract. The authors report on the outcome of leptospirosis with its various ocular manifestations. The association of ocular manifestations with serological reactions including various antigen tests is emphasized. The incidence of leptospirosis in various inflammatory ocular conditions is analysed and discussed.

Introduction

Leptospirosis is caused by spirochetes and is usually accompanied by fever with a diphasic manifestation. The predilection sites are kidney, liver and meninges, however, various ocular manifestations can be observed during the course of the disease.

In the first phase of the infection, conjunctival hyperemia and diffuse subconjunctival hemorrhages may occur. Subsequent to an acute or chronic anterior uveitis, panuveitis and multifocal choroiditis may be encountered; rarely, an optic neuritis is observed. Ocular findings may also present in seroconverted patients as the only clinical evidence of the infection.

Geographical and local factors may play an important role in the epidemiology of this disease.

At our hospital, we have studied the incidence and distribution of leptospirosis in Southern Italy since 1962. In 1989 (5), we have determined an incidence of leptospirosis in 12% of 87 uveitis patients studied.

In the present report, we wish to further clarify the role of leptospirosis for uveitis of uncertain or unknown etiology.

Study

From 1988 to 1991, 97 subjects (51 male and 46 female) with a mean age of 37 years, ranging from 17 to 68 years, were investigated. In 33 subjects, clinical evidence for acute or recurrent anterior uveitis was found; in 16 a multifocal choroiditis was present and 31 patients showed subconjunctival hemorrhages or conjunctival hyperemia.

This last group of patients was composed of butchers and peasants, the high-risk category. None of the patients evaluated had had a positive history of leptospirosis.

In all of these patients, a complete ophthalmologic work-up and serological tests for leptospirosis were performed. Martin-Pettit agglutination tests for specific antibody identification was carried out by using the following serotypes as antigens:
L.icterohaemorrhagicae (Bianchi 1),
L.copenhageni (Vinberg),
L.canicola (Alarik),
L.pomona (Mezzano),
L.betaviae (Pavia 1),
L.grippotyphosa (Moskva),
L.bratislava (Riccio 2),

L.australis (Ballico),
L.zanoni (Zanoni),
L.saxkoebing (Mus 24),
L.sejroe (Topo 1),
L.castellonis (Castellon 3),
L.tarassovi (Mitis Johnson),
L.poi (Poi),
L.lora (Riccio 37),
L.hardjo (Hardjo prajitno),
L.autumnalis (Akiyami 1,
L.patoc (Patoc 1) and
L.andamana (CH 11).

In each test, a titer of 1:100 was considered positive and in such cases, further titations were done. The control group consisted of 158 clinically healthy age- and sex-matched subjects.

Results

Agglutination tests were positive for L.pomona in 3.4%, L.icterohaemorrhagiae in 2.2%, L.hardjo in 2.2%, L.andamana in 2.2%, L.sejroe in 1.1%, L.canicola in 1.1% and L.poi in 1.1% of the patients (Tab.1).

Serum antibody titers of 11 seropositive patients are shown in Table 2.

Out of 33 patients with recurrent acute anterior uveitis, six were seroconverted (two for L.hardjo 1:100, one for L.canicola 1:100 and one for L.icterohaemorrhagiae 1:500).

Out of 11 patients with sequelae of prior uveitis, three were seroconverted for Leptospires: one for L.andamona 1:100 and for L.sejroe 1:500, one for L.poi 1:100 and one for L.pomona 1:100.

Out of the high-risk group, two patients exhibited antibody titers for L.andamona 1:100 and L.icterohaemorrhagiae 1:100.

In 16 patients with multifocal choroiditis, no seropositives could be detected.

No evidence for leptospirosis seroconversion was found in the control group.

In Table 3, differences in the clinical manifestations of the various patient groups are shown. A higher percentage was found for patients with a history of uveitis, particularly anterior uveitis.

Discussion

Eleven out of 97 patients studied had serological evidence for leptospirosis. Seropositivity may have been induced by previous contact with the microorganism with a subsequent clinically "silent" infectious disease.

These data may be most pertinent to those patients suffering from uveitis or sequelae of it. In these two groups, the highest percentages of seroconversion were observed. In 31 patients with conjunctival hyperemia and subconjunctival hemorrhages, only two cases were seropositive, while those patients with choroiditis were not.

These data support our feeling that despite improved lifestyles and social conditions, leptospirosis still has to be considered in certain ocular inflammatory conditions that quite often go unrecognized. We therefore suggest that serological work-ups of patients suffering from uveitis of uncertain etiology should include leptospirosis.

Table 1. Serum positivity tested with different serovars

No.	PATIENTS	L.I.H.	CANICOLA	POMONA	POI	HARDJO	SEJROE	ADAMANA
1	P.U.						1:500	1:100
6	C.H.							1:100
9	A.U.					1:100		
10	C.H.	1:100						
11	A.U.	1:500 1:100						
14	P.U.				1:100			
17	P.U.			1:100				
22	A.U.			1:100				
26	A.U.		1:100					
31	A.U.			1:100				
33	A.U.					1:100		

P.U. = PREVIOUS UVEITIS C.H. = CONJUNCTIVAL HEMORRAGE A.U. = ANTERIOR UVEITIS

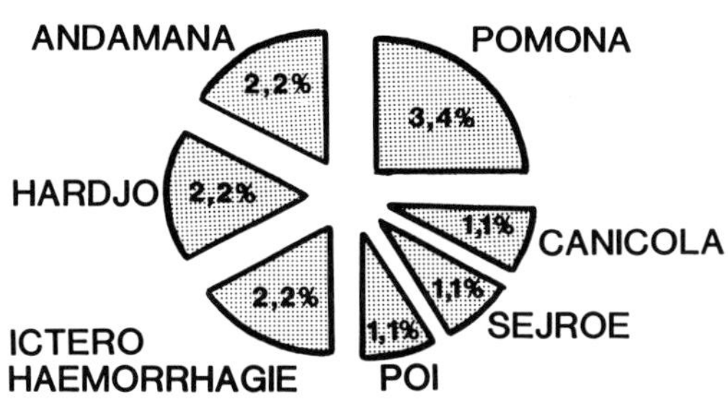

Fig.1. Most frequent agglutinated Serotype

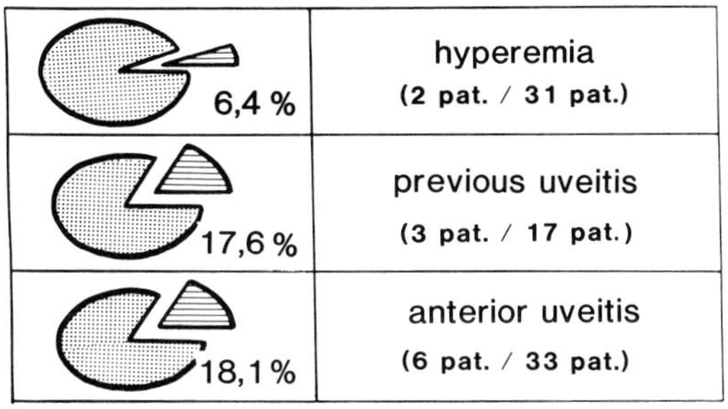

Fig.2. Serum positivity = 11 patients

References

1. Austoni M, Moro F (1952) La uveite quale manifestazione della sindroma oculo-inflammatoria della leptospirosi. Giorn Mal Inf Par 4:339
2. Battistini A (1966) Leptospire Uveitis. Clinical Contribution. Ann Ottal 92/2:77-83
3. Barkay S, Garzozoi H (1984) Leptospirosis and Uveitis. Ann Ophthalmol 16:164-168
4. Beeson PB, Han Key DD, Coger CF (1951) Leptospiral Iridocyclitis: Evidence of Human Infection with L.pomonae in the USA. J Am Med Ass 145:229
5. Castagna I, Piparo R, Dolci S et al (to be published) Inzidenza delle Leptospirosi in Una Indagine Sierologica e Biomicroscopia Oculare Nell'Italia Meridionale. Atti Societa Oftalmologica Mediterranea
6. Cimbal O (1952) Chronische Leptospiren Uveitis. Klin Mbl Augenheilk 119:649
7. David R, Barkay S (1976) Anterior Uveitis and Leptospirosis. Ann Ophthalmol 8:985-962
8. Gutman I, Walsh JB, Knapp AB (1983) Cotton-Wool Spots as a Sign in Leptospirosis. Ophthalmologica 187:133-136
9. Hager G, Mochmann M, Burmeister E (1962) Ocular Disease During and After Leptospiral Infections. Klin Mbl Augenheilk 140:845-854
10. Hegyessy G (1970) Relative Incidence of Eye Complications Accompanying Leptospirosis in Hungary. Szemeszef 107:133-142
11. Imai Y, Suzuki A, Watanabe T et al (1971) Statistical Observation of Endogenous Uveitis for Ten Years in the Department of Ophthalmology, Tohoku University. Clin Ophthalmol 23:736-742
12. Ioli A, Nicosia A (1962) Indagnie Sierologica e Biomicroscopia Oculare ai Fini del Riconoscimento di Leptospirosi in Provincia di Messina. Rivista Italiana de Igiene XXII 6:437-446
13. Pietruschka G, Hergt R (1974) Leptospirosis Uveitis. Klin Mbl Augenheilk 165:279-285
14. Remky H, Metzelberger H (1965) Leptospiral Infections and Uveitis. Klin Mbl Augenheilk 147:1-11
15. Sakharova NM (1962) Early and Late Disease of the Eye in Leptospirosis. Voprosy Oftalmologii 144-153
16. Tarkkanen A, Raitta C (1964) Leptospiral Uveitis. Ophthalmologica 148:91-97

Uveitis in Endemic Syphilis

Khalid F. Tabbara

Abstract. Bejel or non-venereal endemic syhilis, a treponemal infection, is still endemic in many parts of the world including Saudi Arabia.

As in venereal syphilis, man is the reservoir of infection for the endemic form. Transmission is by direct body contact among children and adults. The onset of the disease, however, is usually in childhood. Primary lesions are seldom observed and the late stages may lead to skin and bony changes. Late neurologic and caridovascular lesions are uncommon and congenital transmission is unknown. Although the systemic findings of endemic syphilis have been elucidated, the ocular manifestations have not been previously outlined. We, therefore, decided to study the ocular findings of eight patients with endemic

syphilis. The diagnostic criteria included a positive serology to Treponema pallidum, skin or bone changes, and absence of primary lesion or neurologic involvement. All patients were nomadic or seminomadic and had not travelled out of the Kingdom of Saudi Arabia. All patients had positive serologic tests for Bejel. There were 5 male and 3 female patients with age range of 31-62 years and a mean age of 48 years.
Clinical examination revealed uveitis in 8 patients, optic atrophy in 6, and chorioretinal scars in 4 patients. In four patients who underwent intraocular surgery, two aqueous specimens showed positive antibodies for Treponema pallidum.

Introduction

There are three major genera of spirochetes:
1) Treponema,
2) Borrelia, and
3) Leptospira.

The pathogenic forms of Treponema include
- Treponema pallidum (the causative agent of syphilis),
- Treponema pallidum endemicum (the causative agent of bejel),
- Treponema pertenue (the causative agent of yaws),
- Treponema carateum (the causative agent of pinta) and
- Treponema paraluis-cuniculi (the causative agent of rabbit syphilis).

There are other forms of Treponema which are non-pathogenic and form a part of the normal oral flora including Treponema macrodentium and Treponema vincentii. The Treponema makes up a group of interrelated organisms that are separated by differences in the types of disorders they produce. The infections caused by Treponemas is known collectively as treponematoses. The Treponematoses behave similar in many ways with respect to the elicited immune response. Treponematoses can be differentiated in four major groups. Syphilis is divided into venereal and non-venereal forms including bejel, yaws and pinta.

It is speculated that species of treponema have their origin in tree-living monkeys in tropical Africa. Man may have become infected with Treponema and served as the main host reservoir for this infection for thousands of years. The Treponema was carried through the Bering strait with the migration of primates to the Americas causing yaws or pinta in their new home. The inhabitants of the dry hot regions of Northern Africa developed a non-venereal form of syphilis, bejel, which is transmitted by bodily contact among adults.

Bejel occurs in parts of East Africa, the Near East and South East Asia. The disease has also been reported in Yugoslavia. Prior to mass treatment under the supervision of the WHO, patients with non-venereal syphilis made up as much as 5% of the population. Active infection, however, has been almost eradicated. The prevalence of the disease has been decreasing in many parts of the world including Saudi Arabia. The current patchy distribution of the disease is predominantly related to inadequate health services and to an increase in the atypical and subclinical form of the disease.

Clinicians are largely not familiar with this entity. Furthermore, the disease cannot be differentiated from venereal syphilis on serologic grounds. All available serologic assays for syphilis would be positive in patients with non-venereal syphilis. Similar to venereal syphilis, man is the only reservoir of the infection.

The onset of the disease is in early childhood, and the infection is usually transmitted via non-venereal routes: by intimate skin contact, kissing, and the use of common fomites or drinking vessels. Familial transmission is common. Congenital transmission has not been reported.

The main objective of this study is to report the major ocular findings among 8 patients with non-venereal syphilis.

Patients and Methods

A total of 8 patients with bejel were included prospectively in this study. Each patient underwent complete ophthalmological evaluation including biomicroscopy, ophthalmoscopy, visual acuity testing, and tonometry. X-rays of the lower extremities were performed and blood for luetic serology was requested on each patient.

Other causes of uveitis were ruled out by the history, clinical examination, and appropriate laboratory testing. The diagnosis of bejel was based on all of the following:

1) the absence of a history of a primary lesion,
2) the presence of reactive syphilitic serology by specific tests for syphilis,
3) the lack of history of promiscuity,
4) the absence of cardiovascular or neurologic findings and
5) the radiological evidence of osteoperiostitis of the tibia.

Results

Five male and three female patients with a mean age of 48 years (range:31-62 years) were examined.

- All patients had evidence of anterior uveitis (Fig.1) with posterior synechiae.
- A fibrovascular membrane in the pupillary area was noted in two patients.
- Four patients had clinical evidence of chorioretinitis. One patient had destruction of his nasal cartilage. None of the patients had cardiovascular or neurologic findings. All patients had radiologic evidence of osteoperiostitis of the tibia or fibula with cortical thickening and osteolytic lesions. One had gumma of the lower tibia.

All patients had a reactive syphilis serology by Treponema pallidum hemagglutination test and FTA-ABS test. All active ocular lesions responded to benzathine penicillin 2.4x106 IU once every week for three weeks.

Discussion

Bejel remains to be an endemic disease in many parts of the world including Saudi Arabia. The disease is common among nomads but rare among urban communities (1). The disease cannot be differentiated from syphilis on serologic grounds. It is of crucial importance to be familiar with this entity. Venereal diseases carry certain social stigmata, and mistaking non-venereal disease with a venereal entity may carry serious social consequences.

The uveitis and chorioretinitis associated with bejel do respond to systemic penicillin. Routine serologic testing for syphilis is man datory for patients presenting with uveitis in endemic areas.

Bejel is a preventable and curable cause of uveitis. Early diagnosis and prompt treatment with penicillin may prevent irreversible damage to the ocular structure. The current moral standards in Saudi Arabia may help in hindering the transmission of venereal syphilis, but facilitated communication by air travel with sexual contacts of Saudis abroad may contribute to an increase in venereal syphilis in the future.

It remains to be shown whether bejel affords protection against venereal syphilis.

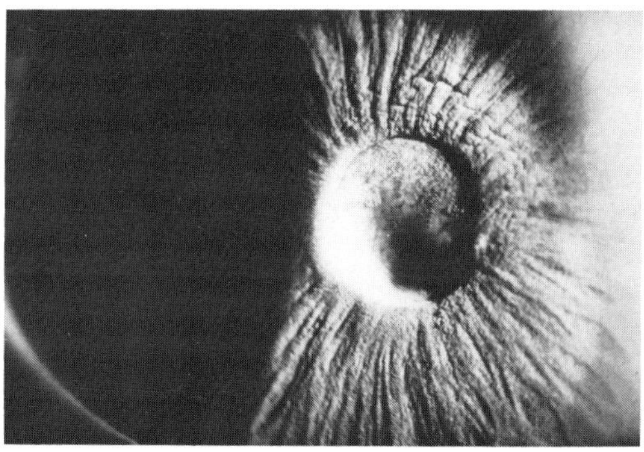

Fig.1. Posterior synechiae, pupillary membrane and cataract are shown in a patient with bejel.

References

1. Pace JL, Csonka GW (1984) Endemic Non-Venereal Syphilis (Bejel) in Saudi-Arabia. Br J Ven Dis 60:293-297
2. Pace JL (1983) Trepanematosis in Saudi Arabia. Saudi Med J 4:211-220
3. Tabbara KF, Al-Kaff A, Fadel T (1989) Ocular Manifestations of Bejel. Ophthalmolgy 96:(7)1087-1091

Viral

Acute Retinal Necrosis: Laboratory Diagnosis

Aize Kijlstra, Joke H. de Boer, Leny Luyendijk

Abstract. Laboratory diagnosis of the Acute Retinal Necrosis Syndrome is focussed on the fact that it is now accepted that this disease is caused by a reactivation of latent neurotropic viruses of the herpes group.
Determinations of viral antibody titers in acute and convalescent sera are generally not informative. Since therapy must often be started before results of cultures are available, rapid detection of locally produced anti-Herpes Virus antibodies or cell associated viral antigens can be a precious tool in the diagnosis of ocular viral infection. Intraocular synthesis of IgG antibodies against Herpes Simplex Virus or Varicella Zoster Virus is considered as an indirect proof of uveoretinal infection. To prove the validity of this hypothesis we have compared local viral antibody production in three patient groups, namely the Acquired Immmunodeficiency Syndrome with retinitis, toxoplasma

retinochoroiditis and the Acute Retinal Necrosis. Paired serum and vitreous/aqueous samples were tested for total immunoglobulin G levels and antibodies to Herpes Simplex Virus, Cytomegalovirus, Varicella Zoster Virus, Epstein-Barr Virus and toxoplasma using an immunofluorescence technique.

Seven out of 20 Acute Retinal Necrosis patients tested showed evidence of local antibody production against Herpes Simplex Virus or Varicella Zoster Virus whereas none of the 12 toxoplasma patients were positive. Two out of 26 Acquired Immmunodeficiency Syndrome patients tested had a positive response against Varicella Zoster Virus or Herpes Simplex Virus.

Negative results in the Acute Retinal Necrosis group were probably due to massive blood-retinal barrier breakdown leading to leakage of IgG into the eye thereby masking local antibody production as determined by the Goldmann-Witmer coefficient.

The Polymerase Chain Reaction to detect viral nucleic acids in combination with the immunologic detection of viral antigens and antibodies will hopefully provide highly sensitive and specific results in the near future.

Introduction

The Acute Retinal Necrosis Syndrome is a serious blinding disease which is considered to be caused by viruses of the Herpes group (5).

The disease was first described by Urayama (13) in Japan and is characterized by a necrotizing retinitis, vasculo occlusive retinal arteritis, vitritis, panuveitis and retinal detachment. Viruses which have been implicated in Acute Retinal Necrosis include Varicella Zoster Virus, Herpes Simplex Virus, Cytomegalovirus and Epstein-Barr Virus. Of 26 eyes with Acute Retinal Necrosis studied in Japan, five were due to Herpes Simplex Virus Type 1, 11 to Varicella Zoster Virus and 10 were unknown (9).

It is now accepted that most cases Acute Retinal Necrosis are caused by a recrudescence of a latent infection with either Herpes Simplex Virus or Varicella Zoster Virus. Evidence for this theory was obtained in a study showing intrathecal antibody production against these viruses in Acute Retinal Necrosis (1).

Diagnosis

A number of intraocular diseases show certain features in common with the Acute Retinal Necrosis and should be thought of in the differential diagnosis (5). A number of serological laboratory tests may help in the differential diagnosis (Tab.1).

Since viruses are implicated in Acute Retinal Necrosis laboratory diagnosis is mainly directed towards a direct or indirect proof of the viral cause of the disease.

Isolation and culture of the virus, by taking a chorioretinal biopsy, vitreous or aqueous sample is a time consuming technique which may often be negative. Varicella Zoster Virus can be cultured but is a relatively labile Virus which is easily destroyed if not adequately stored or transported to the laboratory. Culbertson and coworkers were the first to report a positive culture for Varicella Zoster Virus from a vitreous sample taken from enucleated eyes of patients with Acute Retinal Necrosis (4). Since Acute Retinal Necrosis may have a rapid progressive course and the time period needed to culture this virus may take weeks, this approach may not be satisfactory for a fast routine diagnostic screening.

Identification of viruses in biopsy material by electron microscopy is also a procedure too laborious and time consuming to be considered as a routine test. Inclusion bodies and Herpes-like particles habe been observed in the retina of Acute Retinal Necrosis patients by light and electron microscopy (3).

Histological and cytochemical techniques to identify the virus in biopsy specimens have improved markedly since the advent of specific immunological probes such as monoclonal antibodies. Varicella Zoster Virus antigens were first reported in the Western literature by Culbertson and coworkers (4) in blind enucleated eyes. Varicella Zoster Virus antigens were also detected in cells from vitreous aspirates in two out of four patients tested by Soushi and coworkers (10). Since indentification of viral antigens in infected cells by immunohistochemistry only takes a few hours, this procedure is recommended for rapid diagnosis of uveitis of unknown etiology (10).

Detection of viral antigens in ocular specimens using either Enzyme-Linked Immunosorbent Assays or radioimmunoassays has not yet been reported.

Indirect proof of a viral cause may be obtained by determining local antibody production against the viral species suspected of causing the disease. Determination of acute and convalescent serum viral titers against Herpes Simplex Virus, Varicella Zoster Virus and Cytomegalovirus are generally not informative (3). Elevated intraocular Varicella Zoster Virus antibody levels have now been reported by various groups (8,11,12).

Since Acute Retinal Necrosis is considered a reactivation of latent neurotropic viruses, certain authors have suggested to first determine local antibody production in the central nervous system by taking a cerebrospinal fluid tap (1).

In the Netherlands the participants of the Dutch Uveitis Study Group have investigated the usefulness of local antibody determination in aqueous humor or vitreous taps. The results show that a positive test result is obtained in 35% of cases investigated indicating the need for additional improvement of laboratory tests. As suggested by others (10), a combination of viral antigen and antibody detection may improve the reliability of the laboratory test.

Patients and Methods

The department of Ophthalmo-Immunology of the Netherlands Ophthalmic Research Institute serves as a national diagnostic center for the laboratory diagnosis of uveitis.

Aqueous or vitreous with paired serum samples were tested for total IgG, albumin and for antibodies against toxoplasma gondii, Herpes Simplex Virus, Varicella Zoster Virus, Epstein-Barr Virus and Cytomegalovirus as described below. Details of the techniques have been published elsewhere (2,7,8).

Total immunoglobulin (IgG) and albumin levels were determined in serum and aqueous using radial immunodiffusion (Mancini). Serum was tested in a 1:200 dilution and aqueous undiluted or 1:2 diluted. Agar

(Difco laboratories) 1.5% plates containing a 1:100 dilution of anti human-IgG precipitating antiserum (Central Laboratory of the Red Cross Bloodtransfusion Service, Amsterdam) were used for this purpose. Various dilutions of a normal human serum known to contain 10mg/ml were used as a standard. Albumin was measured with commercially available radial immunodiffusion plates (LC-partigen, Behringwerke, Marburg, Germany).

The fixed cell immunofluorescence technique (Gull Laboratories, Salt Lake City, Utah, USA) available as a ready for use test kit served as a quantitative detection method for antibodies against Cytomegalovirus, Herpes Simplex Virus, Epstein-Barr Virus and Varicella Zoster Virus respectively. Serial two-fold dilutions of serum (starting point 1:16) and aqueous (starting point undiluted) were put on top of the reaction sites of the 10-well slides with the fixed virus-infected human fibroblast cells. Slides were placed in a moist chamber and incubated at room temperature for 30 minutes. After rinsing and drying the procedure was repeated with a goat anti-human FITC labeled heavy-chain specific IgG. If antibodies to the virus are present they will bind to the antigen substrate and not rinse off. Subsequently, when fluorescinated anti-human IgG is added to the reaction site, it will bind to the antibodies, causing the virus infected cells to fluoresce when viewed through a fluorescence microscope. The reaction was positive when approximately 10% of the cells in each field exhibited a greenish fluorescence. The remaining uninfected cells are stained red and serve as a control. The titer was the highest dilution which produced a positive reaction. Alltogether the mentioned tests required no more than 50 - 100 μl of material and could be performed within a few hours. The reading of the radial immunodiffusion plates was performed after 24 hours and is the rate limiting step in the whole procedure.

Antibodies detected in the aqueous can originate from the peripheral blood or from within the eye. Intraocular synthesis of antibodies is considered to have taken place if the relative amount of specific antibodies compared to the total immunoglobulin level found in the aqueous exceeds that measured in a paired serum sample.

Theoretically a coefficient above 1.0 would indicate a local antibody production within the eye. In view of the variability in the results of the various measurements, an antibody coefficient above 3.0 is considered significant.

The results of the vitreous and aqueous testing in the three patient groups is represented in Table 2. Of the 20 patients with a clinical diagnosis of Acute Retinal Necrosis five had a positive coefficient indicating local antibody production against Varicella Zoster Virus (Tab.2). Three out of 20 patients had local antibody production against Herpes Simplex Virus. These three cases were found after investigating a vitreous aspirate. One of these patients also had a positive test for Varicella Zoster Virus. In total therefore a positive test result was obtained in 7 (35%) cases. Local Cytomegalovirus, Epstein-Barr Virus or toxoplasma antibody production was found in none of the cases of Acute Retinal Necrosis tested. In three out of 12 patients a positive test result was obtained for Varicella Zoster Virus using an aqueous sample. Two positive

Varicella Zoster Virus tests results were obtained from a vitreous sample.

In the toxoplasma chorioretinitis group no local antibody synthesis was detected against Cytomegalovirus, Epstein-Barr Virus or Varicella Zoster Virus whereas 28 of the fourty samples tested showed a positive antibody coefficient for toxoplasma. Of the AIDS patients tested most of the positive results were obtained for Cytomegalovirus.

Discussion

Determination of local intraocular Herpes virus antibody production is an important diagnostic tool in suspected cases of the Acute Retinal Necrosis Syndrome. As we have experienced it may be decisive concerning therapeutic measures in these patients (2). The time point when an aqueous tap is taken during the course of the disease may be quite important. If aqueous is obtained in the late stages of the disease there is a good chance that due to severe inflammation a blood aqueous barrier breakdown may have caused prominent serum leakage into the vitreous and aqueous. In that case the antiviral titer in the aqueous/vitreous is not a true reflection of the intraocular antiviral antibody production and determination of the local synthesis of specific antibodies as determined by the Goldmann-Witmer calculation becomes impossible.

Of the seven Acute Retinal Necrosis patients showing local intraocular antibody production in this study, six had a higher anti-Varicella Zoster Virus or anti-Herpes Simplex Virus antibody titer in the eye as compared to the blood. In one patient no antibodies were detectable in serum whereas the vitreous aspirate showed a titer of 1:64 against Herpes Simplex Virus. This remarkable phenomenon of higher antibody titers in the eye has been observed earlier in horses suffering from leptospirosis uveitis (6).

In one Acute Retinal Necrosis patient we found a positive antibody coefficient for both Herpes Simplex virus as well as Varicella Zoster Virus whereby very high titers were found for Varicella Zoster Virus. A similar finding has been reported by others (12) and may be explained by an antibody response against cross-reacting antigens.

Direct proof of specific intraocular infection would involve the detection of the virus itself or its antigens in the aqueous sample. Future diagnostic procedures will include detection of the presence of virus DNA or RNA using Polymerase Chain Reaction techniques. In view of the fact that in Acute Retinal Necrosis one is dealing with latent viruses it may be advisable to analyse RNA to eliminate false positive results. Combination of modern molecular biological techniques with the classical immunologic detection of viral antigens and antibodies will be the future laboratory test to confirm a suspected diagnosis of the Acute Retinal Necrosis Syndrome.

Table 1. Differential Diagnosis of Acute Retinal Necrosis

	Laboratory Test
cytomegalovirus retinitis	local antibody production
toxoplasma	local antibody production
sarcoid	ACE/lysozyme
lymphoma	cytology
retinoblastoma	DNA testing
toxocariasis	local antibody production
syphilis	serology

Table 2. Local Antibody Production in the Eye

Diagnosis	CMV[1]	HSV[1]	VZV[1]	EBV[1]	TOXO[1]
Retinitis and AIDS 12/41	1/26	1/25	1/22	2/31	
Acute Retinal Necrosis	0/12	3/20	5/20	0/15	0/8
Toxoplasmosis	0/6	0/12	0/12	0/5	28/40

[1] CMV=Cytomegalovirus, HSV=Herpes Simplex Virus, VZV=Varicella Zoster Virus, EBV=Epstein-Barr-Virus, TOXO=Toxoplasmosis. Numbers indicate patients with a coefficient larger than three compared to total numbers of patients tested. Sufficient material was not always available for all the tests.

References

1. Azazzi el M, Samuelsson A, Linde A et al (1991) Intrathecal Antibody Production Against Viruses of the Herpes- virus Family in Acute Retinal Necrosis Syndrome. Am J Ophthalmol 112:76-82
2. Baarsma GS, Luyendijk L, Kijlstra A et al (1991) Analysis of Local Antibody Production in the Vitreous Humor of Patients with Severe Uveitis. Am J Ophthalmol 112:147-150
3. Culbertson WW, Blumenkranz MS, Haines H et al (1982) The Acute Retinal Necrosis Syndrome. Part 2. Histopathology and Etiology. Ophthalmology 89:1317-1325
4. Culbertson WW, Blumenkranz MS, Pepose JS et al (1986) Varicella Zoster Virus is a Cause of the Acute Retinal Necrosis Syndrome. Ophthalmology 93:559-569
5. Duker JS, Blumenkranz MS (1991) Diagnosis and Management of the Acute Retinal Necrosis (ARN) Syndrome. Surv Ophthalmol 35:327-343
6. Goldmann H, Witmer R (1954) Antikörper im Kammerwasser. Ophthalmologica 127:323-330
7. Kijlstra A, van den Horn GJ, Luyendijk L et al (1990) Laboratory Tests in Uveitis. New Developments in the Analysis of Local Antibody Production. Doc Ophthalmol 75:225-231
8. Luyendijk L, van den Horn GJ, Visser OHE et al (1990) Detection of Locally Produced Antibodies to Herpes Viruses in the Aqueous of Patients with Acquired Immune Deficiency Syndrome (AIDS) or Acute Retinal Necrosis Syndrome. Curr Eye Research 9S:7-11
9. Matsuo T, Morimoto K, Matsuo N (1991) Factors Associated with Poor Visual Outcome in Acute Retinal Necrosis. Br J Ophthalmol 75:450-454
10. Soushi S, Ozawa H, Matsuhashi M et al (1988) Demonstration of Varicella Zoster Virus Antigens in the Vitreous Aspirates of Patients with Acute Retinal Necrosis Syndrome. Ophthalmol 95:1394-1398

11. Suttorp-Schulten MS, Zaal MJ, Luyendijk L et al (1989) Aqueous Humor Tap and Serology in Acute Retinal Necrosis. Am J Ophthalmol 108:327-328
12. Takano S, Seki F, Okitsu Y et al (1990) Herpes Viral Antibodies of Intraocular Fluid in Acute Retinal Necrosis (ARN). Ocular Immunology Today 146-150
13. Urayama A, Yamada N, Sasaki T et al (1971) Unilateral Acute Uveitis with Retinal Periarteritis and Detachment. Jpn J Clin Ophthalmol 25:607-619

Polymerase Chain Reaction in the Diagnosis of the Acute Retinal Necrosis Syndrome

Jürgen Gerling, Hans-Martin Seuffert, Wolfgang Schrader and Lutz Hansen

Abstract. The Acute Retinal Necrosis Syndrome is a disease entity, which occurs at an increasing frequency comprising peripheral vaso-occlusive retinitis, papillitis and anterior uveitis. The disease is supposed to be caused by alpha Herpes group viruses. Because of the progressive course of the disease including retinal detachments and peripheral retinal shrinkage, an early diagnosis and therapy is important and essential for the post-treatment results.
In all patients with the clinical features of the Acute Retinal Necrosis Syndrome local antibody synthesis in the anterior chamber of the eye and the vitreous should be controlled (Herpes Simplex Virus, Varizella Zoster Virus; IgA- and IgG-ELISA). The diagnosis of Acute Retinal Necrosis Syndrome due to an intraocular viral infection can be established by elevated virus antibody titers in the intraocular fluids compared to serum or by an elevated Goldmann-Witmer coefficient. Both methods have specific disadvantages.
The most sensitive test to prove the existence of intraocular virus DNA is the polymerase chain reaction. We have performed polymerase chain reaction in the course of the disease and present our results in three patients. With respect to the small amount of specimens and the low concentration of the virus in the intraocular fluids this copy process is much more successful than a direct virus detection method employing electron microscopy.

Introduction

The Acute Retinal Necrosis Syndrome is a disease of the posterior segment of the eye. It was first mentioned in 1971 in Japan (17). In the 1980s when the syndrome was more frequently seen it became more and more evident that herpes viruses cause this devastating disease (1,5,6,8,10). Although it is typical for the disease to affect clinically healthy patients, reports on Acute Retinal Necrosis in immunosuppressed patients have recently been published (3,4).

Acute Retinal Necrosis Syndrome typically starts with a peripheral retinitis. Ophthalmoscopically, retinal lesions appear as confluent areas of retinal whitening that may vary from small patches to broad zones. Retinal vasculitis (Fig.1) primarily affects the arteries and is severe and obliterative in nature. Further signs of the Acute Retinal Necrosis Syndrome are a vitritis, a papillitis (Fig.2) and an anterior uveitis. Fig.3 shows the anterior segment of a 12 year old patient with Acute Retinal Necrosis. Fourteen days after the initial symptoms large endothelial precipitates and an aqueous flare in the anterior chamber of the eye could be found. Because of the typical course of the disease Acute Retinal Necrosis has been classified into four different stages (7).

Retinal detachment caused by proliferative vitreoretinopathy may develop later in the course of the disease in about 80% of the eyes (2).

Since the syndrome is a severe disease it has become obvious that an early diagnosis based on clinical symptoms and an immediate therapy are essential for post-treatment results. A medical therapy with Acyclovir and Prednisolon and a peripheral photocoagulation should be performed as early as possible. Surgical treatment (encircling band, pars plana vitrectomy, silicone oil, photocoagulation) should be added at the first signs of proliferative vitreoretinopathy.

However, we face the important problem to start treatment merely on the clinical diagnosis without confirmation of the causative agent. Therefore, the clinical diagnosis should be supported by laboratory methods as early as possible.

Methods established so far are
- electron microscopy (5),
- viral cultures (6,11) and
- antibody titers (5,13,15).

We have also performed the polymerase chain reaction (14) from intraocular fluids.

Patients and Methods

In three patients with the clinical diagnosis of Acute Retinal Necrosis Syndrome we have attempted to establish the diagnosis by electron microscopy, antibody titers and polymerase chain reaction of intraocular fluids. Viral cultures were not performed because they rarely grow (8).

Undiluted aqueous humor and vitreous were aspirated under sterile conditions twice in the course of the disease. In both samples we tried to detect viral particles by electron microscopy.

Antibody studies of the serum were applied as following: Treponema pallidum hemagglutination, Candida-IgG hemagglutination and IgM immunofluorescent antibody tests, Toxoplasmosis complement binding reaction, immunofluorescent antibody tests and immunohemagglutination, HIV agglutination tests, Cytomegalovirus Enzyme-Linked-Immunosorbent-Assays (ELISA)(IgG and IgM) and Epstein Barr Virus immunofluorescent antibody tests (IgG and IgM), Herpes Simplex Virus ELISAs (IgA), Herpes Simplex Virus immunofluorescent antibody tests (IgG) and Varicella Zoster Virus ELISAs (IgA) and Varicella Zoster Virus immunofluorescent antibody tests (IgG).

Antibody studies for intraocular fluids included the same tests for Cytomegalovirus, Epstein Barr Virus, Herpes Simplex Virus, and Varicella Zoster Virus.

Another method to confirm the presence of a viral agent is the polymerase chain reaction. The test has been introduced in 1985 (14) and is an in vitro enzymatic cyclic amplification of genetic material (18). With the polymerase chain reaction it is possible to detect very small amounts of DNA particles (less than 100) in small specimens (Fig.4).

A cycle begins with heat denaturation of the DNA at 94°C for one minute. In a second step the temperature of the sample is reduced to 55°C for another minute. This allows a specific primer, HSV-01 and 02-Plasmid pFR 106 to anneal and to hybridize to opposite strands of the target sequence. Thus, the primers are oriented with their 3'ends pointing towards each other. In a third phase (72°C for two minutes) the thermostable enzyme Taq-DNA-polymerase, isolated from the thermophilic bacterium Thermus aquaticus, amplifies the genetic sequence before another cycle begins. The heat denaturation of the DNA is the initial step again.

Each of the 36 cycles used in our experiment doubles the amount of the DNA fragment produced in the previous cycle. With this method it is possible to get a billionfold copy of DNA within a few hours. The sample is finally analyzed by a polyacrylamide gel electrophoresis.

Results

Patient 1

Patient K.K., a 57 year old healthy male, was admitted with a stage 2 Acute Retinal Necrosis Syndrome featuring a confluent necrotizing retinitis, vasculitis and moderate vitritis six days after onset of the first symptoms. Physical and serological examinations were unremarkable. Six weeks and 10 weeks after the initial symptoms we performed electron microscopy of the vitreous specimen and antibody ratios of the vitreous to the serum. At this time polymerase chain reaction was not available for viral diagnostics.

On both occasions, electron microscopy was negative but the diagnosis could be confirmed by a highly (> >4:1) elevated Herpes Simplex Virus Enzyme-Linked-Immunosorbent-Assay (IgA) in the vitreous compared to serum. The remaining titers were within normal limits.

Patient 2

Patient S.B., a 12 year old otherwise healthy female, was admitted with a stage 3 Acute Retinal Necrosis Syndrome exhibiting necrotizing retinitis, vitritis, papilledema and anterior segment inflammation 14 days after onset of the first symptoms. Physical and serological examinations were unremarkable. At admission, a diagnostic vitrectomy and an anterior chamber tap were performed before initiation of the virustatic treatment. After 6 weeks of medical treatment a second vitrectomy was required for therapeutic reasons.

Electron microscopy of the vitreous specimens was negative both times. The antibody ratio was determined for the vitreous and the aqueous humor compared to the serum level. Herpes Simplex Virus IgG immunofluorescent antibody test showed a slight (2:1) elevation with 1:640 in the vitreous compared to 1:320 in the serum. This marginal elevation could not definitely confirm our clinical diagnosis. The result of the polymerase chain reaction two weeks after the initial symptoms is shown in Fig.6. Lane one of the gel electrophoresis shows the negative control indicating that the reaction has not been contaminated with external

DNA. Lane 10 shows the marker of 123 base pairs. Five and six were not used in this experiment. In 7, 8 and 9 different concentrations of Herpes Simplex Virus plasmid pFR 106 can be identified. Lanes two and three are samples of vitreous and aqueous humor (lane four) from our patient. It also shows Herpes Simplex Virus pFR 106 in the vitreous and aqueous humor.

A similar result for both fluids was obtained 6 weeks later.

Patient 3

Patient M.H., a 68 year old healthy female, was admitted with a stage 4 Acute Retinal Necrosis Syndrome with necrotizing retinitis, vitritis, papilledema, anterior segment inflammation and retinal detachment 6 weeks after the onset of the first symptoms. Physical and serological examinations were normal. A vitrectomy had to be performed 8 weeks after the initial symptoms because of proliferative vitreoretinopathy.

While electron microscopy was negative, Varicella Zoster Virus Enzyme Linked Immunosorbent Assay (IgA) showed a fourfold elevation in the vitreous compared to serum. Polymerase chain reaction for Herpes simplex was negative while polymerase chain reaction for Varicella Zoster Virus was positive in the anterior chamber fluid and in the vitreous.

Discussion

The Acute Retinal Necrosis Syndrome is a severe ophthalmologic disease that has caused a high percentage of blindness in those times when no antiviral drugs had been at hand. Nowadays an early diagnosis based on the clinical symptoms and an immediate therapy may improve the post-treatment results and prevent blindness. As treatment usually starts without confirmation of the causative agent, it is important to get laboratory results as quickly as possible. Therefore, application of new diagnostic procedures may be necessary. It remains to be seen if an anterior chamber tap as recommended by Suttorp-Schulten and coworkers (16) or a diagnostic vitrectomy should be preferred.

It is well known that a viral culture although it may directly show the virus is not worthwhile for clinical application, because it often fails (8). Similar experiences have already been made with electron microscopy. It is a time-consuming method that also often fails to detect a viral agent. In our patient we could not find a virus in any of our three subjects by these methods.

The indirect method of specific antibody testing in the serum and in intraocular fluids has shown intraocular antibody titer elevations in all three patients. This method does not prove the virus directly but persistent and definite intraocular antibody titer elevations as in the first and third cases strongly support the clinical diagnosis. On the other hand, slight elevations of IgG as in the second case should not be considered valuable for the confirmation of a diagnosis. The demonstration of intraocular antibody synthesis by the Goldmann-Witmer ratio (19) should be preferred if possible. It has the disadvantage that even larger amounts of intraocular specimens are needed.

Polymerase chain reaction is reported to show Varicella Zoster Virus in clinical cases of Acute Retinal Necrosis (9,12(this work)) and we were able to demonstrate Herpes Simplex Virus oligonucleotides in the anterior chamber and the vitreous at different stages of the Acute Retinal Necrosis Syndrome. It is a direct proof, because intraocular DNA is amplified and it is a relatively fast method. Even small amounts of DNA are sufficient to achieve a positive result, which is especially important for the diagnosis of intraocular infection. However, one has to take into account that control studies of patients without retinitis are necessary.

From our results and other studies we may conclude that after the clinical diagnosis of an Acute Retinal Necrosis Syndrome has been made polymerase chain reaction and antibody testing are the appropriate laboratory methods to start with. Both methods together help to ensure adequate treatment at an early stage of the disease.

Additionally, the incidence of retinitis is increasing considerably for example in the acquired immunodeficiency syndrome. Even simultaneous infections by more than one microorganism may occur. In this respect polymerase chain reaction and antibody testing seem to become important tools to establish the correct diagnosis.

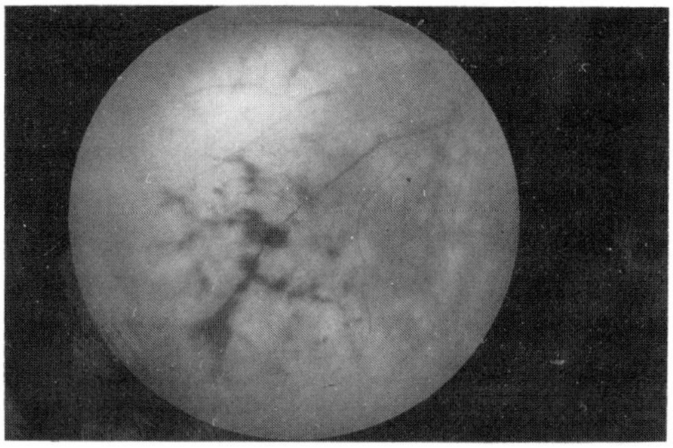

Fig.1. Peripheral retinitis and retinal vasculitis (stage 1) in a 57 year old patient with Acute Retinal Necosis 6 days after initial symptoms.

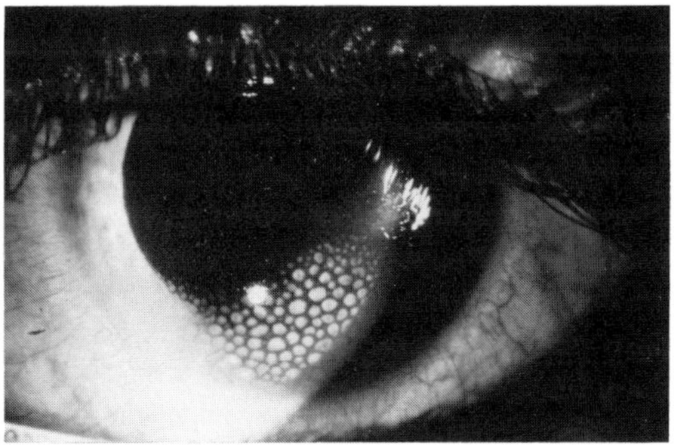

Fig.2. Iridocyclitis with large endothelial precipitates in a 12 year old patient 14 days after initial symptoms.

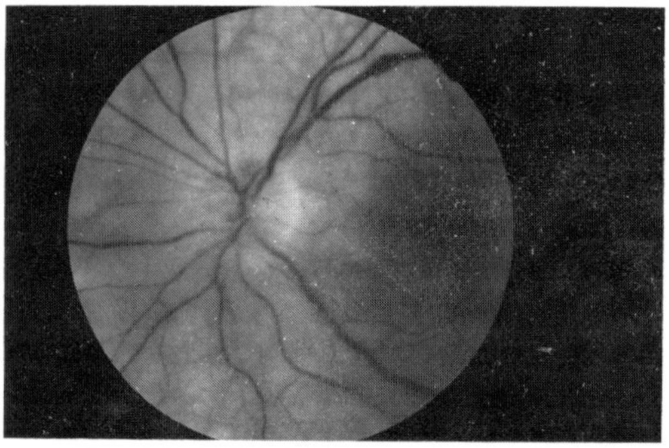

Fig.3. Papillitis with beginning vitritis in stage 2 of the disease.

Patient	Antibody vitreous/serum	PCR (aqu. humor, vitreous)	EM
K.K.	HSV -IgA-ELISA >>4/1	*	—
S.B.	HSV-IgG-IFT 2/1	++ HSV	—
M.H.	VZV -IgA-ELISA 4/1	– HSV	—

Fig.5. Three patients with Acute Retinal Necrosis. Laboratory testing. On the left the antibody concentration of the vitreous and the serum is given as a ratio. It shows elevated intraocular titers for all three patients. In one patient (*) polymerase chain reaction was not performed, because the method was not yet available. Electron microscopy was negative in all three patients.

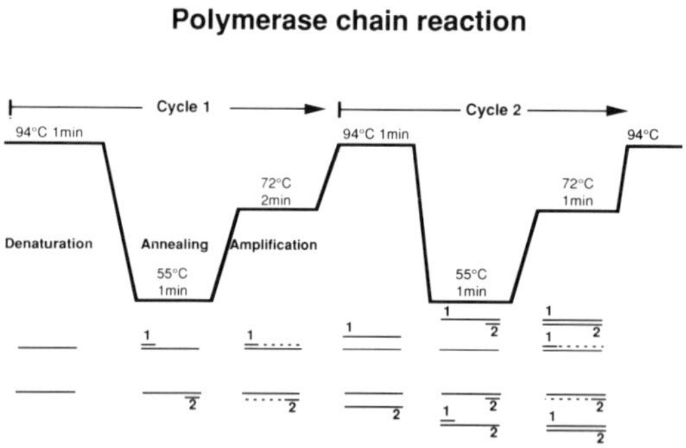

Fig.4. Polymerase chain reaction. The upper line shows the duration of three different phases of the polymerase chain reaction and the course of reaction temperatures. Two identical cycles are shown. In the lower part of the figure the amplification and amount of DNA-sequences is presented. The specific primers 1 und 2 are necessary to anneal in 3`5`and 5`3`direction.

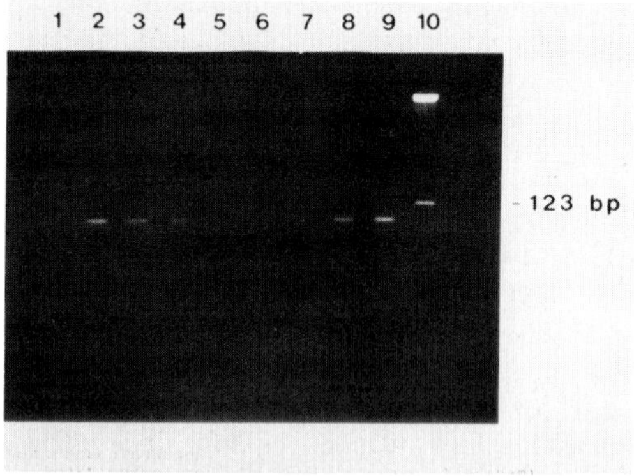

Fig.6. Result of the gel electrophoresis after polymerase chain reaction from patient S.B. Lane 1 shows the negative control, indicating that the reaction was not contaminated with external DNA. Lane 10 gives the marker (123 base paires) indicating correct work-out of the electrophoresis. Five and 6 were not used in this experiment. In 7,8 and 9 different concentrations of a well known sequence of Herpes simplex DNA can be identified. Lanes 2,3,4 are samples of aqueous humor and vitreous from our patient and show the typical Herpes simplex band (see 7 to 9). This result was obtained at two different stages of the disease.

References

1. Blumenkranz MS, Culbertson WW, Clarkson JG et al (1986) Treatment of the Acute Retinal Necrosis Syndrome with Intravenous Acyclovir. Ophthalmology 93:296-300
2. Clarkson JG, Blumenkranz MS, Culbertson WW (1984) Retinal Detachment Following the Acute Retinal Necrosis Syndrome. Ophthalmology 91:1665-1668
3. Chambers RB, Derick RJ, Davidorf FH et al (1989) Varizella-Zoster Retinitis in Human Immunodeficiency Virus Infection. Arch Ophthalmol 107:960-961
4. Chess J, Marcus DM (1988) Zoster-Related Bilateral Acute Retinal Necrosis Syndrome as Presenting Sign in AIDS. Ann Ophthalmol 20:431-435
5. Culbertson WW, Blumenkranz MS, Haines H et al (1982) The Acute Retinal Necrosis Syndrome. Part 2: Histopathology and Etiology. Ophthalmology 89: 1317-1325
6. Culbertson WW, Blumenkranz MS, Pepose JS et al (1986) Varizella Zoster Virus is a Cause of the Acute Retinal Necrosis Syndrome. Ophthalmology 93:559-569
7. Duker JS, Blumenkranz MS (1991) Diagnosis and Management of the Acute Retinal Necrosis (ARN) Syndrome. Surv Ophthalmol 35:327-343
8. Freeman WR, Thomas EL, Rao NA et al (1986) Demonstration of Herpes Group Virus in Acute Retinal Necrosis Syndrome. Am J Ophthalmol 102:701-709
9. Garweg J, Fenner T, Winter R et al (1991) The Diagnostic Tool of the PCR in the Diagnosis of the Acute Retinal Necrosis Syndrome. Fortschr Ophthalmol 88 (Suppl. II):389
10. Holland GN, Togni BI, Briones OC et al (1987) A Microscopic Study of Herpes Simplex Virus Retinopathy in Mice. Invest Ophthalmol Vis Sci 28:1181-1190
11. Lewis ML, Culbertson WW, Post JD et al (1989) Herpes Simplex Virus Type 1. A Cause of the Acute Retinal Necrosis Syndrome. Ophthalmology 96:875-878
12. Nishi M, Hondo R, Mori S et al (1991) The Use of Polymerase Chain Reaction (PCR) for the Detection of Varicella Zoster Genome in Acute Retinal Necrosis. Invest Ophthalmol Vis Sci 32/4:987, A1569 Suppl
13. Pepose JS, Stewart JA, Grose C (1986) ARN: Serologic Studies and Further Characterization of the Virus. Invest Ophthalmol Vis Sci 25:12A Suppl
14. Saiki RK, Scharf S, Faloona F et al (1985) Enzymatic Amplification of ß-Globin Genomic Sequences and Restriction Site Analysis for Diagnosis of Sickle Cell Anemia. Science 230:1350-1354
15. Soushi S, Ozawa H, Matsuhashi M et al (1987) Positive Varicella-Zoster-Virus Antigen in the Vitreous of a Case with Acute Retinal Necrosis Syndrome. Jpn J Ophthalmol 41:199-202
16. Suttorp-Schulten MSA, Zaal MJW, Luyendijk L et al (1989) Aqueous Chamber Tap and Serology in Acute Retinal Necrosis. Am J Ophthalmol 108:327-328
17. Urayama A, Yamada N, Sasaki T et al (1971) Unilateral Acute Uveitis with Retinal Periarteritis and Detachment. Jpn J Clin Ophthalmol 25:607-619
18. White TJ, Arnheim N, Erlich HA (1989) The Polymerase Chain Reaction. Trends in Genetics 5:185-189
19. Witmer R (1978) Clinical Implications of Aqueous Humor Studies in Uveitis. Am J Ophthalmol 86:39-44

Acute Retinal Necrosis: What We Know from the Mouse

Sally S. Atherton

Abstract. Although Acute Retinal Necrosis has been reported in a small number of immunocompromised individuals, Acute Retinal Necrosis is a blinding disorder observed usually in immunocompetent patients. Both Varicella Zoster Virus and Herpes Simplex Virus have been recovered in ocular specimens from acute Retinal Necrosis patients. The von Szily mouse model of Herpes Simplex Virus type 1-induced retinal necrosis appears to be appropriate to study the virologic and immunologic contributions to the pathogenesis of Acute Retinal Necrosis. In this model, injection of Herpes Simplex Virus type 1 into the anterior chamber of one eye of the mouse leads to retinal necrosis in the uninoculated eye within 10-14 days. Both virus and host factors are important in the pathogenesis of Acute Retinal Necrosis. Development of retinal necrosis requires a mouse strain that is susceptible to Herpes Simplex Virus type 1 and a high titer of virus ($>10^5$ plaque forming units) in the uninoculated eye. The extent and speed of virus replication and the ability of the virus to enter (neuroinvasiveness) and replicate (neurovirulence) in the central nervous system are also important factors in the development of Acute Retinal Necrosis. The ability to mount an immune response to the virus influences the retinal necrosis, and both the microscopic appearance and timing of the retinal necrosis are markedly different when euthymic and athymic mice are compared. Following anterior chamber inoculation of Herpes Simplex Virus type 1, the process leading to Acute Retinal Necrosis cannot be reversed (for example, by administration of virus-specific immune effector cells) later than 24 hours after virus inoculation.
These results from the mouse model of Acute Retinal Necrosis suggest one reason why treatment is difficult in human patients with Acute Retinal Necrosis is that the process leading to Acute Retinal Necrosis is established soon after virus infection, days to perhaps weeks, before retinal involvement and the beginning of symptoms.

Introduction

Acute retinal necrosis is a blinding disorder that usually occurs in apparently healthy, immunocompetent individuals (24), although a limited number of cases of Acute Retinal Necrosis have been reported in patients with the acquired immunodeficiency syndrome (12). In humans, Acute Retinal Necrosis is caused by several members of the herpesvirus family - Herpes Simplex Virus type 1, Varicella Zoster Virus, Herpes Simplex Virus type 2 and Cytomegalovirus (8, 10, 16, 18, 21). Clinically, Acute Retinal Necrosis is characterized by choroidal and retinal arteritis, necrotizing retinitis, and vitritis. Other common features of Acute Retinal Necrosis are anterior segment inflammation, optic neuritis and retinal tears resulting in late retinal detachment (11,23). Most cases of Acute Retinal Necrosis are unilateral,

unilateral, although about one third of patients have bilateral disease (7).

Acute Retinal Necrosis Model

Retinal necrosis, which shares some features with Acute Retinal Necrosis in humans, can be induced experimentally in rabbits and mice. In 1924, von Szily reported that injection of Herpes Simplex Virus into one eye of a rabbit produced retinal necrosis in the uninoculated, contralateral eye (26). In 1984, Whittum and her colleagues observed the same phenomenon in mice and reported that uniocular anterior chamber inoculation of Herpes Simplex Virus type 1 (KOS strain) in euthymic BALB/c mice produced retinal necrosis of the uninoculated contralateral eye 8-10 days later (28). In mice, anterior chamber inoculation of Herpes Simplex Virus type 1 produces massive inflammation of the anterior segment of the injected eye; the retina of the inoculated eye is not destroyed, although retinal folding and mild to moderate vitritis are observed in the posterior segment (28).

After uniocular anterior chamber inoculation of 1-2x10^4 plaque forming units of Herpes Simplex Virus type 1 (KOS) in BALB/c mice, the titer of virus in the injected eye peaks 2-3 days after inoculation (3). Between day 1 and day 2 p.i., virus leaves the injected eye and spreads to the central nervous system via parasympathetic fibers of the oculomotor nerve that supply the iris and the ciliary body. Once in the brain, virus travels via neural pathways and enters the optic nerve of the uninoculated eye around day seven after inoculation (25). The virus travelling in the optic nerve comprises the latter of the two waves of virus recovered from the contralateral eye; virus in this latter wave arrives in the contralateral eye coincident with the development of acute retinitis (3,6). Acute retinitis proceeds rapidly to retinal necrosis, often within 24 hours of onset. Following uniocular anterior chamber inoculation of Herpes Simplex Virus type 1, the microscopic features of the progressive retinitis in the uninoculated eye include inflammation, vasculitis, hemorrhage, schisis and loss of the retinal architecture (5,6,28).

BALB/c mice inoculated with the KOS strain of Herpes Simplex Virus type 1 via the anterior chamber route make a virus-specific cytotoxic T cell response to the virus as well as virus-specific neutralizing antibody (27). Anterior chamber inoculation of the KOS strain of virus in BALB/c mice also induces anterior chamber-associated immune deviation, the hallmark of which is suppression of the delayed type hypersensitivity response to the virus (27). To date the link, if any, between the development of anterior chamber-associated immune deviation and retinitis in the contralateral eye remains controversial. One requirement for the induction of anterior chamber-associated immune deviation is that the virus must be able to replicate to high titer ($>5\log_{10}$ plaque forming units/ml) in the injected eye within the first 24 hours following anterior chamber inoculation (4). However, anterior chamber-associated immune deviation is not always induced following injection of Herpes Simplex Virus type 1 into the anterior chamber. Using several virus-strain/mouse-strain combinations, we have demonstrated that induction of the anterior chamber-associated immune deviation after anterior chamber inoculation of Herpes Simplex Virus type 1 is neither an exclusive feature of a particular strain of virus nor a distinguishing characteristic of an individual mouse strain. The outcome of anterior chamber inoculation of Herpes Simplex Virus type 1 (either induction of anterior chamber-associated immune deviation or establishment of virus-specific delayed type hypersensitivity responsiveness) depends on both the strain of the injected virus and on the strain of the mouse host (4).

In any viral infection such as Acute Retinal Necrosis, the outcome of the infection depends on a variety of host and viral factors. One advantage of an animal model is that individual host and viral factors that contribute to the pathogenesis of a disease can be identified and studied. Individual strains of mice vary tremendously in their resistance or susceptibility to Herpes Simplex Virus type 1 infection, irrespective of the route by which Herpes Simplex Virus type 1 is administered. Resistance to Herpes Simplex Virus type 1 is multifactorial and is not linked to the mouse major histocompatibility complex, H-2 (17). In the von Szily model, resistance to retinal necrosis following anterior chamber inoculation of Herpes Simplex Virus type 1 is dominant (21). The Igh-1 locus, whose gene products control both the constant and variable regions of immunoglobulin heavy chains, appears to play a role in determining susceptibility to retinitis in different strains of mice, and mice that differ at the Igh-1 locus also differ in their susceptibility to retinal necrosis following anterior chamber inoculation (20).

The original description of the von Szily model in mice was perhaps fortuitous in that the experiments were performed in BALB/c mice which are among the most susceptible to Herpes Simplex Virus type 1 infection. Following uniocular anterior chamber inoculation of the KOS strain of Herpes Simplex Virus type 1, the incidence of retinal necrosis in BALB/c mice varies between 70% and 100% (6,27). When C57BL/6 mice, a strain that is among the most resistant to Herpes Simplex Virus type 1 infection, are injected with the same dose of the KOS strain of Herpes Simplex Virus type 1 via the anterior chamber route, retinal necrosis is not observed in the uninoculated eye (15). Virus recovery studies from C57BL/6 mice inoculated with the KOS strain of Herpes Simplex Virus type 1 via the anterior chamber route revealed only low titers of virus in the injected eye, the central nervous system and the contralateral eye at any time after injection (15). In vitro, cells from C57BL/6 mice are restricted in their ability to support Herpes Simplex Virus type 1 virus replication (1), so some of the restriction of virus replication and the resistance to retinal necrosis observed in C57BL/6 mice may be attributable to the inability of the cells of the injected eye or central nervous system to be infected and/or to support virus replication.

In mice, development of retinal necrosis is linked to a high titer of Herpes Simplex Virus type 1 in the uninoculated eye at the time when acute retinitis becomes maximal (8-10 days after inoculation). In BALB/c mice inoculated with the KOS strain of Herpes Simplex Virus type 1, an average titer of $5.57 \log_{10}$ plaque forming units/ml 8-10 days after inoculation correlates with retinal necrosis (6). Although C57BL/6 mice are resistant to retinal necrosis following inoculation of the KOS strain of Herpes Simplex Virus type 1, anterior chamber inoculation of SC16, a more virulent strain of Herpes

Simplex Virus type 1, produces retinal necrosis in 71% of C57BL/6 mice, and high titers of virus (>5$\log_{10}$ plaque forming units/ml) are recovered from the uninoculated eyes at day 10 after inoculation (4). These results demonstrate that the resistance of C57BL/6 mice to virus infection and retinal necrosis can be overcome by infecting resistant strains of mice with a more neurovirulent strain of Herpes Simplex Virus type 1. Taken together, the results from the BALB/c and the C57BL/6 mice suggest that if a sufficiently high titer of virus reaches the uninoculated eyes of Herpes Simplex Virus type 1-resistant mice, retinal necrosis (such as is observed in BALB/c mice infected with the KOS strain of Herpes Simplex Virus type 1) will also occur in resistant mice.

The results of the experiments using C57BL/6-SC16 also suggest that the virulence of an individual strain of Herpes Simplex Virus type 1 influences both its ability to replicate and its ability to spread through the central nervous system to the contralateral eye. We are using the mouse model to document the extent of virus replication and to trace the intraocular routes of neural spread following inoculation of the KOS strain of Herpes Simplex Virus type 1 (which is neuroinvasive but relatively non-neurovirulent) and the H129 and RE strains of Herpes Simplex Virus type 1 (both of which are neuroinvasive and highly neurovirulent). It has been demonstrated previously when BALB/c mice are injected with KOS via the anterior chamber route, none of the animals dies from viral encephalitis, and virus is cleared from all ocular and central nervous system sites around day 14 after inoculation (3,28). In contrast, anterior chamber inoculation of neurovirulent strains of virus such as H129 and RE in BALB/c mice results in viral encephalitis and death of all of the mice by day eight after inoculation, a time when virus titers are significantly elevated in all ocular and central nervous system sites in H129- and RE-infected mice above those observed in KOS-infected animals (Fig.1) (Vann and Atherton, unpublished observations).

Our current studies to trace the route of viral spread after anterior chamber inoculation from the injected eye to the central nervous system and from the central nervous system to the retina have revealed several critical differences between the relatively avirulent KOS strain and the neurovirulent viruses, H129 and RE. For these studies, we used wild type KOS, H129 or RE to complement RH116 a TK mutant of Herpes Simplex Virus type 1 that contains the E.coli gene for ß-galactosidase (13). RH116 and one of the three wild type virus are coinjected into the anterior chamber of BALB/c mice. At intervals after infection, animals are sacrificed and the eyes and brains are removed. Each tissue is frozen and sectioned using a cryostat. The tissue sections are reacted with 5-bromo-4-chloro-3-indolyl-ß-D-galactopyranoside, a chromogenic substrate for ß-galactosidase and examined for bluestained cells indicative of virus infection (25).

Our tracing and virus recovery studies revealed differences between the relatively non-neurovirulent KOS strain of Herpes Simplex Virus type 1 and the neurovirulent H129 and RE strains of Herpes Simplex Virus type 1 in terms of the sites of central nervous system infection, the timing of virus spread to infected sites in the central nervous system, and the extent of virus replication at a particular site. Although it was initially hypothesized that virus entered the central nervous system via the optic nerve of the injected eye (3), our recent experiments and those of other investigators have demonstrated that following anterior chamber inoculation of Herpes Simplex Virus type 1, virus leaves the injected eye by two, non-optic nerve routes: (1) the trigeminal sensory nerves that supply the anterior segment and (3) the parasympathetic fibers of the oculomotor nerve that supply the iris and the ciliary body (19,25).

Also, both KOS and the more neurovirulent viruses (H129 and RE) follow the same sensory nerves, after reaching the ipsilateral trigeminal ganglion, the neurovirulent viruses are able to spread from the ganglion into the second order sensory neurons of the nucleus of the spinal trigeminal tract in the brainstem. In contrast, KOS reaches the trigeminal ganglion but is unable to spread into the trigeminal nucleus of the brainstem. It has been suggested by other investigators that the DNA polymerase of certain strains of Herpes Simplex Virus type 2 is defective, thereby preventing the spread of virus to the central nervous system after corneal inoculation (9). Perhaps the same mechanism accounts for the apparent inability of KOS to enter the brainstem. The ability of the neurovirulent viruses to reach the brainstem, whereas KOS does not, may be one reason why H129- and RE-infected mice die from encephalitis and KOS-infected mice survive.

The second route by which KOS, RE, and H129 leave the injected eye is by the parasympathetic component of the third cranial nerve, and irrespective of virus strain, virus is first detected in the ipsilateral ciliary ganglion at 48 hours after inoculation. From the ciliary ganglion, virus travels via axonal transport to the ipsilateral Edinger-Westphal nucleus. From this nucleus, virus spreads to the hypothalamus and to the visual system. From the Edinger-Westphal nucleus, virus spreads to the suprachiasmatic nuclei of the hypothalamus, and we hypothesize that the timing of virus spread from the Edinger-Westphal nucleus to the suprachiasmatic nuclei is important in determining whether one or both retinas will be affected. In H129- and RE-infected mice, virus is first detected in the ipsilateral suprachiasmatic nucleus at day three after inoculation and in the contralateral nucleus at day four after inoculation; in contrast, KOS is slower and virus is not detected in the ipsilateral suprachiasmatic nucleus of KOS-infected mice until day five after inoculation and in the contralateral nucleus until day seven after inoculation. In KOS-infected mice, virus reaches the optic nerve of the contralateral eye by direct spread from the ipsilateral suprachiasmatic nucleus around day seven after inoculation. In H129- or RE-infected mice, virus enters both optic nerves at day five after inoculation and these mice develop bilateral retinitis. The difference in timing of virus entry into the suprachiasmatic nuclei observed between mice infected with H129 or RE and KOS may be the reason mice infected with the neurovirulent strains of Herpes Simplex Virus type 1 develop bilateral disease. In either unilateral or bilateral retinitis, the optic nerve provides the conduit through which virus is transported to the eye to infect the retina (25) (Vann and Atherton, unpublished observations).

In these tracing studies, differences in timing of virus entry into central nervous system sites and qualitative differences in the number of virus-infected cells were observed throughout the course of infection when frozen sections of ocular and central nervous system tissues from H129- and RE-infected mice were compared with tissues from KOS-infected animals. The impression of a qualitative difference in the number of virus-infected cells in frozen sections was confirmed by virus recovery studies in which the growth of virus in both eyes and in the brain was compared for all three strains (Fig.1). The speed with which H129 and RE replicate and spread probably contributes to their virulence, since by replicating faster, they are able to reach critical sites in the central nervous system (ipsilateral trigeminal sensory ganglion and both suprachiasmatic nuclei) before an immune response can be made to the virus.

We hypothesize that one reason why BALB/c mice infected with KOS do not have retinal necrosis in the inoculated eye is because the immune response to the virus is established in time for it to limit virus spread from the contralateral suprachiasmatic nucleus into the optic nerve of the injected eye. Neurovirulent strains of Herpes Simplex Virus type 1 gain access to both optic nerves at least two days before KOS enters the optic nerve of the contralateral eye. In mice infected with H129 or RE, early entry of these viruses into central nervous system sites and high titers of virus in the central nervous system are likely to be the major factors which contribute to death of the animals eight days following anterior chamber inoculation.

In spite of treatment, most patients with Acute Retinal Necrosis experience severe and permanent visual loss from a variety of sequelae. Studies using the von Szily mouse model of Acute Retinal Necrosis have demonstrated that retinal necrosis can be prevented by immunologic or pharmacologic intervention within the first 24 - 48 hours following anterior chamber inoculation of virus. Intravenous administration of virus-specific, in vitro restimulated immune effector cells within 24 hours of anterior chamber inoculation of KOS protects mice from retinal necrosis in the uninoculated eye (14). Likewise, passive transfer of monoclonal antibody against glycoprotein D (a viral glycoprotein known to be involved in neuroinvasiveness) within 24 hours of virus inoculation into the anterior chamber also prevents retinal necrosis in the uninoculated eye (2). Virus recovery results from the experiments to study the effect of passive transfer of virus-specific immune effector cells or glycoprotein D monoclonal antibody on development of retinal necrosis suggest that the interaction between virus-specific immune effector cells or passively-transferred antibody occurs both in the injected eye and in the central nervous system. Virus titers in the inoculated eye after day 1 and the central nervous system of treated animals were significantly lower than the titers of virus recovered from control animals that received only an inoculation of virus into the anterior chamber.

Protection by immune effector cells or antibody appears to prevent retinitis either by (1) preventing the spread of virus from the inoculated eye or (3) by limiting the replication and/or spread of virus in the central nervous system, so that virus is unable to reach the uninoculated eye. Preliminary studies from our laboratory have also demonstrated that treatment with the antiviral agent Acyclovir can prevent retinal necrosis of the drug is administered within the first two days following inoculation of KOS into the anterior chamber. We have not treated animals at later times, so we do not know if Acyclovir alters the course of disease once the virus has reached the central nervous system.

Discussion

These results indicate that specific immune effector mechanisms or antiviral therapies are limited in what they can accomplish. In mice and in human patients with Acute Retinal Necrosis following primary infection by the virus, the host's own immune response may be mobilized too late for it to have any effect on the spread of the virus. In patients with Acute Retinal Necrosis due to viral reactivation, pre-existing antiviral immunity may be insufficient to prevent virus replication and spread from the site of latency. In Acute Retinal Necrosis due to virus reactivation, there may be an additional problem related to accessibility of immune effector modalities as virus spreads from the site of reactivation to an ocular site, and virus transported intra-axonally to the eye may not be accessible to either cellular or humoral immune effector mechanisms in the early stages of the reactivated disease. Furthermore, these results suggest that for any antiviral therapy to be effective in Acute Retinal Necrosis, such therapy should be administered early in the course of the disease before the onset of retinal symptoms. However, in Acute Retinal Necrosis, by the time the retinal symptoms occur, the viral infection is well-established.

In summary, both virus and host factors play a role in the mouse model of Acute Retinal Necrosis, and it is likely that the immune response of the host and the virulence of the infecting virus also influence the spread of virus and the development of Acute Retinal Necrosis in human patients. Knowledge of routes of virus spread from the mouse model may provide insight into the mechanism of Acute Retinal Necrosis in humans. Many patients with Acute Retinal Necrosis have anterior uveitis, and most patients also have evidence of optic nerve involvement.

By extrapolation from the mouse, we hypothesize that the following sequence of events might occur in human Acute Retinal Necrosis. Herpesvirus infection results in mild anterior uveitis, either as a result of a primary or a reactivated infection from the corresponding trigeminal ganglion. Once in the anterior segment, probably the vast majority of eyes with herpetic anterior uveitis resolve the disease, and the virus returns to latency in the trigeminal ganglion. In patients destined to develop Acute Retinal Necrosis, the virus does not go to the trigeminal ganglion but, instead, travels via the parasympathetic component of the oculomotor nerve to the central nervous system. Once the virus reaches the central nervous system, it enters the optic pathway of one or both eyes following the route described for the mouse model and then travels to the retina via the optic nerve. As in the mouse, it is possible that, in humans, the virus may be arrested at one of several sites in the central nervous system either by cell-mediated immune mechanisms and/or by antibody of sufficiently high titer and affinity. The development of Acute Retinal Necrosis in human patients might therefore be viewed as a failure of the host to control either a primary or a reactivated infection with Herpes virus.

Future studies using the mouse model will be needed to identify sites of interaction between the virus and passively administered immune effectors or between the virus and antiviral agents. The results of these types of studies may aid in design of therapies specifically targeted to sites of ocular and central nervous system infections.

Acknowledgement

This work was supported by EY-06012.

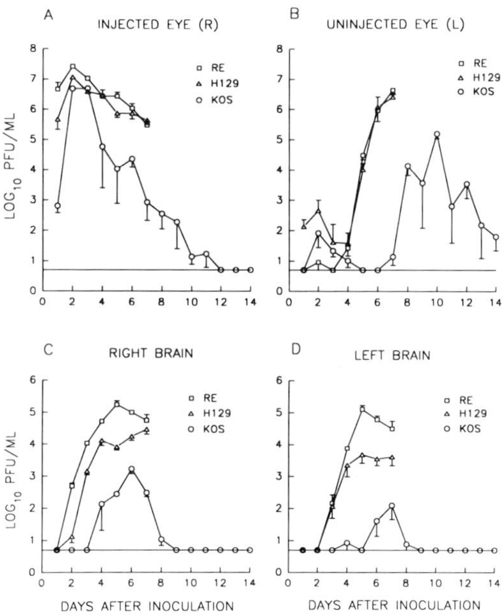

Fig.1.
Recovery of virus from the injected eye (A), uninjected eye (B), ipsilateral (right) brain hemisphere (C), and contralateral (left) brain hemisphere (D) of BALB/c mice inoculated with 10^4 plaque forming units of KOS (o-o), H129 (^-^), or RE (#-#) via the anterior chamber route. Four mice from each group were sacrificed at each time point, and the amount of virus in each specimen was determined (in duplicate) by plaque assay on monolayers of Vero cells.
The amount of virus at each time point is the mean virus titer (expressed as Log_{10} plaque forming units/ml +- S.E.M.) of all samples harvested at that time. The solid line indicates the lower limit of virus detection.

References

1. Abghari SZ, Stulting RD, Nigida SM et al (1986) Comparative Replication of HSV-1 in BALB/c and C57BL/6 Mouse Embryo Fibroblasts in Vitro. Invest Ophthalmol Vis Sci 27:909-914
2. Atherton SA (to be published) Protection from Retinal Necrosis by Passive Transfer of Monoclonal Antibody Specific for Herpes Simplex Glycoprotein D. Curr Eye Res
3. Atherton SS, Streilein JW (1987) Two Waves of Virus Following Anterior Chamber Inoculation of HSV-1. Invest Ophthalmol Vis Sci 28:571-579
4. Atherton SS, Kanter MY, Streilein JW (1991) ACAID Requires Early Replication of HSV-1 in the Injected Eye. Curr Eye Res 10S:75-80
5. Cousins SW, Altman NH, Atherton SS (1989) Schisis Contributes to Necrosis in Experimental HSV-1 Retinitis. Exp Eye Res 48:745-760
6. Cousins SW, Gonzalez AR, Atherton SS (1989) Herpes Simplex Retinitis in the Mouse: Clinicopathologic Correlations. Invest Ophthalmol Vis Sci 30:1485-1494
7. Culbertson WW, Blumenkranz MS (1984) The Acute Retinal Necrosis Syndrome. In: Blodi FC (ed) Herpes Simplex Infections of the Eye. Churchill Livingstone, New York, pp.77-89
8. Culbertson WW, Blumenkranz MS, Pepose JS et al (1986) Varicella Zoster Virus is a Cause of the Acute Retinal Necrosis Syndrome. Ophthalmology 93:559-569
9. Day SP, Lausch RN, Oakes JE (1988) Evidence that the Gene for Herpes Simplex Type 1 DNA Polymerase Accounts for the Capacity of an Intertypic Recombinant to Spread from Eye to Central Nervous System. Virology 163:166-173
10. Duker JS, Nielsen JC, Eagle RC et al (1990) Rapidly Progressive Acute Retinal Necrosis Secondary to Herpes Simplex

Virus Type 1. Ophthalmology 97:1638-1643
11. Fisher JP, Lewis ML, Blumenkranz M et al (1982) The Acute Retinal Necrosis Syndrome Part 1: Clinical Manifestations. Ophthalmology 89:1309-1316
12. Friberg TR, Jost BF (1984) Acute Retinal Necrosis in an Immunosuppressed Patient. Am J Ophthalmol 98:515-517
13. Ho DY, Mocarski ES (1988) ß-Galactosidase as a Marker in the Peripheral and Neural Tissues of the Herpes Simplex Virus-Infected Mouse. Virology 167:279-283
14. Igietseme JU, Calzada PJ, Gonzalez AR et al (1989) Protection of Mice from Herpes Simplex Virus-Induced Retinitis by In Vitro-Activated Immune Cells. J Virol 63:4808-4813
15. Kielty D, Cousins SW, Atherton SS (1987) HSV-1 Retinitis and Delayed Hypersensitivity in DBA/2 and C57BL/6 Mice. Invest Ophthalmol Vis Sci 28:1994-1999
16. Lewis ML, Culbertson WW, Post JD, et al (1989) Herpes Simplex Virus Type 1: A Cause of the Acute Retinal Necros is Syndrome. Ophthalmology 96:875-878
17. Lopez C (1975) Genetics of Natural Resistence to Herpes Simplex Infections in Mice. Nature 258:152-153
18. Mahjoub SB, Ganley JP, Misra RP et al (1989) Isolation of a Herpes Simplex Virus Type 2 that is Retinovirulent in Mice. Curr Eye Res 7:687.695
19. Margolis TP, LaVail J, Setzer PY et al (1989) Selective Spread of Herpes Simplex Virus in the Central Nervous System after Ocular Inoculation. J Virol 63:4756-4761
20. Opremczak EM, Foster CS, Hemady R et al (1989) Chorioretinal Disease Patterns in Congenic Mice Following Intraocular Inoculation with HSV 1. Invest Ophthalmol Vis Sci 30:1041-1046
21. Pepose JS, Whittum-Hudson JA (1987) An Immunogenetic Analysis of Resistance to Herpes Simplex Virus Retinitis in Inbred Strains of Mice. Invest Ophthalmol Vis Sci 28:1549-1552
22. Rungger-Brändle E, Roux L, Leuenberger PM (1984) Bilateral Acute Retinal Necrosis (BARN): Identification of the Presumed Infectious Agent. Ophthalmology 91:1648-1658
23. Sergott RC, Belmont JB, Savino PJ et al (1985) Optic Nerve Involvement in the Acute Retinal Necrosis Syndrome. Arch Ophthalmol 103:1160-1162
24. Urayama A, Yamada N, Sasaki T et al (1971) Unilateral Acute Uveitis with Periarteritis and Detachment. Jpn J Clin Ophthalmol 25:607-619
25. Vann VR, Atherton SS (1991) Neural Spread of Herpes Simplex Virus after Anterior Chamber Inoculation. Invest Ophthalmol Vis Sci 32:2462-2472
26. von Szily A (1924) An Experimental Endogenous Transmission of Infection from Bulbus to Bulbus. Klin Mbl Augenhlkd 75:593-602
27. Whittum JA, Niederkorn JY, McCulley JP et al (1983) Intracameral Inoculation of Herpes Simplex Type 1 Induces Anterior Chamber Associated Immune Deviation. Curr Eye Res 2:691-697
28. Whittum JA, McCulley JP, Niederkorn JY et al (1984) Ocular Disease Induced in Mice by Anterior Chamber Inoculation of Herpes Simplex Virus. Invest Ophthalmol Vis Sci 25:1065-1073

Acute Retinal Necrosis - Clinical Features and Clinical Diagnosis

Eva-Maria Fabricius

Abstract. Acute retinal necrosis begins with a mild anterior uveitis and episcleritis. Fleecy-white spots of periarteriolar sheathing and arteriolar occlusion develop several days later, followed by milky-white, confluent areas of necrotizing retinitis throughout the periphery of the retina (Stage 1).
Decreased visual acuity is caused by vitritis and frequently by papillitis (Stage 2).
After 4-12 weeks the retinitis recedes from its posterior margin leaving behind atrophic retina with occluded vessels (Stage 3). Within the following weeks, retinal tears develop at the junction of necrotic and unaffected retina leading to retinal detachment in >75% of cases (Stage 4).
Further complications include proliferative vitreo-retinopathy and neovascularization causing blindness in 64% of the eyes affected by the acute retinal necrosis. In one third of the cases, the fellow eye becomes involved within weeks to years ("Bilateral Acute Retinal Necrosis Syndrome").
A mild type of the Acute Retinal Necrosis may occur.
The Acute Retinal Necrosis is usually caused by Varicella Zoster Virus or Herpes Simplex Virus, but atypical cases of Cytomegalovirus-, toxoplasmic and syphilitic retinitis may have a similar appearance. In exceptions, the acute retinal necrosis can involve the posterior retina first.
The diagnosis is made by repeated fundoscopy with dilated pupils and the patient's history and physical examinations to establish dermatitis, encephalomyelitis or neuritis. Vascular occlusion can be made visible by fluorescein angiography and retinal detachment by ultrasonography. Invasive procedures to identify organisms or antibodies include paracentesis, vitrectomy, aspiration of subretinal fluid and chorioretinal biopsies.

Introduction

The Acute Retinal Necrosis Syndrome is a distinct clinical entity featuring a combination of retinal vasculitis, retinal necrosis, vitritis, anterior segment inflammation and late retinal detachment (Fig.1).

The "syndrome of uveitis, retinal arteriitis and retinal detachment" was first described by Urayama and coworkers in 1971. The authors noted a similarity in appearance between confirmed viral infections of the posterior segment such as neonatal Herpes Simplex Virus retinitis and cases of the Acute Retinal Necrosis Syndrome. Hayasaka called this disease "Kirisawa's uveitis" in 1983, and since then the syndrome was thus mentioned in the Japanese literature. Various other names were found by several authors such as "peripheral retinal necrosis and total retinal detachment of vascular origin" by Martenet in 1976 or "necrotizing vaso-occlusive retinitis" by Willerson in 1977, until Young and Bird in 1978 coined the term "Acute Retinal Necrosis Syndrome" resp. "Bilateral Acute Retinal Necrosis" (4,5).

Etiology and Pathogenesis

The Acute Retinal Necrosis Syndrome usually occurs as a result of secondary reactivation of latent Varicella Zoster Virus or of Herpes Simplex Virus type 1 or 2; only in a very few cases it may also occur in the course of primary infection with these viruses (3,8,9,12).

The pathogenesis of Acute Retinal Necrosis Syndrome is not completely clear. In addition to the cytopathogenic effects of the virus on retina and pigment epithelium and occlusion of retinal and choroidal arterioles with subsequent ischemia of the retina, other factors seem to have an influence on the development of this special pattern of posterior segment inflammation.

Contrasting the high contamination rate of man with viruses of the Herpes family to the rareness of the Acute Retinal Necrosis Syndrome (7), some kind of immunogenetic predisposition with specific HLA types may perhaps explain an individual's propensity to develop an Acute Retinal Necrosis Syndrome.

Furthermore, an immunologic modulation of virus-induced pathologic features is derived from T-lymphocytes (17). Finally, it is hypothesized that the Acute Retinal Necrosis Syndrome is caused by relatively recent mutations of the Herpes virus family, however, this has not yet been proven by restriction endonuclease patterns (16).

Complications and Visual Outcome

Despite various modalities of treatment, the Acute Retinal Necrosis Syndrome continues to be a devastating ocular disease. Retinal detachment occurs in three quarters of the eyes affected by the Acute Retinal Necrosis Syndrome, and two thirds of the eyes become blind (visual acuity: 20/200 or less). In cases of early treatment, blindness may be reduced to one third or even one half of the diseased eyes. One third of the patients suffer from bilateral involvement, although an interval of weeks or years may pass before the fellow eye is affected (4).

Clinical Features

Prodromal symptoms of the Acute Retinal Necrosis Syndrome ("Stage 0") are characterized by mild to moderate ocular and periorbital pain, "red eye" with episcleritis or scleritis and pericorneal hyperemia, mild to moderate anterior uveitis, frequently elevated intraocular pressure and, in immunodeficient patients, a simultaneous viral keratitis.

A staging of the course of the Acute Retinal Necrosis Syndrome has revealed to be useful, esp. in the view of the prophylaxis and treatment of retinal detachment (2)(Tab.1).

Stage 1 is characterized by initial necrotizing retinitis developing several days after the onset of the prodromal symptoms.

Stage 1A bears the manifestations of a discrete areas of peripheral retinitis with fleecy, white, small patches of retinal necrosis as well as narrowing and sheathing of arterioles (Fig.2).

In Stage 1B confluent areas of peripheral retinitis and frequently papillitis are typical. The entire periphery is involved with milky-white areas with geographic margins and partially preserved transparency. The retinitis spreads to the posterior pole with pseudopode-like projections. Phlebitis and hemorrhages are less prominent features in the early Acute Retinal Necrosis Syndrome. "Fingerprints" of necrosis may precede the confluent zones directed towards the posterior pole (Fig.3).

Stage 2 is characterized by complete retinal necrosis and vitreous opacification. There are extensive areas of retinal necrosis. A hazy view of the posterior segment from the standpoint of the examining ophthalmologist and floaters and blurred vision noted by the patient are caused by a cellular inflammatory reaction and the debris from the necrotic retina in the vitreous. Contributing to the decreased visual acuity, cystoid macular edema and optic neuropathy develop frequently. Optic neuropathy is due to either infiltration by inflammatory cells or to thrombotic arteriolar occlusion of the nutritive optic nerve vessels, or to localised exsudates within the optic nerve sheath. A non-prominent, fleeting, serous retinal detachment may occur, and more or less extensive hemorrhages may be seen. The vessels are often attenuated. The intraocular pressure is frequently reduced in this phase (Fig.4).

In Stage 3, regression of retinal necrosis, which means a disappearing intraocular inflammation, may occur 4-12 weeks following the onset of symptoms. Since the disease is self-limited on many occasions, the retinitis recedes from its posterior margin (located in the anterior retina) leaving behind the destroyed atrophic retina with granular pigmentation and occluded vessels. The peripheral retina primarily involved is left scarred exhibiting pseudopode-like projections similar to those seen in the inflamed retina of Stage 1B. Visual acuity may improve, because the vitreous cavity clears up due to condensation, and the vitreous base contracts. Without specific treatment, the intraocular inflammation subsides as soon as the host's immune system controls the infecting virus, or if there is no more retinal tissue left to destroy (Fig.5).

In Stage 4, retinal detachment occurs two to three months after the onset of the disease in up to 75% of the Acute Retinal Necrosis Syndrome.

In Stage 4A, acute retinal tears lead to a rhegmatogenous retinal detachment accompanied by proliferative vitreoretinopathy and vitreous fibrosis causing traction detachment. Large, irregularly shaped, multiple tears develop at the junctions of necrotic and unaffected or scarred retina.

In Stage 4B, the acute stages of retinal detachment are followed by a chronic course. The vitreous becomes more cloudy due to necrotic debris stemming from the retinal tissue and examination of the fundus may be obscured. Thus, in some cases, retinal detachment can only be diagnosed by the use of ultrasound. More unusual sequelae of the Acute Retinal Necrosis Syndrome consist of neovascularisation of the retina, optic disc and iris sometimes accompanied by intraocular hemorrhage. In the end, the globe becomes phthisical (Fig.7).

Atypical Manifestations of the Acute Retinal Necrosis Syndrome

As proposed by Matsuo and coworkers in 1988 (11), a "mild type" of the Acute Retinal Necrosis Syndrome exists, which is slowly progressive and self-limited without retinal detachment accompanied by a well-

-preserved visual acuity. It is assumed that such a mild course may coexist with a primary Varicella Zoster Virus (or Herpes Simplex Virus) infection such as chickenpox (12), especially if the patient is in an immunocompromised state. It should also be kept in mind that patients with chickenpox and ocular symptoms may suffer from the Acute Retinal Necrosis Syndrome. Further correlations with systemic diseases have not yet been completely evaluated in these mild courses.

Those cases of the Acute Retinal Necrosis Syndrome, which have a good visual outcome, are associated with an abortive retinal arteriitis limited to exudates or no apparent arteriitis at all on initial examination. This group also has low levels of circulating immune complexes and normal electroretinograms (13). It is assumed that additional clinical factors play a role such as the presence of complete posterior vitreous detachment before onset of the disease, which might be important for a good visual outcome. Furthermore, the differences in severity of the disease could be attributed to different virulence patterns of Herpes viruses and a variable degree of the host's immune response. The effects of early Acyclovir treatment have not yet been clearly proven by controlled studies, however, we have had the impression that in some patients Acyclovir really seems to act beneficial on the course of the disease (Fig.8).

In certain cases, the Acute Retinal Necrosis Syndrome may start in the perimacular or peripapillary areas of the posterior pole. The appearance of the whitish necrotic areas is similar to the socalled "Arcuate Neuroretinitis" (9). The necrosis progresses along the paramacular or peripapillary nerve fibers causing early visual impairment (Fig.9). Immediate intravenous Acyclovir treatment may result in an excellent outcome as we have reported earlier in a patient with a recent human immunodeficiency virus infection (5). Therapeutic success in this case has not only been limited to the retinitis, but also extended to a simultaneous encephalitis. The patient has regained a good visual acuity, hearing (which had been impaired) and consciousness within one week. The retinitis has resolved leaving only a small focus of paramacular scarring in the right eye - as can also be visualized in the late phase fluorescein angiogram (Fig.11) - and some attenuated peripapillary arterioles and macular pigmentation in the left eye. Both visual fields, however, show permanent dense inferior arcuate scotomas corresponding to the nerve fiber loss caused by the healed focuses of Acute Retinal Necrosis . In view of the underlying acquired immunodeficiency, which had been expected to progress, we have decided to apply oral Acyclovir to the patient on a long-term treatment regimen, and thus, he has been well until now for three years without any recurrence. This patient's disease may also be accounted for a mild type of the Acute Retinal Necrosis Syndrome.

In a third type, patchy, necrotic lesions can be found disseminated over the entire fundus as shown in a child suffering from a Herpes Simplex Virus encephalitis as well. Visual functions have not been possible to assess, because of the severe central nervous damage.

Recently, we have become acquainted with the so-called "Outer Retinal Necrosis" as a distinct form unique to immunosuppressed individuals and patients with the acquired immunodeficiency syndrome (6). It is characterized by little inner retinal involvement, sparing of vessels, little intraocular inflammation and a rapid course. The macula may appear like a cherry-red spot within the deep white retinal lesions. This may be the result of central artery occlusion rather than diffuse edema. Almost all of the cases reported have been related to episodes of zoster dermatitis, and Varicella Zoster Virus has been recovered from chorioretinal specimens and vitreous aspirates in some of these cases. Until now, it has not been clarified why Varicella Zoster manifests itself in the eye in this way. This type of the Acute Retinal Necrosis Syndrome suggests that the host's immune response may play a role in the pathogenetic process as we have already mentioned. The augmented B-cell response known to occur in patients with the acquired immunodeficiency syndrome may induce an immune complex-mediated response to the proliferating virus (6,10,14). In this disease entity, the ophthalmologist should particularly be aware of an underlying human immunodeficiency virus infection and human immunodeficiency virus antibody testing is demanding (Fig.10).

Differential Diagnosis

The differential diagnosis of the Acute Retinal Necrosis Syndrome includes retinal whitening of most diverse etiology, above all necrotizing retinitis of a different etiology such as cytomegalovirus infection, toxoplasmosis, syphilis or retinal vasculitis of various etiologies, tumors such as large cell lymphomas and retinoblastomas, initial bacterial or fungal endophthalmitis, acute arterial occlusion with retinal infarction as caused by embolization of the ophthalmic artery or its retinal branches and Berlin's edema in retinal contusion (4).

Although we think that the differential diagnosis of necrotizing retinitis and other forms of retinal whitening can be made by means of clinical examinations in 70-80% of cases, there are some cases left, in which the differential diagnosis may be really difficult. Particularly, cytomegalovirus retinitis in immunodeficient patients as well as toxoplasmic or syphilitic retinitis may appear similar to the Acute Retinal Necrosis Syndrome (Tab.2).

Clinical and Laboratory Diagnosis

The diagnosis of the Acute Retinal Necrosis Syndrome is based on the clinical appearance, but should also be supported by evaluation for evidence of systemic infections and - in certain cases - by an appropriate analysis of intraocular specimens (4). The clinical diagnosis of Acute Retinal Necrosis is made by repeat funduscopy with dilated pupils.

Evidence of systemic infection is sought by evaluation of the patient's history and a physical examination to exclude dermatitis, encephalomyelitis or neuritis that may be caused by Herpes Simplex or Varicella Zoster Virus.

Work-up of intraocular specimens to establish a definite etiology is warranted in only a very few cases. Particularly in atypical forms of the Acute Retinal Necrosis Syndrome, histopathologic confirmation of the infecting organism is needed in order to make the best choice of therapy. Intraocular probes are obtained by paracentesis, vitrectomy, puncture of subretinal fluids or chorioretinal biopsy. The material is used for culturing virus, identification of viral antigens or viral DNA genomic sequences (which may be amplified by using the Polymerase Chain Reaction) or for antibody immunofluorescent studies to assess local Varicella Zoster Virus and Herpes Simplex Virus antibody production.

Serum titers of viruses are usually unrevealing, because the syndrome is most commonly associated with a local ocular reactivation subsequent to a prior systemic viral infection. Even positive IgG titers will not assist in the initial management of the ocular disease in view of the high contamination of man with Herpes Simplex Virus or Varicella Zoster Virus, and convalescent sera can be drawn only six to eight weeks after the onset of symptoms. In a few cases, a primary Herpes Simplex Virus or Varicella Zoster Virus infection can be detected by elevated IgM titers. Serum titers for viral seroconversion are useful when compared to those of intraocular fluids proving local antibody production.

Additional diagnostic methods utilized to identify pathological processes in the course of the disease include fluorescein angiography, ultrasound and electroretinography, but these methods are not suitable to establish a diagnosis of Acute Retinal Necrosis Syndrome or to prove its etiology. Fluorescein angiography may be useful to verify arteriolar obstruction, leakage phenomena due to vasculitis and optic neuropathy as well as window defects caused by retinal pigment epithelium alterations in the recovery phase. Ultrasound is invaluable for detecting the presence of a retinal detachment when the degree of vitritis precludes an ophthalmoscopic examination of the posterior segment. Ultrasonography can also be helpful in diagnosing an enlargement of the optic nerve sheath indicating optic neuritis, but the sensitivity of this procedure is rather poor. Pathologic electroretinographic findings are usually dependent on the amount of retinal tissue affected and are mainly suggestive of inner retinal malfunction. Sometimes, however, these changes can be detected in the healthy fellow eye as well and are therefore particularly interesting for scientific evaluations.

Therapy

Therapeutic trials with Acyclovir may lend relatively convincing evidence of an Acute Retinal Necrosis Syndrome caused by Herpes Simplex Virus or Varicella Zoster Virus whereby healing of the retinal lesions is observed within two to four weeks compared to untreated cases, which show spontaneous scarring after 6-12 weeks. Unfortunately, however, Acyclovir has no apparent effect on the high incidence of subsequent retinal detachment (1).

Table 1. Stages of the Acute Retinal Necrosis

Stage 1:	Necrotizing retinitis
A:	Discrete areas of peripheral retinitis
B:	Confluent areas of peripheral retinitis, cystoid macular edema
Stage 2:	Vitreous opacification / organization
Stage 3:	Regression of retinal necrosis, pigmentation, condensation and contraction of the vitreous base
Stage 4:	Retinal detachment
A:	Acute retinal tears or detachment with traction, proliferative vitreoretinopathy
B:	Prolonged retinal detachment

Table 2. Differential diagnosis of the Acute Retinal Necrosis syndrome

- Necrotizing retinitis, different etiologies (cytomegalovirus, toxoplasmosis, syphilis)
- Retinal vasculitis
- Intraocular tumors (large cell lymphoma, retinoblastoma)
- Bacterial or fungal endophthalmitis
- Acute arterial occlusion with retinal infarction (embolization of the ophthalmic artery or its retinal branches)
- Contusion of the retina

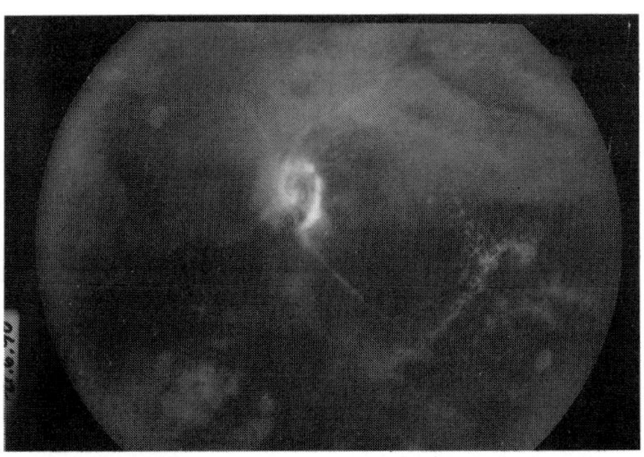

Fig.1. Full-blown Acute Retinal Necrosis with retinal vasculitis, retinal necrosis, vitritis, hemorrhages and serous retinal detachment.

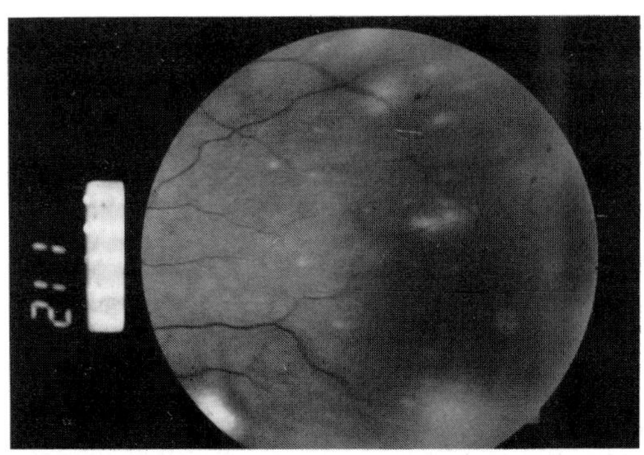

Fig.2. Stage 1A of the Acute Retinal Necrosis: Fleecy, white, small patches of retinal necrosis distributed all over the fundus periphery, mainly related to small retinal vessels.

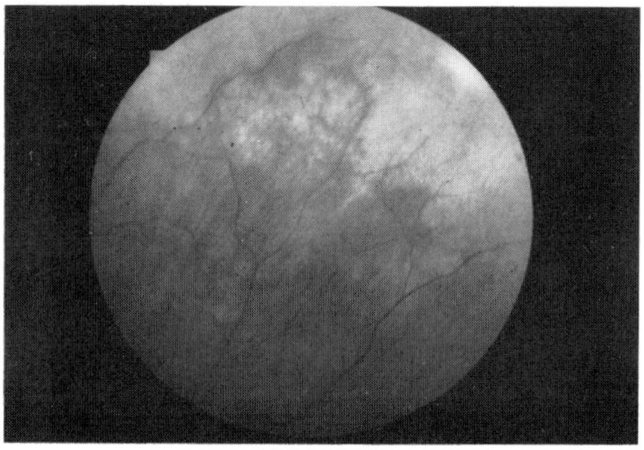

Fig.3. Stage 1B of the Acute Retinal Necrosis: Confluent areas of peripheral necrosis with milky-white areas, geographic borderlines and partially preserved transparency.

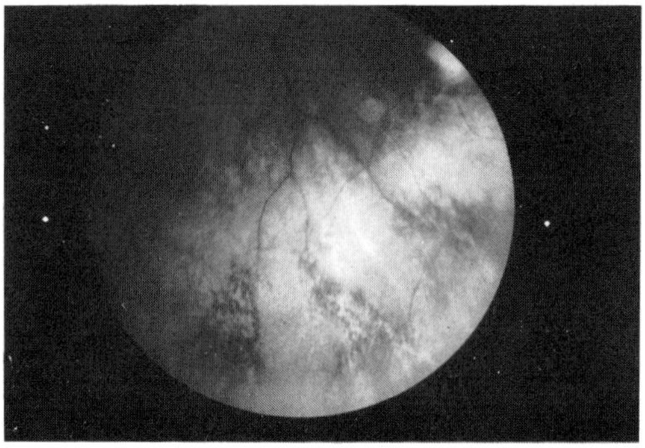

Fig.5. Stage 3 of the Acute Retinal Necrosis: Regression of the necrotising retinitis by receding from its posterior margin leaving behind destroyed atrophic retina with granular pigmentation. The scarred, primarily involved peripheral retina shows pseudopode-like projections similar to those seen in the inflamed retina of Stage 1B.

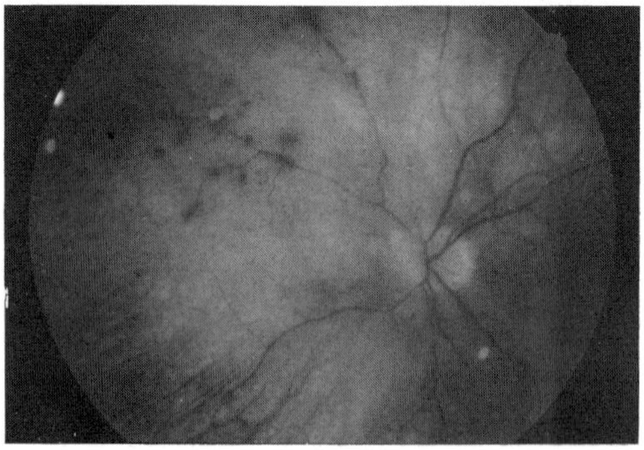

Fig.4. Stage 2 of the Acute Retinal Necrosis: Extensive retinal necrosis with serous retinal detachment, attenuated arteries, vitritis and hemorrhage.

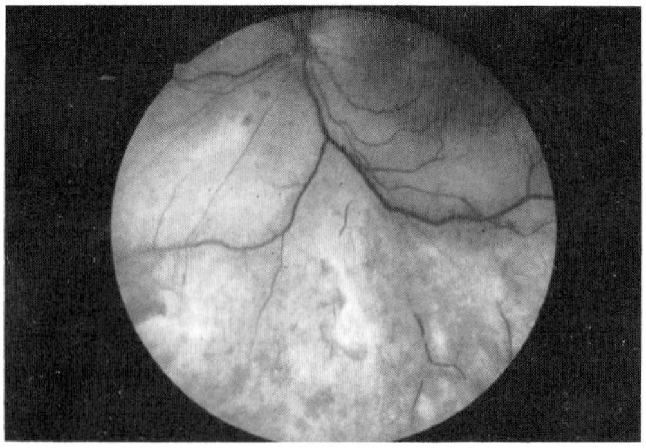

Fig.6. Stage 4A of the Acute Retinal Necrosis: Large, irregularly shaped, multiple tears at the junction of necrotic and scarred or unaffected retina leading to acute rhegmatogenous retinal detachment.

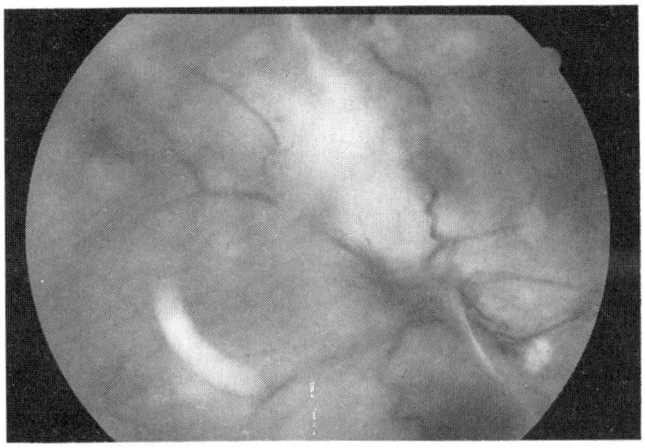

Fig.7. Stage 4B of the Acute Retinal Necrosis: Chronic retinal detachment, vitreous opacification.

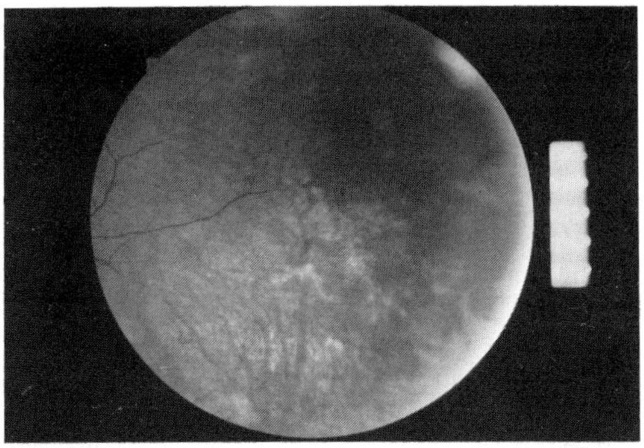

Fig.8. Mild type of Acute Retinal Necrosis (self-limited) with scarred fundus periphery, without visual impairment and without retinal detachment.

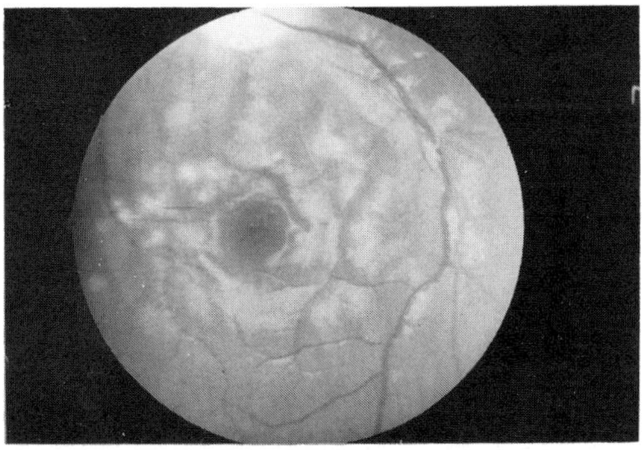

Fig. 9. Atypical form of the Acute Retinal Necrosis in a child suffering from a Herpes Simplex Virus encephalitis: White, patchy necrotic lesions distributed over the entire fundus, attenuated arteries, retinal edema, optic atrophy.

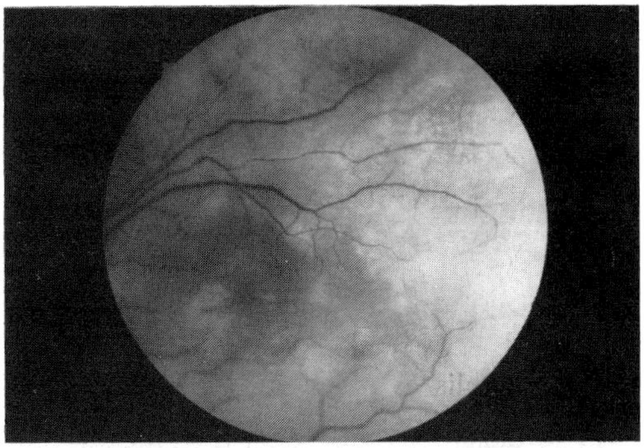

Fig.10. Atypical form of the Acute Retinal Necrosis appearing as "Outer Retinal Necrosis" in a patient with the Acquired Immunodeficiency Syndrome two weeks after the onset of a herpes zoster ophthalmicus with deep white retinal lesions, little inner retinal involvement, relative sparing of the retinal vessels, little intraocular inflammation, rapid deterioration.

References

1. Blumenkranz MS, Culbertson WW, Clarkson JG et al (1986) Treatment of the Acute Retinal Necrosis Syndrome with Intravenous Acyclovir. Ophthalmology 93:296-300
2. Carney MD, Peyman GA, Goldberg MF et al (1986) Acute Retinal Necrosis. Retina 6:85-94
3. Culbertson WW, Blumenkranz MS, Pepose JS et al (1986) Varicella Zoster Virus is a Cause of the Acute Retinal Necrosis Syndrome. Ophthalmology 93:559-569
4. Duker JS, Blumenkranz MS (1991) Diagnosis and Management of the Acute Retinal Necrosis Syndrome. Surv Ophthalmol 35:327-343
5. Fabricius EM, Lipp T, Kaboth W (1990) Akute Retinanekrose und Herpesenzephalitis: Schlüsselrolle des Augenarztes bei der Diagnostik opportunistischer Infektionen bei AIDS, erfolgreiche Therapie mit Acyclovir (Zovirax[R]). Klin Mbl Augenheilk 196:160-165
6. Forster DJ, Dugel PU, Frangieh GT et al (1990) Rapidly Progressive Outer Retinal Necrosis in the Acquired Immunodeficiency Syndrome. Am J Ophthalmol 110:341-348
7. Holland GN, Cornell PJ, Park MS et al (1989) An Association Between Acute Retinal Necrosis Syndrome and HLA-DQw7 and Phenotype Bw62,DR4. Am J Ophthalmol 108:370-374
8. Lewis ML, Culbertson WW, Post JD et al (1989) Herpes Simplex Virus Type 1. A Cause of the Acute Retinal Necrosis Syndrome. Ophthalmology 96:875-878
9. Margolis T, Irvine AR, Hoyt WF et al (1988) Acute Retinal Necrosis Syndrome Presenting with Papillitis and Arcuate Neuroretinitis. Ophthalmology 95:937-940
10. Margolis TP, Lowder CY, Holland GN et al (1991) Varicella Zoster Virus Retinitis in Patients with the Acquired Immunodeficiency Syndrome. Am J Ophthalmol 112:119-131
11. Matsuo T, Nakayama T, Koyama T et al (1988) A Proposed Mild Type of Acute Retinal Necrosis Syndrome. Am J Ophthalmol 105:579-583
12. Matsuo T, Koyama M, Matsuo N (1991) Acute Retinal Necrosis as a Novel Complication of Chickenpox in Adults. Br J Ophthalmol 75:450-454
13. Matsuo T, Morimoto K, Matsuo N (1991) Factors Associated with a Poor Visual Outcome in Acute Retinal Necrosis. Br J Ophthalmol 75:450-454
14. Nussenblatt RB, Palestine AG (1991) Human Immunodeficiency Virus, Herpes Zoster and the Retina. Am J Ophthalmol 112:206-207
15. Pepose JS, Hilborne LH, Cancilla PA et al (1984) Concurrent Herpes Simplex and Cytomegalovirus Retinitis and Encephalitis in the Acquired Immunodeficiency Syndrome. Ophthalmology 91:1669-1677
16. Pepose JS, Biron K (1987) Antiviral Sensitivities of the Acute Retinal Necrosis Syndrome Virus. Curr Eye Res 6:201-205
17. Whittum-Hudson JA, Pepose JS (1987) Immunologic Modulation of Virus-Induced Pathology in a Murine Model of Acute Herpetic Retinal Necrosis. Invest Ophthalmol Vis Sci 28:1541-1548

Acute Retinal Necrosis Syndrome: Systemic Features

Rudolph M. Franklin

Abstract. Typical cases of Acute Retinal Necrosis syndrome have occurred temporarily related to skin lesions and central nervous system abnormalities. Vesicular skin lesions associated with both Varicella Zoster and Herpes Simplex Virus infections have been observed frequently, and support the herpetic etiology of Acute Retinal Necrosis. The occurrence of herpetic skin lesions in immunocompetent as well as immunoincompetent Acute Retinal Necrosis patients suggests viral as opposed to host factors as an explanation for the disease. The occasional headache and stiff neck as well as the cerebrospinal fluid pleocytosis and acute optic neuritis occurring in conjunction with some cases of Acute Retinal Necrosis implicates the central nervous system as another involved organ. Since the herpes viruses are neurotrophic, this further supports the herpetic etiology for Acute Retinal Necrosis.

Introduction

The Acute Retinal Necrosis Syndrome is primarily an ocular disease, which consists of intraocular inflammation, retinal arteritis, peripheral necrotizing retinitis, optic neuritis, and often retinal detachment (8).

The etiologic agent responsible for this ocular condition has been demonstrated to be a virus of the Herpes group including Varicella Zoster (5,25), Herpes Simplex Virus type 1 (7,14), and even evidence for Cytomegalovirus and Herpes Simplex Virus type II has been forthcoming (16,21).

In the reported cases several systemic abnormalities have been observed associated temporarly with the ocular abnormalities. Although many different systemic abnormalities have been associated with individual cases of Acute Retinal Necrosis, several systemic disease aspects have appeared frequently. As will be demonstrated in this review,

- over 25% of Acute Retinal Necrosis cases manifest a dermatitis consistent with a Herpes group virus, and
- in another group of cases central nervous system abnormalities can be seen.

This review will summarize these associations and attempt to relate them to the ocular disease.

Dermatologic Associations with Acute Retinal Necrosis

A review of the available Acute Retinal Necrosis cases, which numbers approximately 100 cases, shows 25 cases associated with a zoster dermatitis (2, 3, 6, 9, 10, 11, 12, 13, 17, 22, 29) and three cases related to an Herpes Simplex Virus type 1 dermatitis (15, 19, 28). Fourteen of these cases occurred in immunocompetent patients and six cases with similar dermatologic lesions have been described in various forms of immunoincompetent patients (Tabs.1 and 2). Another eight cases of Acute Retinal Necrosis have occurred associated with chickenpox (Tab.3).

A careful review of these cases demonstrates no consistent distribution of the dermatitis relative to the eye involved with Acute Retinal Necrosis nor with the severity of the ocular changes. In almost all cases the skin lesions appeared within several weeks prior to the onset of Acute Retinal Necrosis, although several cases demonstrated a longer interval. In one case the dermatitis occurred 17 months after the retinitis. In the cases of chickenpox-associated Acute Retinal Necrosis, the ocular lesions presented between five days and 28 days after the onset of the dermatitis.

Central Nervous System Associations with Acute Retinal Necrosis

Central nervous system signs and symptoms have been a prominent manifestation of reported cases of Acute Retinal Necrosis, especially
- headache and
- neck stiffness (1,16,20).

In addition, instances of
- hearing loss,
- cranial nerve palsy, and
- stroke

have been seen in certain cases (3,24,28,29).

In some reports, cerebrospinal fluid analyses were reported. In only one of the reported cases has the fluid been normal (26). In ten cases the cerebrospinal fluid examination has been abnormal, usually showing between five to 50 cells per cubic millimeter, of which the majority, 80% to 100%, were mononuclear cells (3,5,20,23,24,26,28). None of the cerebrospinal fluid samples were found positive by culture for any organism.

Additional information regarding the optic nerve supports a central nervous system involvement in Acute Retinal Necrosis, and it is reviewed here only for its relevance to the systemic involvement in Acute Retinal Necrosis. The optic nerve has been shown involved by computed tomograhy scan in at least six different instances (24) and of course disc edema is a prominent feature of the ocular manifestations of Acute Retinal Necrosis (8).

Discussion

The systemic manifestations of Acute Retinal Necrosis fall into two broad categories, dermatitis and central nervous system alterations.

The dermatological lesions are typical of the vesicular lesions seen with Herpes Simplex Virus type 1 and Herpes Simplex Virus type 2 as well as the dermatome type involvement characteristic of the Varicella Zoster Virus. The temporal involvement of the skin and nervous system in the above reviewed Acute Retinal Necrosis cases with lesions typical of the herpes group of viruses appears more than coincidentally. It seems likely that the ocular manifestation is but one clinical manifestation of a systemic viral infection which is either not expressed in all patients or is expressed in varying degrees.

The central nervous system involvement in Acute Retinal Necrosis occurs in over 10% of reported cases. It is well established that the Herpes Simplex Virus type 1 group of viruses, especially Herpes Simplex Virus type 1 and Varicella Zoster Virus, can involve the central nervous system often as an encephalitis or as a cerebral vasculitis. Although these clinical manifestations do not often appear associated with the ocular findings in Acute Retinal Necrosis, it certainly seems possible that the herpetic etiology of the ocular manifestations in Acute Retinal Necrosis can be extended to involve the central nervous system, in this instance, as a meningitis.

It is interesting that Herpes zoster ophthalmicus is rarely associated with Acute Retinal Necrosis (4). Herpes zoster ophthalmicus is characterized by intense ocular pain and panuveitis but without the typical peripheral retinitis of Acute Retinal Necrosis. This suggests that reactivation and nerve transmission to the retina is not responsible for Acute Retinal Necrosis, or the retina should be involved frequently in Herpes zoster ophthalmicus.

Another reason to question neuronal latency and reactivation is the lack of consistent ipsilateral involvement. Of the cases reviewed above, approximately one-third demonstrated dermatitis on the opposite side of the face from the retinitis, or dermatitis at sites other than the face.

It seems that viremia is a more reasonable explanation for viral spread in Acute Retinal Necrosis. This would explain the ocular disease in the presence of a distant dermatitis. Support for this is the observation of transient viremia during reactivation and dissemination with Varicella Zoster Virus infection (4). Chickenpox also represents a Varicella Zoster Virus viremic disease, and has now been observed associated with Acute Retinal Necrosis. Viremia may be the best explanation for Acute Retinal Necrosis, but does not explain why a retinitis is infrequently observed with Varicella Zoster Virus and Herpes Simplex Virus infections. Evidence argues against a change in the viral genome, at least for Varicella Zoster Virus (18), and thus host factors, possibly genetic or immunologic, may eventually yield the answer (27).

Table 1. Association of dermatitis and ARN

Author	Cases	Interval[1]	Dermatome
Browning et al (8) 7	5d-3mos	Trunk (4),	1 (3) (2 of 3 ipsil)
Yeo et al.(9)	2	3-6 weeks	V1, V2(ipsil contra)
Jampol (10)	1	17 mos[2]	V1 (ipsil)
Schwartz et al.(11)		7 wks.	V1 (ipsil)
Ludwig et al.(19)		2 wks.	V1, HSV-1 (ipsil)
Willerson et al. (20)	1	2 days	lip, HSV-1 (contra)
Peyman et al. (21)		? mos.	eyelids,HSV-2(ipsil)

[1] Interval - time from onset of dermatitis to ARN; Ipsil - ipsilateral; contra - contralateral
[2] ARN predated dermatitis

Table 2. Association of dermatitis and ARN with Immunoincompetence

Author	Cases	Interval[1]	Dermatome
Jabs et al. (12)	3	4 wks. (2)	V1(bilat),V3(ipsil)
		3 mos.	V1,V2,T12,C1 (bilat)
Freeman et al. (13)	1	4 wks.	V1 (ipsil)
Friberg and Jost (14)	1	4 wks.	T2 - T4
Brown et al. (15)	1	? days	V1 (ipsil)

[1] Interval - time from onset of dermatitis to ARN
Ipsil - ipsilateral; contra - contralateral

Table 3. Association of Chickenpox with ARN

Author	Cases	Interval[1]
Culbertson et al. (16)	4	5-28 days
Matsuo et al. (17) 3	3 wks.	
Kelly & Rosenthal (18)	1	2 wks.

[1] Interval - time from onset of dermatitis to ARN; Ipsil - ipsilateral;contra - contralateral

References

1. Ando F, Kato M, Goto S et al (1983) Platelet Function in Bilateral Acute Retinal Necrosis. Am J Ophthalmol 96:27-32
2. Brown RM, Mendis U (1973) Retinal Arteritis Complicating Herpes Zoster Ophthalmicus. Br J Ophthalmol 57:344-346
3. Browning DJ, Blumenkranz MS, Culbertson WW et al (1987) Association of Varicella Zoster Dermatitis with Acute Retinal Necrosis Syndrome. Ophthalmology 94:602-606
4. Cobo LM, Faulks GN, Liesegang T et al (1986) Oral Acyclovir in the Treatment of Acute Herpes Zoster Ophthalmicus. Ophthalmology 92:763-770
5. Culbertson WW, Blumenkranz MS, Pepose JS et al (1986) Varicella Zoster Virus is a Cause of the Acute Retinal Necrosis Syndrome. Ophthalmology 93:559-569
6. Culbertson WW, Brod RD, Taylor BC et al (1991) Chickenpox-associated Acute Retinal Necrosis Syndrome. Ophthalmology 98:1641-1645
7. Duker JS, Nielsen J, Eagle RC et al (1990) Rapidly Progressive, Acute Retinal Necrosis (ARN) Secondary to Herpes Simplex Virus, Type 1. Ophthalmology 97:1638-1643
8. Duker JS, Blumenkranz MS (1991) Diagnosis and Management of the Acute Retinal Necrosis (ARN) Syndrome. Surv Ophthalmol 35:327-343
9. Freeman WR, Thomas EL, Rao NA et al (1986) Demonstration of Herpes Group Virus in Acute Retinal Necrosis Syndrome. Am J Ophthalmol 102:701-709
10. Fribert TR, Jost BF (1984) Acute Retinal Necrosis in an Immunosuppressed Patient. Am J Ophthalmol 98:515-519
11. Jabs DA, Schachat AP, Liss R et al (1987) Presumed Varicella Zoster Retinitis in Immunocompromised Patients. Retina 7:9-13
12. Jampol LM (1982) Acute Retinal Necrosis. Am J Ophthalmol 93:254-255
13. Kelly SP, Rosenthal AR (1990) Chickenpox Chorioretinitis. Br J Ophthalmol 74:698-699
14. Lewis ML, Culbertson WW, Post JD et al (1989) Herpes Simplex Virus Type 1. A Cause of the Acute Retinal Necrosis Syndrome. Ophthalmology 96:875-878
15. Ludwig IH, Zegarra H, Zakov ZN (1984) The Acute Retinal Necrosis Syndrome. Possible Herpes Simplex Retinitis. Ophthalmology 91:1659-1665
16. Margolis T, Irvine AR, Hoyt WF et al (1988) Acute Retinal Necrosis Syndrome Presenting with Papillitis and Arcuate Neuroretinitis. Ophthalmology 95:937-940
17. Matsuo T, Koyama M, Matsuo N (1990) Acute Retinal Necrosis as a Novel Complication of Chickenpox in Adults. Br J Ophthalmol 74:443-444
18. Pepose JS, Biron K (1987) Antiviral Sensitivities of the Acute Retinal Necrosis Syndrome Virus. Curr Eye Res 6:201-205
19. Peyman GA, Goldberg MF, Uninsky E et al (1984) Vitrectomy and Intravitreal Antiviral Drug Therapy in Acute Retinal Ne-

crosis Syndrome. Arch Ophthalmol 102:1619-1621
20. Price FW, Schlaegel TF (1980) Bilateral Acute Retinal Necrosis. Am J Ophthalmol 89:419-424
21. Rungger-Brandle E, Roux L, Leuenberger PM (1984) Bilateral Acute Retinal Necrosis (BARN) Identification of the Presumed Infectious Agent. Ophthalmology 91:1648-1657
22. Schwartz JN, Cashwell F, Hawkins HK et al (1976) Necrotizing Retinopathy with Herpes Zoster Ophthalmicus; a Light and Electron Microscopical Study. Arch Pathol Lab Med 100:386-391
23. Sergot RC, Belmont JB, Savino PJ et al (1985) Optic Nerve Involvement in the Acute Retinal Necrosis Syndrome. Arch Ophthalmol 103:1160-1162
24. Sergot RC, Anand R, Belmont JB et al (1989) Acute Retinal Necrosis Neuropathy. Arch Ophthalmol 107:692-696
25. Soshi S, Ozawa H, Matsuhashi M et al (1988) Demonstration of Varicella-Zoster Virus Antigens in the Vitreous Aspirates of Patients with Acute Retinal Necrosis Syndrome. Ophthalmology 95:1394-1398
26. Sternberg P, Knox DL, Finkelstein D et al (1982) Acute Retinal Necrosis Syndrome. Retina 2:145-151
27. Streilein JW (1990) Anterior Chamber Associated Immune Deviation: the Privilege of Immunity in the Eye. Surv Ophthalmol 35:67-73
28. Willerson D, Aaberg TM, Reeser FH (1977) Necrotizing Vasoocclusive Retinitis. Am J Ophthalmol 84:209-219
29. Yeo JH, Pepose JS, Stewart JA (1986) Acute Retinal Necrosis Syndrome Following Herpes Zoster Dermatitis. Ophthalmology 93:1418-1422

- Parasitic: Toxoplasmosis

Toxoplasmosis: Current Concepts in Parasitology

H.M. Seitz

Abstract. Toxoplasma gondii has a worldwide distribution and a low host specificity.
It is an obligatory intracellular parasite destroying its host cell during multiplication. Parasite cysts are formed in tissues, which are the source for infection if they are eaten by potential new hosts. Apart from this asexual way of reproduction, a sexual phase exists in the intestine of the cat, which is the final host for T. gondii.
In humans, the infection is usually not associated with any serious disease. No treatment is normally required. For immunodeficient hosts, such as the HIV-infected or the fetus, the infection is dangerous. Ocular involvement is believed to be the late sequela of a fetal infection in most cases.

Introduction

"Toxoplasma" derives from the Greek words "toxon" for bow and "plasma" for structure. The species name "gondii" refers to the small rodent, in which the parasite was discovered: the North African gundi (Ctenodactylus).

Parasitology

Toxoplasma gondii is an obligate intracellular protozoon belonging to the phylum Apicomplexa. The members of this taxon possess an apical complex, which is an arrangement of subcellular elements as polar rings, a conoid and rhoptries. This complex is important for the penetration of the parasite into its host cells. Usually, the cells of the reticular endothelial system are infected, but principally many other cell types can also serve as a habitat for the parasite. Within the cytoplasm of its host cell the toxoplasmas are enclosed in a parasitophorous vacuole. Here they multiply in a peculiar way, which is called endodyogeny. Two daughter parasites develop within the mother cell, which finally fades away. After about 6-10 cell cycles the host cell is completely filled with parasites and destroyed. The liberated parasites enter new host cells.

In addition to the described rather fast multiplication, the parasite may show a slower reproduction leading to another type of parasite accumulation, the Toxoplasma cyst. These cysts may contain thousands of parasites. Their special feature is the cyst wall which is a rather thick structure, composed of several membranes. Preferably, these cysts seem to develop in neural tissue and in muscle cells. Parasites persist for many years in these cysts and are protected against the immunological defence and also against chemotherapeutics. We have reason to believe that the drugs we use for treating toxoplasmosis do not penetrate into the cysts in a sufficient way.

Man is an intermediate host of T. gondii, since he supports only asexual multiplication. The final hosts are cats and cat-like animals. Within the intestine of the cats, the parasite differentiates into male and female cells, fertilization occurs and after some further development the sexual products, the so-called oocysts, are excreted in the faeces of the cat. The excretion lasts about 2-3 weeks. Thus several millions of these oocysts are deposited with the cat faeces. Under suitable circumstances they can persist for more than one year. If they are taken up orally with soil-contaminated food as vegetables, fruits or salad, or eaten by herbivorous animals, they become infected as new intermediate hosts.

In its asexual phase T. gondii has a very low host specificity. The infection is widespread in mammals and birds. Man can be infected as described by eating oocyst-contaminated food. Another, probably more important, way is eating undercooked meat containing cysts. In Europe probably pork and mutton are the usual sources of infection. As judged by the presence of antibodies against T. gondii, in Germany at the age of 40 about half of the population is infected, in France the prevalence is even higher.

Usually, no clinical symptoms develop in infected humans. Swollen lymph nodes, particularly in the neck region are relatively frequent. They may persist for weeks or a few months. During primary infection a solid immunity develops protecting the individual against later infections, as long as not a severe immunosuppression takes place.

The clinical significance of toxoplasmosis comes from the danger that the parasite may infect the fetus during pregnancy, if the mother experiences her primary infection during the pregnancy. Depending on the stage of the pregnancy and probably the number of parasites crossing the placenta the newborn may show no symptoms at all, minor symptoms or severe damage. Early in pregnancy the placenta is a more effective barrier against the parasites than later in pregnancy. One of the organs often involved in prenatal infection is the eye, the retina in particular. More and more evidence accumulates that most cases of toxoplasmotic retinochorioretinitis, or may be even all cases, originate from prenatal infections.

Usually it is not possible to demonstrate the parasite directly. Diagnosis depends on finding antibodies in the serum of the patient. IgM as well as IgG antibodies develop about 7-10 days after the infection. There are a number of methods suitable as antibody tests. Of particular reliability is the Dye Test (Sabin-Feldman Test). Unfortunately do the titers in the blood not correlate well with the activity of the infection in the eye. So the diagnosis of ocular toxoplasmosis is normally made by the recognition of the typical retinal lesions during funduscopy. In special cases a confirmation is possible by a comparative determination of total antibodies in serum and the fluid of the anterior chamber. A high level of antibody in the eye indicates a local production and an acive process in the eye.

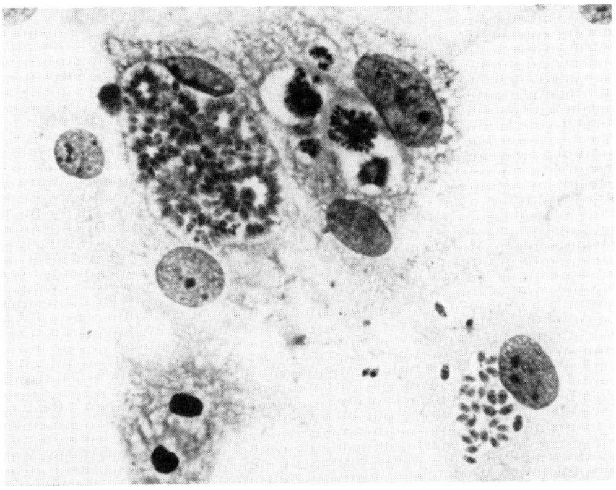

Fig.1. Toxoplasma gondii in cell culture. The cells of the monolayer show various degrees of infection.

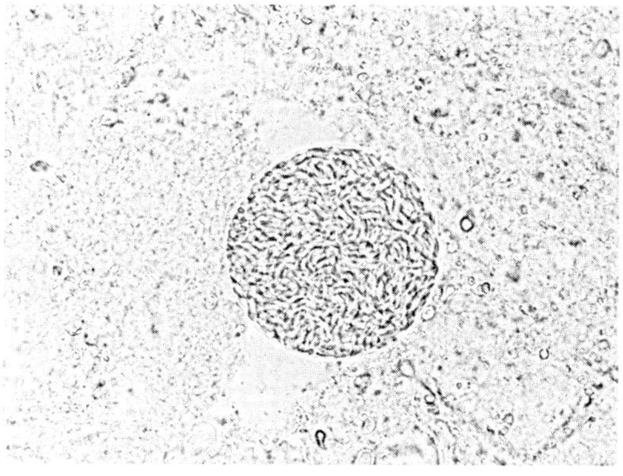

Fig.2. Toxoplasma cysts from a mouse brain containing probably thousands of individual parasites. The mouse was inoculated for diagnostic purposes with the cerebrospinal fluid from a newborn with hydrocephalus.

Histopathology of Ocular Toxoplasmosis

W. Richard Green

Abstract. Toxoplasma gondii is an obligate intracellular protozoan parasite with almost universal geographic distribution.

Up to 50% of the population in the United States and higher in some European countries have been infected by the organism. Most infections are asymptomatic or transient and are not recognized. Ocular toxoplasmosis is a common cause of ocular inflammatory disease.

Congenital and acquired forms of the disease are recognized. Most cases occurring in adolescents and adults are due to reactivation of congenital infections.

While the incidence of ocular involvement in acquired disease is very low, there appears to be increasing disease with ocular involvement associated immunosuppression. The retinitis in association with immunosuppression is apt to be more extensive and may be confused with retinitis due to other causes.

Introduction

Toxoplasma gondii may cause congenital and acquired retinochoroiditis.

Epidemiology

In a study of 15000 women, Desmonts and coworkers (6) had observed that 16% of pregnant women had no protective antibodies and were susceptible to toxoplasmosis. The risk was greatest for young women foreigners living in France. Frequency of acquired toxoplasmosis was 8 per 1000. No overt or latent congenital toxoplasmosis was observed when maternal infection preceded pregnancy. Of the 24 cases of acquired toxoplasmosis in pregnancy the off-spring were followed and 12 were unaffected and subsequent serologic reactions were negative. Two died and presumably had congenital toxoplasmosis. Ten survived and had congenital toxoplasmosis - nine were latent and one had ocular involvement.

These results confirmed the classical opinion that congenital toxoplasmosis follows an infection acquired by the mother during pregnancy.

In 1989, Koppe and Rothova of the Netherlands described a prospective study that was begun in 1964 (14). Of 1821 women who had seroconverted for toxoplasmosis during pregnancy, 10 babies had congenital toxoplasmosis and four of the 10 children had evidence of retinitis and all four had recurrences over 20 years. Five more infected children developed retinitis. Of 10 children that were questionably infected, three subsequently developed retinitis.

A control group of 117 patients who were not congenitally infected were followed and 56% contracted toxoplasmosis and were seropositive by age 15 years. None developed retinochoroiditis.

Congenital Ocular Toxoplasmosis

In congenital ocular toxoplasmosis there may be solitary or multiple lesions, which often heal with marked scarring (Fig.1). We obtained the eyes of a 16 day old female the product of a pregnancy complicated by lymphadenopathy during the seventh month. The child had diffuse intracranial calcification and early hydrocephalus. Both eyes had retinal neovascularization and extensive retinitis due to toxoplasmosis (Fig.2).

Recurrence of congenital toxoplasmosis is the most common form of ocular toxoplasmosis and accounts for up to 50% of cases in some uveitis clinics. Most typically the new areas of retinitis develop adjacent to old healed lesions (Fig.3) presumably from encysted dormant organisms.

Histopathology

There is an acute inflammatory cell infiltrate in the retina with variable involvement of the vitreous. The organisms are present in the retina which becomes necrotic (Fig.4,5). The organisms may also be identified by a fluorescent antibody technique (21). An obliterative arteritis may be present (4,18) (Fig.6). A variably intense inflammatory reaction involves the anterior segment with lymphocytic and sometimes granulomatous infiltration in the iris and angle and synechia may develop keratic precipitates with large mononuclear cells are often present (Fig.7).

It is in the eyes with recurrent disease that Helenor Campbell Wilder first observed organisms in the retina in adults and juvenile patients (27). In many of the 53 eyes there was an intense adjacent granulomatous choroiditis and scleritis (Fig.8). When such lesions involve the peripheral retina the scleritis may be evident externally as noted in this case reported by Schuman and coworkers (24).

A variant of probable recurrent disease with multifocal punctate outer retinal lesions (Fig.9) has been reported by Friedman and Knox (8), Doft and Gass (7), and Matthews and Weiter (16).

Thus congenital toxoplasmosis results in recurrences in adolescents and adults. Furthermore, acquired toxoplasmosis seems not to result frequently in ocular involvement.

Acquired Ocular Toxoplasmosis

Acquired ocular toxoplasmosis, however does occur. Only 2-3% of patients with acquired systemic toxoplasmosis have ocular involvement. Saari and coworkers reported a 33-year-old patient who developed systemic toxoplasmosis a few days after exposure to nasal secretions of infected cows (23). The patient developed rhinitis, sore throat, muscular pains, fatigue and headache. He developed retinochoroiditis 11 days after exposure.

Michelson and coworkers reported the case of a 43-year-old woman who developed systemic toxoplasmosis and retinitis documented by recovery of the organism from a lymph node (17).

Akstein and coworkers studied 37 persons who developed acute systemic toxoplasmosis and were thought to have acquired the disease as the result of aerosolization of oocysts from infected cats in a riding stable (1). After four years of follow-up, only one person had developed ocular disease. This study shows that some sporadic cases of toxoplasma retinitis are due to acquired toxoplasmosis.

In contrast to the foregoing generalization, which are true for most areas such as Western Europe and North America, there are reports of observations of multiple sibling involvement in apparent congenital ocular toxoplasmosis (3,15). Silveira and coworkers observed that some families in Southern Brazil have a high incidence of acquired toxoplasmosis (25). These authors concluded that the incidence of acquired subclinical toxoplasmic infection that causes late or recurrent retinitis is probably more frequent than previously noted.

The association of ocular toxoplasmosis with pigmentary retinopathy (26) and Fuchs' heterochromic iridocyclitis (2,5) are curious and require additional investigation to determine if this is a causal relationship.

Toxoplasmosis in Immunodeficiency

An apparent increasing number of cases of ocular toxcoplasmosis have been associated with immunosuppression including long-term corticosteroid therapy (19), chemotherapy for Hodgkin's disease (11), following chemotherapy for lymphoma (28) and irradiation and chemotherapy for lymphoma, after bone marrow (20) and renal transplantation, and with the acquired immune deficiency syndrome (9,10,13).

This is the appearance of the large area of retinitis in the case reported by Nicholson and Wolchok (19) (Fig.10). Numerous proliferative forms are present in the retina at the margin of the lesion. Cysts with organisms were present in the area of the retinalpigment epithelium.

Toxoplasmic retinochoroiditis in the immunodeficient host has more extensive tissue destruction, may be more difficult to diagnose and treat, may have a single lesion in one or both eyes, have multifocal lesions or diffuse areas of retinal necrosis (12,22). Most lesions do not arise from borders of old healed lesions. Organism may also involve iris, choroid, vitreous. The disease responds to standard antiparasite therapy but continued therapy is probably necessary to prevent reactivation.

In Fig.11a-c, the ophthalmoscopic view of a patient with the acquired immunodeficiency syndrome and retinitis is given. When first seen the patient was considered to have retinitis to be due to Cytomegalovirus. A smaller lesion was present in the left eye. An area of partial healing with fibroglial scarring of the retina was present in the lesion of the right eye (Figs.11c,12a). Numerous toxoplasma cysts were present in adjacent retina in the right eye (Fig. 12 b,c) and the left eye.

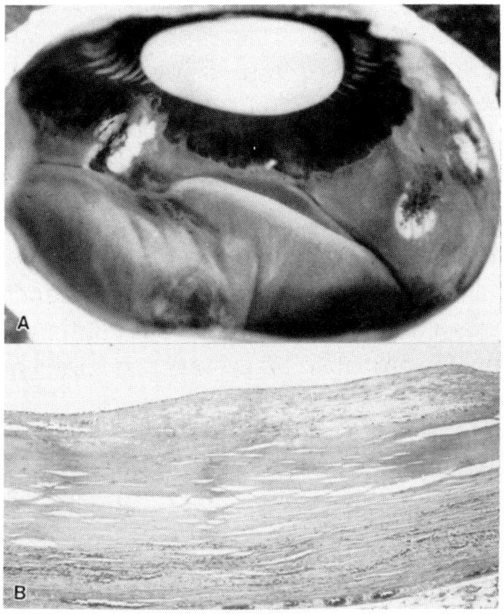

Fig.1. Congenital toxoplasmosis. A: Gross appearance of multiple healed retinochoroidal lesions. B: Scar of congenital toxoplasmosis lesion has total replacement of retina and choroid by a dense fibrous connective tissue (Hematoxylin/Eosin x110)

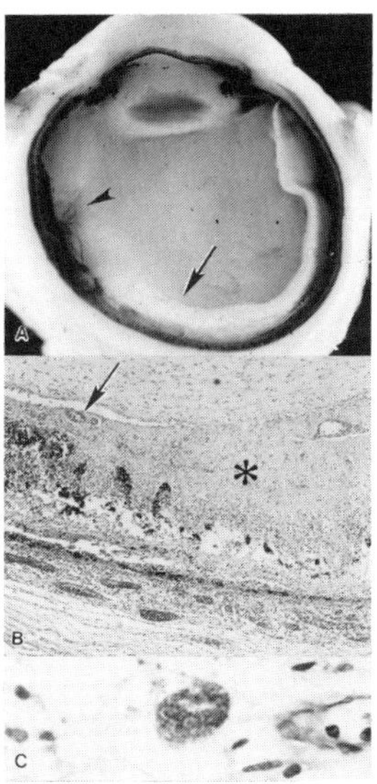

Fig.2. Congenital toxoplasmosis. A: Gross appearance of extensive area of retinal necrosis (arrow) and retinal neovascularization (arrrowhead). B: Area of junction of necrotic retina (asterisk) and relatively preserved retinal (arrow) (Hematoxylin/Eosin x50)
C. Toxoplasma cyst in necrotic area of retina (Periodic Acid-Schiffx750)

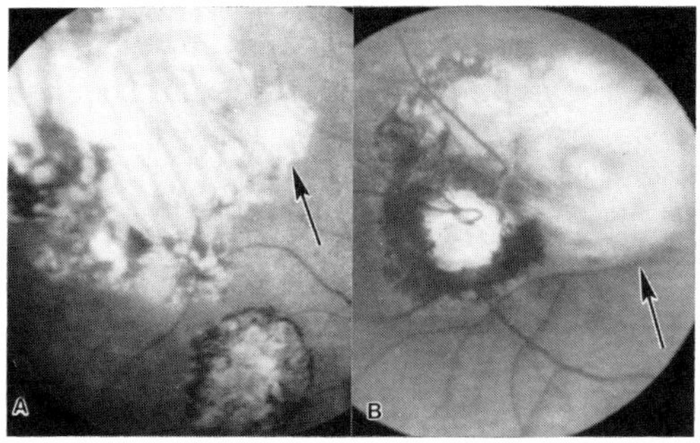

Fig.3. A and B: Examples of recurrent toxoplasma retinochoroiditis (arrows) adjacent to healed retinochoroidal scars.

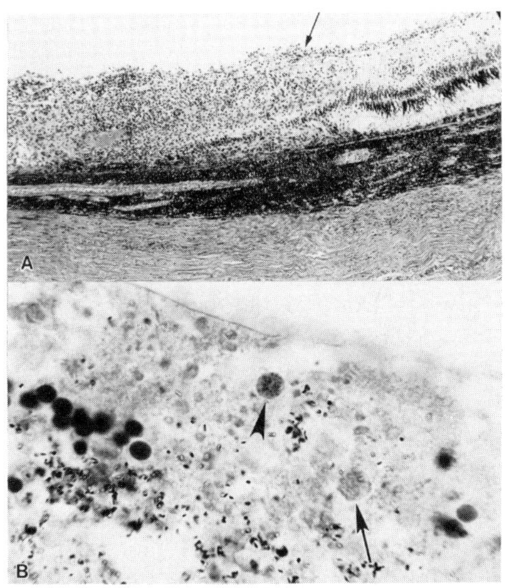

Fig.4. Recurrent toxoplasmosis. A: Area of acute retinitis (left of arrow). Acute and chronic inflammatory cells are present in the overlying vitreous, the retinal pigment epithelium is destroyed and there is an intense lymphocytic infiltrate in the subjacent choroid (AFIP 754058) (Hematoxylin/Eosin x90). B: Area of necrotizing retinitis with necrotic (arrow) and viable (arrowhead) cysts of Toxoplasma gondii (Periodic Acid-Schiff x525)

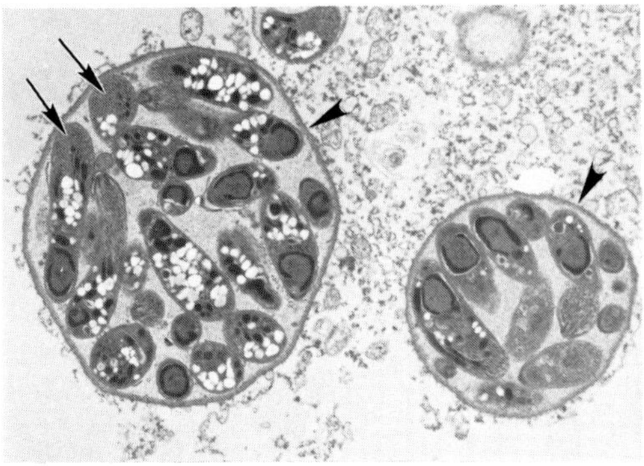

Fig.5. Ultrastructural appearance of toxoplasma cyst from the retina with a two-layered cyst wall (arrowheads) containing numerous oval or crescent-shaped organisms containing toxonemes (arrows), a nucleus and vacuoles (rhoptries) (x6500).

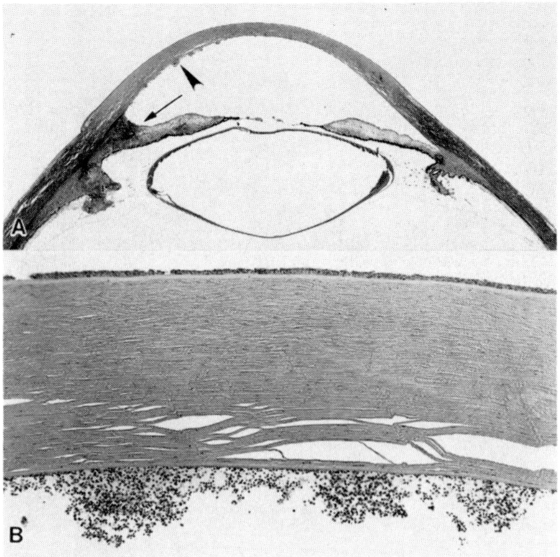

Fig.7. A: Anterior segment of eye with active toxoplasma retinochoroiditis (Fig.4) with large keratic precipitates (arrowhead) and obstruction of the anterior chamber angle inferiorly by inflammatory cells (arrow) (AFIP 754058) (Hematoxcylin/Eosin x6.5). B. Large keratic precipitates composed of large mononuclear inflammatory cells (Hematoxylin/Eosin x90)

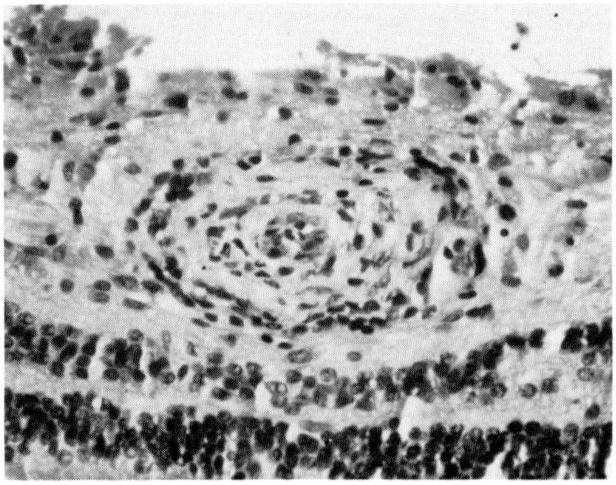

Fig.6. Obliterative arteritis near an area of toxoplasma retinitis (Hematoxylin/Eosin x328).

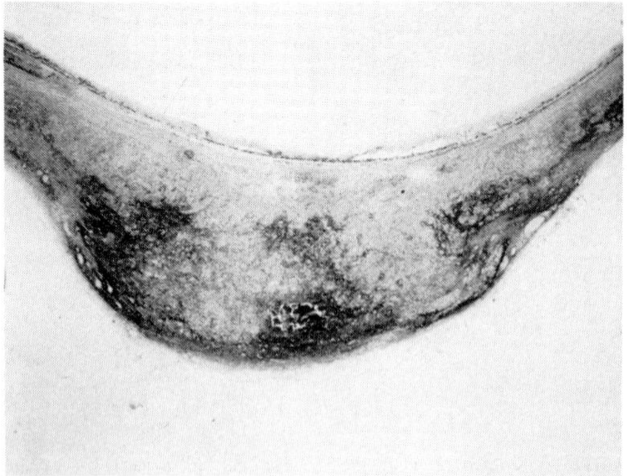

Fig.8. Surgically enucleated eye with acute retinitis due to toxoplasma. The retina is partially necrotic and there is an intense granulomatous inflammatory infiltrate in the choroid, sclera and episclera (AFIP 70313) (Hematoxylin/Eosin x15)

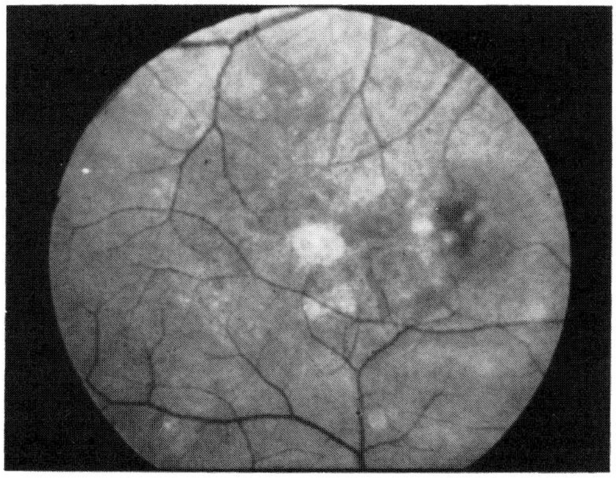

Fig.9. Deep punctate retinitis involving the outer aspect of the retina (Photo courtesy of Dr.David L. Knox).

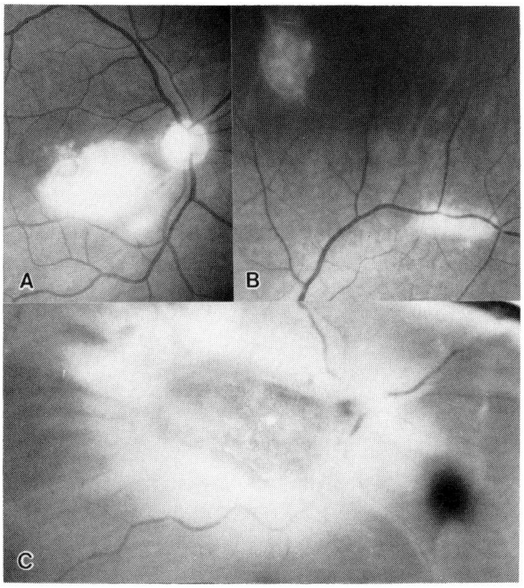

Fig.11. Ophthalmoscopic appearance of acute retinitis in right (A) and left (B) and the gross appearance of the lesion in the right eye (C) of a 42-year-old man with acquired immune deficiency.

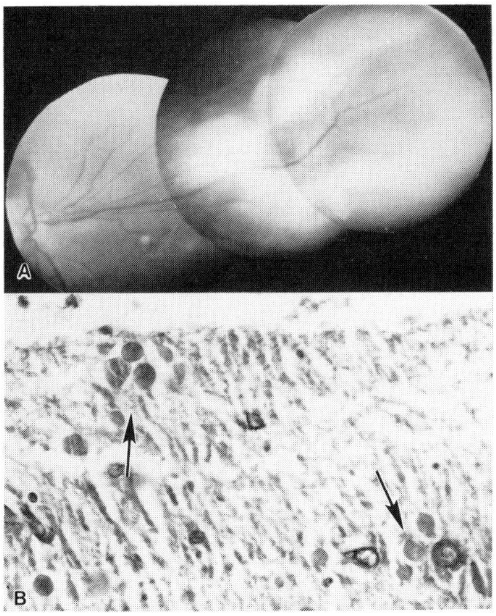

Fig.10. A: Composite photograph illustrating an extensive area of retinochoroiditis. B: Area of necrotic retina with numerous toxoplasma cysts (arrows) (hematoxylin and eosin x 525) (From: Nicholson DH and Wolchok EB (1976) Arch Ophthalmol 94:248-254.

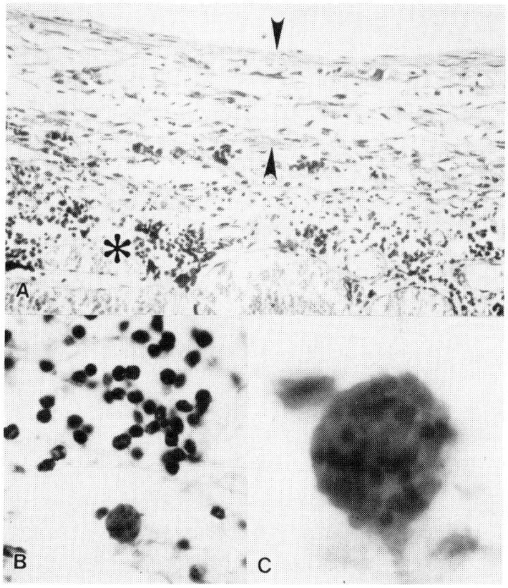

Fig.12. A: Post mortem examination of the lesion of the right eye of patient illustrated in figure 11 discloses an area where the retina is replaced by a fibrocellular scar (between arrowheads) and a moderate lymphocytic infiltrate is present in the choroid (asterisk) (Hematoxylin/Eosin x137) B: An area of active retinitis adjacent to the scarred area has toxoplasma cysts (Periodic Acid-Schiff x325). C: Higher power of toxoplasma cysts (Periodic Acid-Schiff x1300)

References

1. Akstein RB, Wilson LA, Teutsch SM (1982) Acquired Toxoplasmosis. Ophthalmology 89:1299-1302
2. Arffa RC, Schlaegel TF Jr (1984) Chorioretinal Scar in Fuchs' Heterochromic Iridocyclitis. Arch Ophthalmol 102:1153-1155
3. Asbell PA, Vermund SH, Hofeldt AJ (1982) Presumed Toxoplasmic Retinochoroiditis in Four Siblings. Am J Ophthalmol 94:656-663
4. Braunstein RA, Gass DM (1980) Branch Artery Obstruction Caused by Acute Toxoplasmosis. Arch Ophthalmol 98:512-513
5. de Abreu MT, Belfort R Jr, Hirata PS (1982) Fuchs' Heterochromic Cyclitis and Ocular Toxoplasmosis. Am J Ophthalmol 93:739-744
6. Desmonts G, Couvreur J, Ben Rachid MS (1965) Le toxoplasme, la mère et l'enfant. Extraits des Arch. Francaises de Pediatrie 22:1183-1199
7. Doft BH, Gass DM (1985) Punctate Outer Retinal Toxoplasmosis. Arch Ophthalmol 103:1332-1336
8. Friedmann CT, Knox DL (1969) Variations in Recurrent Active Toxoplasmic Retinochoroiditis. Arch Ophthalmol 81:481-493
9. Grossniklaus HE, Specht CS, Allaire G et al (1990) Toxoplasma gondii Retinochoroiditis and Optic Neuritis in Acquired Immune Deficiency Syndrome. Ophthalmology 97:1342-1346
10. Heinemann MH, Gold JMW, Maisel J (1986) Bilateral Toxoplasma Retinochoroiditis in a Patient with Acquired Immune Deficiency Syndrome. Retina 6:224-227
11. Hoerni B, Vallat M, Durand M et al (1978) Ocular Toxoplasmosis and Hodgkin's Disease. Arch Ophthalmol 96:62-63
12. Holland GN (1989) Ocular Toxoplasmosis in the Immunocompromised Host. Int Ophthalmol 13:399-402
13. Holland GN, Engstrom RE, Glasgow BJ et al (1988) Ocular Toxoplasmosis in Patients with the Acquired Immunodeficiency Syndrome. Am J Ophthalmol 106:653-667
14. Koppe JG, Rothova A (1989) Congenital Toxoplasmosis. Int Ophthalmol 13:387-390
15. Lou P, Kazdan J, Basu PK (1978) Ocular Toxoplasmosis in Three Consecutive Siblings. Arch Ophthalmol 96:613-614
16. Matthews JD, Weiter JJ (1988) Outer Retinal Toxoplasmosis. Ophthalmology 95:941-946
17. Michelson JB, Shields JA, McDonald PR et al (1978) Retinitis Secondary to Acquired Systemic Toxoplasmosis with Isolation of the Parasite. Am J Ophthalmol 86:548-552
18. Morgan CM, Gragoudas ES (1987) Branch Retinal Artery Occlusion Associated with Recurrent Toxoplasmic Retinochoroiditis. Arch Ophthalmol 105:130-131
19. Nicholson DH, Wolchok EB (1976) Ocular Toxoplasmosis in an Adult Receiving Long-Term Corticosteroid Therapy. Arch Ophthalmol 94:248-254
20. Pauleikhoff D, Messmer E, Beelen DW et al (1987) Bone-Marrow Transplantation and Toxoplasmic Retinochoroiditis. Graefe's Arch Clin Exp Ophthalmol 235:239-243
21. Rao NA, Font RL (1977) Toxoplasmic Retinochoroiditis. Arch Ophthalmol 95: 273-277
22. Rehder JR, Burnier M Jr, Pavesio CE et al (1988) Acute Unilateral Toxoplasmic Iridocyclitis in an AIDS Patient. Am J Ophthalmol 106:740-741
23. Saari M, Vuorre K, Neiminen H et al)176) Acquired Toxoplasmic Chorioretinitis. Arch Ophthalmol 94:1485-1488
24. Schuman JS, Weinberg RS, Ferry AP et al (1988) Toxoplasmic Scleritis. Ophthalmology 95:1399-1403

25. Silveira C, Belfort R Jr, Burnier M Jr et al (1988) Acquired Toxoplasmic Infection as the Cause of Toxoplasmic Retinochoroiditis in Families. Am J Ophthalmol 102:352-364
26. Silveira C, Belfort R Jr, Nussenblatt R et al (1989) Unilateral Pigmentary Retinopathy Associated with Ocular Toxoplasmosis. Am J Ophthalmol 107:682-684
27. Wilder HC (1952) Toxoplasma Chorioretinitis in Adults. Arch Ophthalmol 48: 126-136
28. Yeo JH, Jakobiec FA, Iwamoto T et al (1983) Opportunistic Toxoplasmic Retinochoroiditis Following Chemotherapy for Systemic Lymphoma. Ophthalmology 90:885-898

Toxoplasmosis: Current Concepts and Therapeutic Options in Brazil

Rubens Belfort Jr., CM. Silveira, MC. Martins, MT. Abreu, M. Burnier Jr.

Abstract. Ocular toxoplasmosis comprises 50% of all uveitis cases in Brazil, often in multiple siblings.

Over 150 families with multiple affected siblings have now been identified and active ocular lesions have been diagnosed in 29 individuals with serological evidence of acquired infection with T.gondii. All of them presented with a typical retinochoroiditis and had IgM circulating antibodies to Toxoplasma at the time of the onset of the uveitis or in the past (up to 3 years before); 72.3% of the patients had less than 30 years of age, IgM serum levels were lower than 1:64 in 41% of the cases.

A recent household survey performed by us in the region in 1044 individuals has shown an overall prevalence of ocular toxoplasmosis in adults as high as 20%. This also cannot be explained by congenital infections alone.

The incidence of acquired undiagnosed toxoplasmic infection that causes late necrotizing retinochoroiditis in normal hosts or immunosuppressed individuals (acquired immunodeficiency syndrome patients) is much more frequent than classically believed. The experience with different antitoxoplasmic agents has shown that recurrences are higher in acquired immunodeficiency syndrome patients and that the rates are similar independently of the specific drugs used.

Introduction

Ocular Toxoplasmosis is the most common cause of retinal inflammation in non immunocompromised patients. It is also the most important and frequent cause of uveitis in several countries. T.gondii is a intracellular protozoan parasite that is ubiquitous in nature and produces one of the most common infections of humans (8,12,13).

Epidemiology

Cats are pivotal in the transmission of toxoplasmosis. Epidemiologic data indicate that most cats become infected in nature soon after they are weaned and that the infection is higher in female animals. Results of epi demiologic studies have been inconclusive in linking human infection to the presence of cats in the household of infected people as well as to link the presence of the cysts in the soil to human infections. However, results of epidemiologic studies based on the shedding of oocysts by cats and the cultural habits and rates of this infection in the general population indicate the cat is involved and important in the epidemiologic aspects of toxoplasmosis. Epidemiologic data suggest the ingestion of tissue cysts in undercooked or uncooked meat is probably the most important cause of infection (5).

The importance of beef in the transmission of T.gondii infection to people is probably not important according to several authors and this has also been our experience (7). Fresh pork and raw sausages may be the main meat source of T.gondii in several countries, followed by lamb, sheep and even chicken (5,7,9). To prevent infection hands should be washed thoroughly with soap and water after handling meat. All cutting boards, sinks and other materials should be washed because the stages of T.gondii in meat are killed by water. Meat of any animal should be cooked at 70°C. Pregnant women should avoid contact with cats, soil and raw meat. Pet cats should be fed only dry canned or cooked food. The cat litter should be emptied daily to prevent the ovulation of the cysts and only with gloves, preferably not by pregnant women, children or seronegative people (5).

Various strains of T.gondii exist and they differ in their virulence to man. It is possible that the pathogenicity to the eye also differs, some strains being more destructive and others forming more cysts and leading to more recurrences.

Classically the strains have been differentiated almost exclusively according to their virulence to different animals. The DNA technology has allowed the initiation of the characterization of organisms from different sources such as the eye, brain, food and different species of animals. The results will probably be important in a better understanding of the pathogenicity of these organisms.

Toxoplasmosis comprises approximately 50% of all uveitis seen in Brazil (8).

Familial ocular toxoplasmosis seen notably in the southern part of the country (Erexim, Alto Uruguay region), where the incidence of ocular toxoplasmosis is definitely higher and accounts for 70 to 90% of the uveitis cases seen in rural areas (14). A household survey conducted recently in the area showed that more than 20% of the population has a toxoplasmic scar in the retina, a finding that cannot be explained by congenital infections alone (6).

This region of the world constitutes a natural laboratory for the study of ocular toxoplasmosis. The abnormally high prevalence of the disease has helped us to understand mechanisms that are also present in other regions though difficult to appreciate.

We now know that ocular toxoplasmosis does not reflect a congenital infection in almost all cases as it was considered in the past (13).

Congenital toxoplasmosis is considered to occur in the fetus only when the mother acquires the primary infection during the pregnancy or in the preceded months. Subsequent siblings are thought to be protected by the mother's acquired immunologic defense mechanisms. Therefore one would not expect siblings of a child with ocular toxoplasmosis to be at risk of contracting the same ocular disease (8,10,13).

Acquired ocular toxoplasmosis can nevertheless affect several members of a family as has been recognized. Various familial patterns of ocular toxoplasmosis have been noted. We have now seen more than 150 families where ocular toxoplasmosis follows this familial pattern. A large number of mothers that presented with ocular toxoplasmosis several years before the pregnancy, later had their children found to have ocular toxoplasmosis. Ocular toxoplasmosis in these families affected two to 9 siblings and has been identified also in three successive generations of female patients in some of the families (14).

T.gondii cysts have been identified in the retina of enucleated eyes from three non-twin siblings with ocular toxoplasmosis as well as been identified by PCR (3). The T.gondii antigen has been also demonstrated by the analysis of aqueous humor of some patients using the Polymerase Chain Reaction. It has been detected in three patients during the amplification of the B1 gene (4).

We have recently reported 29 cases of ocular toxoplasmosis acquired postnatally: All patients presented with a typical retinochoroiditis and had IgM antibodies to T.gondii at the time of the onset of the uveitis or in the past (up to three years before); 35% were male, 62% were unilateral, 17.2% of the patients had less than 10 years and 55.1% had between 10 and 30 years of age. IgM serum levels were ephemeral and lower than 1/64 in 41% of the cases (16).

Uveitis often appears months to years after the infection and the clinical and laboratorial differentiation between both forms is usually impossible since the clinical picture can be the same. At the time the uveitis presents the patient has usually low titers of circulating specific IgG antibodies and has no IgM antibodies for toxoplasmosis. The final diagnosis would depend on previous clinical and serologic information not frequently available.

According to our clinical experience following more than one hundred of cases of acquired toxoplasmosis the ocular recurrences are more frequent in the first years after the infection and this could explain partly the higher frequency of the disease in the first decades of life.

It seems therefore that the acquired T.gondii infection as well as the congenital form can present an early or late ocular onset, and the incidence of acquired subclinical infection that causes late or recurrent necrotizing retinochoroiditis is probably much more frequent than previously believed.

Clinical and Laboratorial Diagnosis

Currently the diagnosis of ocular toxoplasmosis is only presumptive based mainly on the clinical evaluation of a lesion in the fundus and positive serologic results for T.gondii antibodies.

The classical clinical presentation of an active lesion is that of a fresh, white, elevated focus of necrotizing retinochoroiditis near an old pigmented scar (satellite lesion). This lesion can vary greatly in size, is usually oval or circular and considered to be more frequently located posterior to the equator. The preference for the posterior pole and the macula is not clearly understood. Classically there is much exudation of cells into the vitreous. The anterior segment of the eye may also become involved. This is assumed to be a hypersensitivity phenomenon, since actual infection of the anterior segment by T.gondii has been demonstrated only in the acquired immunodeficiency syndrome in a single patient (11). Direct optic nerve involvement and scleritis can also occur as well as secondary vasculitis and branch occlusion. Curious associations with Fuchs' heterochromia (1) as well as with unilateral pigmentary retinopathy resembling unilateral retinitis pigmentosa (15) have been reported.

The Sabin-Feldman dye test and the indirect immunofluorescent antibodies tests are still the mainstay for the diagnosis. Any titer of antibodies may be significant. Western Blots may gradually become more valuable if present technical problems are resolved. The Enzyme Linked Immunosorbent Assays may be more sensitive than the classic tests, especially when dealing with low titers. However, before introduction as a routine procedure, Enzyme Linked Immunosorbent Assays still need further investigations (10).

In atypical cases, evaluation of the aqueous humor and comparison with respective serology may provide evidence of specific antibody formation in the eye especially if more antibody per unit of gamma globulin can be detected in the aqueous humor than in the serum. Demonstration of a local intraocular antibody production may enable the specific diagnosis of the uveitis. The possibility of monoclonal activation of resident cells by nonspecific factors has decreased the clinical importance of this test.

Treatment

The treatment of ocular toxoplasmosis has not really changed in the last 20 years. It depends on the location, size and severity of retinitis (5). The patient with a vision-threatening lesion (lesions menacing the macula, the optic nerve and the papillomacular bundle) needs every form of treatment that can help preserve vision.

High dosage of oral systemic corticosteroids are mandatory in this situation but they should not be used without concurrent treatment with antitoxoplasmic drugs. Periocular injections of depot corticosteroids can cause the worsening of the disease in some patients and should not be used unless in unusual circumstance that would justify the risk. Again, it should not be used without simultaneous treatment with antitoxoplasmic drugs.

Therapy with Pyrimethamine and sulfonamides produce the better results.

In spite of being effective in the treatment of experimental ocular toxoplasmosis, Clindamycin did not resist the test of time. It does not affect the rate of recurrences and is inferior to the old regimen.

The combination of Pyrimethamine and sulfonamides with other antitoxoplasmic agents such as Clindamycin has no scientific basis and probably increases the side-effects without benefitting the patient.

Being usually benign and self-limited, ocular toxoplasmosis is a classic example of an ocular disease where a randomized clinical trial is urgently required to help ophthalmologists in its management.

The experience gained in the management of patients with ocular toxoplasmosis in the acquired immunodeficiency syndrome has shown that they usually have less vitreous involvement and more recurrences than normal hosts. Also, the anterior chamber reaction tends to be non-granulomatous. It has also confirmed the classic impression that the association of Pyrimethamine and sulfonamides leads to better results and the association with other anti-toxoplasmic drugs, in spite of very common application in some countries, does not improve the results. Until now, we have not seen any patient with acquired immunodeficiency syndrome and ocular toxoplasmosis in whom the classic combination of Pyrimethamine and Sulfonamide has not resulted in control of the infection or had recurrences under this treatment, but we have had several patients that have developed recurrent retinitis during the treatment with Spiramycin or Clindamycin. The response to the classic antimicrobial treatment is usually quick and better than that observed in non-immunosuppressed patients stressing the possible role of immune mechanisms and secondary autoimmunity of the ocular disease in normal hosts. Most of these patients require maintenance of the treatment to avoid a recurrence of the retinal disease.

A common problem is the presence of iatrogenic complications, some of them with ocular involvement (2) that require the use of other medications. Efficient anti-toxoplasmic cysticidal drugs with low toxicity for normal and immunosuppressed hosts are necessary and will probably become available in the future.

References

1. Abreu MT, Belfort R Jr, Hirata PS (1982) Fuchs' Heterochromic Cyclitis and Ocular Toxoplasmosis. Am J Ophthalmol 39:739-744
2. Belfort R Jr, Smet MD, Whitcup SM et al (to be published) Ocular Complications of Stevens Johnson Syndrome and Toxic Epidermal Necrolysis in Patients with AIDS. Cornea
3. Brézin AP, Egwuagu CE, Burnier M Jr et al (1990) Identification of Toxoplasma Gondii in Paraffin Embedded Sections by the Polymerase Chain Reaction. Am J Ophthalmol 110:599-604
4. Brézin AP, Silveira CM, Thulliez P et al (1991) Aqueous Humor Analysis in Ocular Toxoplasmosis.N Engl J Med 324:699-700
5. Dubey JP (1986) Toxoplasmosis. J Am Vet Med Assoc 189:166-170
6. Glasner PD, Silveira CM, Martins MC et al (1991) The Prevalence of Ocular Toxoplasmosis in a Rural Population in Southern Brazil. Int Ophthalmol Vis Sci (supl)32:681
7. Martins MC, Silveira CM, Jamra LF et al (1990) Isolamento de Toxoplasma gondii de carnes e derivados, provenientes de regiao endemica de toxoplasmose ocular. Arq Bras Oftal 53:60-66
8. Orefice F, Belfort R Jr (1987) Uveitis. Roca, Sao Paulo
9. O'Connor GR (1975) Ocular Toxoplasmosis. Jap J Ophthalmol 19:1-24
10. Pavésio CEN (1991) A Contribution to the Study of Toxoplasma Gondii. (Thesis) Escola Paulista de Medicina, Sao Paulo, Brazil
11. Rehder JR, Burnier M Jr, Pavésio CEN et al (1988) Acute Unilateral Toxoplasmic Iridocyclitis in an AIDS Patient. Identification of the Toxoplasma Gondii Cysts in the Iris. Am J Ophthalmol 106:740-741
12. Remington JS, Desmont G (1990) Toxoplasmosis. In: Remington JS, Klein JD (eds) Infectious Diseases of the Fetus and the Newborn Infant. Saunders, Philadelphia pp 90-195
13. Schlaegel TF Jr (1978) Ocular Toxoplasmosis and Pars Planitis. Grune & Stratton, New York/San Francisco/London
14. Silveira CM, Belfort R Jr, Burnier M Jr et al (1988) Acquired Toxoplasmic Infection

as the Cause of Toxoplasmic Retinochoroiditis in Families. Am J Ophthalmol 106:362-364

15. Silveira CM, Belfort R Jr, Nussenblatt R et al (1989) Unilateral Pigmentary Retinopathy Associated with Ocular Toxoplasmosis. Am J Ophthalmol 107:682-684
16. Silveira CM, Martins MC, Tagliari EI et al (1991) Clinical Characterization of Acquired Ocular Toxoplasmosis. Final Program 95th Ann Meeting American Academy Ophthalmol. Scientific Poster 137:113

Current Concepts in the Management of Ocular Toxoplasmosis in the USA

Gary N. Holland

Abstract. The treatment of ocular toxoplasmosis is based on an understanding of disease mechanisms that include retinal necrosis caused by proliferation of organisms; hypersensitivity reactions to Toxoplasma gondii that result in iridocyclitis, retinal vasculitis, and retinal edema; and the self-limited course of recurrent infections in otherwise healthy individuals. Usual therapy consists of one or more antiparasitic drugs in combinations with systemic corticosteroids, but the most effective combination of agents has never been determined.

A survey of physician members of the American Uveitis Society showed a diversity of opinion regarding the indications for treatment and drugs used. Most treat patients with large, posterior lesions that have caused a severe vitreous reaction and decreased vision; in contrast, small anterior lesions not affecting vision may not be treated. Most American Uveitis Society members treat patients with one of four drug regimens: pyrimethamine/sulfadiazine/prednisone (32%); pyrimethamine/sulfadiazine/clindamycin/prednisone (27%); sulfadiazine / clindamycin / prednisone (16%); or clindamycin / prednisone (6%).

Therapy may need to be modified and prolonged in immunocompromised patients.

Use of adjunctive therapies (photocoagulation, cryotherapy, vitrectomy) is uncommon and their benefits remain uncertain.

Introduction

Toxoplasma gondii remains the most common cause of infectious retinitis in otherwise healthy individuals, yet its treatment has remained a subject of controversy after more than three decades of study. Furthermore, the emergence of acquired immunodeficiency syndrome (AIDS) and other immunodeficiency states have required modifications in traditional therapeutic approaches. The purpose of this review is to summarize concepts about disease pathophysiology upon which treatment recommendations have been based, and to identify various treatment strategies currently used by specialists in the field of uveitis.

Disease Pathophysiology

In the United States and other industrialized nations of the Western Hemisphere, the vast majority of ocular toxoplasmosis cases are thought to be due to recurrence of congenital Toxoplasma gondii infection. Foci of inflammation almost always arise at the borders of old retinochoroidal scars, assumed to be the residua of congenital disease. In some other areas of the world, however, newly-acquired Toxoplasma gondii infections may make up a much higher percentage of ocular toxoplasmosis cases than heretofore recognized. Such is the case in southern Brazil (Rubens Belfort,Jr. personal communication, 1991).

Much of our current understanding of the pathophysiology of recurrent ocular toxoplasmosis stems from various animal studies. Extrapolating from experiments by Frenkel, who used the related parasite Besnoitia jellisoni, it is assumed that recurrent toxoplasmic retinochoroiditis results from breakdown of encysted organisms within scars (6). Cyst breakdown could result in disease by at least two mechanisms: hypersensitivity reactions alone to exposed Toxoplasma gondii antigens, or a tissue-destructive infection of adjacent retinal tissues by live, reactivated parasites. The relative importance of these potential disease mechanisms in the pathogenesis of recurrent ocular toxoplasmosis is not fully understood. Studies using a nonhuman primate model of ocular toxoplasmosis have shed some light on this subject, however. Inoculation of live parasites onto the retina of a healthy nonimmune monkey will produce a self-limited focus of retinochoroiditis that is clinically and histopathologically similar to human disease (1). In contrast, intravenous and intraocular injection of Toxoplasma gondii antigen in previously infected animals does not produce recurrent necrotizing retinochoroiditis (14). Also, intraocular inoculation of live Toxoplasma gondii organisms or Toxoplasma gondii antigen in previously immunized animals does not produce necrotizing retinochoroiditis (23). It is assumed therefore that tissue invasion and destruction of cells by live organisms plays a major role in the pathogenesis of recurrent disease (16). The factors that lead to breakdown of cysts and reactivation of parasites remain to be elucidated. Inflammatory reactions in response to the parasites cause secondary problems, including cystoid macular edema, vitritis, anterior chamber inflammation, and retinal vasculitis (15).

Treatment

The synergistic combination of pyrimethamine and sulfadiazine was recommended by Eyles and Coleman in 1953 for the treatment of toxoplasmosis (4). (Because pyrimethamine affects dihydrofolic acid metabolism by inhibition of dihydrofolate reductase, folinic acid is also given to patients receiving pyrimethamine to prevent bone marrow suppression.) Subsequent reports have provided conflicting information regarding the efficacy of various antimicrobial drugs.

A number of other antimicrobial agents have demonstrated either in vitro or in vivo efficacy against Toxoplasma gondii, including various other sulfonamides (sulfamerazine, sulfamethazine, and sulfapyrazine), clindamycin and the tetracyclines. Agents are generally used in combination because of a perception that lesions respond incompletely to any given agent. Interest in the use of clindamycin stems from the fact that the drug appears to be concentrated in ocular tissue and can penetrate cyst walls (21). Animal experiments have shown that clindamycin treatment reduces the number of, although it does not eliminate, tissue cysts (13), but there is no good clinical evidence to support the concept that clindamycin prevents recurrences (12).

Corticosteroids are used in combination with antimicrobial drugs to reduce the inflammatory reactions that can potentially further damage the eye. Without concurrent antiparasitic therapy, however, the suppression of immune defense mechanisms by corticosteroids may lead to overwhelming Toxoplasma gondii infection, which may even lead to loss of the eye (19).

There have been very few prospective, controlled studies of drug therapy for ocular toxoplasmosis. It is difficult to assess the relative efficacy of various drugs without such studies, since toxoplasmic retinochoroiditis tends to be self-limited even without treatment. In a prospective, but non-randomized study, Rothova and associates found no difference in the time to healing between three patient groups: one group treated with pyrimethamine, sulfadiazine, and prednisone; one group treated with clindamycin, sulfadiazine, and prednisone; and one group left untreated (18).

Adjunctive therapies for active ocular toxoplasmosis have been advocated by some investigators, but experience with non-medical treatments is limited, and their contribution to the management of ocular toxoplasmosis remains uncertain. Laser photocoagulation is the most frequently used nonmedical modality, with the presumed goal of encircling an active lesion with photocoagulation scars, thereby limiting cell-to-cell spread of infection (7,20,22). Cryotherapy has been advocated as a means of destroying lesions within active foci of disease (2). Vitrectomy has been used for severe or persistent vitreous inflammation, as a means of eliminating inflammatory mediators that may perpetuate disease (5).

The Immunocompromised Host

The immunocompromised host presents special problems in the diagnosis and management of ocular toxoplasmosis (9). It is generally believed that toxoplasmosis occurs with increased frequency in patients on immunosuppressive drugs and in patients with diseases characterized by defects in cell-mediated immunity including Hodgkin's disease and the acquired immunodeficiency syndrome. Animal studies suggest, however, that immunodeficiency alone is insufficient stimulus for reactivation of encysted organisms. Immunosuppression of nonhuman primates by total lymphoid irradiation, which produces a prolonged suppression of cell-mediated immunity, does not lead to reactivation of healed toxoplasmic scars (8). Clinical evidence also tends to support this conclusion; despite the severe defects in cellular immunity associated with the acquired immunodeficiency syndrome, toxoplasmic retinochoroidal scars and cysts may be seen in these patients without evidence of reactivation. Although toxoplasmosis is the most common nonviral intracranial infection in patients with the acquired immunodeficiency syndrome, ocular toxoplasmosis is uncommon. When it does occur, ocular infections are not seen adjacent to old scars, suggesting that they may be due to acquired disease or to organisms newly disseminated to the eye.

Patients with acquired immunodeficiency syndrome have been reported to have a variety of clinical lesions, including single foci of retinochoroiditis in one or both eyes, multifocal lesions, or diffuse areas of retinal necrosis (10). Left untreated in acquired immunodeficiency syndrome patients or in other immunocompromised hosts, toxoplasmic retinochoroiditis will progress to widespread tissue destruction. As stated above, the majority of lesions seen in acquired immunodeficiency syndrome patients do not arise from the borders of preexisting scars, which may led to problems in accurately diagnosing a toxoplasmic infection. Toxoplasma gondii may infect iris, choroid, and vitreous, tissues that are not usually infected in the immunocompetent host (17).

Ocular lesions appear to respond to standard antiparasitic drugs in immunocompromised hosts, but the most effective treatment regimens have yet to be determined. Histopathologic studies show little retinal inflammation; therefore antiinflammatory drugs, such as oral corticosteroids, probably have no role in the management of infection. In patients with acquired immunodeficiency syndrome, pyrimethamine use is sometimes avoided because of preexisting bone marrow suppression, and corticosteroid use is avoided to prevent further suppression of host immune defenses. Other considerations include the high incidence of sulfonamia allergies among patients with the acquired immunodeficiency syndrome and the fact that zidovudine (an antiretroviral agent used to treat many patients with the acquired immunodeficiency syndrome) has been shown to be antagonistic to pyrimethamine, which might lead to treatment failures if both agents were used concurrently (11).

Like many infections in immunocompromised patients, toxoplasmosis may reactivate if therapy is discontinued. Maintenance therapy with lower, suppressive doses of antimicrobial agents is therefore usually recommended for patients with the acquired immunodeficiency syndrome. Clindamycin is commonly used for this purpose, although there are no studies confirming that it is a better maintenance drug than other agents.

The American Uveitis Society Survey

Because there is a lack of data clearly supporting the superiority of one specific drug or drug combination for the treatment of ocular toxoplasmosis, clinicians use many different therapeutic regimens. To delineate current practices in the management of ocular toxoplasmosis, the American Uveitis Society conducted a comprehensive survey of its membership in 1990 (3). A detailed questionnaire was distributed to the 85 physician-members of the American Uveitis Society requesting information regarding their

- indications for treatment of ocular toxoplasmosis; their
- preferred therapeutic regimens; their
- experience with adjunctive, nonmedical therapies; and
- how they alter their management, if at all, in special situations, such as ocular toxoplasmosis in pregnancy, in newborns, and in immunocompromised patients.

An exellent response rate of 85% was achieved.

Only 6% of respondents treat all cases of ocular toxoplasmosis, regardless of findings. For those who do not treat every case, decisions regarding therapy are based on the patient's

- visual acuity, the
- location of lesions, the
- amount of vitreous reaction and the
- character of the lesion.

The majority consider the following factors to be absolute indications for treatment regardless of other findings:

- a drop in visual acuity below 20/200;
- lesions located adjacent to the optic nerve head, maculopapillary bundle, or fovea; and
- lesions associated with a severe vitreous inflammatory reaction.

Respondents were more likely to treat patients with

- multifocal lesions,
- patients with acquired infections, and
- patients whose lesions have persisted for longer than one month, but even these factors would not lead to treatment in every case, according to most respondents.

In contrast, most respondents do not treat patients with ocular toxoplasmosis if they

- retain good visual acuity or if
- lesions are located in the far peripheral retina.

Situations where there was the greatest disagreement between respondents regarding indications for treatment were lesion size smaller than 1 disc diameter; lesions location outside the major vascular arcades, but posterior to the equator; and the presence of only a mild to moderate vitreous inflammatory reaction.

Respondents identified 8 different antimicrobial agents that are utilized in the initial treatment of ocular toxoplasmosis. They are used in 15 different drug combinations, but only four treatment regimens were cited by more than one respondent.

- "Classic therapy" (pyrimethamine, sulfadiazine, oral corticosteroids), the most frequently used regimen, is preferred by 32%.
- "Quadruple therapy" (pyrimethamine, sulfadiazine, clindamycin, and oral corticosteroids) used by 27% of respondents, was almost as popular.
- The combination of sulfadiazine, clindamycin, and oral corticosteroids is used by 16%, and
- clindamycin and oral corticosteroids alone is used by 6%.

The preferred dosages and duration of therapy for these regimens can be found in the published results of the survey (3).

Nearly all respondents use oral corticosteroids in the management of ocular toxoplasmosis. They are divided, however, on the best time to initiate therapy. Half begin oral corticosteroids simultaneously with antimicrobial agents, while half wait 24 to 48 hours to allow the antimicrobial agents to reach therapeutic levels in the blood. The majority of respondents base the duration of oral corticosteroids use on the patient's clinical response.

Adjunctive therapies (laser photocoagulation, cryotherapy, and vitrectomy) have been used by a third of American Uveitis Society members, but are generally reserved for unusual situations, such as intolerance to all oral medications or the persistence, despite medical therapy of active lesions that are adjacent to the fovea or other visually-important structures.

Indications for treatment and preferred drug regimens differ in special clinical situations for most respondents. Most will treat recurrent ocular toxoplasmosis in pregnant women to preserve vision, but will alter their drugs of choice, usually by excluding pyrimethamine, since its effect on the fetus is unclear. It was agreed by those who have treated active neonatal ocular toxoplasmosis that they treat all cases, regardless of lesion characteristics. Repondents were more likely to treat ocular toxoplasmosis in immunocompromised patients than in otherwise healthy patients, but still, only 30% stated that they would treat any patient, regardless of retinal findings or visual acuity. If patients are treated, most agreed that some form of antiparasitic drug should be continued for the duration of the immunocompromised state, even after the lesion has become quiescent, to prevent reactivation.

The American Uveitis Society survey demonstrated that considerable controversy continues to exist regarding the indications for treatment, and that there is a lack of consensus on preferred medical management. Most respondents agree, however, that therapy should be tailored to the specific patient's clinical situation. The results of this survey will help to identify important treatment questions and other areas of concern that can be addressed in future clinical studies.

Conclusions

Antiparasitic drugs are the mainstay of therapy for ocular toxoplasmosis in all patients, based on current concepts regarding the pathogenesis of retinal lesions.

Corticosteroids also play an important role in the treatment of otherwise healthy patients by controlling destructive inflammatory reactions associated with infection, but should be used with caution, if at all, in patients with underlying immune system disorders. The best antiparasitic agents, drug combinations, and dosing schedules remains a subject of debate. Although nearly all uveitis specialists believe that available drugs provide at least some treatment benefit, it is widely acknowledged that current therapies are far from perfect, and some studies have even raised questions regarding the extent to which treatment really helps patients with ocular toxoplasmosis.

It is hoped that in the future, prospective, well-designed clinical trials will provide a better understanding of this very important clinical problem.

References

1. Culbertson WW, Tabbara KF, O'Connor GR (1982) Experimental Ocular Toxoplasmosis in Primates. Arch Ophthalmol 100:321-323
2. Dobbie JG (1968) Cryotherapy in the Management of Toxoplasma Retinochoroiditis. Tr Am Ac Ophthalmol Oto 72:364-376
3. Engstrom RE, Holland GN, Nussenblatt RB et al (1991) Current Practices in the Management of Ocular Toxoplasmosis. Am J Ophthalmol 111:601-610
4. Eyles DE, Coleman N (1953) Synergistic Effect of Sulfadiazine and Daraprim against Experimental Toxoplasmosis in the Mouse. Antib Chemo 3:483-490
5. Fitzgerald CR (1980) Pars Plana Vitrectomy for Vitreous Opacity Secondary to

Presumed Toxoplasmosis. Arch Ophthalmol 98:321-323

6. Frenkel JK (1961) Pathogenesis of Toxoplasmosis with a Consideration of Cyst Rupture in Besnoitia Infection. Surv Ophthalmol 6:799-825
7. Ghartey KN, Brockhurst RJ (1980) Photocoagulation of Active Toxoplasmic Retinochoroiditis Am J Ophthalmol 89:858-864
8. Holland GN, O'Connor GR, Diaz R et al (1988) Ocular Toxoplasmosis in Immunosuppressed Nonhuman Primates. Invest Ophthalmol Vis Sci 29:835-842
9. Holland GN (1989) Ocular Toxoplasmosis in the Immunocompromised Host. Int Ophthalmol 13:399-402
10. Holland GN, Engstrom RE, Glasgow BJ et al (1988) Ocular Toxoplasmosis in Patients with the Acquired Immunodeficiency Syndrome. Am J Ophthalmol 106:653-667
11. Israelski DM, Tom C, Remington JS (1989) Zidovudine Antagonizes the Action of Pyrimethamine in Experimental Infection with Toxoplasma Gondii. Antimicrob Ag Chemother 33:30-34
12. Lakhanpal V, Schocket SS, Nirankari VS (1983) Clindamycin in the Treatment of Toxoplasmic Retinochoroiditis. Am J Ophthalmol 95:605-613
13. McMaster PRB, Powers KG, Finerty JF et al (1973) The Effect of Two-Chlorinated Lincomycin Analogues against Acute Toxoplasmosis in Mice. Am J Trop Med Hyg 22:14-17
14. Newman PE, Ghosheh R, Tabbara KF et al (1982) The Role of Hypersensitivity Reactions to Toxoplasma Antigens in Experimental Ocular Toxoplasmosis in Nonhuman Primates. Am J Ophthalmol 94:159-164
15. O'Connor GR (1970) The Influence of Hypersensitivity on the Pathogenesis of Ocular Toxoplasmosis. Trans Am Ophthalmol Soc 68:501-547
16. O'Connor GR (1983) The Roles of Parasite Invasion and of Hypersensitivity in the Pathogenesis of Toxoplasmic Retinochoroiditis. Ocular Inflamm Ther 1:37-46
17. Rehder JR, Burnier M, Pavesio CE et al (1989) Acute Unilateral Toxoplasmic Iridocyclitis in an AIDS Patient. Am J Ophthalmol 106:740-741
18. Rothova A, Buitenhuis HJ, Meenken C et al (1989) Therapy in Ocular Toxoplasmosis. Int Ophthalmol 13:415-419
19. Sabates R, Pruett RC, Brockhurst RJ (1981) Fulminant Ocular Toxoplasmosis. Am J Ophthalmol 92:497-503
20. Spalter HF, Campbell CJ, Noyori KS et al (1966) Prophylactic Photocoagulation of Recurrent Toxoplasmic Retinochoroiditis. Arch Ophthalmol 75:21-31
21. Tabbara KF, O'Connor GR (1975) Ocular Tissue Absorption of Clindamycin Phosphate. Arch Ophthalmol 93:1180-1185
22. Theodossiadis GP, Koutsandrea C, Tzonou A (1989) A Comparative Study Concerning the Treatment of Active Toxoplasmic Retinochoroiditis with Argon Laser and Medication (Follow-up 2-9 Years). Ophthalmologica 199:77-83
23. Webb RM, Tabbara KF, O'Connor GR (1984) Retinal Vasculitis in Ocular Toxoplasmosis in Nonhuman Primates. Retina 4:182-188

- Parasitic: Other

Successful Thiabendazole Therapy of Patients with Diffuse Unilateral Subacute Neuroretinitis

J. Donald M. Gass

Abstract. Diffuse unilateral subacute neuroretinitis (DUSN) is a recently described endemic disease associated with severe visual loss in the south-eastern and mid-western United States as well as the Caribbean and Latin America. Recent finding of a case in Bavaria suggests that its distribution may be worldwide. It is caused by a single nematode that may wander in the subretinal space for many months or years. It is at least five times more common than Toxocariasis in the south-eastern United States. Until recently, the only effective treatment has involved the difficult, time-consuming biomicroscopic detection of the worm followed by photocoagulation. This report concerns our recent experience with a new therapeutic technique that employs oral administration of an anti-helminthic agent and serial fundus photography to detect early destruction of the worm.

Introduction

Diffuse subacute neuroretinitis (DUSN) is an infectious disease with protean manifestations caused by a single nematode that may wander in the subretinal space for four years or longer (1,2). It most frequently affects children or young adults and often causes profound loss of vision in one eye. During its early stages the patient typically develops acute visual loss, mild to moderate vitreitis, optic disc swelling, and recurrent crops of evanescent, multifocal, gray-white lesions at the level of the outer retina (Fig.1A and 2A). The nematode is always found near these lesions which are typically clustered in only one segment of the fundus. These active lesions disappear in one to two weeks as the nematode moves elsewhere in the eye (Fig.1B). Less than one percent of these lesions are of sufficient intensity to cause a visible chorioretinal scar. Failure to recognize and photocoagulate the nematode results in severe permanent loss of vision, optic atrophy, narrowing of the retinal arteries, and marked focal as well as diffuse degenerative changes in the pigment epithelium and retina (Fig.1C and 2B). The nematode often assumes an "S-shaped" (Fig.2A and 3A) or coiled (Fig.1A and 3B) configuration. Occasionally extensive retinal perivascular exudation simulating that seen in sarcoidosis and other conditions occurs.

The facts that active outer retinal lesions are always confined to one area of the fundus, that they disappear within 7 to 10 days usually leaving no visible scar, and that the nematode is always found in proximity to these lesions, suggest that they are caused by material left behind by the nematode as it migrates in the subretinal space.

DUSN is prevalent in the southeastern United States, Caribbean area, and probably Latin America. With greater awareness of the disease, it probably will prove to be endemic in other parts of the world. In this regard I was shown recently a patient that presented with a subretinal nematode at the eye clinic at Erlangen.

Our initial experience with orally administered antihelminthic agents suggested that they were ineffective in eradication of the nematode (2). Three patients, each with a motile nematode, were hospitalized and in each case administration of either one or both thiabendazole and diethylcarbamazine failed to immobilize the nematode. We concluded therefore in 1983 that the drugs were unable to penetrate the blood-retinal barrier and that photocoagulation was the only effective treatment which, in our experience, has resulted in complete and permanent inactivation of the disorder. Locating the nematode which varies in size from 400 to 1000 microns in length, however, can be difficult, time consuming, and requires multiple patient visits. It was because of this that we considered a second trial of thiabendazole when we could not find the nematode in patients with a moderately severe vitreitis, in the hope that the blood-retinal barrier in such cases might permit the drug to reach the nematode.

We now have preliminary evidence that thiabendazole is effective in the treatment of some patients with DUSN, particularly those with a moderate degree of vitreitis, and we have used a photographic technique for early detection of success of treatment (4). We theorized that if the drug was successful in penetrating the blood-retinal barrier and if the multiple focal areas of retinitis are caused by substances left in the subretinal space by the nematode, that we should observe one week after the treatment two fundus changes: firstly fading or disappearance of the multiple foci of retinitis, and secondly, the appearance of a new intense focus of retinitis at the site of the dead or incapacitated nematode.

The following protocol was used in three patients. A fundus map was made on the day of the treatment. Thiabendazole was given orally for two to four days. Indications of successful treatment included:

1) at one week fading of the multifocal areas of retinitis, and appearance of a new focus of intense retinitis,
2) development in four to six weeks of a focal chorioretinal scar at the site of the post-treatment retinitis and lessening of the vitreitis, and
3) six months after treatment no evidence of new lesions and complete inactivity of the disease.

Case Reports

Case 1. A 10-year-old boy was seen five months after rapid development of loss of vision in the left eye. Visual acuity was 7/200. His right eye was normal. In the left eye he had multiple atrophic scars in the periphery of the fundus as well as diffuse changes in the retinal pigment epithelium. There was a moderate vitreitis. In the superonasal quadrant there were multiple active outer retinal lesions. No nematode was found. When he returned two weeks later, the active lesions noted previously had faded and there were new lesions in the juxtapapillary area (Fig.4A). Because of the moderately intense vitreitis, he was given thiabendazole. Six days later the multifocal active lesions surrounding the optic disc had faded and there was a new intense focus of retinitis in the temporal part of the macula (Fig.4B).

There was rapid resolution of the vitreitis and the appearance of a chorioretinal scar at the site of the post-treatment retinitis (Fig.4C). None of the other active lesions present at the time of treatment caused chorioretinal scars.

Case 2. A 16-year-old boy presented with a three-month history of blurred vision in the right eye. His visual acuitiy was 20/40. He had an afferent pupillary defect and 2+ vitreous cells. There were multiple peripheral chorioretinal scars, mild disc edema, and a cluster of focal active outer retinal lesions in the inferior macular region (Fig.5A). Within one of these lesions there was a suggestion of a nematode. During one hour of observation, however, no movement occurred. Because this patient still had good visual acuity we elected to give him thiabendazole rather than risk further observation. One week later the multiple foci of retinitis had faded and there was a new intense focus of retinitis with marked narrowing of the overlying retinal artery (Fig.5B). There was rapid disappearance of all activity and a scar formed at the site of the post-treatment retinitis (Fig.5C).

Discussion

DUSN is a common and yet frequently misdiagnosed disorder in the southeastern United States where it is estimated to be at least five times more prevalent than ocular toxocariasis (4). During its early stages when associated with active outer retinal lesions it may be mistaken for acute posterior multifocal placoid pigment epitheliopathy, multiple evanescent white dot syndrome, multifocal choroiditis and panuveitis syndrome (pseudo-presumed ocular histoplasmosis), Behcet's disease, and sarcoidosis. When active outer retinal lesions are not present and the optic disc is swollen, a misdiagnosis of papilledema or non-specific papillitis may be made. Pallor of the optic disc during the later stages of the disease may be incorrectly attributed to diseases affecting the intraorbital optic nerve or posterior optic pathways. The optic atrophy, retinal arterial narrowing and widespread pigment epithelial changes seen in the later stages of the disease may simulate those caused by ophthalmic artery obstruction, trauma, and tapetoretinal dystrophies.

DUSN caused by a nematode twice the size of the one found in the southeastern United States is endemic in the north midwestern United States (Fig.6) (2,3,5). It causes a more coarse derangement of the pigment epithelium and is easier to find biomicroscopically. The identification of both of these nematodes is unknown. Leading suspects include Ancylostoma caninum, the common dog hookworm, in the case of the smaller nematode, and Baylisascaris, an intestinal parasite of raccoons, in the case of the larger nematode.

To date we have given thiabendazole to four patients with DUSN because we were unable to find the nematode. In three there was complete resolution of the inflammation. In the forth patient with minimal vitreous inflammation, the therapy was unsuccessful, but subsequently the nematode was found and destroyed with laser. The recommended dose of thiabendazole is 10mg/lb. given two times a day for two to four successive days. The daily dose should not exceed 3 grams. Frequent side effects include nausea, vomiting, anorexia, and mild central nervous system disturbances such as dizziness, drowsiness, or headache. Less frequent adverse reactions include liver damage, hematuria and seizures. Although there is evidence that thiabendazole can enter the aqueous and vitreous of a minimally inflamed human eye (6), it apparently does not reach the subpigment epithelial space in concentrations sufficient to kill the nematode causing DUSN in patients with only mild to moderate vitreitis. Because of its side effects, thiabendazole is recommended only in patients with the typical findings of DUSN and only when the nematode cannot be found. Photographic mapping of the fundus prior to beginning treatment for comparison with the fundus appearance one week later is helpful in detection of early evidence of successful treatment. We are plannig a trial of Ivermectin, a drug with minimal side effects, in lieu of thiabendazole in patients with DUSN. While it has proven effective in humans with onchocerciasis, a filarial disease, it may not be effective in DUSN, since the nematode is probably not a filaria. In patients with minimal vitreous inflammation, we also plan to try a scatter pattern of laser photocoagulation in the vicinity of the active foci of retinitis just prior to beginning oral therapy in order to increase access of the drug to the nematode.

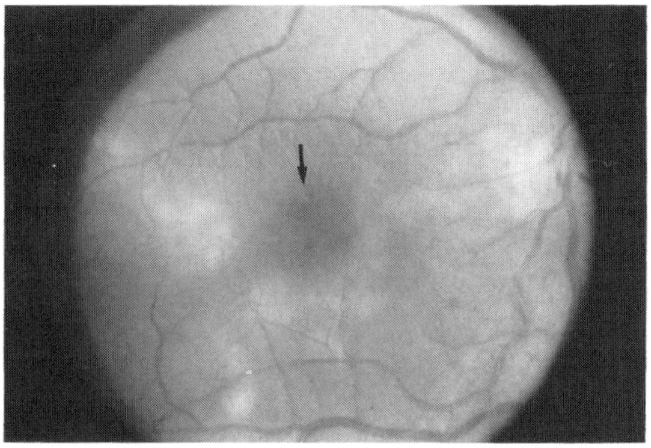

Fig.1. Natural Course of DUSN in a Girl with Acute Onset of Visual Loss
A. Coiled nematode (arrow) in vicinity of multiple foci of active outer retinitis in a girl.

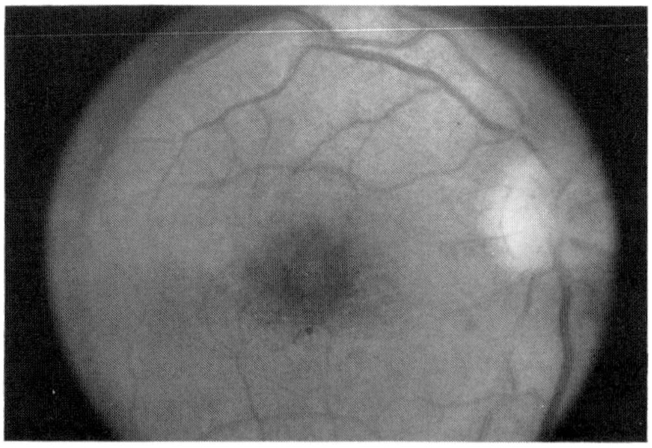

B. One month later, worm and active lesions no longer evident. Visual acuity 20/100.

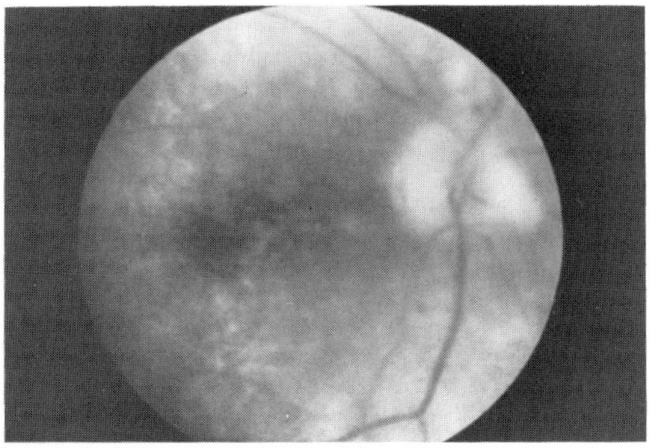

C. Twenty-eight months later, visual acuity counting fingers only. Note optic atrophy, retinal vessel narrowing, and pigment epithelial changes typical of late stages of DUSN (1).

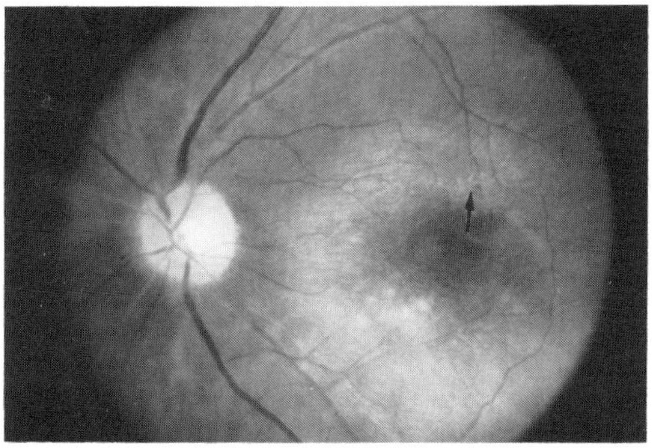

Fig.2. Natural Course of DUSN in a Young Boy with Acute Visual Loss
A. "S"-shaped subretinal nematode (arrow) and multi-focal outer retinitis.

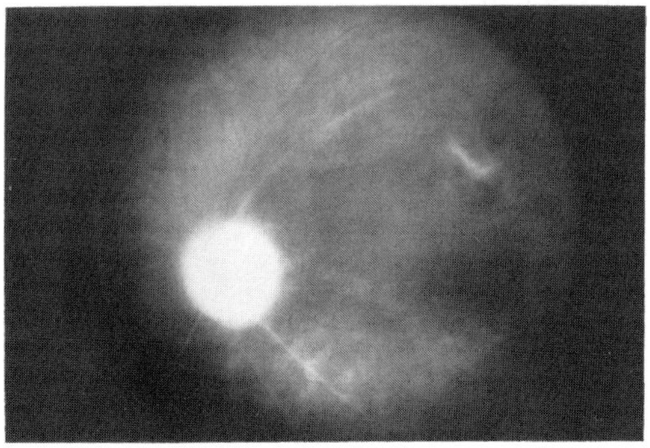

B. Twelve years later, visual acuity counting fingers only.

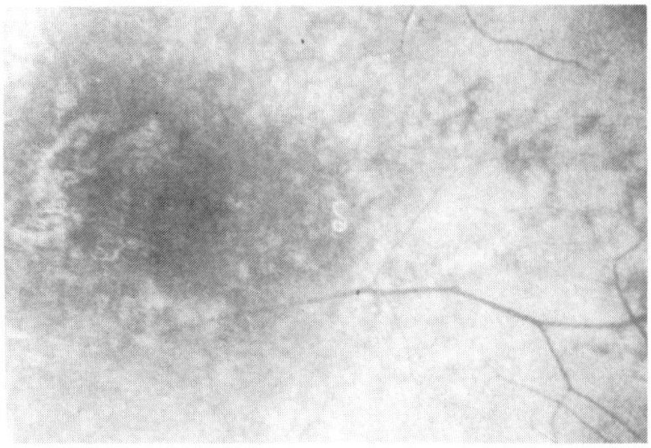

Fig.3. Movement of Subretinal Nematode
A. "S"-shaped configuration

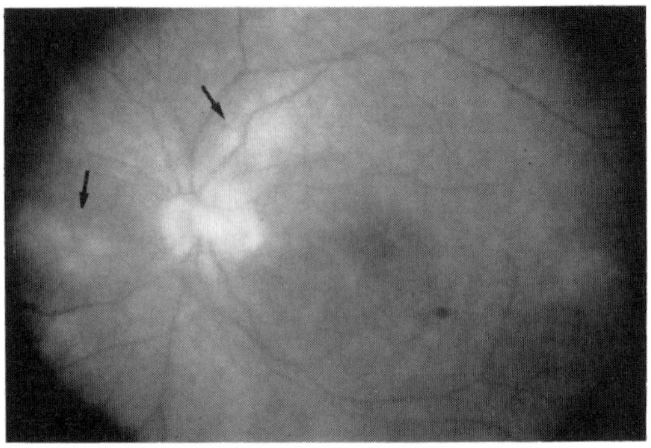

Fig.4. Case 1
A. Active outer retinal lesions (arrows) in juxtapapillary area.

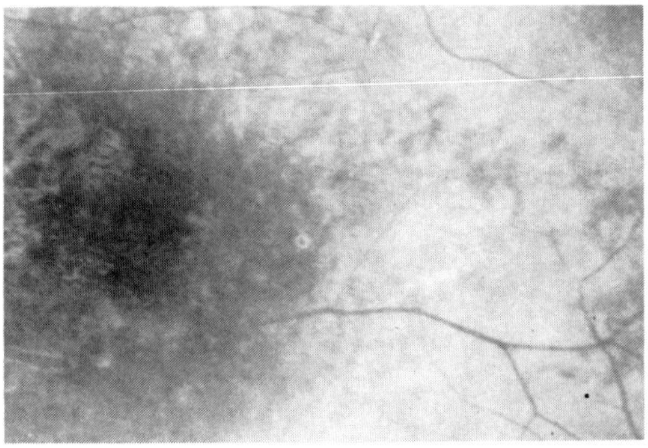

B. Coiled position

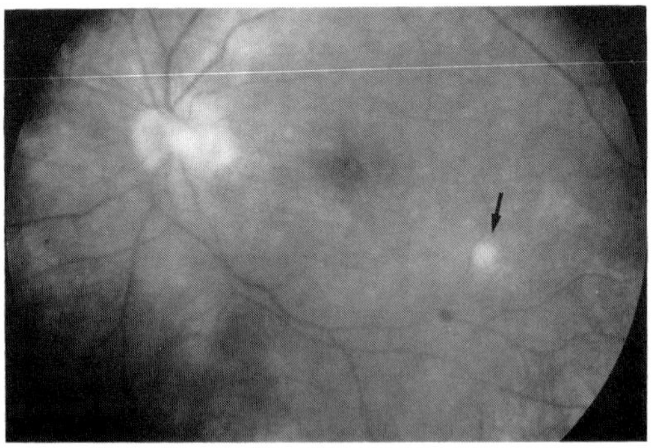

B. One week post-treatment. Note fading of pretreatment lesions and new intense focus of retinitis (arrow).

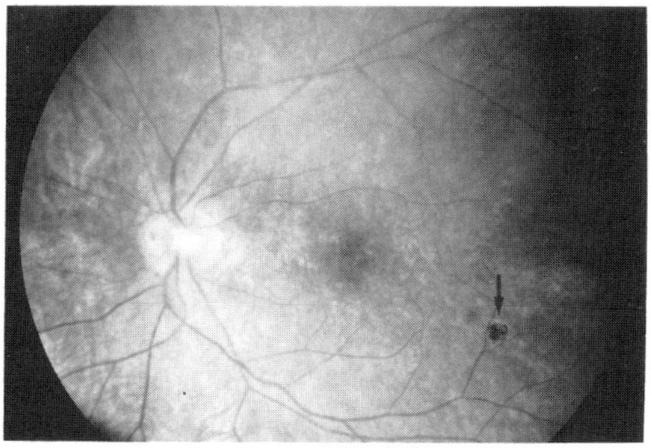

C. Several months later, note focal chorioretinal scar (arrow) at site of post-treatment retinitis and absence of scars caused by pre-treatment foci of retinitis (4)

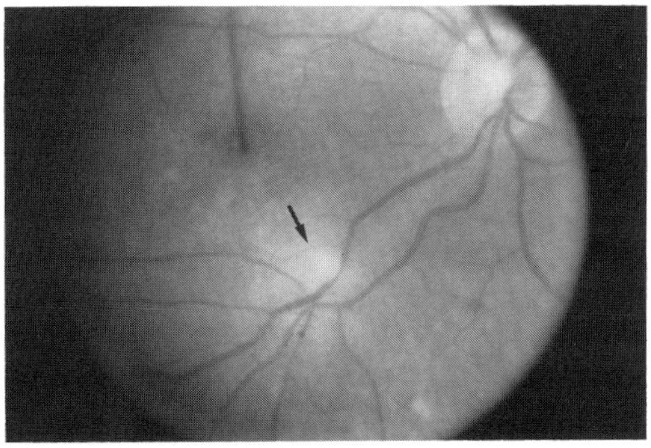

B. One week post-treatment. Note intense focus of retinitis and narrowing of overlying retinal artery (arrow)

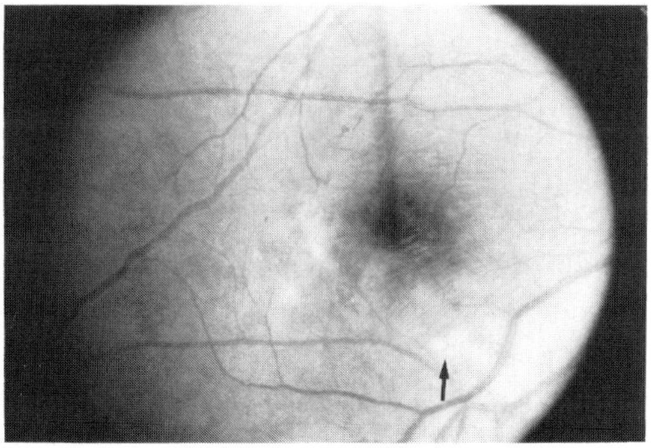

Fig.5. Case 2
A. Active foci of retinitis. Note evidence of worm in one of the lesions (arrow)

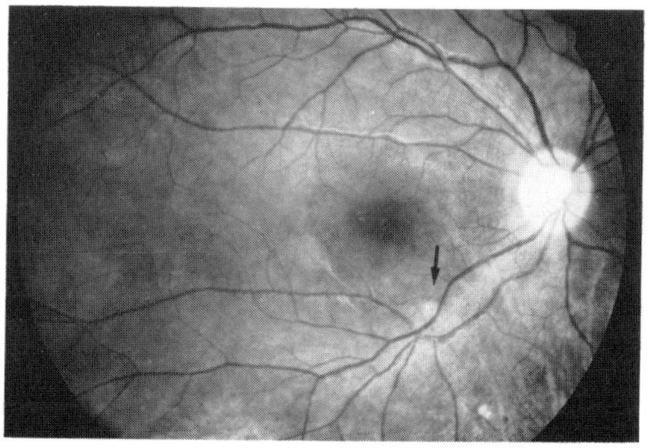

C. Several months later, note scar (arrow) at site of post-treatment retinitis (4)

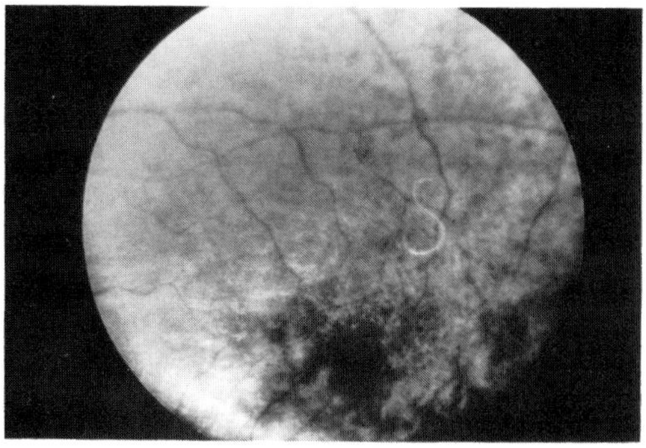

Fig.6. Larger Nematode Causing DUSN in Patient from Chicago area. Note coarse mottling of pigment epithelium.

References

1. Gass JDM, Gilbert WR.Jr, Guerry RK et al (1978) Diffuse Unilateral Subacute Neuroretinitis. Ophthalmology 85:521-545
2. Gass JDM, Braunstein RA (1983) Further Observations Concerning the Diffuse Unilateral Subacute Neuroretinitis Syndrome. Arch Ophthalmol 101:1689-1697
3. Gass JDM (1987) Stereoscopic Atlas of Macular Diseases. Diagnosis and Treatment.3rd ed St.Louis, CV Mosby.pp.470-475
4. Gass JDM, Calanan DG, Bowman CB (to be published) Thiabendazole Therapy in Diffuse Unilateral Subacute Neuroretinitis. Arch.Ophthalmol.
5. Kazacos KR, Raymond LA, Kazacos EA et al (1985) The Raccoon Ascarid. A Probable Cause of Human Ocular Larval Migrans. Ophthalmology 92:1735-1744
6. Maguire AM, Farbin MA, Connor TB (1990) Ocular Penetration of Thiabendazole. Arch Ophthalmol 108:1675

VI. SEXUALLY TRANSMITTED DISEASES

- Epidemiology

Epidemiology of Sexually Transmitted Diseases

Anton Luger

Abstract. The world-wide incidence of major bacterial and viral sexually transmitted diseases has been estimated at over 125 million cases per year by the WHO in 1990.
Syphilis: 2-4 cases per 100000 population are reported in Germany and Austria, but 22/100000 in the USA. The trend shows an increase in the USA, Great Britain and the Netherlands, but a decrease in most other European countries. (Fig.1)
Gonorrhea: 25-30 cases per 100000 population are registered in Germany and Austria, 288/100000 in the USA, 55/100000 in Finland, 36/100000 in Norway, 33/100000 in Denmark and 13/100000 in Sweden. The general trend is downwards in the Northern hemisphere. (Fig.2)
C.trachomatis: Approximately 4 million new cases per year occur in the USA. The incidence ranges between 10%-30% in sexually active young women in Belgium, Norway, Sweden, Germany, USA and Canada.
4%-34% of pregnant women are infected.
Chancroid: Less than 100 cases per year are reported from Great Britain, 37 cases per year in Germany, 2000-5000 between 1985-1989 and 2653 in 1990 in the USA.
Genital Herpes: Approximately 25 million cases have been estimated in the USA. The incidence rose by 15 fold from 1966-1984 in the USA and by 5 fold from 1971-1985 in Great Britain.
Human Papilloma Virus: About one million new cases per year are observed in the USA. In Great Britain, the incidence increased from 30/100000-260/100000 population during 1970-1988.
Hepatitis B: 200000 new infections occur annually in the USA. The incidence is 3.8-32.6/100000 population. Hepatitis B-antibodies are found in 7200-10000/100000 inhabitants.
Human Immunodeficiency Virus Infections: 371803 cases have been reported from almost 200 countries to the WHO until July 5,1991. (Fig.3) The progression of propagation slightly decreases in homo- and bisexual men, but increases in drug addicts and heterosexual contacts.

Introduction

The new concept of Sexually Transmitted Diseases encompasses infections with more than 24 pathogens belonging to the groups of bacteria, viruses, protozoa, fungi, and ectoparasites. Nonsexual transmission of most of these organisms is an infrequent occurrence.

All of the epidemiological data on Sexually Transmitted Diseases emerge from reports of physicians. The correctness of the collected figures depends on the accuracy and completeness of this notification. In most industrialized countries, reporting of Sexually Transmitted Diseases is mandatory by law, but it is limited to the classical venereal diseases (syphilis, gonorrhea, chancroid and lymphogranuloma venereum). However, world-wide experience shows that even in countries with the best-functioning public health systems, only 20% to 25% of the respective infections come to the cognizance of the authorities. Yet, in spite of all inefficiencies, the figures can well indicate trends in the incidence, may point out risk groups and disclose the reservoir of infection. In addition, extrapolation of computerized documentation of Sexually Transmitted Diseases clinics and other public health institutions as well as voluntary reports from private physicians selected on a random basis, permit further precise estimates on the incidence of various infections in the few countries, where such methods are feasible, e.g. USA, Great Britain or Scandinavian countries.

The situation is quite different with infections by the human immunodeficiency virus, which have to be reported since the early 1980s. The severe course and the serious complications of treatment usually require hospitalization and thus, hardly any case can escape registration in industrialized countries.

Generally the prevalence of Sexually Transmitted Diseases is much higher than expected. The figures for the USA are presented in Tab.1.

The WHO (6) considers 8 major Sexually Transmitted Diseases: ---Four bacterial diseases: gonorrhea, chlamydial infections, syphilis and chancroid and

-Four viral contagions: genital herpes simplex, condylomata acuminata, hepatitis B and acquired immunodeficiency syndrome.

The world-wide incidence of major bacterial and viral Sexually Transmitted Diseases is estimated at over 125 million cases yearly (about 6.8 million in the USA) (WHO 1990). However, there are great differences in the incidences between industrialized and developing countries; furthermore, within the Northern hemisphere, and even within one country (e.g. the USA) the number of infections and the trends of spread may vary largely in various areas and in certain groups of the population, distinct by age or race or behavior (12).

Syphilis

The epidemiology of syphilis provides a very good example for trends in the incidence and spread of several other Sexually Transmitted Diseases (Tab.1) and therefore, it is worthwhile to look somewhat more into the details of this disease.

The incidence of syphilis had been high during and after World War II everywhere, then decreased dramatically and had almost disappeared by the end of the nineteen-fifties. Figures of infections increased again during the nineteen-sixties and new peaks were reached in the nineteen-seventies, followed by a steady decline to as few as 2-4 cases per 100000 population in Germany and Austria

- in Germany:

1986:4.5

1987:3.0

1988:2.0

1989:1.6

1990:data not available (12/08/1991),

- in Austria:
1986:4.7
1987:4.8
1988:3.3
1989:3.5
1990:2.7

In heterosexual men and women, a slight upward trend has been noted in Great Britain, in Canada and the Netherlands (6,12).

In the USA (7), the number of reported cases of primary and secondary syphilis has almost doubled from 1986 to 1990,

- in the USA:
1986: 27537
1987: 34008
1988: 39673
1989: 43989
1990: 52600

In 1990, the incidence of early syphilis was 22/100000 population (1982: 14.6/100000; 1985: 11.4/100000; 1989: 18.4/100000).

However, in white men a steady decrease from 10.3/100000 (1982) to 3.2/100000 (1989) was noted.

In white females, the figures rose between 1981 and 1984 from 0.2/100000 to 2.0/100000, stayed around the same level until 1987 and since then rose again to reach 3.0/100000 (16).

In black men, a decrease from 101.9/100000 (1982) to 71.5/ 100000 (1985) was followed by a continued increase to 147.4/100000 (1989) and estimatedly 181/100000 (1990).

A similar trend occurred in black women: 47.8/100000 (1982) to 37.5/100000 (1985) to 98.7/100000 (1989) to about 114.5/100000 (1990) (7,16).

Age groups with the highest incidence are 30-34 years for men and 20-24 years for women. The male to female ratio dropped between 1982 and 1989 from 7.9 to 1.6 in whites, from 4.4 to 2.5 in Hispanics and from 2.1 to 1.6 in Blacks (16). It is obvious that this decrease occurred because of a change in the sexual behavior with the impending danger of the acquired immunodeficiency syndrome (1).

Congenital syphilis seemed to have disappeared in the United States until the early 1980ies but then, figures of reported cases rose from 342 in 1986 to 1747 in 1989 and estimates for 1990 indicate 3264 cases (7). However, the last figure is not comparable to reports in previous years, because the case definition has been changed. Nevertheless, the upward trend is still substantial and is in clear relation to the incidence of early syphilis in women. The characteristics of mothers of syphilitic newborns compared to mothers of healthy infants are shown in a study performed in New York City between 1986 and 1989 (Tab.2) (3). The control mothers matched the case-mothers in hospital delivery as well as in the data of birth and race/ethnicity. 71% were Blacks, 22% Hispanics, 5% non-Hispanic white and 3% of unknown other race.

It is obvious, that congenital syphilis occurred more frequently in children of unmarried, less educated and drug using mothers without prenatal care (Tab.2).

Homosexual men are no longer at highest risk nor has the reservoir of infection remained with them, but both have transgressed to the group of drug addicts. This trend is world-wide and is also clearly shown in a recent study from Amsterdam (Tab.3 (10)).

Table 3 shows that the incidence of early syphilis rose from 11% to 56% in heterosexual men and dropped from 76% to 12% in homosexual and bisexual men from 1985 to

1988. An increase from 8% to 25% was observed in female prostitutes, from 5% to 11% in non-prostitute women and from 7% to 23% in addicts of hard drugs (10).

A change in the sexual behavior and relations between men and women has been observed in 1991 in Amsterdam with the imminent threat of heterosexual transmission of human immunodeficiency virus (9): the number of high-risk contacts has decreased and the use of condoms has increased, particularly in contacts with casual acquaintances (9).

Late syphilis is rather rare in the USA, but a slight increase in the incidence of neurosyphilis has been observed.

The general increase of syphilis in the USA is attributed to (7,12):

- Crack prostitution: Cocain users exchange sex for drugs and do not respond well to public health control measures,such as partner notification.
- Decreased utilization and access to health care by high-risk groups such as drug addicts and innercity poor.
- Widespread use of antibiotics for penicillin-resistant gonorrhea, which do not treat incubating syphilis (e.g. Spectinomycin).
- Sexually transmitted diseases resources (personnel for case-finding and contact-tracing) have focussed more on AIDS and less on other sexually transmitted diseases programs (Tabs.2,3).

Drug addicts have increasingly suffered from simultaneous infections with the human immunodeficiency virus and T.pallidum. In persons with immunodeficiencies, lesions of early syphilis contain excessive numbers of spirochetes and the manifestations persist much longer than in persons with an intact immune system. The risk of infection is therefore extremely high at contact with such persons. Also, drug addicts usually do not care much for personal hygiene, frequently miss to seek medical treatment and neglect public health advice.

At present, a dramatic increase of endemic treponematoses (yaws and endemic syphilis) takes place in Central-Africa: 2500000 persons suffer from early communicable lesions, of these, 2000000 are children (12).

Gonorrhea

The general trend in the incidence of gonorrhea during the past decades is very similar to that of syphilis, but figures are about ten times higher. In Great Britain the male:female ratio was four in 1950 and less than 1.5 in 1985. The highest incidence among females was in the age group 16-18 years and among males in the age group 20-24 years (6).

In the USA, the incidence reached an all-time high of 473/ 100000 population in 1977, but has dropped steadily since then and holds at 288/100000 population in 1990. There were 812693 cases reported in 1987 and the actual figure was estimated at 1.6 million (7). The incidence dropped to 706600 cases in 1988, rose again to 751100 cases in 1989 and then dropped to 701300 in 1990. The incidence in Blacks is 30fold higher than in Whites. Although a general decrease is noted, the actual situation is different in distinct groups of the population: Studies from several European and North American cities suggest that the incidence of gonorrhea in homosexual and bisexual men has declined precipitously, while the incidence in other groups has changed less. There was a slight increase in US-teenage boys (7). In the USA, 65000 strains of N.gonorrhoeae were resistant to antibiotics which represents an increase from 7.9% of all reported gonococcal cases in 1989 to 9.5% in 1990.

Of all strains examined,

*7.4% were penicillinase-producing,

*4.8% tetracycline-resistant,

*0.9% penicillinase-producing plus tetracycline-resistant. Chromosomally mediated resistance to penicillin was noted in 1%, to tetracycline in 8.8% and to both, penicillin and tetracycline, in 2.9% (7).

In Europe, the incidence has decreased steadily in almost all countries. During 1985-1990, 10-20/100000 population have been reported diseased in Germany and Austria:

Germany: 1985:59.2/100000
1986:43.2/100000
1987:25.3/100000
1988:16.3/100000
1989:12.5/100000

Austria: 1986:56.0/100000
1987:38.9/100000
1988:29.2/100000
1989:23.9/100000
1990:20.8/100000

Respective data for 1989-1990 are 55/100000 in Finland, 36/100000 in Norway, 33/100000 in Denmark and 13/100000 in Sweden. The trend indicates a steady regression in all these countries. The reasons for the decline (in spite of increasing numbers of resistant strains) are the same as for the decrease of syphilis: a change in sexual behavior attributable to prevention measures for the acquired immunodeficiency syndrome (1,5,9,11).

Chlamydia Trachomatis

Trends in the incidence of proven C.trachomatis infections cannot be precisely defined, since in most countries it is not a disease, which must be reported. However, trends in the incidence of non-gonococcal urethritis in men provide a reasonable approximation because the proportion of cases attributable to C.trachomatis infection has remained fairly constant at about 40% (at least in industrialized countries) in various studies during the last decade (6). The number of cases of non-gonococcal urethritis increased steadily during the last years and has become far more common than gonorrhoea, syphilis and chancroid together (1,6). Unlike gonorrhea, chlamydial infections commonly occur in all racial and ethnic groups and in all socio-economic classes. The incidence is related to the number of partners. Young women and women using oral contraceptives seem more susceptible than others (1,6). The probability to become infected at contact with a diseased partner is 40% for women and 32% for men (2). Approximately 75% of infected men and 25% of infected women remain asymptomatic (7). Screening programs in young women, particularly during pregnancy, should be part of routine pelvic examinations (1).

In Great Britain, the incidence of non-gonococcal urethritis has steadily increased and is now four times higher than for gonorrhea in men and more than three times in women. There has been a steep rise in laboratory reports of genital C.trachomatis infection, which probably reflects the wider availability of chlamydial diagnostic testing. Reports of infections with C.trachomatis in women rose over fourfold from 3500 in 1981 to 18500 in 1986 (6).

In other industrialized countries, the prevalence of chlamydial urethral infection ranges from 3-12% among asymptomatic men attending different health facilities to 15-20% of all men seen at sexually transmitted diseases clinics. The prevalence is strongly correlated with younger age and heterosexual rather than homosexual preference. In Sweden, the incidence of chlamydial infections is highest in women aged 20-24 years. However, this may be related to the intensive case finding particularly in young women (6).

In the USA, about four million new cases occur per year; 2.6 million in women and 1.8 million in men (1,2). The incidence of infections in pregnant women ranges at 8% to 12%. Recent reports from Europe (Belgium, Norway, Sweden, Germany), from the USA and Canada have revealed that 10%-30% of young, sexually active women of the age group 15-25 years are infected and about 46% of their male contacts harbor the pathogen in their urethra: at least 25% of the latter have had no clinical symptoms (1,2,15).

During pregnancy, Chlamydia trachomatis has been discovered in the cervix of

- 4% (Austria 1982),
- 10% (Germany 1983),
- 8% (USA 1983),
- 27-37% (USA 1984)
- 7% (Great Britain 1984),
- 6% (Canada 1985),
- 14% (Austria 1986),
- 9.4% (Netherlands 1990),
- 12,2% (Sweden 1991),
- 19% (Sweden 1991),
- 34,4% Turkey1991)

(8,13,15,17,19).

Approximately 35% of the neonates born to infected mothers develop inclusion conjunctivitis and 20% pneumonia compared to 1.4% and 0.8% resp. of offsprings of healthy mothers. 40-80% of cases of pelvic inflammatory disease in women are caused by C.trachomatis. Therefore, chlamydial infections must be reported by law in 40 of the 50 States of the USA and routine checks for C.trachomatis infections should be mandatory in prenatal care.

In developing countries, the prevalence of chlamydial infections in women is similar to industrialized countries while the number of men with urethritis seems to be lower. Since C.trachomatis causes a more indolent infection, male patients are less motivated to seek treatment (6).

Chancroid

The global incidence of chancroid greatly exceeds that of syphilis, particularly in developing countries. It parallels the socioeconomic development, e.g. chancroid has declined markedly in Singapore, but has increased in El Salvador. More than 5000 cases per year are seen in a Special Treatment Clinic in Nairobi. Similar figures have been reported from South Africa, Swaziland and Gambia (6). 36%-57% of the patients have been infected by contacts with prostitutes.

In Great Britain, fewer than 100 cases have been reported annually in the past 15 years and so far, no increase has been observed. In the USA, chancroid had been rare since World War II. Beginning in 1984, however, a series of outbreaks began to appear in the inner city migrant labor populations of Los Angeles, Dallas, Boston, New York City,

New Orleans and several Florida cities. In the USA, 665 cases have been reported in 1984, 2000 in 1985, 5000 in 1987, 4998 in 1988, 4712 in 1989 and 2653 in 1990 (7).

During the last decade, in Germany, figures have ranged under 100 cases per year (1985: 103; 1986: 101; 1987: 51; 1988: 29; 1989:37) and below 50 cases per year in Austria (1980:8, 1981:42, 1982:5, 1983:1, 1984:2, 1985:4, 1986:8, 1987:0, 1988:3, 1989:0 and 1990:2).

Genital Herpes

Generally, genital herpes occurs 7-10 times more frequently than gonorrhea.

In the USA, 200000 to 500000 (7) to 750000 (6) new cases of infections with herpes simplex virus type 2 have occurred per year. A 15fold increase has been noted between 1966 and 1984 and by 1990 with a total of about 20 (6) to 25 million (1) persons infected. Of these, only one quarter to one third have ever had clinical manifestations, but asymptomatic carriers of herpes simplex virus type 2 are frequent sources of infection. A slight but steady decrease has been observed since 1984. Three infants per 10000 births are infected at delivery (7). This incidence has remained unchanged.

In Great Britain, the number of cases has increased from 4000 in 1971 to 20000 in 1985. A slight downward trend has been no ticed since then (6).

Human Papilloma Virus Infections

The epidemiology of Human Papilloma Virus infection is similar to that of genital herpes, except that its magnitude is 3-4fold greater and no decrease has yet been noted. Since genitoanal cancers, in particular cervical cancer, are a major consequence of genitoanal Human Papilloma Virus infections, this makes them very important from the public health point of view.

More than 64 types of Human Papilloma Virus can be distinguished. Types 6 and 11 are associated with exophytic condylomata acuminata, types 16 and 18 (and the less frequently occurring types 31,33,35,39) with invasive genitoanal cancer. Types 41 to 45, 51 to 56 and 59 have recently been detected in tissues from genital lesions, but the pathogenetic significance of these findings is not yet determined (12). Infection with Human Papilloma Virus may occur via abrasions of the skin, via sexual contacts and via an infected birth canal.

In the USA, the annual incidence of new infections is about one million. Human Papilloma Virus is found in approximately 5% of all persons visiting Sexually Transmitted Diseases clinics. In private practice, physicians have noted approximately 220000 first visits for Human Papilloma Virus infections. Screening for Human Papilloma Virus DNA using the polymerase chain reaction technique is a most effective and an essential method for early recognition of a risk for cancer (1) and has revealed an incidence of 5-19% in women consulting family-planning clinics, and an incidence of 27% among females who visited STD clinics. At routine examinations of female college students, Human Papilloma Virus DNA was found 8 times more frequently than clinically overt warts. Human Papilloma Virus DNA could be detected in scrapings of the glans and the prepuce of 8% of male Sexually Transmitted Diseases clinic patients at the age of 16 to 45 years.

Human Papilloma Virus type 16 was identified in specimens from the cervix of 22% of female college students and in 44% of female Sexually Transmitted Diseases clinic patients in Seattle (1). The implication of finding cancer-associated virus in such a high proportion of young women is obviously of great concern.

In the United Kingdom, the incidence of genital warts rose from 30/100000 population in 1970 to 260/100000 in 1988. Human Papilloma Virus infection is now the second most frequently reported Sexually Transmitted Disease in Great Britain subsequent to non-gonococcal urethritis (6).

In Finland, the risk for a woman who is Human Papilloma Virus negative at the age of 19 to contract Human Papilloma Virus infection later in her life is 8% at 20, 37% (cumulative %) at 24, 55% at 29, 66% at 39, 72% at 49 and 79% at 79 years of age (18).

Hepatitis B

This form of hepatitis is very contagious (about 100 times more than the acquired immunodeficiency syndrome). Hepatitis B Virus is transferred parenterally (injection, wounds etc.), by sexual contacts or perinatally.

There are an estimated 200 million carriers of Hepatitis B Virus in the world.

In the United States 23419 cases have been reported in 1989, but an estimated 200000 to 300000 (1) infections occur annually. The incidence is 3.8 to 32.6 cases per 100.000 population in the USA, yet Hepatitis B Virus antibodies can be detected in 7200 to 10000 persons per 100000 population. It is discouraging to note that the overall incidence of hepatitis B has not declined much since 1982, despite a steep decline in high-risk homosexual contacts among men and the availability of an effective hepatitis B vaccine. Of all new hepatitis B infections attributed to known risk factors, the percentage associated with homosexual contacts declined from 21% in 1982 to 9% in 1987. Over the same period, however, the proportions ascribed to heterosexual contacts and intravenous drug abuse both rose from 15% to 22% and from 15% to 28% resp.(1,6).

Worldwide, about 250000 individuals die annually from hepatocellular cancer. 80% of these carcinomas are attributable to chronic Hepatitis B Virus infection. Therefore, each year 200000 persons die as a late sequel of hepatitis B.

Infections with the Human Immunodeficiency Virus

The WHO Weekly Epidemiological Record of July 5th, 1991 indicates 371803 reported cases of the acquired immunodeficiency syndrome. Of these,

- 222717 have occurred in the Americas (USA:179136),
- 92957 in Africa,
- 52195 in Europe,
- 2839 in Oceania
- 1095 in Asia.

The incidence per one million population is

- 499.8 in the USA,

- 175.6 in Switzerland,
- 158 in France,
- 101 in Spain,
- 92 in Denmark,
- 85 in Italy,
- 66 in Germany,
- 45 in Austria,
- 35 in Sweden,
- 33 in Norway,
- 5 in Finland,
- 3 in Yugoslavia,
- 3 in Hungaria,
- 1.2 in Romania,
- 1.1 in Czecoslovakia and
- 0.1 in the Soviet Union (20).

The increase over the figure of the previous year was 400% in the USA in 1984, but has decreased to 40% in 1990 (4). In all continents added up, the respective figure is 72.9% (69.3% in Europe, but more than 100% in Africa).

In Europe, new cases per week occur:
- 87-88 in France,
- 50-51 in Italy,
- 34 in Spain,
- 26-27 in Germany,
- 23-24 in the United Kingdom,
- 13 in Romania,
- 9-10 in Switzerland,
- 7-8 in Portugal,
- 6-7 in the Netherlands,
- 4-5 in Belgium,
- 4-5 in Denmark,
- 2-3 in Greece,
- 2-3 in Austria,
- 2-3 in Yugoslavia and
- 1-2 in Sweden (20).

Homo- and bisexual men represent 55.8% of all cases in the USA, 50% in Europe, 16% in Italy, 49% in Austria, 51% in Switzerland, 72% in Germany and 81% in Great Britain, drug addicts 23% in the USA and 27% in Europe (66% in Italy, 28% in Austria and 3% in Great Britain).

The incubation period may last for 6-9 years.

The average survival time after manifestation of clinical symptoms is 8-14 months. 80% of patients have died by the end of the second year and 95% by the end of the third year.

The incidence is slowly decreasing among homosexual and bisexual men, but rising in drug addicts. Transmission by heterosexual contacts is increasing in the USA and in Europe.

Worldwide, about 5 million persons are infected but without clinical symptoms: in the USA about one million, in Germany 80000-100000 and in Austria around 5000.

The expenses for diagnosing and treating patients suffering from the acquired immunodeficiency syndrome in the USA is estimated at US$ 166500000000 for 1991. The supply with Azidothymidine costs US$ 10000 for one patient per year.

Finally, the epidemiology of two clinical syndromes will be discussed because of the increasingly great importance in public health care (pelvic inflammatory disease) and because it may be of particular interest for ophthalmologists (ophthalmia neonatorum).

Ophthalmia Neonatorum

Pathogens of sexually transmitted diseases are three of the four major agents that cause ophthalmia neonatorum: N.gonorrhoeae, C.trachomatis serovars D-K and Herpes simplex virus type 2; the fourth is chemical irritation by 1% silver nitrate solution (Credé's prophylaxis). Clinical symptoms of neonatal infections by N.gonorrhoeae start by 2-5 days, C.trachomatis infections by 7-12 days, Herpes simplex virus type 2 infections by 8 days to 6 weeks. Chemical irritation is seen within 6-24 hours after birth. Without treatment, corneal damage and scarring develop in 25% of N.gonorrhoeae, 39% of Herpes simplex virus type 2, and extremely rarely in C.trachomatis disease. The incidence and etiologic spectrum of neonatal conjunctivitis differ in various parts of the world depending on the relative prevalence of maternal gonococcal and chlamydial infections and the use of ocular prophylaxis. C.trachomatis replaced N.gonorrhoeae as the most important single causative agent even in developing countries with up to 32% of all cases. Herpes simplex virus type 2 is a rare cause of neonatal ocular disease; in the USA, 4000 cases are reported per year. The transmission rate from an infected mother to the newborn is 30-45% for N.gonorrhoeae and 30% for C.trachomatis.

In industrialized countries, the incidence of neonatal gonococcal conjunctivitis dropped from 10% more than a century ago to 0.3% thanks to the introduction of silver nitrate prophylaxis. In Denmark, Credé's prophylaxis was abandoned in March 1985, resulting in an increase of the incidence of ophthalmia neonatorum by 33% (from 0.3/10000 to 1.0/1.000 live births). In some developing countries, this prophylaxis was discontinued as well and has led to a very high incidence of gonococcal ophthalmia neonatorum with as much as 5% of births in some places. Reintroduction of prophylaxis drastically reduced the incidence by 83% when 1% silver nitrate was used and by 93% when 0.5%-1% tetracycline ointment was applied. The WHO therefore considers it very necessary to reintroduce this prophylaxis and enforce it (6). The original opinion that silver nitrate prophylaxis is completely ineffective to prevent infections by C.trachomatis must be revised; recent studies have suggested that the effect may be fairly equivalent to tetracycline or erythromycin (2).

Pelvic Inflammatory Disease

In the USA each year more than one million women experience an episode of Pelvic Inflammatory Disease, the majority being in the age group 15-24 years. About 300000 women are hospitalized, 250000 suffer from more or less severe late complications such as ectopic pregnancy, tuboovarial abscesses, pyosalpinx, scarring with persistent pain and infertility (12). 24 women die each year from Pelvic Inflammatory Disease. 89% have to undergo surgical treatment, 40.6% on the uterus (27.6% hysterectomy), 32% on the ovaries and 11% on the tubes. In Sweden, Pelvic Inflammatory Disease has been found associated with

- C.trachomatis 40-60% (salpingitis 80%),
- N.gonorrhoeae 15-18%,
- M.hominis 10-15%,
- anaerobes 3-5% and
- unknown 10-15% (6).

The global incidence of Pelvic Inflammatory Disease went up by 50% during the nineteen seventies (in Great Britain by 61%), remained high and, in the USA, a striking increase in hospitalization occurred in young white women under 24 years of age (6). The cost for diagnosis and treatment of Pelvic Inflammatory Disease in the USA in 1990 is estimated at about US$ 2200000000 (2) to 3500000000 (12).

An evaluation of all epidemiological facts concerning the major Sexually Transmitted Diseases may lead to the following conclusions (14):

- The highest prevalence is observed in infections with human papilloma virus.
- The most frequent bacterial infection is due to C.trachomatis.
- The greatest increase has occurred with pelvic inflammatory disease, particularly in ectopic pregnancy.
- The highest resource competition is entailed by infections with the human immunodeficiency virus (WHO 1990).

Table 1. Estimated incidence of the ten most frequent STD in the USA (7,12)

Disease	Estimated No. of infections/year
Bacterial vaginosis	8,000.000
Candidosis	7,000.000
Chlamydia infections	4,000.000
Trichomoniasis	2,500.000
Human papilloma virus infection	1,000.000
Herpes genitalis	724.000
Gonorrea	701.300
Hepatitis B	200.000
Syphilis (all stages)	100.000
AIDS	37.000
Total	24,762.954

Table 2. Comparative evaluation of mothers of syphilitic neonates and mothers of healthy infants (3)

	Case mothers	Control mothers	95% Confidence intervall
n	299	598	
Medicaid	61.0%	56.0%	0.9 - 1.6
Age below 20 years	13.0%	17.0%	0.5 - 1.1
No prenatal care	36.0%	5.2%	3.5 - 7.7
Unmarried	84.0%	65.0%	1.9 - 4.0
No high school graduate	60.0%	39.0%	1.7 - 3.2
Cocain use	28.0%	6.0%	4.2 - 10.5
Any drug use	52.0%	14.0%	4.7 - 9.2

Table 3. Early syphilis in attendants of the STD-Clinics in Amsterdam (10)

	1985		1986		1987		1988	
	n	%	n	%	n	%	n	%
Heterosexual men	16	11	23	22	53	47	62	56
Homo/bisexual men	114	76	69	64	33	30	12	12
Prostitues (women)	12	8	6	6	16	14	24	21
Nonprostitutes (women)	8	5	9	8	10	9	12	11
Total	150	100	107	100	112	100	111	100
Among these: users of hard drugs	11	7	9	8	23	21	26	23

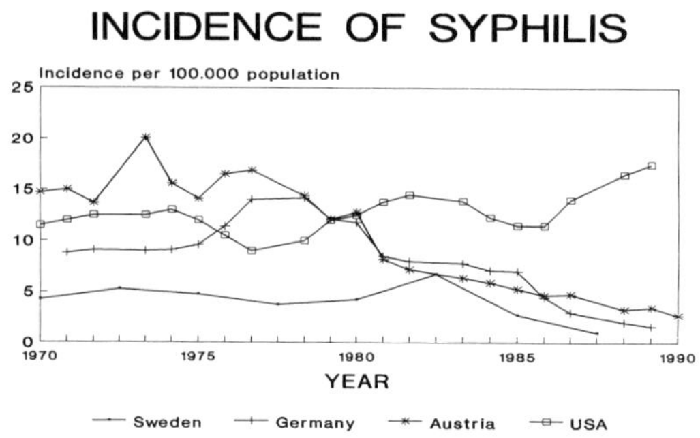

Fig. 1

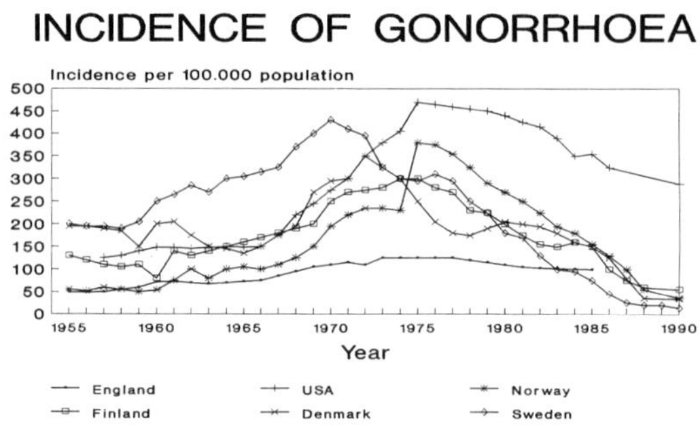

Fig.2

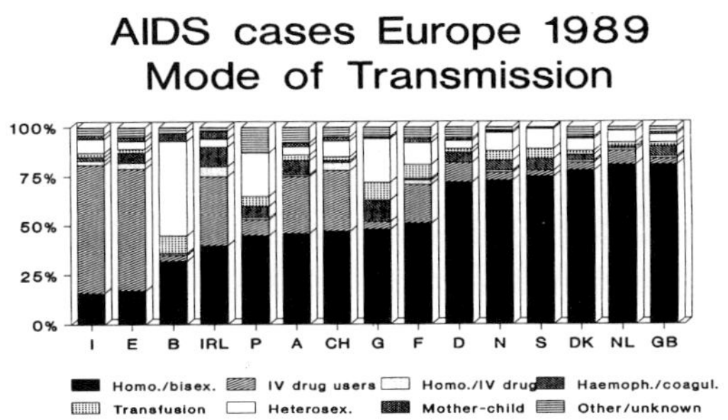

From WHO Weekly Epid.Rec.65,33,1990

Fig.3

References

1. Aral SO, Holmes KK (1991) Sexually Transmitted Diseases in the AIDS Era. Sci Am 264:62-69
2. Cates W, Wasserheit JN (1991) Genital Chlamydia Infections: Epidemiology and Reproductive Sequelae. Am J Obstetr Gynecol 164:1771-1781
3. Centers for Disease Control (1989) Congenital Syphilis New York City 1986-1988. MMWR 48:825-829
4. Centers for Disease Control (1991) HIV/AIDS Surveillance Report 1st April, 1991. CDC Atlanta,GA/USA
5. Danielsson D (1990) Gonorrhea and Syphilis in Sweden - Past and Present. Scand J Inf Dis Suppl 69:69-76
6. DeShryver A, Meheus A (1990) Epidemiology of Sexually Transmitted Diseases: The Global Picture. Bull WHO 68:639-654
7. Drusin L (1991) Report of the Regional Director for North America to the Executive Committee of the International Union against the Venereal Diseases and the Treponematoses, June 1988, April 1989, May 1990 and September 1991.
8. Ertem E, Dereli D, Serter D et al (1991) Screening for Chlamydia Trachomatis in a Turkish Population. Genitourin Med 67:354-355
9. van Haastrecht HJA, van den Hoek JAR, Coutinho RA (1991) Evidence for a Change in Behavior Among Heterosexuals in Amsterdam Under the Influence of AIDS. Genitourin Med 67:199-206
10. van den Hoek JAR, van der Linden MMD, Coutinho RA (1990) Increase of Infectious Syphilis Among Heterosexuals in Amsterdam. Genitourin Med 66:31-32
11. van de Laar MJW, Pickerling J, van den Hoek JAR et al (1990) Declining Gonorrhea Rates in The Netherlands 1976-1988: Consequences for the AIDS Epidemic.Genitourin Med 66:148-150
12. Luger A (1990) Perspectives in Sexually Transmitted Diseases. Chronica Dermatologica (Roma) 3: 355 - 410
13. Luger A (1987) Epidemiologie, Klinik und Therapie der Infektionen mit Chlamydia trachomatis Serotyp D-K. Wien Klin Wchschr 99:1-14
14. Meheus A (1990) Sexually Transmitted Diseases and AIDS. 35th General Assembly of the International Union against the Venereal Diseases and the Treponematoses. London, 5.-11.5.1990.
15. Rahm VA, Odlind V, Pettersson R (1991) Chlamydia Trachomatis in Sexually Active Teenage Girls. Factors Related to Genital Chlamydial Infection: A Prospective Study. Genitourin Med 67:317-321
16. Rolfs RT, Nakashima AK (1990) Epidemiology of Primary and Secondary Syphilis in the United States 1981 Through 1989. J Am Med Ass 264:1432-1437

17. Svensson LO, Mares I, Olsson SE (1991) Detection of C.trachomatis in Urinary Samples from Women. Genitourin Med 67:117-119
18. Syrjänen K, Hakama M, Saarikosi S et al (1990) Prevalence, Incidence and Estimated Life Time Risk of Cervical Human Papillomavirus Infection in a nonselected female Population. Sex Trans Dis 17:15-19
19. Thewessen EAPM, van der Mejden WI, Doppenberg HJAT et al (1990) Screening for Cervical Chlamydia Trachomatis Infections in Two Dutch Populations. Genitourin Med 66:361-366
20. WHO (1991) Weekly Epidemiological Record. 66:109-112

- Bacterial: Syphilis

The History of Ocular Syphilis

Kirk R.Wilhelmus

Abstract. Ocular syphilis was first clearly delineated in the nineteenth century, but case descriptions of eye disease associated with the "great pox" are known from the late fifteenth century. This historical overview of syphilis and the eye illustrates the many pathologic and symbolic aspects of this "great imitator".

The origins of syphilis

How syphilis first came to infect humans is not known. The geography of the various types of human treponematoses suggests a possible relationship linking human migration and microbial disease (22).

The debate lingers whether syphilis in Europe and Asia arose from an endemic source or crossed the Atlantic with the discoverers of the New World (34). Scientific and artistic evidence for a pre-Columbian origin in Europe is slim (28). Since paleopathological investigations have identified skeletal evidence of syphilitic-like disease in prehistoric animals and native humans of North America (2), current theories favor an American origin. Presumably, the sailors (or more likely their aboriginal captives) who returned with Christopher Columbus in 1493 and subsequent convoys introduced syphilis into Spain and Italy.

Clinical reports by Venetian doctors serving at the 1495 battle of the mercenary army in Italy described soldiers with a pustular eruption, some of whom lost their eyesight (5,18). A 1496 woodcut by Albrecht Dürer that illustrates a medical poem on epidemics depicts a knight with a skin rash and possible uniocular disease (Fig.1). Another woodcut from a 1498 medical text also shows disseminated skin lesions, and the possibility of eye disease is suggested by ptosis or eyelid edema (44).

In 1530, Girolamo Fracastoro published a medical poem relating the story of Syphilis, a shepherd who was punished by God with a venereal disease. He fell ill and watched "...the cheerful glories of his eyes decay..". The poem names his illness "syphilis" in memory of its first sufferer. Eye involvement was recognized as one of the many debilitating components of this apparently new disease. Early 16th century painters such as Hieronymous Bosch and Lucas Cranach depicted syphilis as a cause of blindness and other hellish complications (3).

The pustular skin rash and the rapid development of periosteitis and gummas suggest syphilis took a more violent, fulminating course during the Renaissance than is usually seen today. Disease severity seemed to wane somewhat over the next century, but many writers continued to mention a "cold ophthalmia" characterized by pain, tearing and blurred vision (12,13,25). For example, Johannes de Vigo stated, "I have frequently cured several eye diseases which were due to syphilis, especially the ocular inflammation due to cold substances leading to loss of vision" (12). In 1575, Ambroise Paré commented that after dissemination by the blood from a primary chancre, patients would "...lose an eye, and often both, or large portions of their eyelids, and even after they were cured the patients remained hideous to behold, on account of their scarred eyes..." (31). Treatment was prolonged and involved, although cures of ophthalmia due to the "French disease" were claimed using mercury (26).

Descriptions of syphilitic eye disease

Memoirs and literary works during the 16th to 18th centuries alluded to ocular involvement from syphilis. For example, Cellini relates a temporary loss of vision from his venereal disease, and Casanova mentions a syphilitic Bolognese gentleman who apparently had impaired eyesight as his tongue was his only unaffected organ. Depictions of the stigmata of congenital syphilis are also known. For example, Rembrandt's 1665 portrait of Gerard de Lairesse clearly shows the saddle-nose deformity of his contemporary painter.

Syphilis came to be a metaphor for sin and even vengeance. In the 19th century novel Les Diaboliques by Barbey d'Aurevilly, a Spanish duchess sought revenge on her cruel husband by resorting to prostitution and dying of syphilis: "In only a few months she was rotten to the bones. One of her eyes had suddenly jumped from its socket one day, and had fallen at her feet like a large coin. The other had liquified and melted. She had died - but stoically suffering intolerable tortures." Similar moralizing themes also appeared in the visual arts. An 1851 engraving by Rambert shows the effects of syphilis, with lesions affecting the skin, hair, bones, and eyes (Fig.2).

As ophthalmology developed into a speciality, ophthalmic texts were published to classify the diagnosis and treatment of eye diseases. Among the listed causes of ocular inflammation was "venereal ophthalmia" (11,32,35,46), an entity that apparently describes ocular syphilis as well as gonorrheal conjunctivitis. Syphilitic iritis was first well-characterized in the early 19th century (40), and the first accurate textbook description of syphilitic uveitis detailed the signs of intraocular inflammation, iris nodules, and secondary glaucoma (4). Philippe Ricord was one of the first to clearly differentiate gonorrheal and syphilitic eye diseases (36), and he described the eye complications of tertiary syphilis such as diplopia and visual loss (37).

Monographs devoted to venereal eye diseases (9,19,23,24), helped to distinguish the various clinical manifestations. Distinctive eye findings of acquired and congenital syphilis, especially neurosyphilis, were described in several late 19th and early 20th century publications (17,20,21,27,43,45) and collated into comprehensive encyclopedic texts (14,17). Among the distinctive signs were the signe d'omnibus of Alfred Fournier (a white line in the mid-eyebrow), Jonathan Hutchinson's teeth (notching of the upper incisors), and the pupillary changes described by Douglas Argyll Robertson.

As the ocular complications of syphilis were being better recognized, the eyes were also used metaphorically to reflect the tragedy of this disease. For example, after visiting a Norwegian venereal disease clinic, Edvard Munch painted "Heritage" during 1897-1899, depicting a mother and child (Fig.3). He stated that "this face, contracted with despair, had to be painted as I once saw it against the green hospital wall; and I had to paint the inquiring suffering eyes of the child, just the way they appeared out of the pallid yellow little body, as pale as the sheet on which it lay... The child's big eyes peer into the world it unintentionally entered; sick and fearful and inquiring it stares ahead, surprised at the painful life it has entered upon, already asking Why? Why?" (15).

Syphilis in the 20th century

Many of the symptoms of syphilis, including its eye manifestations, are similar to other disease processes, leading William Osler to call syphilis the "great imitator" (29). He advised his students: "Know syphilis in all its manifestations and relations, and all other things clinical will be added unto you" (30). These clinical variations and the risk of developing eye and other complications were assessed in the Oslo (16) and Tuskegee (38) studies on untreated syphilis. These epidemiologic reports identified optic atrophy as the principal cause of permanent visual loss in syphilis.

In the early ophthalmic literature, the role of systemic mercury rather than topical medications was emphasized. Arsenicals, bismuth, iodides, and fever therapy were incorporated into ophthalmologic practice in the early 20th century. Even so, syphilis was reported to be the cause of 10-15% of all cases of blindness in the United States into the 1940s. These sight-threatening consequences of ocular and neuro-ophthalmic syphilis symbolize its virulent effects. To illustrate, African deformity masks that depict syphilitic facies may have been the inspiration for Pablo Picasso's "Les Demoiselles d'Avignon" (39), an oeuvre that can be reinterpreted as an allegory of syphilis. For if the wages of sin is death, then the cost of syphilis is disease, disfigurement, and blindness.

The demonstration of the efficacy of penicillin against early syphilis in 1943 heralded optimism about eradicating this disease. By 1954, the World Health Organization estimated that venereal syphilis had fallen to a recent worldwide low of 20 million. Yet syphilis endures and continues to evolve (10).

Like some other pathogens, an African origin has been postulated. But, as tellingly characterized in the recent Academy Award-winning film "Out of Africa" (33), in which a European woman contracts syphilis from her husband while living in Kenya, the spread of syphilis now depends on community and individual mores that lead to continued transmission. Current estimates are 3-4 times the 1950s figures. This recent resurgence seems directly linked to the illicit drug industry.

In our antibiotic era, neurosyphilis persists (8,42). The acquired immunodeficiency syndrome is recapitulating the historical eyesore of syphilis (6) as it changes the clinical picture. And the spectrum of eye findings of syphilis continues to expand (41,47).

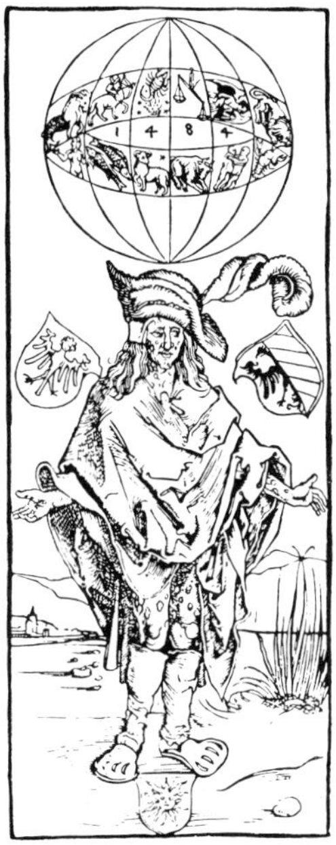

Fig.1. Woodcut illustration attributed to Dürer. The date inscribed in the zodiac derives from the spurious astrological deduction that the first European epidemic of the great pox began on November 25, 1484, during the unlucky conjunction of Saturn and Jupiter and the house of Mars.

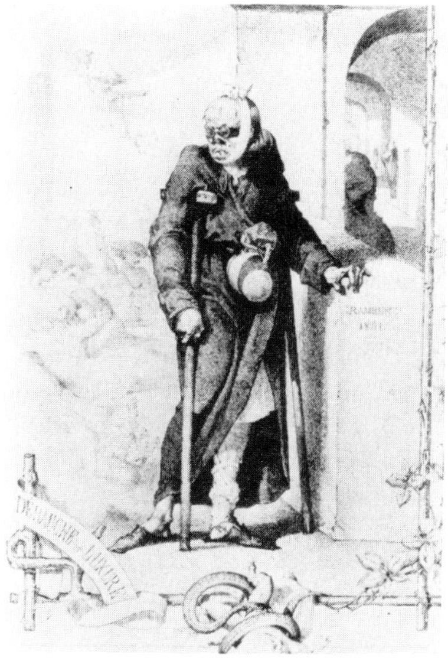

Fig.2. French engraving by Rambert showing a sight-impaired syphilitic leaving behind his former life and family.

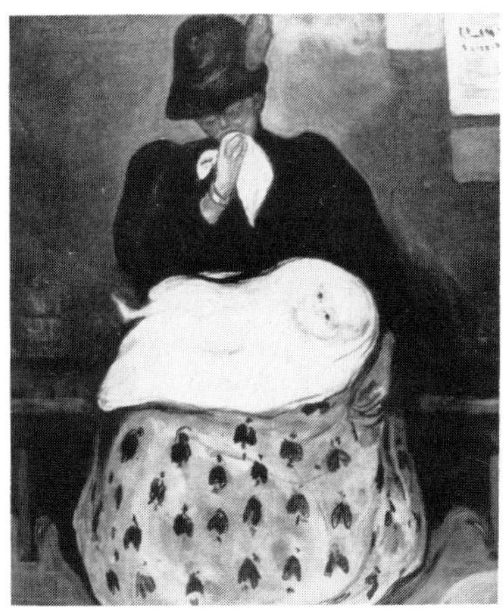

Fig.3. Painting by Munch that was much criticized because of the artist's purposeful linkage of the tragedy of congenital syphilis with the madonna-and-child theme.

References

1. Alexander (1895) Neue Erfahrungen über luetische Augenerkrankungen. Wiesbaden

2. Baker BJ, Armelagos GJ (1988) The Origin and Antiquity of Syphilis: Paleopathological Diagnosis and Interpretation. Curr Anthropol 29:703-720
3. Bax D (1983) Hieronymus Bosch and Lucas Cranach; Two Last Judgement Triptychs; Description and Exposition. North-Holland, Amsterdam
4. Beer J (1813) Die Lehre von den Augenkrankheiten. Vienna
5. Benedicti A (1497) Veronensis Physici Historiae Corporis Humani. Verona
6. Brandt AM (1988) The Syphilis Epidemic and its Relation to AIDS. Science 239:375-380
7. Bull OR (1884) The Ophthalmoscope and Lues. Christiana
8. Burke JM, Schaberg DR (1985) Neurosyphilis in the Antibiotic Era. Neurology 35:1368-1371
9. Camerarii A, Breyer JF (1734) De Ophthalmia Venera. Tübingen
10. Causse G, Meheus A (1988) La lutte contre les maladies sexuellement transmissibles (MST) et les tréponématoses endemiques. World Health Stat Q 41:82-102
11. de Saint-Yves C (1722) Nouveau Traité des Maladies des Yeux. Paris
12. de Vigo J (1514) Patrica Copiosa in Arte Chirurgica. S Guillireti & H Bononiensem, Roma
13. Diaz de Isla R (1539) Tractada Contra el Mal Serpentino. D Roberto, Sevilla
14. Dimmer F (1900) Syphilis des Auges. In: Finger E (ed) Handbuch der Geschlechtskrankheiten. Vienna
15. Eggum A (1984) Edvard Munch. Paintings, Sketches, and Studies. Clarkson N Potter, New York pp. 169-170
16. Gjestland T (1955) The Oslo Study of Untreated Syphilis. Acta Dermatol Venereol 34(suppl):1-318
17. Groeunow A (1904) In: Graefe A, Saemisch T (eds) Handbuch der gesamten Augenheilkunde. Vol XI/1 pp.737-862
18. Grunpeck J (1503) Libellus Josephi Grunpeckii de Mentalagra, alias Morbo Gallico. Venezia
19. Hewson T (1824) Observations on the History and the Treatment of the Ophthalmia Accompanying the Secondary Form of Lues Venera. London
20. Hirschberg J (1885) Netzhaut-Entzündung bei angeborener Lues. Leipzig
21. Hutchinson J (1863) Syphilitic Diseases of the Eye and Ear, Consequent on Inherited Syphilis, London
22. Idse O, Guthe T (1967) The Rise and Fall of the Treponematoses. I. Ecological Aspects and International Trends in Venereal Syphilis. Br J Vener Dis 43:227-243
23. Igersheimer J (1918) Syphilis und Auge. Springer Verlag, Berlin
24. Lawrence W (1830) A Treatise on the Venereal Diseases of the Eye. London
25. Leoniceno N (1497) De Morbo Gallico. A Manutius, Venezia
26. Lusitanus Z (1634) De Praxi Medica Admiranda. Amsterdam
27. Masselon (1883) Choriorétinite Spécifique. Paris
28. Morton RS (1990) Syphilis in Art: An Entertainment in Four Parts. Part 1. Genitourin Med 66:33-40
29. Osler W (1917) The Campaign Against Syphilis. Lancet 1:1789
30. Osler W (1904) Aequanimitas. With Other Addresses to Medical Students, Nurses and Practitioners of Medicine. Blakiston, Philadelphia
31. Paré A (1575) Oeuvres. Le Seizieme Livre Traitant de la Grosse Vérole. Paris
32. Plenck JJ (1777) Doctrina de Morbis Oculorum. Wien
33. Pollack S (director)(1985) Out of Africa. Universal, Los Angeles
34. Quétel C (1990) History of Syphilis. Johns Hopkins University Press, Baltimore
35. Richter AG (1790) Anfangsgründe der Wundarzneikunst. Vol III. Göttingen

36. Ricord P (1842) De l'Ophtalmie Blenorrhagique. Paris
37. Ricord P (1851) Lettres sur la Syphilis. Paris
38. Rockwell DH, Yobs AR, Moore MB Jr (1964) The Tuskegee Study of Untreated Syphilis. The 30th Year of Observation. Arch Intern Med 114:792-798
39. Samaltanos-Stenstrom K (1987) If the Wages of Sin is Death. Critica d'Arte :63-70
40. Schmidt JA (1801) Über Nachstar und Iritis nach Staroperationen. Wien
41. Schwartz B (1969) Syphilis and the Eye. Surv Ophthalmol 14:157-299
42. Simon RP (1985) Neurosyphilis. Arch Neurol 42:606-613
43. Sidler-Huguenin (1902) Die Hereditär-Syphilitischen Augenhintergrunds-Veränderungen. Hamburg & Leipzig
44. Steber B (1498) A Mala Franzos Morbo Gallorum. Wien
45. Terrien F (1905) Syphilis de l'Oeil et de ses Annexes. Paris
46. von Walther P (1810) Abhandlungen aus dem Gebiet der Praktischen Medizin. Landshut
47. Wilhelmus KR (1987) Syphilis. In: Insler MS (ed) AIDS and Other Sexually Transmitted Diseases and the Eye. Grune & Stratton, Orlando,FL pp.73-104

Clinical Features of Syphilis and the Eye

Kirk R. Wilhelmus

Abstract. Syphilis, a systemic infection caused by the spirochete Treponema pallidum, can produce multiple ocular changes. A prospective study over a five-year interval was undertaken to determine the spectrum of syphilitic ocular disease. This information was combined with other reported clinical experiences to illustrate the importance of the eye findings in all stages of syphilis.
Uveitis and optic neuritis are the most common ocular signs of secondary and relapsing syphilis. Typical ocular abnormalities of tertiary syphilis, optic atrophy and pupillary light-near dissociation, are related to central nervous system involvement. Residual stigmata of acquired and congenital syphilis include vascularized corneal scars and chorioretinal pigmentation. Unusual manifestations of syphilis, including posterior segment inflammation and other signs of neurosyphilis, were encountered in patients with human immunodeficiency virus infection.
This review provides a clinical classification scheme that summarizes the inflammatory and degenerative manifestations of ocular syphilis.

Introduction

Syphilis is a systemic infection caused by the spirochete Treponema pallidum (or "pale thread"), so named because of its faint microscopic appearance. The organisms are 10-13µm long and 0.15µm in diameter, just below light microscopic resolution. Treponemes are temperature-sensitive, facultatively anaerobic or microaerophilic bacteria with a doubling time of approximately 30 hours.

T.pallidum can be spread by venereal and nonvenereal routes, commonly known as syphilis and bejel, respectively. While several mammalian species have related spirochetal infections, there is no animal carrier of T.pallidum other than humans. Related, morphologically identical human pathogens are T.pertenue and T.carateum that cause yaws and pinta, respectively. Nonpathogenic treponemes are commensals of the oropharynx, and T.pallidum-like organisms are associated with periodontal disease. Treponemes have not been identified in the normal conjunctiva flora.

The eye may be involved in any of the stages of syphilis, from early disease to late complications. The ocular and neuroophthalmic features of syphilis can best be classified by understanding the clinical stages of T.pallidum infection.

Primary Syphilis

Syphilis is usually acquired by sexual contact. A heterosexual encounter with a person with active syphilis carries a 1-in-3 to 1-in-2 risk of infection. Other means of transmission include direct contact with an infected mucocutaneous lesion, transfusion of fresh blood, and pregnancy (congenital syphilis). Transmission by tear fluid or other ocular routes has not been described.

One exception is a potential oral-ocular route. Several physicians of the late 19th century apparently developed a primary chancre on the eyelid or conjunctiva when examining syphilitic throats (8,13). These lesions resembled a chalazion, a phlyctenule, or Parinaud's oculoglandular syndrome. More bizarrely, sequential cases of primary ocular syphilis occurred from a syphilitic eye care practitioner who removed corneal foreign bodies with her tongue. Cases alleging transmission by opera glasses (8) and other eye-to-eye methods are suspect. Syphilis is not known to be transmitted by corneal transplantation, especially as T.pallidum can probably not survive under the conditions of modern eye-bank storage.

After exposure, the inoculum size and the host's immune status determine the severity and pace of the primary lesion, usually appearing in about three weeks. The primary lesion, or chancre, is a localized skin infection that arises in parallel with dissemination by the lymphatic system and bloodstream. The chancre heals by a localized hypersensitivity-like reaction within 3-6 weeks but can persist longer with concomitant human immuno deficiency virus infection. Regional lymphadenopathy resolves more slowly.

Secondary Syphilis

Despite an effective local immune process, treponemes disseminate and multiply over the next several weeks. About six weeks after the appearance of the primary chancre, the secondary stage begins with low-grade fever, malaise, headache, sore throat, arthralgia, and nontender generalized lymphadenopathy. The most commonly recognized clinical sign is a painless maculopapular skin rash. Usually beginning on the trunk and proximal extremities, syphilis can appear over the entire body including the palms and soles. The eyelids are sometimes affected. Enlarged or coalescent papules, called condyloma lata, may appear in moist areas such as the groin or perineum. Hair follicle involvement may cause temporary, patchy loss of the eyelashes or thinning of the outer half of the eyebrows.

Mucous patches may appear in the oral cavity, genitourinary tract, and conjunctiva, sometimes presenting as a papillary conjunctivitis or a focal, hyperemic conjunctival erosion.

The central nervous system is affected in up to 40% of individuals during secondary syphilis as determined by cerebrospinal fluid analysis of patients without neurologic signs. Usually subclinical, acute meningitis occurs in 1%-2% of patients. Optic neuritis, optic perineuritis, or cranial nerve palsies may be the presenting feature. Approximately 25% of untreated patients develop a relapse of secondary syphilis within four years, frequently presenting with mucous membrane lesions or ocular inflammation. Circulating immune complexes occur in most patients during secondary syphilis and may be involved in the pathogenesis of glomerulo-nephritis as well as anterior uveitis and scleritis.

Anterior uveitis, the most common ocular manifestation of secondary syphilis, occurred in about 5% of cases that went without treatment in the preantibiotic era. While many cases of syphilitic uveitis cannot be distinguished from other cases based on the ocular examination alone, careful general physical examination can show other signs of secondary syphilis. Sometimes associated with the skin rash, iridocyclitis may be the principal clinical sign of relapsing secondary syphilis (4). Beginning as an acute iridocyclitis, the contralateral eye becomes involved in up to one-half of patients. Transient iris roseolae - engorged vascular tufts that probably correspond to the infectious mucocutaneous lesions - may develop in the middle third of the iris that can progress to iris papules (37). These may progress to become vascularized nodules at the pupillary border or near the root of the iris and can lead to sectoral iris atrophy. The severity of anterior uveitis varies from a mild iritis to severe iridocyclitis with hypopyon, vitreitis, and cystoid macular edema.

Episcleritis and scleritis may occur in association with anterior uveitis and can be the principal sign of secondary syphilis. Like the renal disease of secondary syphilis, scleritis is probably related to immune-complex-mediated inflammation. Typically presenting as nodular scleritis, any form of scleral inflammation can occur.

Posterior uveitis may also occur during secondary syphilis. Choroiditis or chorioretinitis may be either diffuse or localized; the focal, placoid type tends to arise adjacent to the disc or macula (10,14). Fluorescein angiography shows early hypofluorescence of the involved area with late staining at the level of the retinal pigment epithelium. About one-half of the cases are bilateral. Progressive inflammation leads to retinal and disc edema, vitreitis, and occasionally secondary exudative retinal detachment. Necrotizing retinitis and other acquired posterior segment changes occur principally in HIV-infected individuals.

Acute meningitis was formerly an unusual condition, occurring principally in patients who received an inadequate dose of arsphenamine, but seems more common in human immunodeficiency virus-infected patients with syphilis. It usually occurs within one year of exposure but not simultaneously with the skin rash. Cranial nerve palsies (III, VI, VII and VIII) generally indicate basilar meningitis. Approximately one-third of patients with acute syphilitic meningitis have increased intracranial pressure with papilledema. Progressive inflammation may lead to vascular occlusion and cerebral infarction with focal neurologic signs.

Inflammatory optic disk swelling may occur from optic neuritis or optic perineuritis that may present with or without other features of meningitis. Optic neuritis tends to be bilateral and can be retrobulbar. Half of affected patients have extension into the peripapillary retina (1). This neuroretinitis is characterized by perivascular lymphocytic inflammation and cellular infiltration into the inner retinal layers. Papillitis with surrounding gray, thickened retina, exudates, and perivascular sheathing are the presenting features. Optic perineuritis is a sign of syphilitic leptomeningitis, distinguished by normal vision and pupillary testing.

Periosteitis and osteitis are characterized by nocturnal pain that increases with heat. Orbital periosteitis tends to involve the orbital roof and the supraorbital rim. Orbital inflammation with proptosis may be the presenting sign of syphilis and can lead to painful hyperplastic, osteophytic nodules or exostoses. Erosion and bony remodeling of the nasal wall may produce chronic dacryocystitis. Bilateral dacryoadenitis has been noted rarely.

Latent Syphilis

Latent syphilis has no actively inflamed clinical manifestations. Ocular stigmata of prior inflammation such as deep corneal ghost vessels or iris synechiae can be the only clue of untreated syphilis. While serologic tests are positive and humoral and cell-mediated immunity can be demonstrated, infection may be quietly progressing.

Early latent syphilis includes the first 2-4 years following secondary syphilis, during the time that relapses most likely occur. Approximately 25% of untreated cases relapse, usually during the first year. Late latent syphilis is defined as the subsequent period of time that may persist indefinitely or evolve to the complications of late syphilis.

Late (Tertiary) Syphilis

Untreated, one third of persons with syphilis develop a clinical sign of the obliterative endarteritis of late syphilis. Approximately one third of these have neurosyphilis, one third progress to cardiovascular complications, and one third develop gummatous disease. In developed countries during the penicillin era, all of these manifestations of syphilis are now rare, although neurosyphilis is still occasionally diagnosed in HIV-infected patients.

Eye signs have been noted in approximately 10% of patients with late syphilis. Approximately 2.5-5% of the cases develop anterior uveitis. Other forms of ocular or periocular inflammation can occur; and neuro-ophthalmic signs, particularly pupillary abnormalities, may be the principal sign of late neurosyphilis.

1.) Neurosyphilis.The term neurosyphilis encompasses the acute meningitis of early syphilis but usually refers to central nervous system involvement during late syphilis that may be asymptomatic or symptomatic. Approximately 3% of symptomatic neurosyphilis is manifest by retinal or optic nerve inflammation. Late symptomatic neurosyphilis includes both inflammatory (meningovascular neurosyphilis) and degenerative (parenchymatous neurosyphilis) components.

Meningovascular neurosyphilis ranges from meningitis to occlusive vasculitis of the central nervous system. Meningitis may be acute, subacute, or chronic. Optic neuritis and neuroretinitis are considered special forms of meningovascular disease. Prolonged inflammation with endarteritis can lead to the abrupt onset of a stroke syndrome or seizure disorder. Vascular involvement may also cause central or branch retinal artery occlusion.

Occlusive vasculitis of the central nervous system can affect the visual pathways and cause visual field defects. For example, hemianopia or quadrantanopia can result from infarction in the region of the middle cerebral artery and is frequently associated with hemiplegia and seizures. Hemianopic visual field defects can also occur with occlusion of the posterior cerebral artery as part of the thalamic syndrome. Posterior inferior cerebellar artery occlusion results in the lateral medullary plate syndrome with ipsilateral Horner's syndrome and vestibular nystagmus. Other brain-stem syndromes may develop from obliterative endarteritis of the vertebrobasilar system. Cortical blindness has also occurred.

Parenchymatous neurosyphilis is the result of postinflammatory neuronal degeneration, particularly of the cerebral cortex, posterior columns, and periaqueductal tissue that produces neuropsychiatric changes, tabes dorsalis, and pupillary abnormalities, respectively. Initial symptoms of parenchymatous neurosyphilis include memory loss, personality changes with depression or delusions, and seizures. The typical neurologic findings of general paresis are sluggishly reacting pupils that later show light-near dissociation and become miotic. Other findings are a lack of facial expression with tremors of the tongue or facial muscles and slurred speech. Neuroimaging may show cortical atrophy and multiple small areas resembling infarctions or demyelinating disease.

Tabes dorsalis is a late neurosyphilitic syndrome with dysfunction of the dorsal roots and posterior columns of the spinal cord. Symptoms and signs include lightning pains, poor bladder control, diminished deep tendon reflexes, and ataxia. Optic atrophy and other features of parenchymatous degeneration may be present.

Various pupillary abnormalities are associated with neurosyphilis. For example, a lesion near the constrictor nucleus can produce both light and near unresponsiveness. More commonly, pupillary light-near dissociation is found in approximately 10% of patients with meningovascular neurosyphilis and most individuals with parenchymatous neurosyphilis. Interruption of the internuncial neurons between the pretectal nuclei and the parasympathetic Edinger-Westphal nuclei produces a diminished or absent light response with a normal near reaction. Miosis is probably due to interruption of the supranuclear inhibitory neurons from the reticular activating system. The complete Argyll Robertson pupil is less than 3mm in diameter with a complete absence of the light response and a normal near response. Pupillary light-near dissociation is the more common finding. Bilateral tonic pupils have also been linked with neurosyphilis (12).

Meningovascular and parenchymatous neurosyphilis are associated with different ocular and neurologic signs but overlap and are somewhat arbitrary elements of progressive central nervous system disease. To illustrate, the optic nerve can be affected by both inflammatory and degenerative processes. In meningovascular neurosyphilis optic neuritis is sometimes the presenting feature. During parenchymatous disease lymphocytic inflammation of the optic nerve sheaths leads to fibrous thickening and adhesions. Subsequent neuronal degeneration begins peripherally and gradually extends toward the center of the optic nerve causing visual field constriction. This progressive optic atrophy usually begins unilaterally but without treatment will almost always involve the other eye. Optic atrophy occurs in 5% of patients with symptomatic neurosyphilis and may be its sole manifestation. Without adequate therapy, progressive visual loss may lead to blindness over the subsequent decade. The visual evoked response can help distinguish primary optic atrophy from optic atrophy following optic neuritis (21), but these processes converge.

Other cranial nerves may be involved in both the meningovascular and parenchymatous forms of late neurosyphilis. Third, fourth, and sixth nerve palsies generally indicate a basilar meningitis. The ophthalmologic features of seventh and eighth cranial nerve involvement include ptosis and vestibular nystagmus, respectively. Ptosis can be due to sympathetic or mesencephalic involvement that, with the compensatory brow wrinkling, produces the characteristic tabetic facies. Supranuclear palsies and even oculogyric crisis have occurred as a result of parenchymatous disease. The paresthesias of tabes dorsalis may also be manifest with trigeminal neuralgia.

2.) Cardiovascular syphilis. Obliterative endarteritis of the vasa vasorum of the aorta may result in aortitis that can cause aortic aneurysm and aortic valvular insufficiency. A similar process may lead to temporal arteritis (40). Ocular manifestations of vasculitis during late syphilis include scleritis, uveitis, and retinal vasculitis.

3.) Gummatous (late benign) syphilis. Formerly the most common late complication of syphilis, gummas are now rarely seen. Before penicillin, approximately 15% of untreated cases developed one or more gummas that would wax and wane or reappear at different sites. These necrotic, granulomatous-like lesions are produced by focal obliterative endarteritis and may occur in any organ including the eye. A gumma of the uveal tract may mimic an intraocular tumor, and gummas have also been reported in the eyelid, lacrimal structures, and orbit. Gummas of the optic nerve (39) and central nervous system, including the optic chiasm, have occurred.

Stromal keratitis occurring during acquired syphilis may be a form of gummatous disease. In contrast to the interstitial keratitis of congenital syphilis, the corneal changes of acquired syphilis are usually unilateral, develop less neovascularization, and are more responsive to penicillin treatment. Corneal findings may vary from deep suppurative inflammation to marginal keratitis (26).

Lens subluxation has occurred after syphilitic uveitis (33) but is usuallly more likely to be due to trauma. Syphilis is not a risk factor for adult-onset cataracts (36).

Congenital Syphilis

Transplacental transmission of T.pallidum may occur throughout pregnancy, principally after the fourth month when the fetal immune system is developed. The risk of fetal infection is most likely if the mother has early syphilis but can still occur in one third with latent syphilis. Maternal serologic screening is required during pregnancy in many developed countries. Testing should be considered in the third trimester for high-risk mothers and at delivery in high-incidence areas. Transmission by the infected birth canal during delivery is unusual but has rarely caused an eyelid chancre, that appeared soon after delivery. Nearly one-half of infected fetuses die before or soon after birth. Some have been found to have various developmental ocular abnormalities including microphthalmia.

Early congenital syphilis, akin to the secondary stage of acquired syphilis, presents with mucocutaneous lesions and osteochondritis. Widespread dissemination results in hepatosplenomegaly, pneumonia, and immunecomplex glomerulonephritis. Infectious foci can lead to the residual stigmata of congenital syphilis. For example, a facial skin eruption along the supraorbital ridges and around the mouth can produce radial scars and rhagades. Rhinitis (snuffles) with osteitis of the nasal bones can lead to a saddle-nose deformity and hypertelorism.

The ocular lesions of early congenital syphilis are also analogous to those found in acquired secondary syphilis. Acute iridocyclitis is the most common eye manifestation and can result in secondary cataract or glaucoma. Multifocal chorioretinitis can occur during infancy that may be subclinical, later recognized as a salt-and-pepper pattern of pigmentary mottling. Optic neuritis and interstitial keratitis have been reported in early congenital syphilis but usually arise later. Spirochetes have been seen pathologically in the cornea during the stromal keratitis of early congenital syphilis.

Without treatment, a latent period ensues. As a result of osteochondritis and perichondritis, bony structural changes arise. The stigmata of congenital syphilis include frontal bossing, supraorbital thickening, sloping skull, short maxilla, arched palate, prominent mandible, sternoclavicular thickening, flared scapula, and sabre shin. Dental abnormalities include peg-shaped upper central incisors (Hutchinson's teeth) and defective first molars (mulberry or Moon's molars). Iridoschisis has been found as an incidental late finding (31).

Nonulcerative stromal keratitis is the most common inflammatory sign of late prenatal syphilis, appearing in 20-50% of cases of untreated congenital syphilis, more commonly in girls than boys. Usually occurring between the ages of 5 to 20 years, the pathogenesis of interstitial keratitis is unclear. One postulated mechanism is that it results from an immunological reaction to treponemal antigens deposited in the cornea, although treponemal invasion of clinically normal cornea has not been adequately documented. Experimental stromal keratitis has not been adequately reproduced by intracorneal injection, but corneal edema with iritis has been noticed following intracameral or intracranial inoculation (25,38). As the cornea contains mutiple phospholipids, including cardiolipin and phosphatidylcholine (35), a cross-reacting autoimmune phenomenon is another possible explanation.

Interstitial keratitis begins with lymphocytic infiltration in the deep stromal layers and is rapidly followed by corneal neovascularization. Variations include sectoral, peripheral, and multifocal infiltrates. Most patients also have an associated anterior uveitis. Bilateral involvement, sometimes separated by several years, occurs in about 80% of cases of stromal keratitis due to congenital syphilis. Without treatment, the corneal inflammation persists for several weeks to months, then spontaneously subsides with residual opacification, alterations of Descemet's membrane and endothelium, and sometimes guttata. Stromal ghost vessels can persist indefinitely and can enlarge or progress in the 5-10% of cases that recur. Approximately 15-20% of individuals with prior stromal keratouveitis are at risk of developing open-angle glaucoma 25-30 years later.

Unlike most other inflammatory components of syphilis, systemic penicillin has no beneficial effect on the course of interstitial keratitis associated with congenital syphilis. Topical corticosteroids and cycloplegic agents are useful in limiting corneal opacification but must sometimes be used for prolonged periods to prevent recrudescences. Corneal transplantation can be performed for residual corneal opacification although allograft rejection may occur. Prior interstitial keratitis accounts for approximately 2-3% of corneal transplants performed in the United States (11).

Other signs of late congenital syphilis include deafness, bilateral knee effusions (Clutton's joints), and gummas of the nasal septum, palate, and throat. Approximately 1-3% of untreated cases will develop anterior uveitis. Late neurosyphilis can occur; pupillary abnormalities, optic neuritis, optic atrophy, and cranial nerve palsies are distinctive ophthalmologic features in these cases. One fourth of untreated children with congenital syphilis have asymptomatic central nervous system infection. But while hydrocephalus, optic atrophy, oculomotor nerve palsy, and other neurologic sequelae were once relatively common, symptomatic late congenital neurosyphilis is now rare.

Syphilis, Human Immunodeficiency Virus Infection and the Eye

The history of syphilis and acquired immunodeficiency syndrome is intertwined (6). Finding one disease should initiate a search for the other. Human immunodeficiency virus infection and other immunocompromised states play an important role in concomitant T.pallidum infection (28). Without a normal host response, recommended penicillin dosages do not assure a cure. Relapses and symptomatic neurosyphilis have occurred in human immunodeficiency virus-seropositive patients following treatment with intramuscular and even prolonged intravenous penicillin.

Human immunodeficiency virus-seropositive individuals are more likely to have serological evidence of prior syphilis than others. One study found that 1.5% of patients with the acquired immunodeficiency syndrome develop neurosyphilis at some point in their disease (20). While antibody production to cardiolipin or treponemal antigens can be impaired in human immunodeficiency virus infection, current serological tests are generally adequate. Seronegative syphilis is an unusual diagnostic dilemma. However, human immunodeficiency virus-seropositive patients, particularly those with a low CD4:CD8 ratio, can lose seroreactivity to a specific test after treatment of syphilis, thus making accurate determination of treatment efficacy problematic.

Treponemal invasion of the central nervous system occurs in many cases of early syphilis, with 15-40% showing cerebrospinal fluid abnormalities despite no symptoms. Even though conventional therapy of early syphilis does not produce effective cerebrospinal fluid levels, subsequent progression to symptomatic early neurosyphilis is unusual unless no or inadequate therapy has been given or if human immunodeficiency virus infection coexists.

While early neurologic or ophthalmologic involvement is not unique to patients with the acquired immunodeficiency syndrome, these complications seem to occur more frequently with human immunodeficiency virus infection. In one study that did not systematically evaluate seropositivity, nearly one-half of patients with symptomatic neurosyphilis were found to have human immunodeficiency virus infection (20). While the various systemic manifestations of early syphilis may not be altered, human immunodeficiency virus infection seems to impair the treatment response of concurrent syphilis and to increase the likelihood of a relapse and early neurosyphilis. As a result of documented relapses in human immunodeficiency virus-seropositive patients treated with conventional single-dose therapy for early syphilis, revised treatment schedules have thus been proposed.

Of reported human immunodeficiency virus-seropositive patients who have eye findings of syphilis, most have had posterior segment inflammation and/or early neurosyphilis (Tab.). Human immunodeficiency virus-infected patients with ocular syphilis or neuro-ophthalmic findings should have cerebrospinal fluid examination, even though interpretation may be difficult because of changes produced by the human immunodeficiency virus and other opportunistic infections. In one study, 16% of patients with the acquired immunodeficiency syndrome who had neuro-ophthalmic findings had evidence of neurosyphilis (15).

Intravenous penicillin treatment for neurosyphilis should be administered to human immunodeficiency virus-infected patients with ocular syphilis. Blood serology and cerebrospinal fluid studies should be reassessed every 3-6 months until normal. Syphilitic uveitis has recurred despite intravenous penicillin therapy (3). Treatment with higher doses or longer duration may be needed for relapses. The development of new diagnostic tests offers opportunities to better assess antibiotic efficacy (29).

Conclusions

Syphilis continues to cause ocular morbidity, being diagnosed in 1 of every 1000 patients in a general ophthalmology clinic (16) and in 2.5% of patients at an urban referral eye center (42). The historical evolution of syphilis and its various eye manifestations illustrate the potent medical and social consequences that this disease has inflicted on mankind. Ophthalmologists will continue to play a key role in determining the diagnosis and prognosis of this "great imitator".

Table Reported cases of ocular or neuro-ophthalmic syphilis in patients with HIV infection[1]

Eye Findings	Age/Sex	Syphilis Stage[2]	Visual Outcome	References
Cranial nerve palsy (VI)	30/M	Neurosyphilis	20 /20 ; 20/20	24
(VII)	34/M	Neurosyphilis	20 /20 ; 20/20	present
Papilledema	26/M	Neurosyphilis	NA	5
	26/M	Neurosyphilis	NA	20
	29/F	Neurosyphilis	NA	20
Optic neuritis or neuroretinitis	23/M	Neurosyphilis	20/100;20/20	27
	27/M	Neurosyphilis	20/ 20;20/20	30
	29/M	Neurosyphilis	20/ 20;20/20	present
	34/M	Neurosyphilis	20/ 25;20/20	27
	46/M	Neurosyphilis	20/ 25;20/20	27
	54/M	Neurosyphilis	20/ 20;20/20	9
Retrobulbar optic neuritis	23/M	Neurosyphilis	NLP;20/20	27
	23/M	Neurosyphilis	NLP;NLP	47
	27/M	Neurosyphilis	NA	20
	33/M	Neurosyphilis	NA	46
Optic perineuritis	26/M	Neurosyphilis	20/ 15;20/15	27
	33/M	Neurosyphilis	20/ 20;20/20	45
Optic nerve gumma	68/M	Neurosyphilis	20/ 15;20/25	39
Retinitis	24/M	Neurosyphilis	20/ 20;20/20	19
	30/M	Neurosyphilis	20/ 15;20/15	19
	31/M	Neurosyphilis	20/ 20;20/20	41
	36/M	Neurosyphilis	20/ 10;20/20	present
	37/M	Neurosyphilis	NA	20
	41/M	Neurosyphilis	20/ 40;20/40	23
	62/M	Neurosyphilis	20/ 20;20/20	27

Eye Findings	Age/Sex	Syphilis Stage[2]	Visual Outcome	References
Chorioretinitis or choroiditis	19/M	Neurosyphilis	20/ 15;20/15	3
	22/M	Neurosyphilis	20/ 15;20/15	3
	23/M	Neurosyphilis	20/ 15;20/15	3
	28/M	Neurosyphilis	NA	2
	29/M	Neurosyphilis	20/ 20;20/20	3
	30/M	Neurosyphilis	20/ 25;20/30	42
	31/M	Neurosyphilis	NA	34
	32/M	Neurosyphilis	20/40;20/200	32
	33/M	Neurosyphilis	NA	17
	35/M	Neurosyphilis	20/70;HM	42
	36/M	Neurosyphilis	20/ 15;20/15	3
	37/M	Neurosyphilis	20/ 20;20/20	3
	37/M	Neurosyphilis	20/ 30;20/25	3
	38/M	Neurosyphilis	NA	18
	39/M	Neurosyphilis	20/50;20/100	3
	41/M	Neurosyphilis	NA	23
	42/M	Neurosyphilis	20/ 20;20/20	14,30
	42/M	Neurosyphilis	20/ 15;20/20	14
	42/M	Neurosyphilis	LP;20/40 22	
	43/M	Neurosyphilis	20/ 20;20/25	3
	45/M	Neurosyphilis	20/ 20;20/20	3
	45/M	Neurosyphilis	NLP;20/15	3
	48/M	Neurosyphilis	NA	20
	49/M	Neurosyphilis	20/ 20;20/20	3
	59/M	Neurosyphilis	20/ 25;20/20	14
Vitreitis	34/M	Relapse	20/20;20/20	27
Anterior uveitis	38/M	Neurosyphilis	20/ 20;20/20	30
	39/M	Neurosyphilis	20/ 30;20/20	27
	39/M	Rellapse	20/ 20;20/20	present

1 Does not include two patients with conjunctivitis occurring during secondary syphilis (20).

2 Diagnosis of neurosyphilis based on clinical findings of central nervous system involvement, including retinal and optic nerve inflammation, and/or abnormal cere-
ospinal fluid changes.

References

1. Arruga J, Valentines J, Mauri F et al (1985) Neuroretinitis in Acquired Syphilis. Ophthalmology 92:262-270
2. Beauvais DA, Michelson JB, Seybold ME et al (1989) Retroviruses and Their Play-Pals. Surv Ophthalmol 34:59-64
3. Becerra LI, Ksiazek SM, Savino PJ et al (1989) Syphilitic Uveitis in Human Immunodeficiency Virus-Infected and Noninfected Patients. Ophthalmology 96:1727-1730
4. Belin MW, Baltch AL, Hay PB (1981) Secondary Syphilitic Uveitis. Am J Ophthalmol 92:210-214
5. Berry CD, Hooton TM, Collier AC et al (1987) Neurologic Relapse After Benzathine Penicillin Therapy for Secondary Syphilis in a Patient with HIV Infection. New Engl J Med 316:1587-1589
6. Brandt AM (1988) The Syphilis Epidemic and its Relation to AIDS. Science 239:375-380
7. Brooks AM, Weiner JM, Robertson IF (1986) Interstitial Keratitis in Untreated Latent (Late) Syphilis. Aust NZ J Ophthalmol 14:127-132
8. Bulkley LD (1889) Unusual Methods of Acquiring Syphilis, with Reports of Cases. JAMA 12:172-176
9. Carter JB, Hamill RJ, Matoba AY (1987) Bilateral Syphilitic Optic Neuritis in a Patient with a Positive Test for HIV. Arch Ophthalmol 105:1485-1486
10. Cunha da Souza E, Jalkh AE, Trempe CL et al (1988) Unusual Central Chorioretinitis as the First Manifestation of Early Secondary Syphilis. Am J Ophthalmol 105: 271-276
11. Eye Banking Statistics (1991) Eye Bank Association of America
12. Fletcher WA, Sharpe JA (1986) Tonic Pupils in Neurosyphilis. Neurology 36:188-192
13. Fournier A (1903) Prophylaxie de la Syphilis. J Rueff,Paris p.239
14. Gass JDM, Braunstein RA, Chenoweth RG (1990) Acute Syphilitic Posterior Placoid Chorioretinitis. Ophthalmology 97:1288-1297
15. Hamed LM, Schatz NJ, Galetta SL (1988) Brainstem Ocular Motility Defects and AIDS. Am J Ophthalmol 106:437-442
16. Harden AF, Wright DJM (1974) Clinical Aspects of Treponema Eye Disease: A Report of 21 Cases. Proc R Soc Med 13:285-290
17. Hungerbühler U, Kulstrunk M, Osusky R (1988) Uveitis luetica bei einem AIDS-Patienten. Schweiz Med Wochenschr 118:1762-1766
18. Johns DR, Tierney M, Felsenstein D (1987) Alteration in the Natural History of Neurosyphilis by Concurrent Infection with the Human Immunodeficiency Virus. New Engl J Med 316:1569-1572
19. Joyce PW, Haye KR, Willis ME (1989) Syphilitic Retinitis in a Homosexual Man with Concurrent HIV Infection: Case Report. Genitourin Med 65:244-247
20. Katz DA, Berger JR (1989) Neurosyphilis in Acquired Immunodeficiency Syndrome. Arch Neurol 46:895-898
21. Kerty E, Eide N, Skjeldal D (1986) Visual Evoked Response in Syphilitic Optic Atrophy. A Case Report. Acta Ophthalmol. 64:535-536
22. Kleiner RC, Najarian L, Levenson J et al (1987) AIDS Complicated by Syphilis Can Mimic Uveitis and Crohn's disease. Arch Ophthalmol 105:1486-1487
23. Levy JH, Liss RA, Maguire AM (1989) Neurosyphilis and Ocular Syphilis Patients with Concurrent Human Immunodeficiency Virus Infection. Retina 9:175-180
24. Mansour AM (1990) Neuro-Ophthalmic Findings in Acquired Immunodeficiency Syndrome. J Clin Neuro Ophthalmol 10:167-174

25. Marra C, Baker-Zander SA, Hook EW II et al (1991) An Experimental Model of Early Central Nervous System Syphilis. J Infect Dis 163:825-829
26. Martinez JA, Sutphin JE (1989) Syphilitic Interstitial Keratitis Masquerading as Staphylococcal Marginal Keratitis. Am J Ophthalmol 107:431-433
27. McLeish WM, Pulido JS, Holland S et al (1990) The Ocular Manifestations of Syphilis in the Human Immunodeficiency Virus Type 1-Infected Host. Ophthalmology 97:196-203
28. Musher DM, Hamill RJ, Baughn RE (1990) Effect of Human Immunodeficiency Virus (HIV) Infection on the Course of Syphilis and on the Response to Treatment. Ann Intern Med 113:872-881
29. Noordhoek GT, Wolters EC, de Jonge ME et al (1991) Detection by Polymerase Chain Reaction of Treponema pallidum DNA in Cerebrospinal Fluid from Neurosyphilis Patients Before and After Antibiotic Treatment. J Clin Microbiol 29:1976-1984
30. Passo MS, Rosenbaum JT (1988) Ocular Syphilis in Patients with Human Immunodeficiency Virus Infection. Am J Ophthalmol 106:1-6
31. Pearson PA, Amrien JM, Baldwin LB et al (1989) Iridoschisis Associated with Syphilitic Interstitial Keratitis. Am J Ophthalmol 107:88-90
32. Radolf JD, Kaplan RP (1988) Unusual Manifestations of Secondary Syphilis and Abnormal Humoral Immune Response to Treponema pallidum Antigens in a Homosexual Man with Asymptomatic Human Immunodeficiency Virus Infection. J Am Acad Dermatol 18:423-428
33. Rapkin JS, Bogorad DD (1986) Bilateral Dislocation of the Crystalline Lens in a Patient with Presumed Syphilitic Uveitis. Henry Ford Hospital Med J 34:207-210
34. Richards BW, Hesburg TJ, Nussbaum JN (1989) Recurrent Syphilitic Uveitis. New Engl J Med 320:62
35. Sachedina S, Greiner JV, Glonek T (1991) Membrane Phospholipids of the Ocular Tunica Fibrosa. Invest Ophthalmol Vis Sci 32:625-632
36. Schwab IR, Armstrong MA, Friedman GD et al (1988) Cataract Extraction. Risk Factors in a Health Maintenance Organization Population Under 60 Years of Age. Arch Ophthalmol 106:1062-1065
37. Schwartz KL, O'Connor GR (1980) Secondary Syphilis with Iris Papules. Am J Ophthalmol 90:380-384
38. Smith JL (1969) Spirochetes in Late Seronegative Syphilis, Penicillin Notwithstanding. Charles C. Thomas, Springfield,IL pp. 137-155, pp.181-221
39. Smith JL, Byrne SF, Cambron CR (1990) Syphiloma/Gumma of the Optic Nerve and Human Immunodeficiency Virus Seropositivity. J Clin Neuro Ophthalmol 10:175-184
40. Smith JL, Israel CW, Harner RE (1967) Syphilitic Temporal Arteritis. Arch Ophthalmol 78:284-288
41. Stoumbos VD, Klein ML (1987) Syphilitic Retinitis in a Patient with Acquired Immunodeficiency Syndrome-Related Complex. Am J Ophthalmol 103:103-104
42. Tamesis RR, Foster SA (1990) Ocular Syphilis. Ophthalmology 97:1281-1287
43. von Walther P (1810) Abhandlungen aus dem Gebiet der Praktischen Medizin. Landshut
44. Wilhelmus KR, Yokoyama CM (1987) Syphilitic Episcleritis and Scleritis. Am J Ophthalmol 104:595-597
45. Winward KE, Hamed LM, Glaser JS (1989) The Spectrum of Optic Nerve Disease in Human Immunodeficiency Virus Infection. Am J Ophthalmol 107:373-380
46. Zaidman GW (1986) Neurosyphilis and Retrobulbar Neuritis in a Patient with AIDS. Ann Ophthalmol 18:260-261
47. Zambrano W, Perez GM, Smith JL (1987) Acute Syphilitic Blindness in AIDS. J Clin Neuro Ophthalmol 7:1-5

- Viral

Virological Aspects of Human Immunodeficiency Virus Infection

Gerhard Jahn and Stephan Stenglein

Abstract. The Human Immunodeficiency Viruses are lentiviruses and belong to the family of retroviruses. Representatives of these pathogenic agents are characterized by induction of immunosuppression and tumors. Infections by Human Immunodeficiency Viruses can provoke most different clinical manifestations including ocular lesions.

Initially, massive virus replication occurs in association with first clinical symptoms of infection (mononucleosis-like disease). After a few days, virus concentration is decreased drastically; however, the virus will forever persist in the infected organism. Many years later, the Human Immunodeficiency Virus (HIV) infection may evolve out of the latent asymptomatic phase into a symptomatic phase with high virus replication rates.

Molecular virologic diagnostic tools applied to the manyfaceted characteristics of HIV have resulted in the identification of regulatory functions and mechanisms of virus replication. These basic findings are most important for any successful prophylaxis and therapy of the Acquired Immunodeficiency Syndrome (AIDS).

Introduction

The Acquired Immunodeficiency Syndrome is caused by infection with the Human Immunodeficiency Virus, a lentivirus belonging to the family of retroviruses. Nearly ten years ago, the appearance of opportunistic infections and otherwise very rare tumors of the skin in young homosexual Americans raised first considerations about a new infectious agent. Speculations about a variety of possible causes of this epidemic-like syndrome soon came up.

In 1983 the first isolation and identification of a lentivirus as the etiological agent of the Acquired Immunodeficiency Syndrome was described by Luc Montagnier and colleagues (2) at the Pasteur Institute in Paris. Subsequently, the virus was termed Human Immunodeficiency Virus type 1 by the International Commission on Taxonomy (5).

Four years later, another human lentivirus denoted Human Immunodeficiency Virus type 2, could be isolated from a West-African patient at the Pasteur Institute (12). This virus may also cause full blown Acquired Immunodeficiency Syndrome although conflicting data exist about the severity of symptoms and the duration of the incubation time for Human Immunodeficiency Virus type 2 infection.

Since the discovery of these two retroviruses associated with the Acquired Immunodeficiency Syndrome, intense international research efforts are going on in the fields of epidemiology, diagnostic possibilities, therapy and prevention. There are already some promising efforts in therapeutical and pro phylactical strategies, a major breakthrough, however, could not be achieved so far. At the beginning of this decade, at least ten million people are worldwide infected with Human Immunodeficiency Viruses.

Taxonomy and Morphology

According to the currently used criteria the family of retroviruses is divided into three subfamilies:
- Oncoviruses
- Spumaviruses
- Lentiviruses
(Members of these subfamilies are shown in Fig.1)
Oncoviruses (e.g. the Human T-Lymphotropic Virus 1) are related to lymphoma, leukemia and sarcoma in man. Thus far, no pathogenic correlate could be found for infections with spumaviruses. The subfamily of lentiviruses comprises the Human Immunodeficiency Virus as well as other mammalian viruses like the visna/maedi virus associated with pneumonia and meningoencephalitis in sheep and goats. Lentiviruses typically display a protracted development of disease as well as a long incubation period. Both in man and in animals they cause chronic degenerative diseases of the hematological and neurological organ systems showing the slow clinical progression mentioned above (14).

Human Immunodeficiency Virus displays the structural features that are typical of retroviruses. The free infectious virion is a spherical particle with a diameter of about 100nm. The icosaedrical inner capsid is surrounded by an outer lipid bilayer derived mainly from the infected host cell, containing certain proteins (e.g. Major Histocompatibility Complex class I and II antigens) of the cell. Virus encoded surface antigens in this envelope are the glycoproteins gp 120 and gp 41, which in part streak through the outer membrane and display a connection to the interior side. Closely under the viral envelope there is the inner membrane of Human Immunodeficiency Virus, made up from the myristoylated protein p17. The prominent constituent of the nucleocapsid is the major structural protein p24. The proteins p7 and p9 are proteolytically cleaved from a precursor molecule (p15) and are attached to the viral RNA. All the core proteins are cleaved from their common precursor protein p55 by a viral protease. Within the nucleocapsid, there are two identical, single-stranded molecules of Human Immunodeficiency Virus-RNA with an approximate length of 10 kilobases (kb). This genomic RNA is associated to certain retroviral enzymes, like the reverse transcriptase and the integrase.

Replication and Regulation of Human Immunodeficiency Virus

In vivo, the most important target cells for an infection with Human Immunodeficiency Virus are the CD4-positive T-lymphocytes and monocytes (15). The virus can adsorb with high affinity to cells displaying this receptor by means of its envelope glycoprotein gp120 (Fig.2). T-helper cells and the monocytes/macrophages exert a central function in immunoregulation and presentation of antigen to certain effector cells of the immune system. This could be an explanation for the observation that infection of these cells by Human Immunodeficiency Virus seems to be the cause of the progressive immunodeficiency leading finally to the full blown Acquired Immunodeficiency Syndrome. A number of different types of cells (e.g. glial cells in the brain, enteric epithelial cells and hemopoetic precursor cells in bone marrow) can also be infected by Human Immunodeficiency Virus (13). The virion is internalised by a receptor-mediated endocytosis or by membrane fusion. The viral RNA as well as certain proteins important for replication, like the reverse transcriptase, are released. This virus encoded enzyme can then start the initial step in the replication of Human Immunodeficiency Virus: the single stranded RNA is converted to a double stranded DNA. Reverse transcriptase first generates an RNA-DNA-hybrid. Another retroviral enzyme, ribonuclease H, degrades the strand of RNA. Subsequently, the generation of double-stranded DNA is again effected by reverse transcriptase. The resulting DNA differs from genomic Human Immunodeficiency Virus-RNA in that it contains "long terminal repeats". These regions in proviral DNA are formed during reverse transcription of Human Immunodeficiency Virus-RNA and are a characteristic feature of retroviruses. The "long terminal repeats" contain different regulatory DNA-sequences for the interaction with host cell factors and viral regulatory proteins. They are also important for the integration of proviral Human Immunodeficiency Virus-DNA into the genome of the host cell mediated by the viral enmzyme integrase. Free nonintegrated Human Immunodeficiency Virus-DNA can also be found in the cytoplasm, where it seems to exist in a circular form, and could be related to the lytic type of host cell infection.

After integration of proviral DNA into the host cell genome, Human Immunodeficiency Virus establishes a persistent type of infection. In viral latency, no replication of virus can be observed over a period of variable duration, whereas in chronic infection Human Immunodeficiency Virus is constantly replicating in small amounts. The respective stage of infection can be influenced by a variety of different viral and cellular factors. Some of them are already characterized concerning their essential properties, while others are currently the object of intense research activities.

One important feature effecting the transition from persistent to lytic type of infection, which is connected with a high production of infectious viral particles, seems to be the general state of activation of a cell. The action of a CD4-positive T-helper cell is positively or negatively regulated by a variety of factors. Certain cytokines like Interleukin-1 or the Tumor Necrosis Factor can effect the activation of a T-cell. Interestingly, this can also be mediated by the action of gene products of certain other viruses, like the Human Herpesvirus 6, Cytomegalovirus (17), or the Human T-Lymphotropic Virus 1. Each of these viruses can coinfect a Human Immunodeficiency Virus-positive organism (21). Thus, the activation of a T-helper cell carrying the Human Immunodeficiency Virus-DNA in its genome can initiate replication of Human Immunodeficiency Virus, resulting in the production of a high number of infectious viral particles and, finally, leading to the lytic destruction of the infected host cell.

Some of these activating elements seem to mediate their effects through certain inducible transcription factors in the host cell.

Here, so called "enhancer-binding proteins", like the nuclear factor kappa B (NF-kB), seem to be important.

Cell activation, however, can also be mediated by some constitutively expressed cell factors, like Sp1 or TFIID. The induction of the nuclear protein NF-kB leads to the regulation of different T-cell genes playing a role in the physiological function of the respective cell, e.g. the Interleukin 1 (IL-1) (19). NF-kB seems to play an important role in reactivating latent proviral sequences of Human Immunodeficiency Virus. This factor binds to the enhancer-element in the Human Immunodeficiency Virus "long terminal repeat", which is positively regulating viral transcription, and is thus effecting the expression of regulatory Human Immunodeficiency Virus-proteins and, subsequently, the activation of latent provirus. In contrast to most other members of the retrovirus family, Human Immunodeficiency Virus type 1 encodes at least 7 regulatory proteins (Tab.1, Fig.3) in addition to the gag-pol-env genes coding for the structural proteins or for those enzymes needed essentially for viral replication.

The prominent feature of Human Immunodeficiency Virus-infection on the molecular pathogenetic level are specific interactions of these regulatory proteins with cellular and viral DNA elements as well as the mechanisms of protein synthesis; most of these interactions are currently only partially understood. For this reason, Human Immunodeficiency Virus is referred to as a "complex retrovirus", and is thus distinguished from the group of "simple retroviruses", where no regulatory proteins have been discovered so far (6). This new view focuses on the molecular mechanism of replication of a retrovirus as the central aspect for classification, whereas the currently used nomenclature is rather considering clinical manifestations and morphological characteristics of viruses.

Two subsequent phases of viral gene expression can be distinguished after activation of integrated Human Immunodeficiency Virus-DNA (7). Initially, Human Immunodeficiency Virus-mRNA transcripts with an approximate length of 2 kilobases (kb) can be found in the cytoplasm of the host cell. They result from multiple splicing (enzymatic removal of non-essential genetic sequences) of genomic Human Immunodeficiency Virus-mRNA, and are coding for the so-called early regulatory proteins tat and nef. Concluding from the currently available data, both are essential factors of viral replication. Tat (transactivator of transcription) effectively increases expression of all retroviral genes. It binds on a viral sequence termed tar (transactivation response element), which is located at the beginning of the Human Immunodeficiency Virus-mRNAs and displays a typical secondary structure. The exact mechanism of tat-interactions with mRNA are not yet fully understood, however, it is commonly accepted that tat should have an important function in initiation or elongation of viral transcription. The mode of action of the second early regulatory protein termed nef (negative factor) is currently subject to reevaluation. Earlier data concerning this myristoylated, probably membrane-associated protein indicated a non-essential or even inhibiting function in the replication of HIV. Now there seems to be evidence for an important positive effect of nef in the viral pathogenesis of Simian Immunodeficiency Virus in rhesus monkeys (18). The role of the vpr (viral protein r) gene product, which is another early protein of Human Immunodeficiency Virus, is still under investigation.

After cytoplasmic expression of early regulatory proteins of Human Immunodeficiency Virus it is mainly the effect of the tat-protein that a high number of genomic mRNA accumulates in the nucleus. To enable the synthesis of structural and regulatory Human Immunodeficiency Virus proteins, this RNA must reach the cytoplasm of the host cell, either as an unspliced gag-pol-mRNA or as a single-spliced env-mRNA. The switch from the first phase with an expression of early regulatory proteins to the second phase, where the generation of retroviral structural proteins takes place, is mediated through another early regulatory protein of Human Immunodeficiency Virus termed rev (regulator of viral expression). This protein, which is essential for the replication of Human Immunodeficiency Virus, seems to exert its function on the posttranslational level, inducing an enhanced cytoplasmic expression of those Human Immunodeficiency Virus mRNAs coding for structural proteins. Its mode of action could be the activation of transport of these mRNAs from the nucleus to the cytoplasm of the host cell, followed by a "down-regulation" of the synthesis of rev. The recognition sequence for the binding of the rev protein is located in the env-sequence coding for the viral envelope, and is denoted rre (rev responsive element).

Following synthesis of structural proteins the assembly of new infectious viral particles starts. The gene products of gag form the nucleocapsid and the env-proteins of Human Immunodeficiency Virus form parts of its envelope. Specific proteins needed for viral assembly are proteolytically cleaved from precursor proteins. The env-precursor gp 160 is cleaved into the glycoproteins gp120 and gp41 by a host-cell protease, whereas the internal structural proteins p24, p17, p9 and p7 are processed from their p55 precursor by a specific viral protease. The mRNA coding for this gene product is also used for the pol-precursor, that is generated through a mechanism of changing the mode of reading the mRNA sequence in ribosomes denoted as frame-shifting. After proteolysis of this precursor, active enzymatic proteins like reverse transcriptase or integrase are formed. The nucleocapsid is assembled in the cytoplasm and contains two identical molecules of Human Immunodeficiency Virus mRNA. During the passage of the host-cell membrane in a process termed budding, the capsid is enveloped by the lipid bilayer of the host cell and specific viral glycoproteins, like gp120 and gp41, are integrated into this envelope. During this final stage of retroviral morphogenesis, two more regulatory proteins denoted vif (virion infectivity factor) and vpu (viral protein u) are important. A role in the process of viral budding (Fig.4,5) is ascribed to vpu, whereas vif seems to be related to the infectivity of free viral particles.

Cell Tropism of Human Immunodeficiency Virus

The Human Immunodeficiency Virus preferentially infects cells expressing the membrane protein CD4 on their surface. CD4 is a glycoprotein belonging to the group of immunoglobulin-like molecules (1), and is also known as the T4-receptor. Its primary biological function is mediation of interactions between T-helper cells and diverse antigen-presenting cells of the human immune system. Here, the CD4-receptor of the T-cell interacts with Major Histocompatibility Complex class II molecules on the surface of the target cell. CD4 is also a specific membrane receptor for infection with Human Immunodeficiency Virus (9). The virus can bind to the T4-receptor with a high affinity through its envelope glycoprotein gp120. The specific epitope mediating the binding of CD4 could be localized in a domain termed V1, which displays a certain sequence homology with hypervariable regions of immunoglobulins.

After binding of Human Immunodeficiency Virus to CD4 the viral particle can be internalized by a fusion of viral and cellular membranes mediated through gp41. A high density of CD4-molecules is found on the surface of T-helper cells, whereas the receptor is expressed in much lesser quantities by macrophages and monocytes. For infection with Human Immunodeficiency Virus, however, a low concentration of CD4 on the surface of a cell seems to be sufficient; these cells (e.g. macrophages) do rarely display a lytic type of Human Immunodeficiency Virus-infection but rather seem to function as a reservoir. In vivo they could be the most important cells permitting reactivation of proviral Human Immunodeficiency Virus-DNA through the activation factors described above. Conversely, after infection of T-cells in-vitro a typical cytopathic effect can often be observed. The formation of multinuclear syncytia (Fig.6,7) seems to be induced by the gp120 of Human Immunodeficiency Virus (20). According to one hypothesis, this effect is induced by gp120 expressed on the surface of infected cells, which can bind to uninfected CD4-positive cells and thereby cause a fusion of cell membranes leading to the formation of multinucleated syncytia. Besides those major target cells like T-helper cells and monocytes/macrophages, the Human Immunodeficiency Virus is also capable of infecting a number of other cell types. Among them are Langerhans-cells in the epidermis, B-lymphocytes, microglial cells in the CNS and intestinal cell types. Knowledge about the importance of these cells in the course of Human Immunodeficiency Virus infection is presently still limited. However, recent interest focuses mainly on the Langerhans-cells, that are supposed to be important in Human Immunodeficiency Virus infection due to their mode of action as recirculating antigen-presenting cells.

Clinical Aspects

Infection with the Human Immunodeficiency Virus results in a slowly progressive degeneration of the immune system and can lead to encephalopathy. The broad spectrum of diseases associated with Human Immunodeficiency Virus infection is pathogenetically related to the increasing insufficiency of immunological functions. This forms the basis for the appearance of opportunistic infections and for the formation of certain types of tumors. In primary infection with Human Immunodeficiency Virus, some patients display a mononucleosis-like syndrome, which appears after approximately two to six weeks. In the majority of cases, however, this type of acute primary infection is not diagnosed. The appearance of specific antibodies against Human Immunodeficiency Virus, i.e. seroconversion can usually be detected after four to twelve weeks. This period is followed by a phase of variable duration, roughly between two to ten years or even longer, where antibodies against viral structural proteins can be detected in serum. During this period, the lymphadenopathy-syndrome and, subsequently, the Acquired Immunodeficiency Syndrome-related complex may develop. There seems to be a relation to continuously increasing replication of virus along with a consecutive decrease of infected T-cells.

With regard to the clinical manifestations of Human Immunodeficiency Virus infection several infectious pathogens are of importance. Frequently, Acquired Immunodeficiency Syndrome-patients suffer from infection with the fungus Pneumocystis carinii. It causes interstitial pneumonia, which is the most frequent opportunistic infection in Acquired Immunodeficiency Syndrome-patients. Pulmonary complications can also be the result of infections with Cytomegalovirus, atypical mycobacteria and Candida albicans. Opportunistic infectious agents in the intestinal tract are cryptosporidiae, Herpes Simplex Virus as well as Cytomegalovirus. A typical and prognostically bad sign in Acquired Immunodeficiency Syndrome-patients is the oral hairy leukoplakia, which has been described to be associated with Epstein-Barr Virus. The central nervous system is also often involved, and a direct neuropathic effect of Human Immunodeficiency Virus is discussed. Interestingly, early in Human Immunodeficiency Virus infection signs of a beginning encephalopathy, the so-called Acquired Immunodeficiency Syndrome-dementia complex, can be observed. In terminally ill Acquired Immunodeficiency Syndrome-patients, the development of a general atrophy of the central nervous system within a short period of time can be diagnosed, which is then dominating the clinical appearance. Opportunistic infections in the central nervous system are cerebral toxoplasmosis, cryptococcal meningitis and fungal abscesses. Also of importance is retinitis caused by Cytomegalovirus. Another special feature of Human Immunodeficiency Virus-infection are tumors of the skin and of the lymphatic system. A variant of Kaposi sarcoma is seen in Human Immunodeficiency Virus-infected patients. This is a neoplasia of the small vessels, appearing on the skin but sometimes involving interior organs, as well. In five to ten percent of Human Immunodeficiency Virus-positive patients the development of Non-Hodgkin Lymphoma is seen, and there is also the possibility of primary lymphomas in the central nervous system. Concerning their pathogenesis, the possible role of the Epstein-Barr Virus is one focus of interest in recent times.

Laboratory Diagnosis of Human Immunodeficiency Virus-Infection

Retroviral infections can be diagnosed either by direct or by indirect methods, the latter being used for routine diagnostic purposes. The so-called "Acquired Immunodeficiency Syndrome-test" is based on the detection of specific antibodies against Human Immunodeficiency Virus in different test procedures (Fig.8). In laboratory routine a serum sample of the respective patient is first tested in the Enzyme Linked Immunosorbent Assay. This test is based on viral antigens coupled to a solid phase, which is in most cases a plastic microtiter-well. Specific antibodies against Human Immunodeficiency Virus in the patient serum can bind to the viral antigen and can be detected in a subsequent enzymatic colour reaction. Enzyme Linked Immunosorbent Assay has a sensitivity of 99.5%, its specificity is about 99.8% (10). Obviously this test assay can be used for routine screening of patient sera. Viral antigen used for the coating of the microtiter-wells can still contain to a certain degree some proteins, e.g. HLA antigens, of its host cell membrane. Some of the patient sera will display antibodies against these nonspecific proteins leading to a false-positive reaction in the Enzyme Linked Immunosorbent Assay. Other serum proteins like the rheumatoid-factor can sometimes lead to a false positive result in a screening test.

Although the quality of this test procedure could be improved by the use of recombinant antigens (11), a positive result in the screening test must be further confirmed. Usually the Western blot system is used as a confirmation test. Here, the specific proteins of Human Immunodeficiency Virus are separated in SDS-polyacrylamide gel-electrophoresis according to their respective molecular weight. In a procedure denoted as blotting they are then transferred to nitrocellulose-membrane, that can be cut into single strips and is then incubated with the single patient sera. In the following enzymatic colour reaction specific antibodies bound to Human Immunodeficiency Virus-proteins can be visualised. The respective size of a detected specific retroviral protein can be identified using control proteins of known molecular weight. By the use of Western blotting the antibody-profile can be obtained. Only those sera showing both a positive result after repeated testing in Enzyme Linked Immunosorbent Assay and a positive result in the Western blot can be classified as Human Immunodeficiency Virus antibody-positive.

In each of the two test systems, a false-negative result may be obtained if a respective patient has not yet developed specific antibodies. In primary infection with Human Immunodeficiency Virus, seroconversion (meaning the appearance of specific antibodies) can usually be diagnosed after four to twelve weeks. Routine testing should be repeated after that period of time, if primary infection with Human Immunodeficiency Virus is suspected. Testing can again be repeated after six and twelve months to exclude any of the rare cases of delayed seroconversion.

In the early phase of primary infection (two to four weeks), Human Immunodeficiency Virus can be detected by direct test procedures such as the p24-antigen-assay or by the isolation of virus in cell culture. Especially in cases of symptomatic primary infection that may be accompanied by a mononucleosis-like syndrome high titers of the major capsid protein p24 as well as high titers of infectious virus can be found in the plasma of infected patients (4). It is of importance that the commonly used routine test systems like the Enzyme Linked Immunosorbent Assay or the Western blot can yield negative results during this period although there is a high titer of infectious viral particles in the blood of the patient. In this situation, testing plasma samples using the p24-antigen assay can be helpful. This is a direct method of testing for Human Immunodeficiency Virus-proteins, where specific antibodies against the major structural protein of Human Immunodeficiency Virus coupled to a solid phase enable the detection of a p24-antigenemia.

Use of the Polymerase Chain Reaction in this symptomatic early phase of Human Immunodeficiency Virus-infection has been described (8). With this method it is possible to detect smallest amounts of Human Immunodeficiency Virus DNA by means of enzymatic gene amplification, but due to contamination there is the possibility of false-positive results. Nevertheless, this new method may be of some advantage in special constellations.

In this context it should be noted that under certain circumstances a "silent" Human Immunodeficiency Virus-infection may rarely occur, where there seem to be no specific antibodies detectable for a relatively long period. This "silent infection" is not detected by the currently used screening tests and can only be diagnosed through special tests like the Polymerase Chain Reaction or by isolation of virus in cell culture.

A further problem is posed by newborns of Human Immunodeficiency Virus-infected mothers. Maternal IgG-antibodies are transplacentally transmitted to the fetus and postnatally detectable up to 15 months in the serum of the child. During this period a supposed infection in a child can only be confirmed by the use of direct test procedures for Human Immunodeficiency Virus.

Diagnostic procedures for the detection of Human Immunodeficiency Virus-infection have reached a higher standard, and their critical use has shown to be very helpful in understanding clinical aspects and pathogenesis of retroviral infections. One special application of virologic diagnosis of Human Immunodeficiency Virus is in the field of transfusion medicine, organ and tissue transplantation including keratoplasty (3).

Under these aspects, a correct and specific viral diagnostic procedure can form an essential preventive measure to avoid transmission of Human Immunodeficiency Virus by tissue transplantation in Ophthalmology.

Regulatory Proteins of HIV-1		
tat	:	transactivator of transcription
rev	:	regulator of viral expression
nef	:	negative factor
vpr	:	viral protein r
vpx	:	viral protein x
vif	:	virion infectivity factor
tnv	:	tnv protein (spliced tat/env/rev)

Table 1. Regulatory proteins of Human Immunodeficiency Virus type 1.

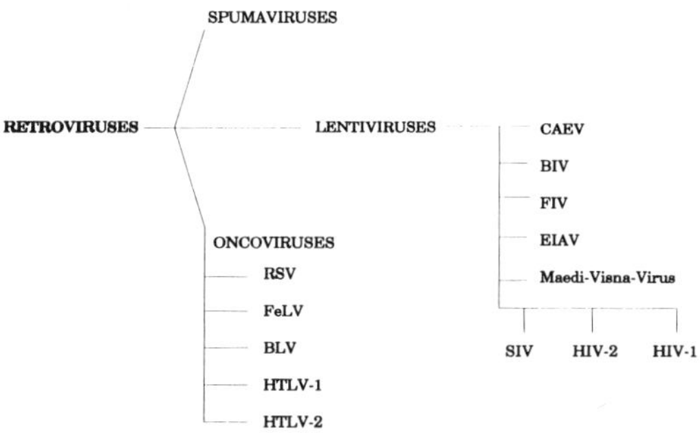

Fig.1. Classification of retroviruses in 3 subfamilies. (RSV: Rous sarcoma virus; FeLV: feline leukemia virus; BLV: bovine leukemia virus; HTLV-1: human T-lymphotropic virus 1; HTLV-2: human T-lymphotropic virus 2; CAEV: caprine arthritis-encephalitis virus; BIV: bovine immunodeficiency virus; FIV: feline immunodeficiency virus; EIAV: equine infectious anemia virus; MVV: maedi visna virus; SIV: simian immunodeficiency virus; HIV-1: human immunodeficiency virus 1; HIV-2: human immunodeficiency virus 2)

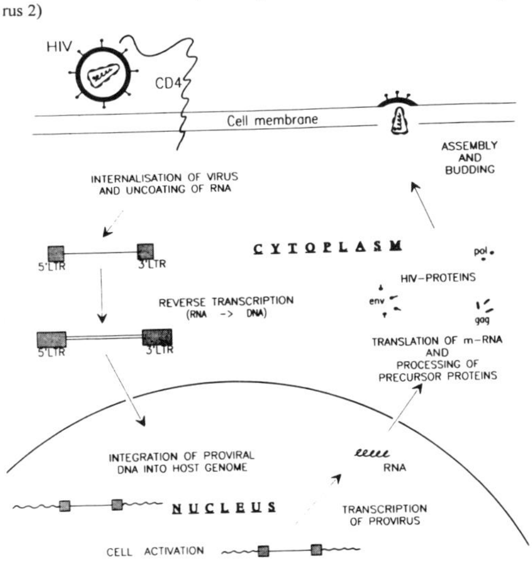

Fig.2. Human Immunodeficiency Virus in a CD4 receptor-positive cell.

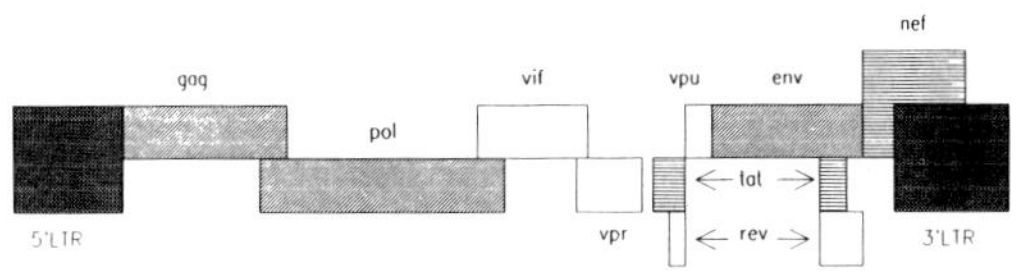

Fig.3. Structure of the Human Immunodeficiency Virus genome showing the coding regions for structural and regulatory proteins. (gag: group antigen; pol: polymerase; vif: virion infectivity factor; vpr: viral protein r; vpu: viral protein u; env: envelope; tat: transactivator of transcription; rev: regulator of viral expression; nef: negative factor; LTR: long terminal repeat).

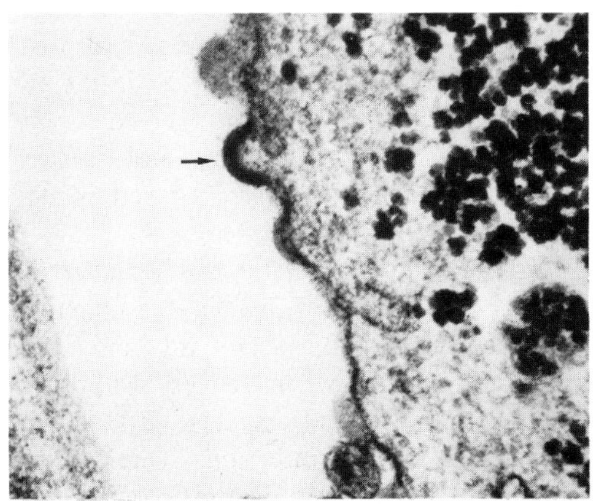

Fig.4. Process of retroviral budding of Human Immunodeficiency Virus at the membrane of the infected host cell as observed in electron microscopy (indicated by arrow).

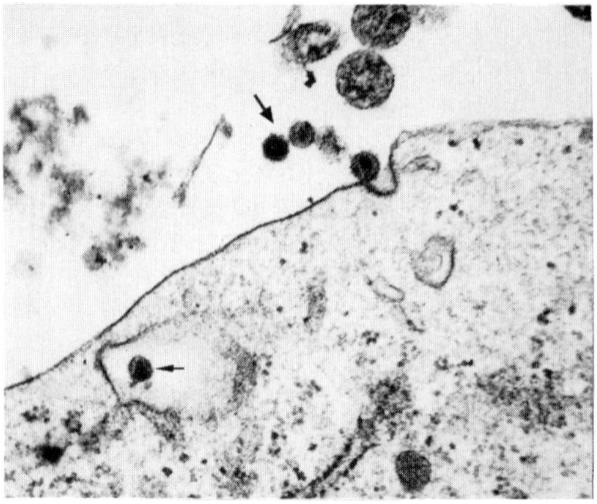

Fig.5. Human Immunodeficiency Virus particle in an infected cell (small arrow) and extracellular viral particles (big arrow).

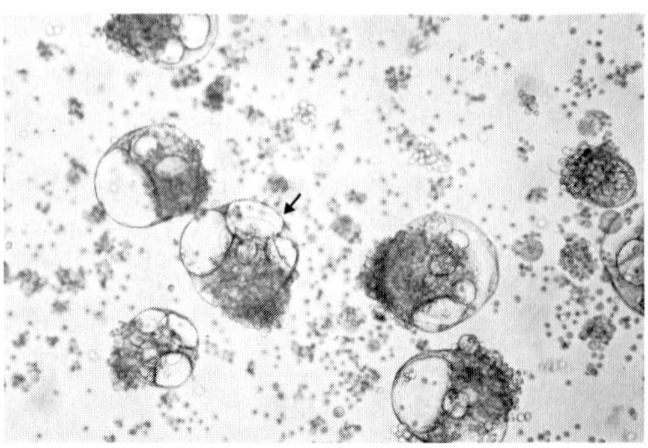

Fig.6. Strong cytopathic effect of Human Immunodeficiency Virus type 1 in a T-cell line in suspension culture. A characteristic feature is the formation of bubbles (arrow) and the development of syncytia.

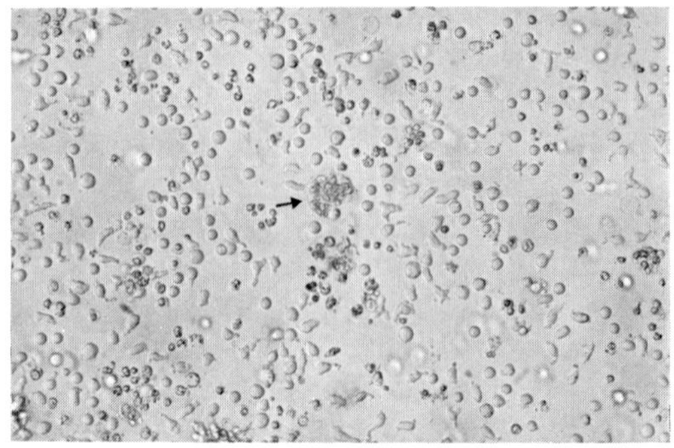

Fig.7. Cytopathic effect of a Human Immunodeficiency Virus type 2 isolate in cell culture.

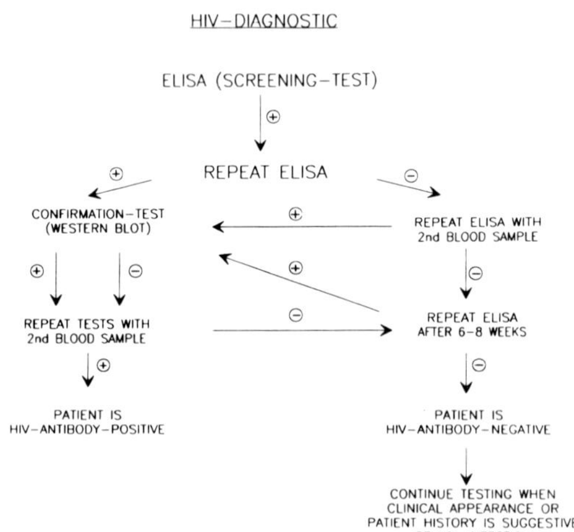

Fig.8. Diagnostic procedures in Human Immunodeficiency Virus infection.

References

1. Arthros J, Deen KC, Chaikin MA et al (1989) Identification of the Residues in Human CD4 Critical for the Binding of HIV. Cell 57:469-481
2. Barré-Sinoussi F, Chermann JC, Rey F et al (1983) Isolation of a T-Lymphotropic Retrovirus from a Patient at Risk for Acquired Immunodeficiency Syndrome (AIDS). Science 220:868-871
3. Bialasiewicz AA, Naumann GOH, Jahn GJ (1988) Virologische Gesichtspunkte bei der Spenderauswahl für allogene Keratoplastik. Klin Mbl Augenheilk 192:634-636
4. Clark SJ, Saag MS, Decker WD et al (1991) Transient High Levels of Viremia in Patients with Primary Human Immunodeficiency Virus Type 1 Infection. N Engl J Med 324:954-960
5. Coffin J, Haase A, Levy J et al (1986) What to Call the AIDS Virus? Nature 321:10
6. Cullen BR (1991) Human Immunodeficiency Virus as a Prototypic Complex Retrovirus. J Virol 65:1053-1056
7. Cullen BR, Greene WC (1989) Regulatory Pathways Governing HIV-1 Replication. Cell 58:423-426
8. Daar ES, Moudgil T, Meyer RD et al (1991) Transient High Levels of Viremia in Patients with Primary Human Immunodeficiency Virus Type 1 Infection. N Engl J Med 324:961-964
9. Dalgleish AG, Beverley PCL, Clapham PR et al (1984) The CD4 (T4) Antigen is an Essential Component of the Receptor for the AIDS Retrovirus. Nature 312:763-767
10. Davey RT Jr, Lane HC (1990) Laboratory Methods in the Diagnosis and Prognostic Staging of Infection with Human Immunodeficiency Virus Type 1. Rev Infect Dis 12:912-930
11. Ellinger S, Mach M, Korn K et al (1991) Cleavage and Purification of Procaryotically Expressed HIV Gag and env Fusion Proteins for Detection of HIV Antibodies in the ELISA. Virology 180:811-813
12. Guyader M, Emerman M, Sonigo P et al (1987) Genome Organisation and Transactivation of the Human Immunodeficiency Virus Type 2. Nature 326:662-669
13. Greene W (1991) The Molecular Biology of Human Immunodeficiency Virus Type 1 Infection. N Engl J Med 324:308-317
14. Haase AT (1986) Pathogenesis of Lentivirus Infections. Nature 322:130-136
15. Haseltine WA (1988) Replication and Pathogenesis of the AIDS Virus. J Acqu Imm Def Sy 1:217-240
16. Imagawa DT, Lee MH, Wolinski SM et al (1989) Human Immunodefiency Virus Type 1 Infection in Homosexual Men who Remain Seronegative for Prolonged Periods. N Engl J Med 320:1458-1462
17. Jahn GJ, Mach M, Fleckenstein B (1988) Cytomegalovirus and AIDS. AIFO 2:59-67
18. Kestler HW III, Ringler DJ, Mori K et al (1991) Importance of the Nef Gene for Maintenance of High Virus Loads and for Development of AIDS. Cell 65:651-662
19. Lenardo MJ, Baltimore D (1989) NF-kB: A Pleiotropic Mediator of Inducible and Tissue-Specific Gene Control. Cell 58:227-229
20. Lifson JD, Reyes GR, McGrath MS et al (1986) AIDS Retrovirus Induces Cytopathy: Giant Cell Formation and Involvement of CD4 Antigen. Science 232:1123-1127
21. Rosenberg ZF, Fauci AS (1989) Induction of Expression of HIV in Latently or Chronically Infected Cells. AIDS Res Hum Retroviruses 5:1-4

Ophthalmic Diseases Associated with Human Immunodeficiency Virus Infection

Gary N.Holland

Abstract. Ophthalmic disorders occur commonly in human immunodeficiency virus-infected individuals.

Most disorders fall into one of four categories: microvascular disease; opportunistic infections; neoplasms; and neuroophthalmic abnormalities related to intracranial or orbital disease. The signs of microvascular disease that occur in the majority of patients are cotton-wool spots and retinal hemorrhages. The cause of microvascular disease remains unknown, but may include immune complexes, direct infection of vascular cells with human immunodeficiency virus, hemorrheologic changes, or a combination of these factors. Cytomegalovirus retinopathy is the most common infection of the eye in patients with acquired immunodeficiency syndrome. A variety of treatment regimens using ganciclovir or foscarnet to improve control of this infection are being studied.

Other important ocular pathogens in patients with acquired immunodeficiency syndrome include varicella- zoster virus, Toxoplasma gondii, and Treponema pallidum.

The conjunctiva and eyelids may be affected by Kaposi sarcoma; treatment with local irradiation may prevent vision-threatening damage to the ocular surface by these neoplasms.

Neuroophthalmic abnormalities include papilledema, optic atrophy, cranial nerve palsies, and visual field defects.

Through early recognition of disseminated infections and intracranial disease, and through treatment of vision-threatening ocular disease, ophthalmologists can contribute to an improved quality of life for patients with human immunodeficiency virus infection.

Introduction

As the acquired immunodeficiency syndrome epidemic spreads world-wide, the spectrum of its ocular manifestations also continues to expand. It is important for ophthalmologists to be familiar with these ophthalmic disorders. Early diagnosis and treatment of the most severe problems can enhance the quality of life for many acquired immunodeficiency syndrome patients by preventing blindness. Furthermore these disorders may be the earliest signs of life-threatening, disseminated infections and neoplasms. The purpose of this review is to summarize the array of ophthalmic problems that may be encountered in the care of acquired immunodeficiency syndrome patients and to highlight factors that may be important in the diagnosis and management of these problems.

Ophthalmic disorders associated with human immunodeficiency virus infection are usually grouped into four broad categories: lesions associated with microvascular disease; opportunistic infections; neoplasms; and neuroophthalmic abnormalities associated with orbital or intracranial disease

(Tab.1). Most of these ophthalmic disorders are not unique to patients with acquired im munodeficiency syndrome. Many, however, were so rare prior to the acquired immunodeficiency syndrome epidemic that they would not have been encountered in the general practice of ophthalmology. Also, the immunosuppression associated with human immunodeficiency virus infection alters the usual clinical presentation and course of other, well-known disorders that can occur in human immunodeficiency virus-infected persons.

Microvascular disease

It is believed that all patients with human immunodeficiency virus infection will eventually develop varying degrees of damage to the retinal microvasculature. Ultrastructural studies have shown damage to retinal capillaries that is similar to the changes observed with diabetic retinopathy (4). In most patients, this damage leads to focal ischemia, resulting in the development of cotton-wool spots, the most common ophthalmic manifestation of human immunodeficiency virus infection (15,20). Other, less frequent disorders presumed to be manifestations of the microvasculopathy include posterior flame-shaped retinal hemorrhages, peripheral blot retinal hemorrhages, and microaneurysms.

Microvascular abnormalities can also be seen in the bulbar conjunctiva, indicating that vascular damage is widespread in patients with human immunodeficiency virus infection (4).

A variety of mechanisms have been hypothesized for the pathogenesis of the microvasculopathy associated with human immunodeficiency virus infection. Immune complex formation (20), human immunodeficiency virus infection of vascular endothelial cells (21), and alterations in blood flow attributed to increased red blood cell aggregation (4) may all contribute to vascular damage and ischemia.

Several studies have found a correlation between the severity of human immunodeficiency virus disease and the prevalence of cotton-wool spots (6,15); the lesions are uncommon among asymptomatic human immunodeficiency virus-infected patients, but occur in the majority of patients with acquired immunodeficiency syndrome. It has been suggested, therefore, that they may represent a poor prognostic sign.

Cotton-wool spots and retinal hemorrhages are usually not associated with any specific visual symptoms. There is growing evidence, however, that patients with human immunodeficiency virus infection have diffuse retinal dysfunction that leads to subtle visual symptoms and that can be identified on electrophysiological testing. It is possible that such changes may be attributable in part to the progressive damage of the retinal vasculature.

Opportunistic Infections

A large number of infectious agents have been shown to infect ocular tissues in patients with human immunodeficiency virus infection (Tab.2). Most are uncommon, despite the frequency of non-ocular infections with the same agents (20). Only cytomegalovirus retinopathy is a common opportunistic pathogen of the eye in patients with acquired immunodeficiency syndrome (AIDS); it is estimated that 20-25% of patients with the acquired immunodeficiency syndrome will develop cytomegalovirus retinopathy during the course of their illness. It is usually a late manifestation of infection, although occasionally it can be the first acquired immunodeficiency syndrome-defining illness (27).

The diagnosis of cytomegalovirus retinopathy is based on clinical findings. The infection is characterized by irregular patches of retinal necrosis with variable amounts of hemorrhage and inflammatory vascular sheathing. The most characteristic feature of a cytomegalovirus retinopathy lesion is the dry-appearing, granular border with little overlying vitreous inflammatory reaction (Fig.1).

Without treatment, cytomegalovirus retinopathy lesions continue to enlarge until the entire retina is destroyed over a several months period. There are currently two drugs used to control cytomegalovirus retinopathy: ganciclovir (10,13) and foscarnet (16). Each inactivates the virus, but neither eliminates virus from the eye. They must therefore be used indefinitely to prevent reactivation and spread of infection, which is made difficult by the fact that both drugs must be administered intravenously. The two drugs have been compared in a National Institutes of Health-sponsored multicenter clinical trial (28). There was no apparent difference in the efficacy of the two drugs for control of cytomegalovirus retinopathy, but there was a statistically significant difference in patient survival. Those who were started on foscarnet therapy had a median survival of approximately 12.6 months, while those who received only ganciclovir had a median survival of approximately 8.5 months. The cause of the differential survival could not be determined. Although it might be a direct effect of the drugs themselves it might also be attributable in part to other uncontrolled factors, including the differential use of antiretroviral agents, such as zidovudine, an agent known to increase survival in patients with acquired immunodeficiency syndrome. Patients receiving ganciclovir were less able to tolerate zidovudine, because both drugs are toxic to the bone marrow, and both result in drug-induced neutropenia. Recent experience shows that patients may tolerate prolonged ganciclovir therapy better with the concurrent use of the growth factors granulocyte-monocyte colony stimulating factor or granulocyte colony stimulating factor, which increase a patient's neutrophil count. The use of such growth factors may allow future patients to use full-dose zidovudine and ganciclovir together. The use of growth factors or newer antiretroviral agents such as didanosine, which does not cause neutropenia, may increase survival among future patients treated with ganciclovir.

In the clinical trial, foscarnet therapy had a greater incidence of side-effects, primarily renal toxicity that required discontinuation of drug administration. Survival among a subgroup of patients with preexisting renal impairment was actually longer with ganciclovir than with foscarnet. The decision to begin treatment with ganciclovir or foscarnet therefore should be based on nonophthalmic factors.

Eventually, cytomegalovirus retinopathy lesions reactivate in all patients and enlarge even with continued intravenous drug therapy. In many cases disease can again be brought under control by temporarily increasing the dose of the antiviral drug if tolerated. The best management of late disease reactivations (repeated "reinductions" with the same drug; alternating ganciclovir and foscarnet; or concurrent use of both medications) is being studied in clinical trials. Even if disease activity cannot be completely eliminated with drug therapy, it is believed that patients receive a therapeutic benefit from continued drug administration by slowing of disease progression.

Some patients cannot tolerate systemic therapy with either ganciclovir or foscarnet because of toxic side-effects. Such patients may benefit from local therapy with repeated intravitreal injections of ganciclovir (2).

Rhegmatogenous retinal detachment is a complication of cytomegalovirus retinopathy that may occur in 50% or more of patients if they survive long enough (14). These detachments are common because of the myriad holes that occur at the borders of normal and necrotic retina. In most cases the retina can be reattached with vitrectomy and silicone oil tamponade, the procedure felt to be most effective by the majority of retina surgeons involved in the care of acquired immunodeficiency syndrome patients (3, 9, 14, 26). Unfortunately, visual results after reattachment have been disappointing. Reasons for poor visual outcome include continued progression of disease, optic atrophy, repeat detachments, and silicone oil-induced cataracts, but in many cases the exact mechanism for continued visual loss is not identified.

Other retinal infections are much less common. Toxoplasmic retinochoroiditis can produce a variety of clinical lesions in patients with acquired immunodeficiency syndrome (11). There may be isolated lesions or disease may be multifocal and bilateral. Eventually lesions enlarge until there is widespread destruction of the retina (Fig.2). In contrast to ocular toxoplasmosis in otherwise healthy individuals, lesions are generally not associated with preexisting retinochoroidal scars, suggesting that ocular toxoplasmosis in most patients is acquired or at least caused by organisms newly disseminated to the eye from nonocular sites. Also in contrast to otherwise healthy patients, infection does not resolve spontaneously. It is therefore recommended that all patients receive antiparasitic therapy. Histopathologic studies have shown little tissue inflammation, suggesting that destruction is primarily due to cell lysis from proliferating organisms. Corticosteroid therapy therefore probably should play no role in the management of this infection in patients with acquired immunodeficiency syndrome. As with cytomegalovirus retinopathy, disease can reactivate when antimicrobial therapy is discontinued; it is recommended that patients continue on chronic therapy with at least one antimicrobial agent, such as clindamycin, if tolerated.

Ocular involvement in patients with syphilis appears to be more common among those who are also human immunodeficiency virus-infected. In these individuals syphilis can cause iridocyclitis without posterior segment disease, but can also result in creamy-yellow, subretinal plaques or an infiltrative retinopathy. Disease will respond to penicillin therapy but conventional doses may be inadequate and recurrences have been described.

Both toxoplasmic retinochoroiditis and syphilitic retinitis can have features in common with cytomegalovirus retinopathy. Both however are usually associated with prominent vitreous and anterior chamber inflammatory reactions and pain; these features help to distinguish the infections from cytomegalovirus retinopathy, which is associated with only minor inflammatory signs.

Patients with acquired immunodeficiency syndrome are at risk for a rapidly progressive necrotizing retinopathy caused by varicella-zoster virus (19). Lesions are characterized by a diffuse, homogeneous retinal opacification without the granular-appearing borders seen with cytomegalovirus retinopathy. In contrast to varicella-zoster virus-associated acute retinal necrosis syndrome (which can also occur in patients with acquired immunodeficiency syndrome) this newly-described "progressive outer retinal necrosis syndrome" is associated with little vitreous or anterior chamber inflammatory reaction, no pain, and can have foveal lesions early in its course. Patients with this syndrome have been treated aggressively with high-dose intravenous acyclovir, but vision has been completely lost in nearly all reported cases.

Choroidal pneumocystosis appears to be a disorder unique to AIDS (5,12,23). It is characterized by multiple, subretinal yellow-white plaques that slowly enlarge over time (Fig.3). Histologic examination of autopsy eyes have shown the plaques to be collections of organisms without an accompanying inflammatory reaction. Lesions will respond to systemic therapy for Pneumocystis carinii.

Retinal and choroidal infections with other agents listed in the table occur rarely, and may be found as an incidental finding at autopsy (20).

Severe infections of the ocular surface may occur in human immunodeficiency virus-infected patients, although they are less common than cytomegalovirus retinopathy (24). Zoster ophthalmicus may occur relatively early in the course of a patient's human immunodeficiency virus infection, and is believed to be a harbinger of further deterioration in the patient's immune status. Im sone cases, patients can be left with a chronic, productive varicella-zoster virus epithelial keratitis, resembling herpes simplex virus epithelial keratitis. Varicella-zoster virus can be cultured from these corneal lesions many weeks after the resolution of cutaneous vesicles, in contrast to the culture-negative chronic keratitis that sometimes occurs in otherwise-healthy individuals with zoster ophthalmicus, which is felt to be immunologic in nature. Varicella-zoster virus epithelial keratitis in human immunodeficiency virus-infected patients responds to topical acyclovir therapy, but not to trifluridine therapy.

Herpes simplex virus epithelial keratitis has been reported in patients with human immunodeficiency virus infection, although there is no indication that it is more prevalent among patients with acquired immunodeficiency syndrome than in the general population. When it does occur, however, it tends to be more prolonged and severe; it is more likely to be adjacent to the corneal limbus; and there is a higher subsequent recurrence rate than in healthy individuals (30). Episodes appear to respond to conventional antiviral therapies.

Fungal and bacterial corneal ulcers have been reported in patients with acquired immunodeficiency syndrome, and are probably related to the same predisposing factors that are seen in healthy individuals, such as epithelial defects, neurotrophic keratitis, or contact lens use (24). These cases emphasize the importance of natural defense mechanisms including normal tear function and an intact corneal epithelium. Acquired immunodeficiency syndrome patients who wear contact lenses therefore should be instructed in the techniques of meticulous contact lens care. Eyelid abnormalities that result in exposure or trichiasis should be corrected immediately.

Corneal microsporidiosis is a previously rare disorder that has been reported in several patients with acquired immunodeficiency syndrome (7,18). The parasite causes a diffuse corneal epitheliopathy without associated corneal inflammation. Patients present with chronically red and irritated eyes and the irregular epithelial surface results in a marked drop in vision. Most attempts at therapy have been unsuccessful although in one reported case, the infection was controlled with epithelial debridement and the new drug itraconazole (29). Microsporidia infect a variety of species, and in many of the reported cases, patients with acquired immunodeficiency syndrome-related corneal microsporidiosis have given a history of owning pet birds.

Neoplasms

Kaposi sarcoma is a common disease among homosexual men with acquired immunodeficiency syndrome. In approximately 20% of patients it will involve the conjunctiva or eyelids (25). Conjunctival lesions may present a cosmetic problem, and bulky conjunctival lesions may cause mild irritation, but they present little or no threat to a patient's vision; they spread slowly and are not invasive. Eyelid margin lesions, on the other hand, can be associated with serious complications. As they progress, eyelid margin lesions may cause entropion formation with trichiasis. Large lesions can also ulcerate and become secondarily infected.

In recent years, very effective chemotherapeutic regimens have been developed for the systemic treatment of Kaposi sarcoma, and therefore eyelid lesions usually do not progress to the point of becoming a management problem. Occasionally, however, eyelid lesions will require local therapy; examples include large lesions that require treatment before chemotherapy has a chance to shrink the lesion, failure of chemotherapy, or isolated eyelid lesions in patients who do not have other lesions requiring chemotherapy. In such cases, local radiation therapy (a total of 2000-3000 centiGrays in 200-300 centi Gray fractions administered over a 2-3 week period) has been shown to be effective in causing regression of tumors, although recurrences are common (25). More recently, investigators have been studying the use of cryotherapy or careful excision of lesions as alternate means of therapy.

Systemic lymphoma is another human immunodeficiency virus-related disorder. Patients may have orbital involvement, with proptosis as the first manifestation (1). Treatment consists of radiation therapy and/or systemic chemotherapy, but the prognosis for the such patients is guarded.

Recently, intraocular lymphoma has been described as a manifestation of acquired immunodeficiency syndrome (22). If the retina is involved, the lymphoma can easily be mistaken for a necrotizing retinopathy.

Neuroophthalmic Abnormalities

A variety of neuroophthalmic abnormalities may occur as early signs of orbital or intracranial disease (8,17). The resulting visual symptoms or ophthalmic signs may bring patients to the attention of an ophthalmologist before other, clinically-apparent neurological problems develop. Visual field defects, for example, may be an early manifestation of progressive, multifocal leukoencephalopathy. Papilledema may be the first sign of an intracranial infection.

Cryptococcal meningitis is the most common cause of papilledema in patients with acquired immunodeficiency syndrome. Patients with cryptococcosis occasionally also develop an unusual syndrome of sudden, severe, bilateral visual loss, with or without papilledema. Its pathogenesis is not fully understood. It occurs in the absence of intraocular Cryptococcus neoformans infection, and is believed to be the result of a retrobulbar or intracranial process.

Other Ophthalmic Disorders

In addition to the well-established manifestations of human immunodeficiency virus infection discussed above, there have been isolated case reports of other ophthalmic disorders in human immunodeficiency virus-infected patients. They include inflammation and tumors of the ocular surface and orbit, and intraocular inflammatory changes (Tab.3). Study of additional cases will be required to determine whether these disorders were simply coincident to the patient's human immunodeficiency virus infection or whether they were causally related to their virus-induced immunosuppression. It is clear, however, that any ophthalmic disease regardless of its underlying cause can have unusual features in an human immunodeficiency virus-infected patient.

Conclusions

With no treatments able to cure human immunodeficiency virus infection and no realistic expectations of an effective vaccine in the near future, the acquired immunodeficiency syndrome epidemic will continue to expand. It will also continue to present diagnostic and therapeutic challenges to the ophthalmic community in the years to come. With regard to the ophthalmic diseases associated with human immunodeficiency virus infection, the following general concepts and principles should be kept in mind:

- Previously rare ocular infections and neoplasms have emerged as frequent manifestations of the acquired immunodeficiency syndrome. Some, such as choroidal pneumocystosis and corneal microsporidiosis, were not identified until several years after the start of the epidemic; it is therefore likely that additional rare disorders will be emerge as the epidemic grows.
- Well-known ocular disorders, such as toxoplasmic retinochoroiditis and herpes simplex virus epithelial keratitis, may be altered in appearance or course by the immunosuppression of human immunodeficiency virus infection. Clinicians should keep this fact in mind when formulating differential diagnosis for lesions that do not fit the classic description of ocular disease.
- Patients and their primary care providers should be taught the signs and symptoms of

intraocular disease, such as floaters, blind spots, and blurring of vision, since it may be impractical to screen all patients with human immunodeficiency virus infection on a regular basis. Patients should seek help from an ophthalmologist immediately if such symptoms develop.

- Early, aggressive, and prolonged therapy will usually be required to control human immunodeficiency virus-related opportunistic infections. For many infections, chronic low-dose antimicrobial therapy will be necessary to prevent reactivation of infection.
- New drugs are being developed that may greatly improve the management of human immunodeficiency virus-related ophthalmic disease. Careful observation of the diseases and their response to treatment in well-designed studies will help to refine the use of such drugs.

Table 1. Ophthalmic diseases associated with human immunodeficiency virus infection

I. Microvasculopathy

A. Retina
- Cotton-wool spots
- Retinal hemorrhages
- Microaneurysms
- Ischemic maculopathy (rare)

B. Conjunctiva
- Changes in vessel structure (dilated capillaries, microaneurysms, isolated vascular fragments, vessel segments of irregular caliber)
- Slowing of blood flow

C. Optic nerve
- Ischemic optic neuropathy (rare)

II. Opportunistic infectious diseases

A. Retinal and choroidal pathogens
- Candida albicans
- Cryptococcus neoformans
- Cytomegalovirus
- Endogenous bacteria
- Herpes simplex virus
- Histoplasma capsulatum
- Mycobacterium avium complex
- Pneumocystis carinii
- Sporotrichum schenckii
- Toxoplasma gondii
- Treponema pallidum
- Varicella zoster virus

Table 1. cont´d

B. Ocular surface/external pathogens
- Candida albicans
- Chlamydia trachomatis, serotype L2 (lymphogranuloma venereum)
- Cytomegalovirus (no reported clinical disease)
- Herpes simplex virus
- Microsporidia sp.
- Molluscum contagiosum
- Varicella zoster virus

III. Neoplasms

A. Kaposi sarcoma (eyelids, conjunctiva)
B. Burkitt lymphoma (orbit)
C. Large cell lymphoma (intraocular tissues)

IV. Neuroophthalmic signs of intracranial disease

A. Cranial nerve palsies
B. Slow saccades
C. Visual field defects
D. Papilledema
E. Pupillary abnormalities
F. Optic atrophy

V. Other reported disorders of uncertain relationship to HIV infection

A. Ocular surface
- Culture-negative keratoconjunctivitis
- Peripheral corneal melting
- Reiter's syndrome
- Atypical conjunctival squamous cell carcinoma

B. Intraocular
- Iridocyclitis
- Retinal vasculitis
- Vitritis
- Choroidal effusion, anterior rotation of ciliary body, and angle closure glaucoma
- Reduced or extinguished electroretinogram

C. Orbit
- Orbital pseudotumor
- Eosinophilic granuloma

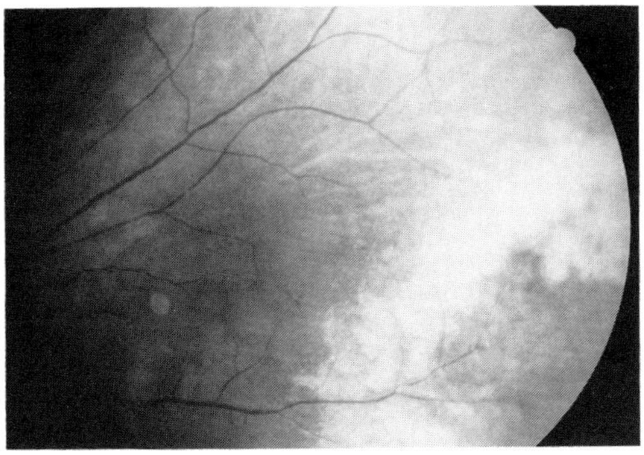

Fig.1. A focus of cytomegalovirus retinopathy in the peripheral retina of a patient with acquired immunodeficiency syndrome. The dry-appearing granular border and lack of overlying vitreous reaction are characteristic features. Other patients can have greater degrees of retinal whitening in the central portions of the lesion and variable amounts of retinal hemorrhage.

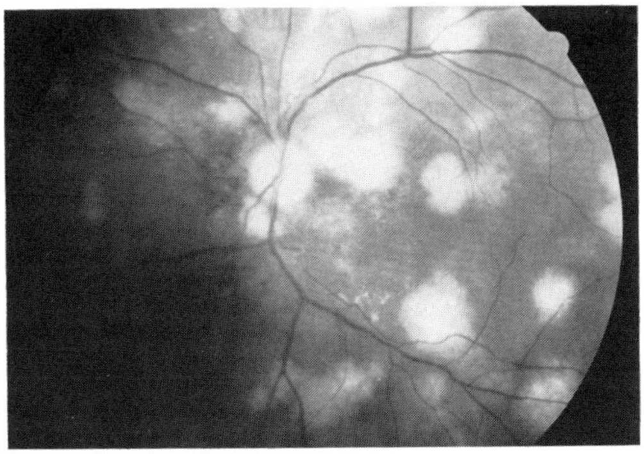

Fig.2. A wedgeshaped area of retinal necrosis caused by Toxoplasma gondii in a patient with acquired immunodeficiency syndrome. The presence of a prominent anterior chamber inflammatory reaction, vitritis, pain, and conjunctival injection helped to distinguish this lesion from cytomegalovirus retinopathy.

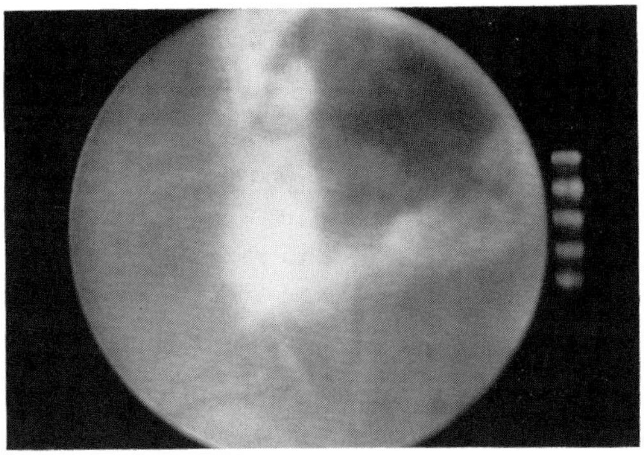

Fig.3. Multifocal subretinal lesions consistent with choroidal pneumocystosis in the left eye of a patient with acquired immunodeficiency syndrome

References

1. Antle CM, White VA, Horsman DE et al (1990) Large Cell Orbital Lymphoma in a Patient with Acquired Immune Deficiency Syndrome: Case Report and Review. Ophthalmology 97:1494-1498
2. Cochereau-Massin I, LeHoang P, Lautier-Frau M et al (1991) Efficacy and Tolerance of Intravitreal Ganciclovir in Cytomegalovirus Retinitis in Acquired Immune Deficiency Syndrome. Ophthalmology 98:1348-1355
3. Dugel PU, Liggett PE, Lee MB et al (1991) Repair of Retinal Detachment Caused by Cytomegalovirus Retinitis in Patients with the Acquired Immunodeficiency Syndrome. Am J Ophthalmol 112:235-242
4. Engstrom RE, Holland GN, Hardy WD et al (1990) Hemorheologic Abnormalities in Patients with Human Immunodeficiency Virus Infection and Ophthalmic Microvasculopathy. Am J Ophthalmol 109:153-161

5. Foster RE, Lowder CY, Meisler DM et al (1991) Presumed Pneumocystis carinii Choroiditis. Unifocal Presentation, Regression with Intravenous Pentamidine, and Choroiditis Recurrence. Ophthalmology 98:1360-1365
6. Freeman WR, Chen A, Henderly DE et al (1989) Prevalence and Significance of Acquired Immunodeficiency Syndrome-Related Retinal Microvasculopathy. Am J Ophthalmol 107:229-235
7. Friedberg DN, Stenson SM, Orenstein JM et al (1990) Microsporidial Keratoconjunctivitis in Acquired Immunodeficiency Syndrome. Arch Ophthalmol 108:504-508
8. Friedman DI (1991) Neuro-Ophthalmic Manifestations of Human Immunodeficiency Virus Infection. Neurol Clin 9:55-72
9. Holland GN (1991) The Management of Retinal Detachments in Patients with Acquired Immunodeficiency Syndrome (Editorial). Arch Ophthalmol 109:791-793
10. Holland GN, Buhles WC, Mastre B et al (1989) A Controlled Retrospective Study of Ganciclovir Treatment for Cytomegalovirus Retinopathy: Use of a Standardized System for the Assessment of Disease Outcome. Arch Ophthalmol 107:1759-1766
11. Holland GN, Engstrom RE, Glasgow BJ et al (1988) Ocular Toxoplasmosis in Patients with the Acquired Immunodeficiency Syndrome. Am J Ophthalmol 106:653-667
12. Holland GN, MacArthur LJ, Foos RY (1991) Choroidal Pneumocystosis. Arch Ophthalmol 109:1454-1455
13. Jabs DA, Enger C, Bartlett JG (1989) Cytomegalovirus Retinitis and Acquired Immunodeficiency Syndrome. Arch Ophthalmol 107:75-80
14. Jabs DA, Enger C, Haller J et al (1991) Retinal Detachments in Patients with Cytomegalovirus Retinitis. Arch Ophthalmol 109:794-799
15. Jabs DA, Green WR, Fox R et al (1989) Ocular Manifestations of Acquired Immune Deficiency Syndrome. Ophthalmology 96:1092-1099
16. Jacobson MA, O'Donnell JJ, Mills J (1989) Foscarnet Treatment of Cytomegalovirus Retinitis in Patients with the Acquired Immunodeficiency Syndrome. Antimicrob Ag Chemother 33:736-741
17. Keane JR (1991) Neuro-Ophthalmologic Signs of AIDS: 50 Patients. Neurology 41:841-845
18. Lowder CY, Meisler DM, McMahon JT et al (1990) Microsporidia Infection of the Cornea in a Man Seropositive for Human Immunodeficiency Virus. Am J Ophthalmol 109:242-244
19. Margolis TP, Lowder CY, Holland GN et al (1991) Varicella-Zoster Virus Retinitis in Patients with the Acquired Immunodeficiency Syndrome. Am J Ophthalmol 112:119-131
20. Pepose JS, Holland GN, Nestor MS et al (1985) Acquired Immune Deficiency Syndrome: Pathogenic Mechanisms of Ocular Disease. Ophthalmology 92:472-484
21. Pomerantz RJ, Kuritzkes DR, de la Monte SM et al (1988) Infection of the Retina by Human Immunodeficiency Virus. N Engl J Med 317:1643-1647
22. Schanzer MC , Font RL, O'Malley RE (1991) Primary Ocular Malignant Lymphoma Associated with the Acquired Immune Deficiency Syndrome. Ophthalmology 98:88-91
23. Shami MJ, Freeman WR, Friedberg D et al (1991) A Multicenter Study of Pneumocystis Choroidopathy. Am J Ophthalmol 112:15-22
24. Shuler JD, Engstrom RE, Holland GN (1989) External Ocular Disease and Anterior Segment Disorders Associated with the Acquired Immunodeficiency Syndrome. Int Ophthalmol Cl 29:98-104

25. Shuler JD, Holland GN, Miles SA et al (1989) Kaposi Sarcoma of the Conjunctiva and Eyelids Associated with the Acquired Immunodeficiency Syndrome. Arch Ophthalmol 107:858-862
26. Sidikaro Y, Silver L, Holland GN et al (1991) Rhegmatogenous Retinal Detachments in Patients with AIDS and Necrotizing Retinal Infections. Ophthalmology 98:129-135
27. Sison RF, Holland GN, MacArthur LJ et al (1991) Cytomegalovirus Retinopathy as the Initial Manifestation of the Acquired Immunodeficiency Syndrome. Am J Ophthalmol 112:243-249
28. Studies in Ocular Complications of AIDS (SOCA) (1992) Research Group in Collaboration with the AIDS Clinical Trials Group (ACTG). Studies of Ocular Complications of AIDS Foscarnet-Ganciclovir Cytomegalovirus Retinitis Trial: 2. Mortality. N Engl J Med 326:213-220
29. Yee RW, Tio FO, Martinez JA et al (1991) Resolution of Microsporidial Epithelial Keratopathy in a Patient with AIDS. Ophthalmology 98:196-201
30. Young TL, Robin JB, Holland GN et al (1989)
31. Herpes Simplex Keratitis in Patients with Acquired Immune Deficiency Syndrome. Ophthalmology 96:1476-1479

Ocular Features of Sexually Transmitted Herpetic Infections

Jay S. Pepose

Abstract. Genital herpes simplex infection is the sexually transmitted disease with the fastest documented increase between 1965 and the onset of the acquired immunodeficiency syndrome epidemic in 1981. Neonatal herpes simplex infection can manifest as keratoconjunctivitis, cataract, optic neuritis or retinitis. In addition, oculo-genital spread of Herpes Simplex Virus Type 2 in adults has been reported.

Sexual transmission and exogenous reinfection is also a significant mode of spread for Cytomegalovirus, which has been isolated from the uterine cervix, semen and saliva. Cytomegalovirus is often found in association with other sexually transmitted diseases, such as chlamydial infections or gonorrhea. Severe ocular manifestations, most prominently retinitis, have been associated with intrauterine and neonatal Cytomegalovirus infection, and may also afflict immunosuppressed adults such as patients with the acquired immunodeficiency syndrome and organ transplant recipients.

Most recently, cell-free Epstein-Barr Virus shedding from the uterine cervix has been demonstrated, raising the specter of venereal, oral-genital and neonatal transmission. In addition, Epstein-Barr Virus-induced infectious mononucleosis is transmitted through exchange of oral secretions. Reported ocular findings in association with Epstein-Barr Virus infection include Sjögren's syndrome, oculoglandular syndrome, conjunctivitis, keratitis, uveitis, papillitis, choroiditis and, rarely, retinitis.

Introduction

In recent years, viral sexually transmitted diseases have taken on increasing prevalence and import. Appreciation of the ophthalmological features of these disorders will lead to an accurate diagnosis and appropriate treatment of the underlying systemic disease, as well as its ocular component. Ocular manifestations of sexually transmitted infections caused by three members of the herpesvirus family are discussed (i.e.Herpes Simplex Virus Type 2, Cytomegalovirus and Epstein-Barr Virus, respectively).

Herpes Simplex Virus Type 2 Infections

From the mid-1960s until the onset of the acquired immunodeficiency syndrome epidemic, genital Herpes Simplex Virus infection was the sexually transmitted disease with the fastest documented increase (6).

Neonatal herpes simplex resulting from maternal infection can manifest as keratoconjunctivitis (Fig.1), microphthalmia, cataract, iridocyclitis, iris atrophy, posterior synechiae, optic neuritis, retinitis, chorioretinal scarring, or encephalitis leading to cortical blindness (18,39). Whereas 80% of neonatal Herpes Simplex Virus infection is caused by Herpes Simplex Virus Type 2, both Herpes Simplex Virus types 1 and 2 have been associated with neonatal keratitis. The frequency of Herpes Simplex Virus infections in newborns is estimated at one in 100000 deliveries (3). Neonatal infection can either remain (1) localized to the skin, eye or mouth, (2) infect the central nervous system with or without skin, eye or mouth involvement, or (3) disseminate to multiple viscera and organs, of which the eye may be one. The reported incidence of keratitis among newborns with Herpes Simplex Virus infections has ranged between 6% to 7% (18,39). Herpes Simplex Virus has been isolated directly from the lens of an infected infant who developed cataracts several months after the acute infection (10). The more common late ophthalmological sequelae following neonatal Herpes Simplex Virus infection include chorioretinal scars (28%) and optic atrophy (22%). These signs are seen predominantly in those children with central nervous system involvement, which is more common in neonates with Herpes Simplex Virus type 2 than type 1. In patients with anterior segment findings alone, visual acuity one to 15 years following neonatal herpetic infection is generally 20/40 or better (18).

Ocular Herpes Simplex Virus Type 2 in adults is thought to be spread predominantly via oculogenital or digitooculogenital routes, (11,16,40-42) although hematogenous dissemination has been proposed (70) in selected cases. Herpes Simplex Virus Type 2 may present with conjunctivitis, blepharitis or keratitis. A number of the cases of Herpes Simplex Virus Type 2 keratitis have been severe, requiring conjunctival flaps or penetrating keratoplasty (11,40). These clinical findings parallel the results of a study in rabbits comparing 8 strains of Herpes Simplex Virus Type 1 and 7 strains of Herpes Simplex Virus Type 2, which showed that primary infection with the type 2 strains resulted in more severe and prolonged keratitis (44,45).

Two cases of Acute Retinal Necrosis Syndrome have corroborative data suggesting Herpes Simplex Virus Type 2 as the etiology, but there is no evidence of sexual transmission linked to the Acute Retinal Necrosis Syndrome (30,51).

The overall frequency of recurrences of genital Herpes Simplex Virus Type 2 appears to greatly exceed that of ocular Herpes Simplex Virus Type 1 (29). It is unclear whether Herpes Simplex Virus Type 2 similarly recurs at a greater frequency than ocular Herpes Simplex Virus Type 1. For ocular Herpes Simplex Virus Type 1, a 32 year natural history study revealed a 9.6% risk of recurrence one year after the initial episode, a 22.9% risk at two years and at 10 years the cumulative incidence of recurrence was 49.5%. The recurrence rate rose with the number of episodes, and there was a trend toward shorter intervals between episodes with increasing number of occurrences (28). During latency, viral replication does not occur, but selected viral transcription has been demonstrated (4,21,69). Several studies have demonstrated that Herpes Simplex Virus Type 1 latency associated transcripts appear to facilitate Herpes Simplex Virus reactivation (24, 27, 68), but are not essential for the establishment or maintenance of latency (27). Herpes Simplex Virus Type 1 latency associated transcripts originate from a region of the genome equivalent to Herpes Simplex Virus Type 1. The type 2 latency associated transcript is transcribed in the same direction and is found in the same cellular location and in a similar proportion of neurons as the type 1 latency associated transcripts (13,36,71). However, the Herpes Simplex Virus Type 2 latency associated transcript has a different open reading frame than type 1 (65), has limited homology with the type 1 latency associated transcripts, and spliced species of latency associated transcripts (69) which are seen during type 1 latency have not been detected in latent Herpes Simplex Virus Type 2 RNA (65). Whether these features contribute to the aforementioned biological differences in the reactivation of Herpes Simplex Virus Type 1 and 2 at different anatomical sites is unclear.

Ocular herpes simplex does not appear to be a common finding in patients with the acquired immunodeficiency syndrome. However, once the keratitis has manifested, its course is generally prolonged and recurrences are frequent, often involving the peripheral cornea (76). The response to standard topical antiviral therapy may be slow and the addition of topical alpha interferon may be useful (34).

Cytomegalovirus Infections

Sexual transmission and exogenous reinfection is also a significant mode of spread for Cytomegalovirus, which has been isolated from the uterine cervix (1), semen (26), and saliva (64). Active Cytomegalovirus infection of the female genital tract has been observed in 4-12% of both pregnant and non-pregnant women (7, 19, 56, 67). Cytomegalovirus is often found in association with other sexually transmitted diseases, such as chlamydial infections or gonorrhea (46). Severe ocular manifestations, most prominently full-thickness necrotizing retinitis (Fig.2), has been associated with intrauterine Cytomegalovirus infection, with postnatal infection following transfusion of blood with high Cytomegalovirus antibody titers, and with pediatric acquired immunodeficiency syndrome (46). Cytomegalovirus infection in utero occurs in 1% of live birth (35000 cases per year in the USA), of which approximately 2% of those infected present with Cytomegalovirus retinitis or optic atrophy (4). The majority of children with symptomatic Cytomegalovirus disease are born to mothers who acquire primary Cytomegalovirus infection during the first trimester (66).

Cytomegalovirus retinitis may also afflict immunosuppressed adults such as patients with the acquired immunodeficiency syndrome (48), patients receiving chemotherapy for malignancies, and organ transplant recipients (17,38). On exceedingly rare occcasions, Cytomegalovirus retinitis has presented in individuals who do not appear to be immunosuppressed (9,20), possibly as a result of primary infection or superinfection. Cytomegalovirus reactivation may also increase with age, in concordance with lower levels of immunocompetence (37). A number of homosexual patients with the acquired immunodeficiency syndrome and women attending a clinic for sexually transmitted diseases have been shown to be infected with multiple strains of Cytomegalovirus (8,63).

Cytomegalovirus infection itself impairs cellular immunocompetence, often further immunosuppressing individuals who are already immunocompromised (25)

The virus is hematogenously spread to the retina during periods of viremia (48), which can result from reactivation of latent Cytomegalovirus or from superinfection. Retinal replication of Cytomegalovirus, visible by ophthalmoscopy, may be a sentinel sign of concurrent active Cytomegalovirus infection of lung, brain and adrenal glands (48).

Cytomegalovirus has been isolated from tears of children with acute lymphocytic leukemia (12) and has also been detected in the iris (50) and conjunctiva of victims with the acquired immunodeficiency syndrome (5). Megalic cells with viral inclusions have been shown in the corneal endethelium of patients with the acquired immunodeficiency syndrome and Cytomegalovirus retinitis (15,58).

Recently, Human Immunodeficiency Virus Type 1 and Cytomegalovirus have been colocalized within retinal tissue of Human Immunodeficiency Virus-infected patients (5, 15, 57, 58, 61) and even within individual retinal cells (61), raising the possibility of direct viral interactions. This finding may explain, in part, the high incidence of Cytomegalovirus retinitis in patients with the acquired immunodeficiency syndrome as compared to other immunocompromised individuals such as organ transplant recipients (49). Potential mechanisms of interaction between Human Immunodeficiency Virus Type 1 and Cytomegalovirus include transactivation of the Cytomegalovirus or Human Immunodeficiency Virus Type 1 promoters by cellular or viral transcription factors, phenotypic mixing or alteration in binding affinity (61).

Human Immunodeficiency Virus Type 1, Cytomegalovirus and Human Herpesvirus 6 have also been demonstrated in the retinas of patients with the acquired immunodeficiency syndrome in varying combinations (55). Human herpes virus 6, the cause of exanthema subitum, appears to be a ubiquitous herpesvirus infecting most individuals early in life (2). The role, if any, that this virus may play in influencing Cytomegalovirus retinitis in certain patients with the acquired immunodeficiency syndrome will require further study.

Concurrent Herpes Simplex Virus and Cytomegalovirus retinitis and encephalitis has been observed in a homosexual man who died of the acquired immunodeficiency syndrome (47), again raising the possibility of viral interactions (43).

Epstein-Barr Virus Infections

Epstein-Barr Virus, another member of the herpesvirus family, is a cause of infectious mononucleosis and may be transmitted through exchange of oral secretions (23). Indeed, Epstein-Barr Virus-induced mononucleosis in adolescents has been referred to be some as "the kissing disease" (60). Most recently, cell-free Epstein-Barr Virus shedding from the uterine cervix has been demonstrated, raising the specter of venereal, oral-genital and neonatal transmission (59).

A broad spectrum of ocular disease has been associated with Epstein-Barr Virus infection. This includes Parinaud's oculoglandular syndrome, dry eye syndromes, conjunctivitis, dendritic and stromal keratitis (Fig.3), uveitis, iridocorneal endothelial syndrome, choroiditis, retinitis, papillitis and ophthalmoplegia (31-33,35,52-54,72-75). The etiologic role of Epstein-Barr Virus in the pathogenesis of many of these findings is uncertain and, in general, few components of Koch's postulates have been met. Many early reports of diverse ocular findings were based solely upon concurrent clinical evidence of infectious mononucleosis or serologic tests not specific for Epstein-Barr Virus infection. Ocular signs listed above were based upon Epstein-Barr Virus-specific serologic testing and/or clinical evidence of Epstein-Barr Virus-like syndromes (31). Epstein-Barr Virus itself has been isolated directly from ocular lesions in a single reported case of dendritic keratitis (74). Epstein-Barr Virus antigens and nucleic acid have been demonstrated in a patient with epithelial and stromal keratitis and in lacrimal gland biopsies from patients with
Sjögren's syndrome (52,54).

Acknowledegement. Supported in part by Public Health Service Grant EY08143-01 from the National Eye Institute.

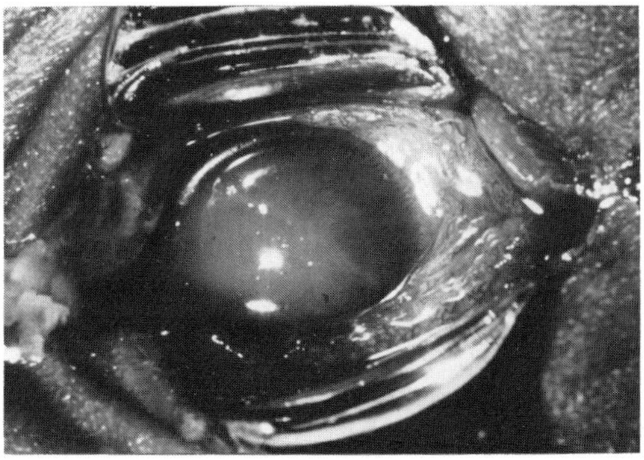

Fig.1. Stromal opacification and conjunctival inflammation in a neonate with ocular herpes simplex type 2 infection.

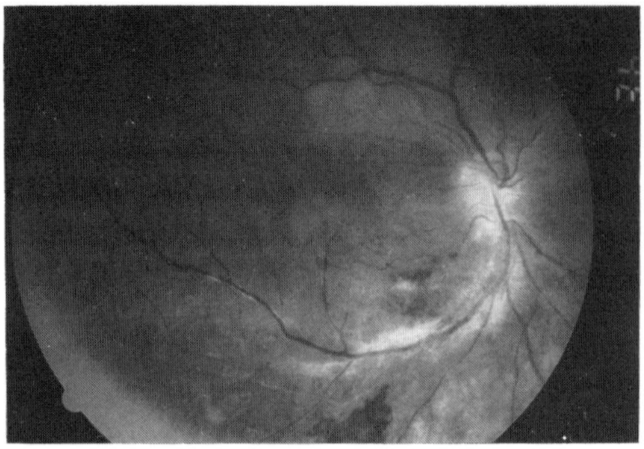

Fig.2. Retinitis, retinal necrosis, intraretinal hemorrhage and sheathing along the inferotemporal vascular arcade are seen in a patient with cytomegalovirus retinitis.

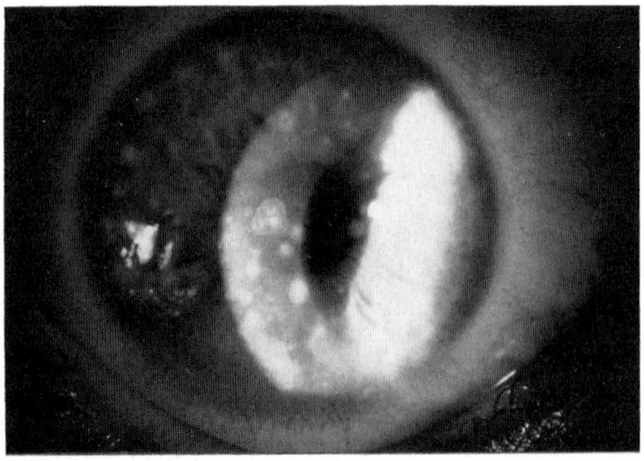

Fig.3. Scattered granular-appearing nummular stromal opacities in a 20 year old woman following infectious mononucleosis (Courtesy of Dr.Alice Y.Matoba)

References

1. Alexander ER (1967) Maternal and Neonatal Infection with Cytomegalovirus in Taiwan. PediatrRes 1:210-215
2. Balachandran N, Tirawatnapong S, Pfeiffer B et al (1991)
3. Electrophoretic Analysis of Human Herpesvirus 6 Polypeptides Immunoprecipitated from Infected Cells with Human Sera. J Infect Dis 163:29-34
4. Baldwin,S, Whitley,RJ (1989) Intrauterine Herpes Simplex Virus Infection. Teratology 39:1-10
5. Britt WJ, Pass RF, Stagno S et al (1991) Pediatric Cytomegalovirus Infection. Transplantation Proc 23 (Suppl):115-117
6. Brown HH, Glasgow BJ, Holland GN et al (1988) Cytomegalovirus Infection of the Conjunctiva in AIDS. Am J Ophthalmol 106:102-104
7. Centers for Disease Control (1986) Genital Herpes Infections - United States, 1966-1984.MMWR 35:402-404
8. Chandler SH, Alexander ER, Holmes KK (1985) Epidemiology of Cytomegaloviral Infection in a Heterogenous Population of Pregnant Women. J Infect Dis 152:248-256
9. Chandler SH, Handsfield HH, McDougall JK (1986) Isolation of Multiple Strains of Cytomegalovirus from Women Attending a Clinic for Sexually Transmitted Diseases. J Infect Dis 155:655-660
10. Chawla HB, Ford HB, Munro JF et al (1976) Ocular Involvement in Cytomegalovirus Infection in a Previously Healthy Adult. Br Med J 2:281-282
11. Cibis A, Burde R (1971) Herpes Simplex Virus Induced Congenital Cataracts. Arch Ophthalmol 85:220-223
12. Colin J, Renard G, Chastel C (1978) Ocular Infection Due to Herpes Simplex Virus Type 2. In: Silverstein AM and O'Connor GR (eds) Immunology and Immunopathology of the Eye. New York, Masson Publishings pp. 279-281

13. Cox F, Meyer D, Hughes WT (1975) Cytomegalovirus in Tears from Patients with Normal Eyes and with Acute Cytomegalovirus Chorioretinitis.Am J Ophthalmol 80:817-822
14. Croen KD, Ostrove JM, Dragovic L et al (1991) Characterization of Herpes Simplex Virus Type 2 Latency-Associated Transcription in Human Sacral Ganglia and in Cell Culture. J Infect Dis 163:23-28
15. Croen KO, Strove JM, Dragovic LJ et al (1987) Latent Herpes Simplex in Human Trigeminal Ganglia: Detection of an Immediate Early Gene "Anti-Sense" Transcript by in Situ Hybridization. New Engl J Med 317:1427-1432
16. Daicker B (1988) Cytomegalovirus Panuveitis with Infection of Corneo-Trabecular Endothelium in AIDS. Ophthalmologica 197:169-175
17. Denis J, Langlois M, Campinichi R (1978) Relationship Between the Clinical Aspects of Ocular Herpes and Antigenic Type. In: Silverstein AM and O'Connor GR (eds) Immunology and Immunopathology of the Eye. New York, Masson Publishing pp. 282-286
18. Egbert PR, Pollard RB, Gallagher JG et al (1980) Cytomegalovirus Retinitis in Immunosuppressed Hosts. II. Ocular Manifestations. Ann Intern Med 93:664-670
19. elAzazi M, Malm G, Forsgren M (1990) Late Ophthalmologic Manifestations of Neonatal Herpes Simplex Virus Infection. Am J Ophthalmol 109:1-7
20. Embil JA, Barner JB, Pereira LH et al (1985) Association of Cytomegalovirus and Herpes Simplex Virus Infections of the Cervix in Four Clinic Populations. Sex Transm Dis 12:224-228
21. Foerster HW (1959) Pathology of Granulomatous Uveitis. Surv Ophthalmol 4:296
22. Gordon YJ, Johnson B, Romanowski E et al (1988) RNA Complementary to Herpes Simplex Type 1 ICPO Gene Demonstrastrated in Neurons of Human Trigeminal Ganglia. J Virol 62:1832-1835
23. Hanna L, Ostler HB, Keshishyan H (1976) Observed Relationship Between Herpetic Lesions and Antigenic Type of Herpesvirus Hominis. Surv Ophthalmol 21:110-114
24. Henle W, Henle G (1973) Epstein-Barr Virus and Infectious Mononucleosis. New Engl J Med 288:263-264
25. Hill JM, Sedarati F, Javier RT et al (1990) Herpes Simplex Virus Latent Phase Transcription Facilitates in Vivo Reactivation. Virology 174:117-125
26. Hirsch MS (1991) Cytomegalovirus and its Role in the Pathogenesis of Acquired Immunodeficiency syndrome. Transpl Proc 23 (Suppl.3):118-121
27. Lang DJ, Kummer JF (1972) Demonstration of Cytomegalovirus in Semen. New Engl J Med 287:711-756
28. Leib DA, Bogard CL, Losz-Nenchak M et al (1989) A Deletion Mutant of the Latency Associated Transcript of Herpes Simplex Virus Type 1 Reactivates from the Latent State with Reduced Frequency. J Virol 63:2893-2900
29. Liesegang TJ (1989) Epidemiology of Ocular Herpes Simplex. Natural History in Rochester, Minnesota, 1950 through 1982. Arch Ophthalmol 107:1160-1165
30. Liesegang TJ, Melton LJ, Daly PJ et al (1989) Epidemiology of Ocular Herpes Simplex. Incidence in Rochester, Minnesota 1950 through 1982. Arch Ophthalmol 107:1155-1159
31. Margolis T, Irvine AR, Hoyt WF et al (1988) Acute Retinal Necrosis Presenting with Papillitis and Arcuate Neuroretinitis. Ophthalmology 95:937-940.
32. Matoba AY (1990) Ocular Disease Associated with Epstein-Barr Virus Infection. Surv Ophthalmol 35:145-150
33. Matoba AY, Jones DB (1987) Corneal Subepithelial Infiltrates Associated with systemic Epstein-Barr Viral Infection. Ophthalmology 94:1669-1671

34. Matoba AY, Wilhelmus KR, Jones DB (1986) Epstein-Barr Viral Stromal Keratitis. Ophthalmology 93:746-751
35. McLeish W, Pflugfelder SC, Crouse C et al (1990) Interferon Treatment of Herpetic Keratitis in a Patient with Acquired Immunodeficiency Syndrome. Am J Ophthalmol 109:93-95
36. Meisler DM, Bosworth DE, Krachmer JH (1981) Ocular Infectious Mononucleosis Manifested as Parinaud's Oculoglandular Syndrome. Am J Ophthalmol 92:722-726
37. Mitchell WJ, Deshmane SL, Dolan A et al (1990) Characterization of Herpes Simplex Virus Type 2 Transcription During Latent Infection of Mouse Trigeminal Ganglia. J Virol 64:5342-5348
38. McVoy MA, Adler SP (1989) Immunologic Evidence for Frequent Age-Related Cytomegalovirus. Reactivation in Seropositive Immunocompetent Individuals. J Infect Dis 60:1-10
39. Murray HW, Knox DL, Green WR et al (1977) Cytomegalovirus Retinitis in Adults: A Manifestation of Disseminated Viral Infection. Am J Med 63:574-584
40. Nahmias AJ, Visintine AM, Caldwell DR et al (1976) Eye Infections with Herpes Simplex Viruses in Neonates.
41. Surv Ophthalmol 21:100-105
42. Neumann-Haefelin D, Sundmacher R, Wochnik G et al (1978) Herpes Simplex Virus Types 1 and 2 in Ocular Disease. Arch Ophthalmol 96:64-69
43. Oh JO, Kimura SJ, Ostler HB (1975) Acute Ocular Infection by Type 2 Herpes Simplex Virus in Adults: Report of Two Cases. Arch Ophthalmol 93:1127-1129
44. Oh JO, Kimura SJ, Ostler HB et al (1976) Oculogenital Transmission of Type 2 Herpes Simplex Virus in Adults. Surv Ophthalmol 21:106-109
45. Ostrove JM, Leonard J, Weck KE et al (1987) Activation of the Human Immunodeficiency Virus by Herpes Simplex Virus Type 1. J Virol 61:3726-3732
46. Oh JO, Moschini GB, Okumoto M et al (1972) Ocular Pathogenicity of Types 1 and 2 Herpesvirus Hominis in Rabbits. Infect Immunol 5:412-413
47. Oh JO, Stevens TR (1976) Comparison of Types 1 and 2 Herpes Virus Hominis Infection of Rabbit Eyes. I. Clinical Manifestations. Arch Ophthalmol 90:473-476
48. Pepose JS (1989) Cytomegalovirus Infections of the Retina. In: Ryan SJ (ed) Retina. CV Mosby Company, St. Louis, pp. 589-596
49. Pepose JS, Hilborne LH, Cancilla PA et al (1984) Concurrent Herpes Simplex and Cytomegalovirus Retinitis and Encephalitis in the Acquired Immune Deficiency Syndrome (AIDS). Ophthalmology 91:1669-1677
50. Pepose JS, Holland GN, Nestor MS et al (1985) Acquired Immune Deficiency Virus Syndrome: Pathogenic Mechanisms of Ocular Disease. Ophthalmology 92:472-484
51. Pepose JS, Laycock KA, Arens MQ et al (1985) Co-factors Associated with Cytomegalovirus Infection of the Retina.In: Usui M and Aoki K (eds) Ocular Immunology Today, Elsevier Science Publishers, Tokyo, pp. 237-240
52. Pepose JS, Newman C, Bach MC et al (1987) Pathologic Features of Cytomegalovirus Retinopathy After Treatment with the Antiviral Agent Ganciclovir. Ophthalmology 94:414-424
53. Peyman G, Goldberg M, Uninsky E et al (1984) Vitrectomy and Intravitreal Antiviral Drug Therapy in Acute Retinal Necrosis Syndrome. Report of Two Cases. Arch Ophthalmol 102:1618-1621
54. Pflugfelder SC, Crouse C, Pereira I et al (1990) Amplification of Epstein-Barr Virus Genomic Sequences in Blood Cells, Lacrimal Glands, and Tears from Primary Sjögren's Syndrome Patients. Ophthalmology 97:976-984

55. Pflugfelder SC, Huang A, Crouse C (1990) Epstein-Barr Virus Keratitis After a Chemical Facial Peel. Am J Ophthalmol 110:571-572
56. Pflugfelder SC, Tseng SC, Pepose JS et al (1990) Epstein-Barr Virus Infection and Immunologic Dysfunction in Patients with Aqueous Tear Deficiency. Ophthalmology 97:313-323
57. Qavi HB, Green MT, Segall GK et al (1989) Demonstration of HIV-1 and HHV-6 in AIDS-Associated Retinitis. Curr Eye Res 8:379-387
58. Reynolds DW, Stagno S, Hosty TS et al (1973) Maternal Cytomegalovirus Excretion and Perinatal Infection. New Engl J Med 289:1-8
59. Schmitt-Gräff A, Neven-Jacob E, Rettig B et al (1990) Evidence for Cytomegalovirus and Human Immunodeficiency Virus Infection of the Retina in AIDS. Virchows Archiv A Pathol Anat 416:249-253
60. Severin M, Hartmann C (1988) Endothelial Alterations in AIDS with Cytomegalovirus Infection. Ophthalmologica 196:7-10
61. Sixbey JW, Lemon SM, Pagano JS (1986) A Second Site for Epstein-Barr Virus Shedding: The Uterine Cervix. Lancet 2:1122-1124
62. Sixbey JW, Nedrud JG, Raab-Traub N et al (1984) Epstein-Barr Virus Replication in Oropharyngeal Epithelial Cells. New Engl J Med 310:1225-1230
63. Skolnik PR, Pomerantz RJ, de la Monte SM et al (1989) Dual Infection of Retina with Human Immunodeficiency Virus Type 1 and Cytomegalovirus. Am J Ophthalmol 107:361-372
64. Slavic HE, Shapiro RA (1981) Fisher's Syndrome Associated with Epstein-Barr Virus. Arch Neurol 38:134-135
65. Spector SA, Hirata KK, Neumann TR (1981) Identification of Multiple Cytomegalovirus Strains in Homosexual Men with Acquired Immunodeficiency Syndrome. J Infect Dis 150:953-956
66. Smith MG (1956) Propagation in Tissue Culture of a Cytopathogenic Virus from Human Salivary Gland Virus Disease. Proc Soc Exp Biol Med 92:412-424
67. Spivack JG, Fraser NW (1987) Detection of Herpes Simplex Virus Type 1 Transcripts During Latent Infection in Mice. J Virol 61:3841-3847
68. Stagno S, Pass RF, Cloud G et al (1986) Primary Cytomegalovirus Infection in Pregnancy. Incidence, Transmission to Fetus, and Clinical Outcome. J Am Med Ass 256:1904-1908
69. Stagno S, Reynolds D, Tsiantos A et al (1975) Cervical Cytomegalovirus Excretion in Pregnant and Non-Pregnant Women: Suppression in Early Gestation. J Infect Dis 131:522-527
70. Steiner I, Spivack JG, Lirette RP et al (1989) Herpes Simplex Virus Type 1 Latency Associated Transcripts are Evidently not Essential for Latency. EMBO J 8:505-511
71. Stevens JG, Wagner EK, Devi-Rao GB et al (1987) RNA Complementary to a Herpesvirus $_q$-Gene mRNA is Prominent in Latently Infected Neurons. Science 235:1056-1059
72. Sumer KD, Sugar J, Levin R (1980) Endogenous Dissemination of Genital Herpesvirus Hominis Type 2 to the Eye. Br J Ophthalmol 64:770-772
73. Tenser RB, Edris WA, Hay KA et al (1991) Expression of Herpes Simplex Virus Type 2 Latency-Associated Transcript in Neurons and Non-Neurons. J Virol 65:2745-2750
74. Tiedeman JS (1987) Epstein-Barr Viral Antibodies in Multifocal Choroiditis and Panuveitis. Am J Ophthalmol 103:659-663
75. Tsai CS, Ritch R, Straus SE et al (1990) Antibodies to Epstein-Barr Virus in Iridocorneal endothelial Syndrome. Arch Ophthalmol 108:1572-1576

76. Wilhelmus KR (1981) Ocular Involvement in Infectious Mononucleosis. Am J Ophthalmol 89:117-118
77. Wong KW, D'Amico DJ, Hedges TR et al (1981) Ocular Involvement Associated with Chronic Epstein-Barr Virus Disease. Arch Ophthalmol 105:788-792
78. Young TL, Robin JB, Holland GN et al (1989) Herpes Simplex Keratitis in Patients with Acquired Immune Deficiency Syndrome. Ophthalmology 96:1476-1479

Epstein-Barr Virus and the Eye: Basic Considerations with Respect to Ocular Diseases

Sally S. Atherton, Stephen C. Pflugfelder, Cecelia A. Crouse

Abstract. Epstein-Barr Virus, a member of the human herpesvirus family, has been associated with infectious mononucleosis, Burkitt's lymphoma, nasopharyngeal carcinoma, and B-cell lymphoproliferation in allograft recipients.

Following primary Epstein-Barr Virus infection, the virus remains latent for the lifetime of the host in the mucosal-associated lymphoid tissue. Two of the mucosal-associated lymphoid tissue structures, the lacrimal gland and corneal epithelium are of special interest, since persistence of virus in these structures supports the idea that this virus may be a cause of ocular disease, either as a result of a primary infection of the ocular mucosal-associated lymphoid tissue or as a result of virus reactivation in these tissues. Recent experimental findings from this laboratoy and from other laboratories have provided further evidence that Epstein-Barr Virus may be a risk factor in some types of ocular disease. Epstein-Barr Virus genomes have been detected at significantly higher frequency in lacrimal gland tissue from patients with Sjögren's syndrome than in lacrimal gland tissue obtained from normal controls.

Using immunohistochemical techniques, we have identified the putative Epstein-Barr Virus receptor (CD21) on corneal epithelium and lacrimal glands; identification of the Epstein-Barr Virus receptor on both lacrimal glands and corneal epithelium suggests that these tissues may be susceptible to Epstein-Barr Virus infection.Current research in our laboratory is focussed on whether ocular mucosal-associated lymphoid tissue-associated Epstein-Barr Virus is in the lytic of latent state, what cell type is infected and if the life-cycle status of the virus correlates with evidence of ocular disease.

Introduction

Epstein-Barr Virus was first discovered in 1964 by Epstein, Achong and Barr when electron microscopic examination of cultured Burkitt's lymphoma tumor cells revealed virus particles whose morphology resembled that of other members of the herpesvirus family (5). Subsequently, the virus was classified as a gamma herpesvirus, and Epstein-Barr Virus is one of the seven known human herpesviruses.

Epstein-Barr Virus is enveloped with an

icosahedral capsid containing a double-stranded linear DNA genome of approximately 172 Kb. In the nucleus of Epstein-Barr Virus-infected cells or Epstein-Barr Virus-containing cell lines, the genome is maintained as a circular episome (11).

Clinical Manifestations

In addition to being associated with over 40% of the cases of Burkitt's lymphoma in endemic areas (Africa), Epstein-Barr Virus is the primary etiologic agent of infectious mononucleosis (8). Besides Burkitt's lymphoma, Epstein-Barr Virus has been linked to several other neoplastic conditions including non-Hodgkin's lymphoma of B-cell origin, Hodgkin's lymphoma, over 90% of cases of undifferentiated nasopharyngeal carcinomas, carcinomas of the parotid glands in Chinese and Eskimos, thymic carcinomas, and B-cell lymphoproliferation in immunosuppressed patients (7,10,12,14, 23). Individuals with the acquired immunodeficiency syndrome exhibit defective T-cell immunity to Epstein Barr-Virus and may have abnormally high numbers of circulating Epstein-Barr Virus-infected B-cells (22). Epstein-Barr Virus genomes have been detected in 40% of non-Hodgkin's lymphomas in acquired immunodeficiency syndrome patients. In acquired immunodeficiency syndrome patients, Epstein-Barr Virus is also associated with oral hairy leukoplakia resulting from Epstein-Barr Virus-induced hyperplasia of the epithelial cells of the tongue (7). Other recent studies have linked Epstein-Barr Virus both to rheumatoid arthritis and to Sjögren's syndrome (1,3,15,19).

In most immunocompetent individuals, primary Epstein-Barr Virus infection results in only a mild upper respiratory infection. A small number of primary Epstein-Barr Virus infections result in clinically apparent infectious mononucleosis characterized by fever, fatigue, pharyngitis, lymphadenopathy, and hepatosplenomegaly. Patients with infectious mononucleosis have increased numbers of $CD8^+$ T-lymphocytes and generally exhibit depressed lymphocyte responses to mitogens and to specific antigens. During infectious mononucleosis, the humoral immune response usually remains intact. Major histocompatibility complex-restricted and perhaps non-major histocompatibility complex-restricted cytotoxic T-cells appear to be important in the control of Epstein-Barr Virus infections (12,17).

Pathogenesis

Primary Epstein-Barr Virus infection establishes viral latency (see below) in a small number of B cells. However, the type of latency in B-cells is quite different from the latency associated with neuronal cells following infections with Herpes simplex Virus; and for example, during immunosuppression, Epstein-Barr Virus reactivates from B-cells and not from cell bodies of sensory nerves. Following primary Epstein-Barr Virus infection, the virus persists at many sites such as the major and minor salivary glands, the oropharyngeal epithelia, the cervical epithelia, the lacrimal gland and the corneal epithelia. Collectively, these sites comprise the mucosal-associated lymphoid tissue (14,16).

In vivo, the usual targets of Epstein-Barr Virus infection are B-cells and epithelial cells, although there is some evidence that the virus may also interact with malignant cells in T-cell lymphomas and with Reed-Sternberg cells in patients with Hodgkin's disease (7). Most of our knowledge of how Epstein-Barr Virus interacts with B-cells is derived from in vitro studies. In a recent review of Epstein-Barr Virus persistence, Rickinson described three different, but related outcomes following Epstein-Barr Virus infection of B-cells (16). Epstein-Barr Virus binds CD21 (the C3d complement receptor) on B-cells which results in:
(1) passive latent infection,
(2) active latent infection, or
(3) lytic infection.

Passive latent Epstein-Barr Virus infection is characteristic of tumor cell biopsies from Burkitt's lymphoma or of early-passage cells derived from Burkitt's lymphoma tissue. During passive latent infection, only one viral gene, Epstein-Barr Virus nuclear antigen 1, is expressed, and there are no detectable virus-induced changes in the proliferative status or in the cell surface markers of these Epstein-Barr Virus-infected cells. Since cells with the passive latent form of infection do not express adhesion molecules such as ICAM-1 and LFA-3 on their surface, the passive latent form of Epstein-Barr Virus infection may facilitate avoidance of the host's virus-specific T-cell response. In addition, since passive latent cells express only one viral protein (Epstein-Barr Virus nuclear antigen 1), the number of target epitopes available for a virus-specific T-cell response is correspondingly lower than if many viral proteins are expressed. Long-term maintenance of passive latent infection does not seem to be favored, and usually, the cells drift toward active latent infection with a concomitant increase in the number of viral genes being expressed.

The active latent form of infection is associated with B-lymphoblastoid cell lines, which have the ability to proliferate indefinitely as a result of being infected with Epstein-Barr Virus in vitro. During active latent infection, eight Epstein-Barr Virus proteins are expressed: six nuclear antigens (Epstein-Barr Virus nuclear antigens 1,2,3A,3B,3C and LP) and two, non-nuclear membrane-associated proteins, latent membrane protein and the terminal protein. Two small, non-polyadenylated, non-capped RNAs (EBER-1 and EBER-2) are also detected in latently infected cells (20). Cells in active latent infection express high surface levels of B cell activation antigens and cellular adhesion molecules and grow in clumps, probably as a result of the increased expression of adhesion molecules. Since lymphoblastoid cell lines form conjugates with activated T-cells via their adhesion molecules, lymphoblastoid cell lines in active latent infection are good targets for Epstein-Barr Virus-specific cytotoxic lymphocytes. Lymphoblastoid cell lines are also good cytotoxic lymphocyte targets, because they express at least eight viral proteins each with a variety of epitopes, and any or all of these epitopes may be recognized by the immune system. It is not yet known if any one of the eight viral proteins expressed during active latent infection functions as an immunodominant protein. If there is an immunodominant protein, it is likely that the epitopes of this protein would be the preferred targets of virus-specific immune responses against Epstein-Barr Virus-infected cells.

The third type of interaction of Epstein-Barr Virus with B- cells is lytic infection. Lytic infection generally occurs in cells which have progressed to the lytic cycle from the active latent form of infection. Without inductions such as occurs following treatment with phorbol ester, only a low frequency of cells (from 1:1000 to 1:1000000 cells) of lymphoblastoid cell lines switch spontaneously from the latent to the lytic cycle. Expression of the BZLF1 gene (an immediate early gene whose product is the ZEBRA protein) seems to be necessary but not sufficient for initiation of the lytic cycle. The ZEBRA protein has been shown to be involved in the switch from the Epstein-Barr Virus latent phase to the lytic phase, and its function may be to transactivate the promoters of several early Epstein-Barr Virus genes, thus moving the virus from the immediate early to the early phase of the replication cycle (13). With the exception of latent membrane protein, most proteins that are expressed during the active latent infection are inhibited early in the lytic cycle. The number of cells entering the lytic cycle from the active latent infection can be increased by treating the lymphoblastoid cell lines with phorbol ester or cross-linking of surface immunoglobulin on lymphoblastoid cell lines using an anti-immunoglobulin antiserum. With the latter treatment, Burkitt's lymphoma cell lines can be induced to proceed from passive latent infection directly to the lytic cycle without an intervening active latent infection.

Most of the knowledge of expression of Epstein-Barr Virus genes during replication has been obtained from studies of latently-infected B-lymphocytes induced into the lytic phase. Like other members of the herpesvirus family, replication of Epstein-Barr Virus during a lytic cycle proceeds via an ordered sequence of events involving expression of immediate early genes, followed by expression of early genes, and finally, by expression of late viral genes. At the beginning of the lytic cycle, the immediate early genes are expressed, and these genes are predominantly latency-associated genes. Several of the immediate early Epstein-Barr Virus mRNAs may function as transactivators of early lytic gene transcription. Immediate early genes induce expression of the early genes. There are at least thirty Epstein-Barr Virus early genes, and although the function of many of these early genes is not known, most of the early genes whose functions have been identified are associated with DNA replications such as DNA polymerase, thymidine kinase, DNA-binding proteins, alkaline reductase and ribonucleotide reductase. Epstein-Barr Virus genes expressed during the late phase of the lytic cycle encode mostly Epstein- Barr Virus structural proteins and proteins that allow for the transport of the virus out of Epstein-Barr Virus infected cells. To date, most of the Epstein-Barr virus late proteins whose functions have been identified are heavily glycosylated and are associated with the outer envelope of the virus particle. A late protein, gp350/220, is the most abundant late gene expressed; it is found in the host cell membrane as well as in the outer envelope of the virus particle. The gp350/220 protein is the predominant envelope protein recognized by antiviral neutralizing antibodies and T-lymphocytes.

Much experimental and clinical evidence supports the ability of Epstein-Barr Virus to infect epithelial cells. However, the interaction of Epstein-Barr Virus with epithelial cells is less well-defined and understood than the interaction of Epstein-Barr Virus with B-cells. This lack of knowledge about the interaction of Epstein-Barr Virus with epithelial cells is attributable in large measure to the lack of a suitable epithelial culture system in which to study the virus. After being placed in culture, most epithelial cells lose their susceptibility to Epstein-Barr Virus infection quite quickly, hindering detailed study of Epstein-Barr Virus infection of epithelial cells. Most of the information about Epstein-Barr Virus infection of epithelial cells has been derived from studies of oral hairy leukoplakia, a lesion produced by Epstein-Barr Virus replication in the epithelium of the tongue of immunosuppressed patients. Overall, from what has been observed, either from tumor specimens or from limited in vitro studies, it appears that latent virus is maintained or remains in association with the less-differentiated epithelium. As the epithelium becomes more differentiated, early and late Epstein-Barr Virus lytic antigens are detected.

Following primary infection, Epstein-Barr Virus has been shown to persist at many sites including the mucosal-associated lymphoid tissue, but the cell type or cell types in which the virus persists in these sites have not been well-defined. The results of early investigations suggested that Epstein-Barr Virus persists only in B-cells, but recent studies suggest that Epstein-Barr Virus may also persist in epithelial cells (16). However, lack of an Epstein-Barr Virus permissive epithelial cell line to study persistence has hampered study of lytic Epstein-Barr Virus infection in epithelial cells. Lacking a suitable cell line, three alternative and complementary approaches to studying the relationships between Epstein-Barr Virus and epithelial cells are to determine:

(1) if epithelial cells possess the receptor for the virus,

(2) if the viral genome is maintained in the epithelial cells, and

(3) if the viral genome is maintained, what viral genes are expressed.

Positive results from these experiments would provide strong circumstantial evidence that Epstein-Barr Virus is able to infect epithelial cells and that the epithelium is a site of viral persistence.

Although there may be more than one receptor for Epstein-Barr Virus on susceptible cells, the predominant cellular receptor for Epstein-Barr Virus appears to be the C3d complement receptor, CD21 (6). Several investigations have demonstrated that Epstein-Barr Virus binds to the Cd3 receptor:

1) treatment of peripheral blood B cells with antibody to Cd3 blocks Epstein-Barr Virus binding,

2) purified Cd3 binds Epstein-Barr Virus, and

3) purified gp350/220 membrane antigen of Epstein-Barr Virus binds C3d.

Epithelial cells of the salivary gland ducts and oropharynx express the Cd3 receptor, and Epstein-Barr Virus has been shown to infect these structures (21). There are many similarities between the external eye and the oropharynx. Both of these sites are lubricated by aqueous secretions from exocrine glands, have cavities lined by non-keratinizing stratified squamous epithelium, and are components of the mucosal-associated lymphoid tissue (9). Because of these similarities, we hypothesize that the lacrimal gland and ocular surface epithelia also express the Epstein-Barr Virus receptor (CD21) and may therefore, like the other tissues which comprise the mucosal-associated lymphoid tissue, be susceptible to Epstein-Barr Virus infection and be sites of Epstein-Barr Virus persistence following primary infection.

Ocular Study

To determine whether the ocular mucosal-associated lymphoid tissue could serve as a site of Epstein-Barr Virus persistence, we examined cells of normal lacrimal glands and ocular surface epithelia for expression of CD21.

Normal lacrimal glands, conjunctiva, limbal and corneal tissues were obtained from normal cadavers within 8 hours of death. The tissues were frozen, embedded in OCT (Tissue Tek^{R}, Naperville, IL,USA), and sectioned for immunohistochemical analysis.

Three monoclonal antibodies reactive for the epitopes expressed on the C3d complement receptor, CD21, were used:
(1) HB-5,
(2) B2, and
(3) OKB7.
The monoclonal antibody, OKB7 has been shown to block attachment of purified Epstein-Barr Virus to B-cells. HB-5 and anti-B2 bind epitopes of CD21 that are different from those recognized by Epstein-Barr Virus and therefore they do not block Epstein-Barr Virus binding.

Positive control tissues for CD21 included:
- frozen sections of normal human tonsil and
- oral mucosa and
- cytospin preparations of CD21-positive Raji cells.

An anti-cytokeratin antibody was used as the positive control antibody, and (NS-1) supernatant from a non-secreting mouse myeloma was used as the negative control antibody.

As we reported previously, a similar pattern of epithelial CD21 expression was noted in the lacrimal gland and ocular surface tissue sections from each of the donors. Staining of suprabasal lacrimal gland ductal epithelium and all ocular surface epithelia, except limbus, was observed with HB-5. Anti-B2 stained lacrimal gland ductal and limbal epithelia, and OKB7 stained only the limbal and the corneal epithelia. The intensity of limbal and corneal epithelial staining with HB-5 and anti B2 appeared to correlate with the level of epithelial differentiation, since the weakest staining was seen in the limbus and basal corneal epithelial cells which are suspected of being the stem and transient amplifying cells, respectively, of the cornea (2). A summary of these results is provided in Table 1 and in Levine and coworkers (9).

Since the cells of the ocular mucosal-associated lymphoid tissue express the Epstein-Barr Virus receptor, the results of the staining studies provided circumstantial evidence that these cells may be susceptible to infection.

Further evidence that the cells of the ocular mucosal-associated lymphoid tissue are susceptible to Epstein-Barr Virus infection was obtained by molecular studies in which the polymerase chain reaction was used to detect the presence of Epstein-Barr Virus genomes in normal human lacrimal gland and corneal epithelia. The polymerase chain reaction method permits the logarithmic amplification of a specific gene sequence by a thermostable DNA polymerase using designated primers flanking the desired gene sequence (18). For these experiments, normal lacrimal gland tissue was obtained from Epstein-Barr Virus-seropositive cadavers, and normal corneal epithelium was obtained from another group of cadavers within 24 hours of death. Lymphocytes were purified from the peripheral blood of Epstein-Barr Virus-seropositive donors. Four Epstein-Barr Virus-containing cell lines were used as positive controls for the polymerase chain reaction, and an Epstein-Barr Virus-negative Burkitt's lymphoma cell line, BL-3, was used as the negative control. After extraction, all DNAs were amplified with ß-globin or HLA-DQR primers to verify the amplifiability of the DNA.

The Epstein-Barr Virus genome was detected by polymerase chain reaction in 32.3% (11/34) of normal lacrimal gland specimens and in 9.4% (3/32) of normal corneal epithelial specimens from Epstein-Barr Virus-seropositive donors (3,4). Interestingly, although the DNA extracted from the lymphocytes of Epstein-Barr Virus seropositive donors was positive for ß-globin amplification, none of the lymphocyte samples from normal Epstein-Barr Virus-seropositive donors amplified Epstein-Barr Virus sequences. This finding suggests that the detection of Epstein-Barr Virus genomes in lacrimal gland samples from Epstein-Barr Virus-seropositive individuals was not due merely to Epstein-Barr Virus-positive lymphocytes trafficking through the lacrimal gland.

Discussion

Taken together, the results from our studies demonstrating the Epstein-Barr Virus receptor on lacrimal gland and ocular surface epithelia and the Epstein-Barr Virus genome in the same tissues suggest that these sites may be sites of Epstein-Barr Virus persistence after primary infection with the virus.

We are currently studying these tissues using immunohistochemistry and in situ hybridization to determine which Epstein-Barr Virus genes are expressed. Epstein-Barr Virus has been shown to be associated with several external ocular diseases and systemic diseases with ocular manifestations, such as Sjögren's syndrome, and our continuing studies to define the interaction of Epstein-Barr Virus with the ocular mucosal-associated lymphoid tissue may provide additional insights into the pathogenetic mechanisms of Epstein-Barr Virus associated ocular diseases.

Acknowledgment

This research was supported by NIH grants EY-06012 (SSA), EY- 08193 (SCP) and EY-02180 (core grant). CAC was supported in part by NEI training grant T32 EY-07021.

Table 1. Reactivity of epithelial cells of the lacrimal gland and ocular surface with anti CD-21 antibodies

	Anti-CD-21 Antibodies[a]		
	HB-5	B2	OKB7
Lacrimal Gland			
- Acini	-	-	-
- Ducts	3+	1+	-
Conjunctiva	3+	-	-
Limbus	-	+/-[b]	2+
Cornea	3+	-	2+

[a] - Intensity of staining graded as follows:
3+ =strong, 2+ =moderate, 1+ =weak, - =no staining
[b] - weak staining of superficial cells only

References

1. Alspaugh MA, Jensen FC, Tan EM (1978) Lymphocytes Transformed by Epstein-Barr Virus. Induction of Nuclear Antigen Reactive with Antibody in Rheumatoid Arthritis. J Exp Med 147:1018-1027
2. Cotsarelis G, Cheng SZ, Dong G, et al (1989) Existence of Slow-Cycling Limbal Epithelial Basal Cells That Can be Preferentially Stimulated to Proliferate: Implications on Epithelial Stem Cells. Cell 57:201-209
3. Crouse CA, Pflugfelder SC, Cleary T et al (1990) Detection of Epstein-Barr Virus Genomes in Normal Human Lacrimal Glands. J Clin Microbiol 28:1026-1032
4. Crouse CA, Pflugfelder SC, Pereira I, et al (1990) Detection of Herpes Viral Genomes in Normal and Diseased Corneal Epithelium.Curr Eye Res 9:569-581
5. Epstein MA, Achong BG, Barr YM (1964) Virus Particles in Cultured Lymphoblasts from Burkitt's Lymphoma. Lancet i:702-703
6. Fingeroth JD, Weiss JJ, Tedder TH et al (1984) Epstein Barr Virus Receptor of Human B Lymphocytes is the Cd3 Receptor of CR2. Proc Natl Acad Sci USA 81:4510-4514
7. Gaffey MJ, Weiss LM (1990) Viral Oncogenesis: Epstein-Barr Virus. Am J Otolaryngol 11:375-381
8. Henle W, Henle G (1973) Epstein-Barr Virus and Infectious Mononucleosis. New Engl J Med 288:263-264
9. Levine J, Pflugfelder SC, Yen M et al (1990) Detection of the Complement (CD21) Epstein-Barr Virus Receptor in Human Lacrimal Gland and Ocular Surface Epithelia. Region Immunol 3:164-170
10. Leyvraz S, Henle W, Chahinian AP et al (1985) Association of Epstein-Barr Virus with Thymic Carcinoma. N Engl J Med 312:1296-1299
11. Lindahl T, Adams A, Bjursell G et al (1976) Covalently Closed Circular Duplex DNA of Epstein-Barr Virus in a Human Lymphoid Cell Line. J Mol Biol 102:511-530
12. Matoba AY (1990) Ocular Disease Associated with Epstein-Barr Virus Infection. Surv Ophthalmol 35:145-150
13. Miller G (1990) The Switch Between Latency and Replication of Epstein-Barr Virus. J Infect Dis 161:833-844

14. Pflugfelder SC, Crouse CA, Atherton SS (to be published) Epstein-Barr Virus and Ocular Disease. In: Robin JB, Meisler DM (eds) Ocular Infectious Disease. Lippincott, Philadelphia
15. Pflugfelder SC, Roussel TJ, Culbertson WW (1987) Primary Sjögren's Syndrome After Infectious Mononucleosis. JAMA 257:1049-1050
16. Rickinson AB (1990) On the Biology of Epstein-Barr Virus Persistence: A Reappraisal. Adv Exp Med Biol 278:137-146
17. Rinaldo CR, Jr (1990) Immune Suppression by Herpesviruses. Ann Rev Med 41:331-338
18. Saiki RK, Scharf S, Faloona F et al (1985) Enzymatic Amplification of ß-Globin Genomic Sequences and Restriction Site Analysis for Diagnosis of Sickle Cell Anemia. Science 230:1350-1354
19. Saito I, Compton T, Fox RI (1989) Detection of Epstein-Barr Virus DNA by Polymerase Chain Reaction in Blood and Tissue Biopsies from Patients with Sjögren's Syndrome. J Exp Med 169:2191-2198
20. Sample J, Kieff E (1990) Transcription of the Epstein-Barr Virus Genome During Latency in Growth-Transformed Lymphocytes. J Virol 64:1667-1674
21. Sixbey JW, Davis DS, Young LS et al (1987) Human Epithelial Cell Expression of an Epstein-Barr Virus Receptor. J Gen Virol 68:805-811
22. Thomas JA, Hotchin NA, Allday MJ et al (1990) Immunohistology of Epstein-Barr Virus-Associated Antigens in B Cell Disorders from Immunocompromised Individuals. Transplantation 49:944-953
23. Wolf H, Zur Hausen H, Becker V (1973) Epstein-Barr Viral Genomes in Epithelial Nasopharyngeal Carcinoma Cells. Nature 244:245-247

Ocular Involvement in Protracted Epstein-Barr Virus Infection

Rolando Tittarelli, Alfonso Giovannini, Enrico Bertelli

Abstract. The authors report four cases of ocular involvement in the course of a protracted Epstein-Barr Virus infection.
The first patient (female, 49yrs.) developed an acute posterior multifocal placoid pigment epitheliopathy 8 months after flu-like symptoms, which had lasted for 8 weeks.
The second patient (male, 11yrs.) was affected by a vitritis dating back 6 months, which had appeared a few weeks after an infectious mononucleosis.
The third and the fourth patients (male, 48yrs.; female, 24 yrs.) both developed an acute plurifocal involvement of the retinal pigment epithelium at the posterior pole in one case resembling a diffuse retinal pigment epitheliopathy.
All four patients showed serological evidence of a protracted active Epstein-Barr Virus infection (positive high titer of Viral Capsid Antigen-IgG, Early Antigen-IgG/IgA) and negative serum titers against other possible etiological agents (Cytomegalovirus and other herpes viruses, Adenovirus). The hypothesis of a possible etiological role of a protracted Epstein-Barr virus infection for these ocular clinical features is in accordance with previous reports.
Although serology cannot provide a definite diagnosis in these cases the authors believe that the well-known epithelial tropism of Ep-

stein-Barr Virus may explain its etiological role.

Introduction

Over the last years, Epstein-Barr Virus has gained increasing attention as a possible etiologic agent of numerous ocular affections.

The detection of ocular manifestations related to Epstein-Barr Virus infections is problematic for two reasons: first of all, systemic infection is often subclinical, secondly, since the culture of virus from the involved tissue is rarely possible from intraocular structures, the diagnosis is based exclusively on the serological findings, that cannot provide a definite diagnosis.

The considerable and encouraging development of diagnostic serology during the past years presently allows a thorough serological characterization of recent, protracted and past Epstein-Barr Virus infections, which is critical to the comprehension and interpretation of any work on the etiologic role of Epstein-Barr Virus in intraocular disease.

Materials and Methods

The spectrum of antibodies that can be presently used to characterize an Epstein-Barr Virus infection with a generally accepted clinical significance are:

Viral Capsid Antigen (IgM):
(VCA)
- Appears at clinical outbreak
- Persists 2 to 6 months
- Best index of 1st infection in course
- Absent in reactivations
- Still detectable in protracted infections

Viral Capsid Antigen (IgG):
- Appears at clinical outbreak
- Persists all life
- Marker of past or active infection

Viral Capsid Antigen (IgA):
- Appears transiently during clinical course of infectious mononucleosis
- Occasionally reported in ophthalmic literature as diagnostic finding

Early Antigen (IgG,IgA) diffuse:
- Peaks 3-4 weeks after clinical outbreak
- Persists 3-6 months
- Indicates more aggressive infectious mononucleosis
- Detectable in Nasopharyngeal Carcinoma
- IgA against Early Antigen-D predicts Nasopharyngeal Carcinoma in populations at risk

restricted:
- Peaks a few weeks after clinical outbreak
- Persists for months, up to one year
- High titers in African Burkitt's Lymphoma
- Signals reactivation in the immunocompromised patient

Epstein-Barr

Nuclear Antigen (IgG):
(EBNA)

- Appears 3-6 weeks after clinical outbreak
- Persists through life
- The later appearance after clinical infectious mononucleosis signals past primary infection

With these premises Epstein-Barr Virus infections may show the following serological patterns:
Acute Infection:

- VCA IgM
- (- VCA IgG)
- (-EA IgG: may be marker of infectious mononucleosis with particularly aggressive clinical course)

Past Infection:

- VCA IgG
- EBNA IgG

Protracted/Chronic Infection:

- VCA IgM
- VCA IgG - IgA
- EA IgG - IgA
- EBNA IgG: Absent or delayed appearance

Review of the Literature

Ocular involvements attributed to Epstein-Barr Virus are not frequent in literature, but encompass a wide variety of manifestations, affecting virtually all parts of the eye.
Tanner (25) in 1952 first distinguished:

1) Manifestations of infectious mononucleosis directly involving the eye and its adnexa
2) Manifestations of infectious mononucleosis involving vision and the neuro-ophthalmologic apparatus

Eye and Adnexa

Conjunctiva :

- Follicular conjunctivitis in the early clinical phase, often unilateral, in 1% to 38% of infectious mononucleosis (8,25)

Cornea:

- Epithelial keratitis; microadenites, subepithelial infiltration (11,28)
- Stromal keratitis;
    1) annular/nummular anterior mild stromal opacities (12,19)
    2) multifocal, peripheral, full-thickness involvement with associated confluent, geographic endothelial precipitates (12)

Uvea:

- Iritis:
- Sporadic cases described (24,25)
- Choroiditis/Chorioretinitis:
- 10 cases of multifocal mainly peripheral choroiditis with pigment epithelial lesions and vitreous cellular infiltrates associated with Epstein-Barr Virus antibodies compatible with recent or continuing Epstein-Barr Virus Infection (26)
- Punctate Outer Retinitis:
- One case with mainly perimacular involvement (20)
- Panuveitis:
- Wong and coworkers (29) describe three patients, affected by panuveitis, with chorioretinal lesions resembling in one case the lesions described by Tiedeman (26)

- One case of bilateral, single sited chorioretinitis, in one eye associated with corneal stromal edema and Koeppe's nodules (10)

Other Localizations

Lacrimal apparatus: Several investigations in the last years have attempted to identify an exposure to Epstein-Barr Virus as a risk factor in the pathogenesis of primary Sjögren's syndrome (2,4,16, 17,21).
Parinaud's ocular syndrome has been reported once during acute infectious mononucleosis (14).

Vision and Neuroophthalmologic Apparatus

Neuroophthalmologic manifestations described in the literature essentially include:

- cranial nerve palsies
- optic neuritis
- IIIrd cranial nerve palsy: 1 case (15)
- Bell's palsy: 1 case (7)
- Fisher's Syndrome: 1 case (22)
- (acute ophthalmoplegia, ataxia, areflexia)
- Guillain-Barré Syndrome: 3 cases (3,5,6) (associated with variable impairments of ocular motility)
- Papilledema 3 cases (1,18,25)
- Unilateral optic neuritis: 1 case (9) and macular edema

Ocular Manifestations Associated with Burkitt's Lymphoma and Nasopharyngeal Carcinoma

In order to provide a complete survey of the ocular manifestations attributed to Epstein-Barr Virus infections, the rare ocular complications described in the course of Burkitt's lymphoma and nasopharyngeal carcinoma, two clinical entities that have been strongly linked to Epstein-Barr Virus infection, should also be considered.
Burkitt's Lymphoma:

- One case of reduced corneal sensitivity and VI nerve palsy in course of Epstein-Barr Virus involving the sphenoidal and ethmoidal sinuses (27)
- One case of proptosis due to massive orbital Burkitt's lymphoma (13)

Nasopharyngeal Carcinoma (53 cases (23)):

- VI nerve palsy 18 cases
- III nerve palsy 7 cases
- IV nerve palsy 4 cases

Less frequently, unilateral proptosis, papilledema and Horner's syndrome, due to involvement of cervical lymph nodes may occur.

Case Reports

During the last two years we have observed four cases of ocular lesions, which in our opinion can be related to the occurrence of a protracted or reactivated Epstein-Barr Virus infection.
Patient 1: The first of these patients is an 11 year old boy, who presented with a marked vitritis in his right eye dating back 6 months. Clinical symptoms (blurred vision) had ap-

peared a few weeks after the resolution of a previously diagnosed infectious mononucleosis.

Visual acuity at admission was 8/10 and continuously improved to 10/10 after three parabulbar administrations of corticosteroids at three weeks' intervals.

In Table 1 we present the development of the serological pattern against Epstein-Barr Virus observed over a period of 18 months.

All other serological investigations performed to rule out other possible etiologic agents yielded negative results. In this first case the history of an infectious mononucleosis immediately drew our attention to the possible etiological role of Epstein-Barr Virus.

In the other three cases, the approach to an etiological diagnosis necessarily followed a much more indirect course, since systemic involvement had been subclinical.

Patient 2: The second patient was a 49 year old female presenting with bilateral acute posterior multifocal placoid pigment epitheliopathy.

A thorough history-taking could only identify mild flu-like symptoms dating back 8 months, which had lasted approximately two months. The patient still reported episodes of fatigue and headache appearing at irregular intervals.

Ocular symptoms included blurred vision and photopsia. Visual acuity nevertheless never dropped below 10/10.

In Fig.1 the fluorescein angiographic picture is given at the time of admission, and in Tab.2 we report the serological pattern detected during 12 months follow-up.

The Viral Capsid Antigen IgM test was not performed at first admission, but the delayed appearance of Epstein-Barr Virus Nuclear Antigen titers and the still detectable titers of IgM five months after admission may in our opinion justify the diagnosis of a protracted infection.

Accurate serologic investigations for other etiologic agents yielded the following positive results:

- Herpes Simplex Virus 1 IgG 1:10
- Toxoplasma IgG 1:80
- all investigations concerning Cytomegalovirus and Adenoviruses

remained negative. The clinical picture resolved permanently after a three months systemic corticosteroid therapy (Dexamethasone 30mg daily for 30 days, then 15mg daily for 30 days and eventually 6mg daily for the last 30 days) with recovery of full visual acuity.

Patients 3 and 4: Patients 3 and 4 were a 48 year old male and a 24 year old female and presented with a multifocal involvement of the retinal pigment epithelium at the posterior pole, presently being inactive.

In Fig.2 and 3 the fluorescein angiographic pictures of these patients 3 and 4 are given. It might be noted, that patient 3 exhibited signs of a diffuse retinal pigment epitheliopathy.

Tab.3 and 4 show the serological findings of these two patients.

Since in both patients the lesions did not present any signs of activity, we chose to follow them without treatment.

Conclusions

We have reported four cases of ocular involvement that we be-lieve related to a protracted Epstein-Barr Virus infection.

The serological findings we have observed clearly outline a protracted infection by Epstein-Barr Virus according to most recent reports concerning the subject.

IgM against Epstein-Barr viral capsid antigen and IgG against early antigen were consistently positive in all cases; in one case we observed a seroconversion in viral capsid antigen IgG. In two cases IgG against Epstein-Barr nuclear antigen became positive a few months after first observation.

Keeping in mind that an etiological diagnosis of ocular manifestations based on serological criteria may only be presumptive, we must nevertheless emphasize the accordance of our findings with many reports, which have contributed to the expanding ophthalmologic recognition of Epstein-Barr virus disease.

If we accept the hypothesis of a possible etiological role of Epstein-Barr Virus in these ocular lesions, different modes of pathogenesis might be suggested: a direct invasion of retinal pigment epithelial cells by Epstein-Barr Virus for the two cases of pigment epithelial involvement, as might be supported by the well-known epitheliotropism of the virus, and an ill-defined immunopathological mechanism, that may explain the vitreous flare (patient 1) and the acute posterior multifocal placoid pigment epitheliopathy (patient 2).

Table 1. Evolution of the serologic pattern against Epstein-Barr virus (Case 1)

	October 1989 (admission)	April 1990	July 1990	May 1991
VCA IgM	not determined	1:160	1:40	-
VCA IgG	1:320	1:640	1:1280	1:640
EA	not determined	1:40	1:5	-
EBNA	1:20	1:10	1:40	1:320
Heterophile AB	+	+	-	-

Table 2. Serological patterns detected during 12 months follow-up (Case 2)

	March 1990 (1st admission)	August 1990	February 1991
VCA IgM	not determined	1:80	-
VCA IgG	1:640	1:320	1:640
EA	1:20	< 1:5	-
EBNA	-	1:40	1:160
Heterophile AB	+	+	+

Table 3. Serological findings (Case 3)

	December 1989 (1st.admission)	June 1990
VCA IgM	1:160	-
VCA IgG	1:80	1:320
EA	1:160	1:80
EBNA	-	1:40
Heterophile AB	+	-

Table 4. Serological findings (Case 4)

	April 1991 (1st.admission)	May 1991
VCA IgM	not determined	1:40
VCA IgG	1:160	1:1280
EA	not determined	1:20
EBNA	1:40	1:40
Heterophile AB	+	+

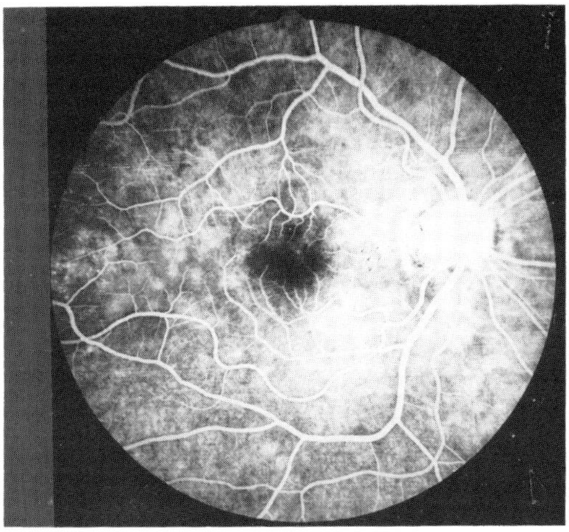

Fig.1. Fluorescein angiography (patient 2)

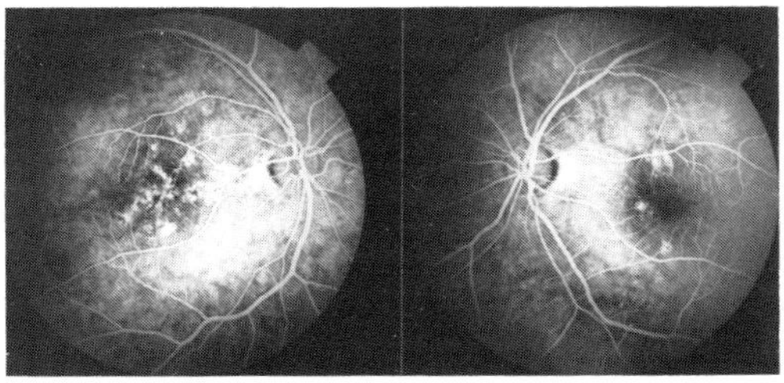

Fig.2. Fluorescein angiography (patient 3)

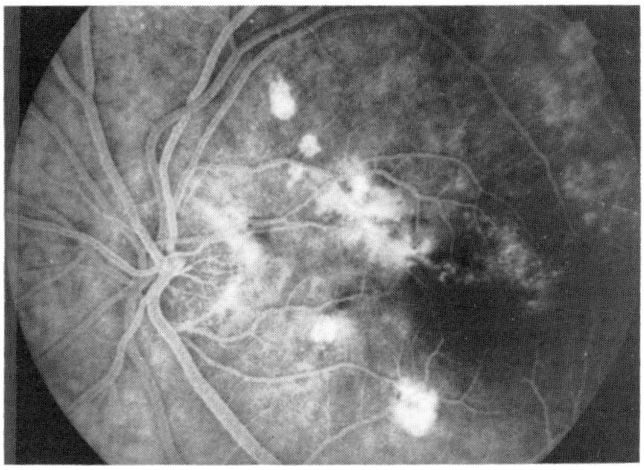

Fig.3. Fluorescein angiography (patient 4)

References

1. Blaustein A, Caccavo A (1950) Infectious Mononucleosis Complicated by Bilateral Papilloretinal Edema. Arch Ophthalmol 43:853-860
2. Crouse CA, Pflugfelder SC, Clearly T et al (1990) Detection of Epstein-Barr Viral Genomes in Normal Human Lacrimal Glands. J Clin Microbiol 28:1026-1032
3. Davie JD, Ceballos R, Little SC (1963) Infectious Mononucleosis with Fatal Neuronitis. Arch Neurol 9:265-270
4. Fox RI, Pearson G, Vaughan JH (1986) Detection of Epstein-Barr Virus Associated Antigens and DNA in Salivary Gland Biopsies from Patients with Sjögren's Syndrome. J Immunol 137:3162-3168
5. Garvin JS (1953) Infectious Mononucleosis with Guillain-Barré Syndrome: Report of a Case. J Am Med Ass 151:293-299
6. Grose C et al (1975) Primary Epstein-Barr Virus Infections in Acute neurologic Disease. N Engl J Med 292:392-401

7. Grose C, Foerin PM, Dye LA et al (1973) Bell's Palsy and Infectious Mononucleosis. Lancet ii:231-238
8. Jones BR, Howie JB, Wilson RP (1952) Ocular Aspects of an Epidemic of Infectious Monocucleosis. Proc Univ Otago Med Sch 30:1-4
9. Karpe G, Wising P (1948) Retinal Changes with Acute Reductions of Vision as Initial Symptoms of Infectious Mononucleosis. Acta Ophthalmol 26:19-29
10. Kelly SP, Rosenthal AR, Nicholson KG et al: (1989) Retinochoroiditis in Acute Epstein-Barr Infection. Br J Ophthalmol 73:1002-1003
11. Matoba AJ, Jones DB (1987) Corneal Subepithelial Infiltrates Associated with Systemic Epstein-Barr Viral Infection. Ophthalmology 94:1669-1671
12. Matoba AY, Wilhelmus KR, Jones DB (1986) Epstein-Barr Viral Stromal Keratitis. Ophthalmology 93:746-750
13. McMoli TE, Ogunmekan AO, Odunjo EO (1980) Orbital Burkitt's Tumor Presenting as Advanced Retinoblastoma. J Pediatr Ophthalmol Strabismus 17(3):147-149
14. Meisler DM, Bosworth DE, Krachmer JH (1981) Ocular Infectious Mononucleosis Manifested as Parinaud's Oculoglandular Syndrome. Am J Ophthalmol 97:722-729
15. Nelhaus G (1966) Isolated Nerve Palsy in Infectious Mononucleosis: A Report of an Unusual Case and Review of the Literature. Neurology 16:221-224
16. Pflugfelder SC, Crese CA, Pereira IC et al (1990) Amplification of Epstein-Barr Virus Genomic Sequences in Blood Cells, Lacrimal Glands and Tears from Primary Sjögren's Syndrome Patients. Ophthalmology 97:976-984
17. Pflugfelder SC, Roussel TJ, Culbertson WW (1987) Primary Sjögren's Syndrome after Infectious Mononucleosis. (Letter) J Am Med Ass 257:1049-1050
18. Piel JJ, Thelander HE, Shaw EB (1950) Infectious Mononucleosis of the Central Nervous System with Bilateral Papilledema. J Pediatr 37:661-668
19. Pinnolis M. McCulley JP, Urman JD (1980) Nummular Keratitis Associated with Infectious Mononucleosis. Am J Ophthalmol 89:791-794
20. Raymond LA, Wilson CA, Linnermann CC et al (1987) Punctate Outer Retinitis in Acute Epstein-Barr Virus Infection. Am J Ophthalmol 104:424-429
21. Saito I, Compton T, Fox RI (1989) Detection of Epstein-Barr Virus DNA by Polymerase Chain Reaction in Blood and Tissue Biopsies from Patients with Sjögren's Syndrome. J Exp Med 169:2191-2198
22. Slavik HE, Shapiro RA (1981) Fisher's Syndrome Associated with Epstein-Barr Virus. Arch Neurol 38:134-135
23. Smith JL, Wheeliss JA (1962) Ocular Manifestations of Nasopharyngeal Tumors. Trans Am Acad Ophthal Otolaryngol 66:659-664
24. Stevens JE, Bayard ED, Heck FJ (1951) Infectious Mononucleosis. Am J Med 11:202-209
25. Tanner OR (1952) Ocular Manifestations of Infectious Mononucleosis. Arch Ophthalmol 51:229-241
26. Tiedeman JS (1987) Epstein-Barr Viral Antibodies in Multifocal Choroiditis and Panuveitis. Am J Ophthalmol 103:659-663
27. Trese MT, Krohel GB, Hepler RS et al (1980) Burkitt's Lymphoma with Cranial Nerve Involvement. Arch Ophthalmol 98:2015-2017
28. Wilhelmus KR (1981) Ocular Involvement in Infectious Mononucleosis. Am J Ophthalmol 91:117-118
29. Wong KW, D'Amico DJ, Hedges III TR et al (1987) Ocular Involvement Associated with Chronic Epstein-Barr Virus Disease. Arch Ophthalmol 105:788-792

- Clamydial

Ocular Features of Oculogenital Chlamydial Infections

Alexander A. Bialasiewicz

Abstract: Chlamydial infections represent the most frequent venereal disease with ocular manifestations. There is no strict clinical classification in adult chlamydial keratoconjunctivitis as is known for endemic trachoma, however, distinct clinical features may be found, which may suggest a similar grading as in endemic trachoma. Thus, follicular conjunctivitis may precede or be associated with epithelial and subepithelial keratitis. Limbal infiltrates that resemble phlyctenules and frank corneal phlyctenules may leave pits similar to Herbert's pits. Persisting infections or multiple reinfections may result in pannus formation and corneal vascularization that rarely will necessitate corneal grafting.

Introduction

The ophthalmologist plays a key role for the establishment of a diagnosis of chlamydial diseases. Chlamydial diseases comprise the "classical" endemic trachoma, oculogenital infections, lymphogranuloma venereum, infections with C.psittaci and C.pneumoniae.

While the clinical diagnosis of endemic trachoma as a disease occurring mainly in underdeveloped tropical countries has been known for more than a thousand years, a new ocular infection resembling trachoma was described in Europe at the end of the 19th century when better microbiological technologies became available (6, 42, 65, 82, 140).

Problems of both ophthalmology and obstetrics and gynecology such as non-gonococcal blennorrhea of the newborn and venereal trachoma-like ocular inflammatory disease were important clinical pacemakers bearing the most significant propulsive effect on the development of better laboratory diagnostic techniques in this field of ophthalmology.

Historical Data

Evidence for inclusion bodies by means of Giemsa stains in conjunctival probes accounted for the most significant laboratory diagnostic achievement in 1907 performed by Stanislaus von Prowazek and Ludwig Halberstaedter (39,46,47,58). Two postulates of Koch could be fulfilled in 1909 when cervical mucus of mothers who gave birth to neonates with non-gonococcal blennorrhea was successfully inoculated in monkeys resulting in conjunctivitis (44, 48, 86, 104, 141). In 1910, these experiments were repeated by Fritsch and Lindner, and they additionally found that male urethral discharge caused symptoms in the conjunctiva of baboons (37).

In the following years, clinical case reports further supported the hypothesis of a sexually transmitted disease reported by von Prowazek and Halberstaedter (137,138). Epidemiologic data concerning the incidence of trachoma, "paratrachoma" and the so-called swimming-pool conjunctivitis were published (4, 18, 25, 26, 34, 40, 59, 63, 96, 105, 112, 115, 117, 125, 126, 147, 148). Although in these years the genuine idea of a sexually transmitted disease had been well established by many researchers (64,92,93), interest faded in the middle of the century and infection in adults was reported only sporadically (49,103). Until these days, ophthalmologists attempted to focus on probable non-sexual modes of transmission, a circumstance, which still contributes to many a misunderstanding in textbooks of ophthalmology and creates treatment failures. In 1910, improved staining techniques (39), work on the infectious entity ("initial forms" (91)) and the stages of chlamydial replication had already been published by ophthalmologists. The spectrum of differential diagnosis in infectious kerato-conjunctivitis enlarged, however, a great number of viral and bacterial pathogens could not yet be detected (5, 34, 83, 94, 156, 158).

Despite successful attempts to grow chlamydiae in cell cultures since 1933 (20, 57, 139, 157), a reliable and systematic approach could not be performed until the end of the 1950ies primarily due to the lack of established detection methods (151). Then, advances in microbiology led to the differentiation of several non-bacterial external infections of the eye caused by Adenovirus (27,77,106,107), Herpes simplex virus (52,88,120,162), Newcastle disease virus (95) or mycoplasmas (35), which exhibited distinctly different features compared with trachoma-like disease (108). In the sixties, interest again focussed on chlamydial disease in the developed countries (72,73,129).

Epidemiology of Chlamydial Infections

Today, chlamydial infections rate as the most frequent sexually transmitted disease in the world (21, 32, 55, 85, 109, 111, 113, 130, 145, 146, 153, 164). In the USA, 3-4 million new cases of chlamydial infections are estimated each year. Up to 62% of gonococcal infections are coinfected with C.trachomatis (70, 130, 153). Ocular involvement in chlamydial infections of non-endemic countries mostly occurs via genito-ocular transfer of infectious material (109); a rare case of eye-to-eye transmission has been reported (72).

Almost exclusively, oculogenital infections are caused by the serovars D through K (159). Oculogenital infections due to serovar B, however, have been reported in Denmark recently (84). More than 90% of female patients with culture-positive chlamydial infections of the eye yield positive cultures from genital sites (74).

In keratoconjunctivitis clinics, oculogenital chlamydial disease may represent 6-19% of bacterial infections (9, 11, 68, 124, 159, 161). Reported incidences have been published in - Great Britain: Viswalingham: 18.6% (out of 2166 patients),

- Denmark: Mordhorst: 18.0% (out of 1001 patients),
- Sweden: Rönnerstam: 15.5% (out of 800 patients),
- Germany: Bialasiewicz: 9.7% (out of 2408 patients),
- Austria: Huber-Spitzy: 6.0% (out of 89 patients).

The most notable reasons for the differing incidences of chlamydial infections in the quoted infectious disease units are promiscuity, particularly simultaneous sex partners

(164), age and neighborhood area (11).- In the area of Erlangen-Nürnberg with its mixed rural/urban population, incidence rates of about 7% culture-positive and 9.7% culture- and IgA-seropositive patients could be stated in 1985-1989. In the sexually active ages of 20 to 30, the incidence was 12.5%.

Coinfections of chlamydiae with conventional bacteria are common and can be detected in one third of patients with chlamydial infections (11). Most frequent isolates include coagulase-negative staphylococci (75%), coagulase-positive staphylococci (50%), hemolysing streptococci (12%) and others (12%). Infected mothers transmit the agent at a rate of 25%-70% (23, 38, 50, 60, 98, 144, 150, 154). English, American and Swedish investigations have found an incidence of chlamydial cervicitis in 3%-37% of regularly screened apparently healthy pregnant women (54, 60, 67, 101, 150, 154). In Germany, similar data have been reported from Tübingen, Würzburg and Kiel (67,101,144). Approximately 18%-50% of exposed neonates will develop blennorrhea, 15%-20% naso-pharyngeal infections, 3%-18% pneumonitis and less than 5% otitis media (1,132,136). In the area of Erlangen-Nürnberg less than 6% of neonatal ocular infections are caused by C.trachomatis (102). Almost one third of patients with ocular chlamydial disease mention a history of post-gonococcal urethritis or cervicitis (11,105). A culture-established diagnosis of ocular C.psittaci infections has only rarely been reported in the literature (71,114). Although the incidence of rhino-conjunctival C.psittaci infections in pet cats is high (>5%) and frequent transmission can be expected, human C.psittaci conjunctivitis probably is underdiagnosed because of the lacking specificity of routine laboratory procedures for this agent (71).

Lymphogranuloma venereum (serovars L_{1-3}) has up to now only- been known cause follicular conjunctivitis in Parinaud's syndrome (3, 45, 89, 90, 134, 155). In the wake of the AIDS epidemic, however, a case report of a patient seroconverted for Human Immunodeficiency Virus has documented bilateral necrotizing corneal ulcers due to C.trachomatis L_2.

Ophthalmologists can only rarely diagnose infection-associated syndromes ("Reiter's") first, since arthralgias/arthritis and genital disease are the presenting symptoms. In Germany, anterior uveitis of C.trachomatis-associated infectious disease is a rare event, which has been observed by us in only two patients from 1985-1992. In women, conjunctivitis may be found in 52% and arthralgias in 72% (33,145,165). Chlamydiae can only be isolated from the conjunctiva as an exception (30,160). Ocular, skin and joint disease are commonly seen as para-infectious events although some reports also point at the existence of elementary bodies in joints (100,110).

Clinical Work-Up of Patients with Oculogenital Chlamydial Disease

Patients complain about an acutely diseased or chronic "red eye", often combined with a blepharitis, foreign body sensation, and photophobia, while itching and burning are mentioned less. Bilateral symptoms can always be found, although some time may elapse before the second eye becomes involved; a feature reported as early as 1928 (16). A complete history of genital diseases and sex partners must be taken by the diagnosing ophthalmologist Additionally, infectious diseases of pets should be evaluated in order to rule out C.psittaci infections (79). History and microbiologic work-up of genital specimens must include the parents of neonates with blennorrhea even when asymptomatic.

Ocular Features

The spectrum of ocular manifestations of C.trachomatis infections often encountered in keratoconjunctivitis clinics in developed countries in adults may include

- conjunctival hyperemia - hyposphagma and tarsal follicles (Fig.1),
- putrid follicular conjunctivitis and accompanying blepharitis,
- papillary conjunctivitis,
- epibulbar follicles,
- superficial epithelial and subepithelial infiltrates (Fig.2,3),
- epithelial defects and infiltration of Bowman's layer,
- corneal phlyctenules,
- corneal vascular pannus, and
- corneal scarring and vascularization accompanied by a mucus-deficiency syndrome (Fig.4)(17, 28, 29, 53, 149).

In some rare cases, long-standing oculogenital chlamydial disease may result in a decrease in visual acuity necessitating lamellar corneal grafting (12, 53). Overall, corneal involvement in oculogenital serovars of C.trachomatis is less severe than in endemic trachoma, and occurs in 35%-80% of primary lesions in adults (10, 28, 29). As has been gathered from experiments in human volunteers, most chlamydial infections will only produce a follicular conjunctivitis after one inoculation (28). Corneal phlyctenular reactions in chlamydial infections are rare and have been defined as pathogen-free accumulations of lymphocytic and monocytic cells (24,62).

The staging for endemic trachoma by the World Health Organization differentiates TF (trachomatous follicular), TI (trachomatous intense), TC (trachomatous cicatrization), TT (trachomatous trichiasis) and CO (corneal opacity) and cannot be transferred completely to oculogenital infections in developed countries. Cicatrization and trichiasis are missing in this spectrum and a chla-mydial epithelial keratitis (E) stage should be added, thus leaving CF (chlamydial follicular), CE (chlamydial epithelial), CI (chlamydial intense) and CO as a useful staging of ocular features of chlamydial infections.

Ocular manifestations of neonatal chlamydial infections are mostly seen in the second week after birth with a range between the 1st-20th day; it occurs rarely if ever later than that. The acute disease presents with a mucopurulent conjunctivitis and blennorrhea without corneal involvement (13,69,133). Untreated, conjunctival papillae will develop and a micropannus may become apparent (66). It is mandatory that the caring physician exclude a coinfection, since this is of utmost importance to prevent loss of vision and destruction of the globe as well as oculogenic septicemia (14). The cornea must be visualized, even if general anesthesia is required (12).

Laboratory Diagnosis

Routine screening methods for the diagnosis of oculogenital chlamydial infections include

- cultivation of conjunctival smears in cell cultures (McCoy,HeLA, BHK etc.),
- direct assays of conjunctival smears (monoclonal antibody direct tests to detect elementary bodies, enzyme immunoassays etc.) and
- tests to detect seroconversion (enzyme-linked immunosorbent assays, indirect immunofluorescent antibody assays, immunoperoxidase techniques etc.) (7, 15, 19, 22, 36, 41, 43, 97, 119, 123, 128, 131, 152).

The sensitivities and specificities of selected tests for the diagnosis of adult oculogenital chlamydial infections compiled from the literature are provided as averages:

- McCoy cell culture (Fig.5): sensitivity: 80%, specificity: 99%
- monoclonal antibody direct test (Fig.6): sensitivity: 100%, specificity: 50%
- enzyme immunoassay: sensitivity: 95%, specificity: 90%
- IgA-IPA (Fig.7): sensitivity: 100%, specificity: 70%
- IgG-IFT (Fig.8): sensitivity: 94%, specificity: 67%

The gold standard of laboratory diagnosis of chlamydial infections of the eye is the cell culture inoculated with conjunctival probes containing infected epithelial cells.

The use of monoclonal antibody direct tests and enzyme immunoassays is indicated in

- neonatal conjunctivitis,
- severe mucopurulent oculogenital keratoconjunctivitis and
- endemic trachoma TI.

The value of these tests for the diagnosis of chronic adult chlamydial oculogenital infections has not been established.

The predictive values for the IgG-detecting methods are unacceptably low.

The IgA-detecting immunoperoxidase test should be reserved for patients with an active salpingitis, whereas in urethritis patients this test is not worthwhile to perform (81).

Therapy

Medical therapy can be initiated after the repective sex partners have been evaluated. According to the recommendations of the Center for Disease Control, systemic doxycyline should be started at 200 mg/d for 7 days (143). In pregnancy, erythromycin is preferred at 2x1 g/d for 7 days and in newborn erythromycin 50 mg/kg/d for 14 days (135,143). In some cases, systemic antibiotic therapy must be prolonged up to 4 weeks.

Medical therapy has been recommended along the lines of in vitro minimal inhibitory concentrations:

- MIC erythromycin: 0.2-10.0μg/ml,
- MIC tetracyclines: 0.2-1.0μg/ml,
- MIC ofloxacin: 0.4-1.0μg/ml
- MIC ciprofloxacin: 0.6-2.5mg/ml,
- MIC rosaramycin: 0.01μg/ml,
- MIC rifamycin: 0.007mg/ml,
- MIC sulfamethoxazole: 0.5-4.0μg/ml,
- MIC penicillin G: 1.0->50.0μg/ml
- MIC amoxycillin: 15μg/ml

Systemic therapy may be supplemented by topical chlamydia-effective antibiotics and anti-inflammatory ointment.

Problems after "cure" (meaning the persistence of clinical symptoms with negative isolation attempts) most often include a post-infectious dry eye the syndrome, caused by a loss of goblet cells with resulting mucin deficiency (87). Artificial tears are sufficient to treat this transient unpleasant condition.

Surgical therapy is seldom required, but may include lamellar keratectomy and lamellar keratoplasty for visual rehabilitation (12) as well as modified lacrimal drainage and lid surgery (31).

Comment

The ophthalmologist plays a key role in the diagnosis of chlamydial infections that can be elaborated through a genuine cooperation with a bacteriologist and a virologist. The diagnosis is important from the standpoint of preventive medicine, since chlamydial infections are the most frequent cause of infectious female infertility, can cause salpingitis, and increased morbidity in pregnancy (61, 99, 163) as well as prostatitis (80) and epididymitis with possible subsequent infertility in man (8, 56, 75). Chronic chlamydial infections have been suspected to increase the risk of cervical neoplasia (55,116). Maternal -neonatal transmission may result in pneumonitis (118, 150) or otitis media (51) as well as blennorrhea and in untreated cases vision-threatening vascular pannus (66, 121, 133, 136, 154).. Pregnant women with a culture-established chlamydial infection should be cured before giving birth (135).

Diagnosis of chlamydial infections may prevent antibiotic or various other therapeutic unnecessary interventions including gynecologic surgery and is therefore of utmost economic importance. Expenses for the treatment of undiagnosed chlamydial infections are estimated at almost 1 billion US$ every year (111), and may be expected acvcordingly for other developed countries.

A mutual cooperation between ophthalmologists, dermato-venerologists, gynecologists, urologists, rheumatologists, microbiologists and virologists should be sought to improve the diagnostic strategies and facilitate specific treatment (127).

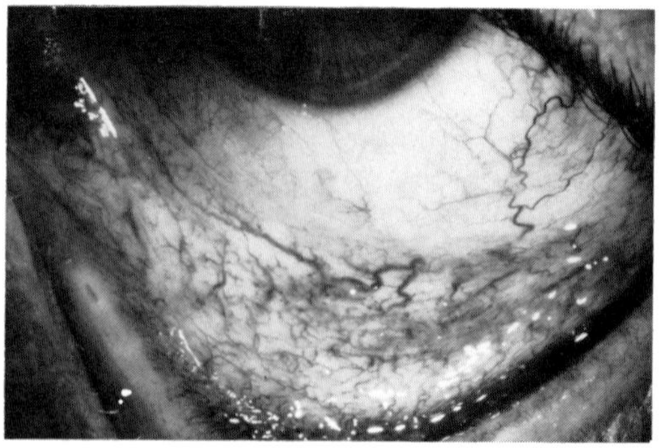

Fig.1 Follicular conjunctivitis in oculogenital chlamydial infection.

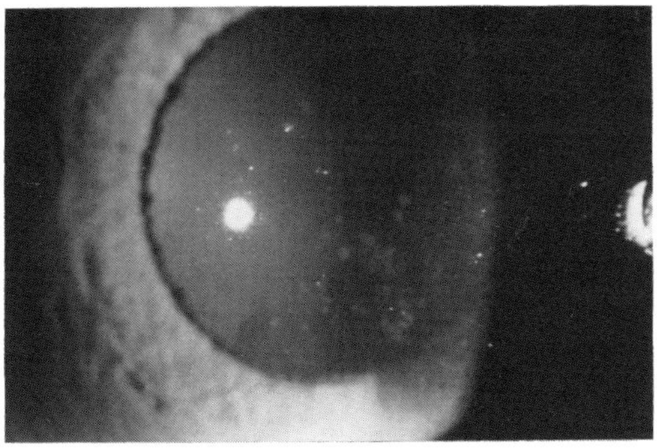

Fig.2 Epithelial irregularly shaped corneal infiltrates in oculogenital chlamydial infection.

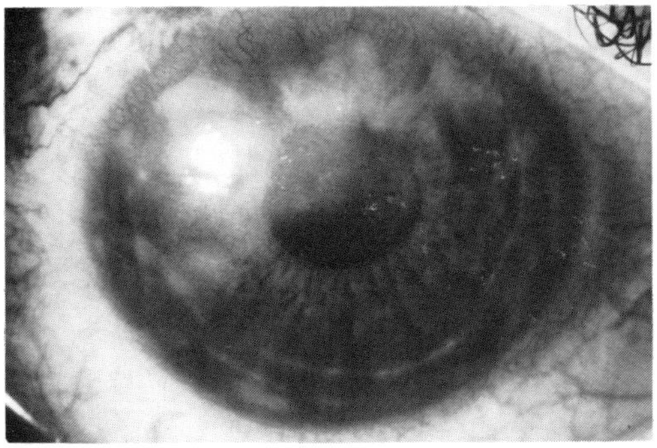

Fig.4
Corneal vascular pannus and corneal scarring in a patient with a five-year history of oculogenital chlamydial infection.

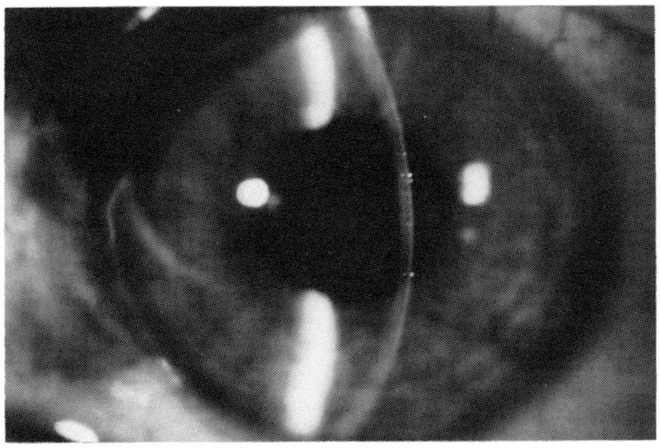

Fig.3 Subepithelial corneal infiltrates in oculogenital chlamydial infection.

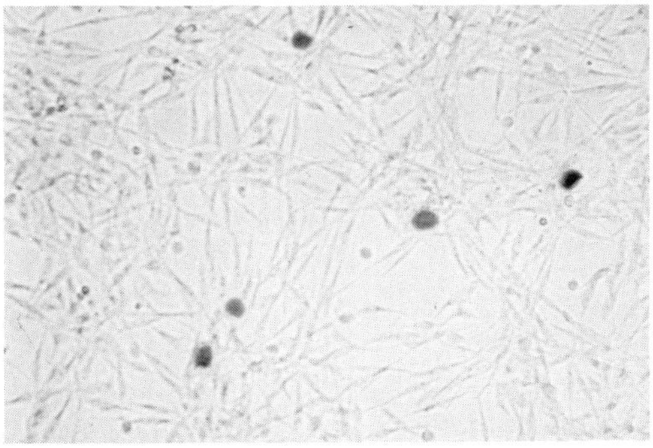

Fig.5 Iodine-stained C.trachomatis inclusion bodies in McCoy cell culture.

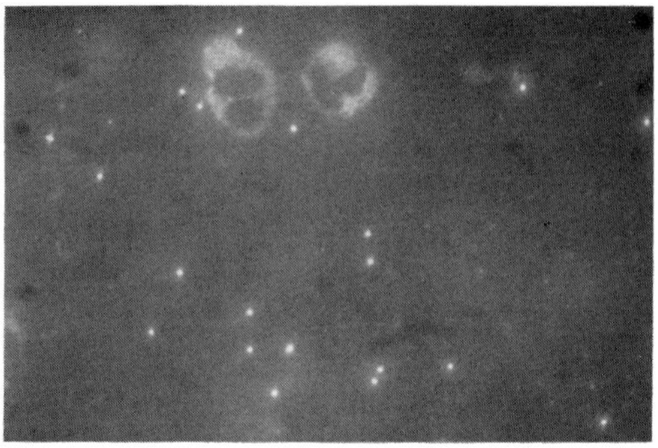

Fig.6 Elementary bodies stained green by fluorescent monoclonal antibody direct test.

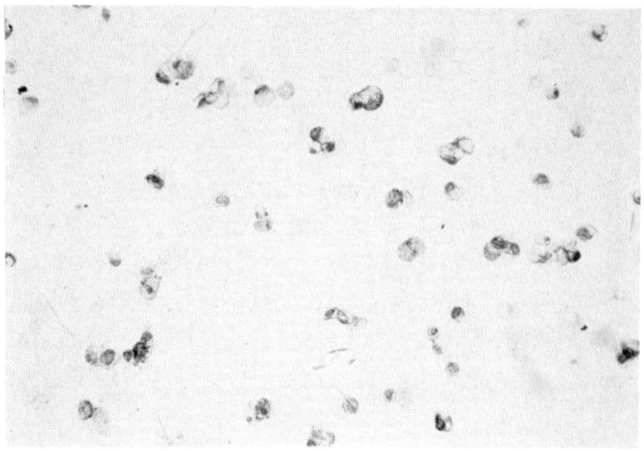

Fig.7 Black-stained inclusion bodies incubated with patient serum containing chlamydia-specific IgA antibodies.

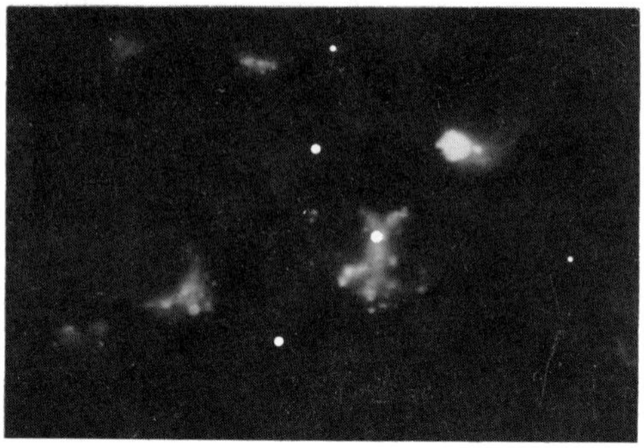

Fig.8 Indirect immunofluorescent assay with chlamydia-specific IgG antibodies marking inclusions.

References:

1. Alexander ER, Harrison HR (1983) Role of C.Trachomatis in Perinatal Infections. Rev Inf Dis 5/4:713-719
2. 2.Amor BA (1983) Chlamydia and Reiter Syndrome. Br J Rheumatol 22/2:156-160
3. Appelmans M (1938) Conjonctivite Infectieuse de Parinaud Causé par le Virus de la Maladie de Nicolas-Favre. Ophthalmologica 96:321-332
4. Aust O (1929) Beiträge zur Trachomforschung. Graefes Arch. Ophth 123:93
5. Bartels R (1911) Ein Beitrag zur Augeneiterung der Neugeborenen. Kl Mbl Augenhlkd 69:537-561
6. Becker N, Meyer N (1954) Conjunctivitis follicularis ohne Trachomsymptome (1876) zitiert nach L.Poleff
7. Bell TA, Kuo CC, Stamm WE et al (1984) Direct Fluorescent Monoclonal Antibody Stain for Detection of Infant Chlamydia

Trachomatis Infections. Pediatrics 74/2:224-228
8. Berger RE, Alexander ER, Harnisch JP et al (1979) Etiology, Manifestations and Therapy of Acute Epididymitis: Prospective Study of 50 Cases. J Urol 121:750-754
9. Bialasiewicz AA, Barthelmeß S, Lang GK et al (1984) Zur Abklärung infektiöser äußerer entzündlicher Augenerkrankungen. Klin Mbl Augenhlkd 185:274-276
10. Bialasiewicz AA, Junkenitz A, Jahn GJ (1985) Korneale Symptomatik bei chlamydienbedingten Keratokonjunktivitiden. Klin Mbl Augenhlkd 187:36-39
11. Bialasiewicz AA, Jahn GJ (1986) Epidemiology of Chlamydial Eye Infections in a Mixed Rural/Urban Population of West Germany. Ophthalmology 93/6:757-762
12. Bialasiewicz AA, Jahn GJ (1986) Mehrjähriger Verlauf einer okulogenitalen Chlamydieninfektion. Klin Mbl Augenhlkd 190:50-52
13. Bialasiewicz AA, Jahn GJ (1986) Neugeborenenblennorrhoe. Z Prakt Augenhklkd 7:172-183
14. Bialasiewicz AA, Deeg KH (1986) Gruppe B Streptokokken-Panophthalmie bei Neugeborenen-Sepsis. Klin Mbl Augenhlkd 189:251-253
15. Bialasiewicz AA, Radtke U, Jahn GJ (1986) Diagnostik von okulären Chlamydieninfektionen durch Direktnachweis: Klin Mbl Augenhlkd 191:106-109
16. Blatt N (1928) Einseitiges Trachom. Klin Mbl Augenhlkd 81:810-822
17. Blenk H, Jahn GJ, Bialasiewicz AA et al (1982) Einseitige Keratitis, verursacht durch einen C.trachomatis-Subtyp. Graefes Arch Ophth 218:301-303
18. Botteri A (1912) Klinische, experimentelle und mikroskopische Studien über Trachom, Einschlußblennorrhoe und Frühjahrskatarrh. Klin Mbl Augenhlkd 50/1:653
19. Bowie B, Holmes KK (1979) C.Trachomatis. In: Mandell GL, Gordon-Douglas R, Bennett JE (eds) Principles and Practice of Infectious Diseases. Wiley Publications. New York pp.1464-1476
20. Braley AE (1949) Experimental Studies of Inclusion Blennorrhea: Isolation of a Virus. Arch Ophthalmol 41/2:151-171
21. Burns DCM, Darougar S, Finn FN et al (1975) Isolation of Chlamydia from Women Attending a Clinic for Sexually Transmitted Disease. Br J Ven Dis 51:314-318
22. Cevenini R, Rumpianese F, Donati M et al (1983) A Rapid Immunoperoxidase Assay for the Detection of Specific IgG-Antibodies to C. Trachomatis. J Clin Pathol 36:353-356
23. Chandler JW, Alexander IR, Pfeiffer TA et al (1977) Ophthalmia Neonatorum Associated with Maternal and Chlamydial Infections. Trans Am Ac Ophthalmol Otolaryngol 83:302-308
24. Cohen C (1909) Über die Phlyktaene bei Erwachsenen. Klin Mbl Augenhlkd 60:405-416
25. Comberg W (1920) Über Badconjunctivitis. Z Augenhlkd 44:13
26. Comberg W (1925) Bemerkungen über die Einteilung der Einschlußkrankheiten mit besonderer Berücksichtigung klinisch verwandter Bindehautleiden. Z Augenhlkd 56:109
27. Dawson CR, Darrell R (1963) Infections Due to Adenovirus Type 8 in the United States. New Engl J Med 268:1031
28. Dawson CR, Jawetz E, Hanna L et al (1966) Experimental Inclusion Conjunctivitis in Man. Am J Epidemiol 84/3:411-425
29. Dawson CR, Thygeson P, Wood R et al (1967) Keratitis and Other Complications in Volunteers Infected with Inclusion Conjunctivitis Agents. Rev Intern Trach 1:7-14
30. Dawson CR, Schachter J, Ostler H et al (1971) Inclusion Conjunctivitis Syndrome in a Married Couple. Arch Ophthalmol 83:300-306

31. Denig A (1911) Transplantation bei chronischem trachomatösen Pannus. Z Augenhlkd 125:278
32. Dunlop MC, Vaughan-Jackson JD, Darougar S (1972) Chlamydial Infection: Incidence in Non-Specific Urethritis. Br J Ven Dis 48:425-458
33. Editorial: (1985) Is Reiter's Syndrome Caused by Chlamydia? Lancet I:317-319
34. Engelking E (1925) Die Schwimmbadconjunctivitis in ihren Beziehungen zum Trachom, zur Einschlußblennorrhoe und zur Gonorrhoe. Klin Mbl Augenhlkd 74:622
35. Erm HG, Woolrich RL, Cheng KH et al (1966) Isolation of Mycoplasma Organisms from the Human Eye. AJO 62/3:1125
36. Evans RT, Taylor-Robinson D (1982) Development and Evaluation of an Enzyme-Linked Immunosorbent Assay (ELISA), Using Chlamydial Group Antigen to Detect Antibodies to C.Trachomatis. J Clin Pathol 35:1122-1128
37. Fritsch H, Hofstetter A, Lindner K (1910) Experimentelle Studien zur Trachomfrage. Graefes Arch Ophth 76/3:547-558
38. Frommell GT, Rothenberg R, Wang SP et al (1979) Chlamydial Infections of Mothers and their Infants. J Ped 95:28-32
39. Gallenga C (1910) Zur Färbung der Prowazek-Halberstaedterschen Trachomkörper. Klin Mbl Augenhlkd 68/1:195-196
40. Gebb H (1914) Experimentelle Untersuchungen über die Beziehungen zwischen Einschlußblennorrhoe und Trachom. Z Augenhlkd 31:475
41. Gerhard-Fsadni D, Krech T, Hofman N et al (1985) Nachweis von C. trachomatis mit monoklonalen Antikörpern: Empfindlichkeit und Spezifität. Labormed 9:156
42. Gilbke T (1896) Der akute epidemische Schwellungskatarrh und sein Erreger: eine klinische und bakteriologische Untersuchung. Graefes Arch Ophth 62/4:97-150
43. Gordon FB, Quan AL (1965) Isolation of the Trachoma Agent in Cell Culture. Proc Soc Exp Biol Med 118:354-359
44. Groenow A (1901) Augenentzündungen der Neugeborenen in klinischer und bakteriologischer Hinsicht. Graefes Arch Ophth 52:1-71
45. Guze PA, Bayer AF, Anthony BF et al (1981) Spectrum of Human Chlamydial Infections. West J Med 135:208-225
46. Halberstaedter L, v.Prowazek F (1907) Zur Ätiologie des Trachoms. Dtsch Med Wchschr 32:1285-1287
47. Halberstaedter L, v.Prowazek F (1907) Über Zelleinschlüsse parasitärer Natur beim Trachom. Arbeiten aus dem Kaiserlichen Gesundheitsamte 26:44-47
48. Halberstaedter L, v.Prowazek F (1909) Über Chlamydozoenbefunde bei Blennorhoea neonatorum nongonorrhoica. Berl Klin Wchschr 46:1838
49. Hamburger FA (1934) Die Rolle des Einschlußvirus am Auge des Neugeborenen und am Genitale der Frau. Graefes Arch Ophth 133:90
50. Hammerschlag MR, Anderka M, Semine DZ et al (1979) Prospective Study of Maternal and Infantal Infection with C.Trachomatis. Pediatrics 64:142-148
51. Hammerschlag MR, Hammerschlag P, Alexander ER (1980) The Role of C.Trachomatis in Middle Ear Effusions in Children. Pediatrics 66/4
52. Hanna L, Davids E, Coleman VR (1957) Studies on Herpes Simplex. The Significance of Isolating Herpes Simplex Virus from the Eye. AJO 43/2:126-131
53. Hanna L, Jawetz E, Dawson CR et al (1982) Longtime Clinical Microbiological, and Immunological Observations of a Volunteer Repeatedly Infected C.Trachomatis. J Clin Microbiol 16/5:895-900
54. Hardy PH, Hardy JB, Nell EE et al (1984) Prevalence of sic STD Agents among Pregnant Innercity Adolescents and Pregnancy Outcome. Lancet II:333-337
55. Hare MJ, McCoq MA, Finn RN (1983) Chlamydial Infection of the Lower Genital Tract of Women. Br Med Bull 39:138-144

56. Harnisch JP, Berger RE, Alexander ER (1977) Etiology of Acute Epididymitis. Lancet I:819-821
57. Harrison RW, Julianelle LA (1937) Studies on the Infectivity of Trachoma: Cultivatibility of the Infectious Agent in Tissue Culture. AJO 20:360
58. Haupt M (1903) Über gonorrhoische und nichtgonorrhoische Bindehautentzündungen bei Neugeborenen. Klin Mbl Augenhlkd 60/1: 447-471
59. Hegner CA (1911) Über die Histologie der experimentell erzeugten Einschlußconjunctivitis. Klin Mbl Augenhlkd 49/1:440
60. Heggie AD, Lumicao GG, Stuart LA et al (1981) C.Trachomatis Infections in Mothers and Infants. Am J Dis Child 135:507-511
61. Henry-Suchet J, Catalan F, Lofredo V et al (1980) Microbiology of Specimens Obtained by Laparascopy from Controls and from Patients with Pelvic Inflammatory Disease or Infantility with Tubal Obstruction: Chlamydia Trachomatis and Ureaplasma Urealyticum. Am J Obstet Gyn 138:1022-1025
62. Hertel E (1898) Anatomische Untersuchungen eines Falles von phlyktänulärer Keratoconjunctivitis. Graefes Arch Ophth 46/3:630-638
63. Herzog H (1910) Über die Ätiologie des Trachoms. Ber Dtsch Ophth Ges 36:240
64. Heymann B (1910) Über die Fundorte der Prowazek'schen Körperchen. Berl Klin Wchschr 47:663
65. Hirsch G (1897) Die Art der Ausbreitung des Trachoms im Rheinisch-Westfälischen Industriebezirk. Graefes Arch Ophth 43/3:706-713
66. Hobson D, Rees E (1983) Chlamydial Infections in Neonates and Older Children. Br Med Bull 39:128-132
67. Hoyme UB (1983) Chlamydia trachomatis - Epidemiologische Daten aus der Univ.-Frauenklinik Tübingen. Geburtsh u Frauenhlkd 43:363-365
68. Huber-Spitzy V, Stary A, Grabner G et al (1985) Klinik, Diagnose und Therapie der okulären Chlamydieninfektion. Klin Mbl Augenhlkd 187:363-365
69. Jahn GJ, Bialasiewicz AA (1983) Massive Blennorrhoe beim Neugeborenen durch einen Subtyp von Chlamydia trachomatis. Klin Mbl Augenhlkd 183/6:467-470
70. Jahn GJ, Bialasiewicz AA, Jenisch A et al (1984) The Importance and Frequency of Mixed Infections with C.Trachomatis and Mycoplasmas in Acute Gonococcal Urethritis. S Afr Med J 65:462-467
71. Jahn GJ, Bialasiewicz AA (1985) Keratokonjunktivitis durch Chlamydia psittaci. Klin Mbl Augenhlkd 188:47-49
72. Jones BR (1964) Ocular Syndromes of TRIC Virus Infections and the Possible Genital Significance. Br J Ven Dis 40:3-18
73. Jones BR (1964) Genital Trachoma. Rev Int Trach 41:425-438
74. Jones BR, Alhussain K, Dunlop E (1965) Infection of the Eye and Genital Tract by TRIC Agent: Ocular Syndromes Associated with Infections of the Genital Tract by TRIC Agent. Rev Int Trach Patrol Ocul Trop Subtrop 42:27-43
75. Kaufmann RD, Wiesner PJ (1974) Nonspecific Urethritis. New Engl J Med 291:1175-1177
76. Keat A, Thomas BJ, Taylor-Robinson D (1983) Chlamydial Infection in the Etiology of Arthritis. Br Med Bull 39:169-174
77. Kendall EJC, Riddle RB, Tuck HA et al (1957) Pharyngo-Conjunctival Fever. School Outbreaks in England during the Summer 1955 Associated with Adenovirus 3,7 and 14. Br Med J 131:5037
78. Kousa M, Saikku T, Richmond S et al (1978) Frequent Association of Chlamydial Infection with Reiter's Syndrome. Sex Trans Dis 57-61
79. Kraus H (1982) Die Bedeutung von Rickettsien und Chlamydien bei kleinen Haustieren als Erreger von Zoonosen. Berl Klin Wchschr 95:480

80. Kraus H, Schiefer HG, Weidner W et al (1983) Significance of C.Trachomatis in a Bacterial Prostatitis. Zbl Bakt Hyg Abt 1 Originalien A 254:541-551
81. Krech T (1986) Chlamydieninfektionen: Schnellerer Nachweis und gezielte Therapie. Dt Ärztebl 93:394-404
82. Kroner T (1884) Zur Ätiologie der Ophthalmo-Blennorrhoea neonatorum. Zbl Gyn 41:643-645
83. Krückmann E (1930) Einige Mitteilungen über den sog. Frühjahrskatarrh. Ber Dtsch Ophth Ges p. 308
84. Kuo CC, Wang SP, Holmes KK et al (1983) Immunotypes of C.Trachomatis Isolates. Inf Immunol 41/2:815-818
85. Ladany S, Sarov I (1985) Recent Advances in C.Trachomatis. Eur J Epidemiol 1/4: 235-256
86. Lang E (1896) Über die sog. Spätinfektion der Ophthalmo-Blennorrhoea neonatorum. Arbeiten aus dem Gebiet der Geburtshilfe und der Gynäkologie. Festschrift für C.Ruge, Berlin. pp.136-142
87. Leedham-Green C (1894) Über die Bedeutung der Becherzellen der Conjunctiva. Graefes Arch Ophth 60/1:1-21
88. Lenette E, van Allen A (1957) The Laboratory Diagnosis of Herpetic Infections of the Eye. AJO 33/2:118-125
89. Levaditi C, Bollack J, Basch G (1936) Desvignes: Conjonctivite avec Adenopathie du Virus de la Maladie de Nicolas-Favre (Lymphogranoulomatose à Localisation Oculaire). Bull Soc Franc Derm 43:1238-1243
90. Levaditi C, Schön R, Renier LL (1936) Reproduction Experimentale de la Conjonctivite Lymphogranoulomateuse (Maladie de Nicolas-Favre) chez les Chimpanzee. Cr Acad Sci Paris 203:828-830
91. Lindner K (1910) Die freie Initialform der Prowazek'schen Einschlüsse. Graefes Arch Ophth 76/3:559-567
92. Lindner K (1911) Gonoblennorhoe, Einschlußblennorrhoe und Trachom. Graefes Arch Ophth 78:245
93. Lindner K (1925) Gibt es ein genitales Trachom? Wiener Med Wchschr 75:2488
94. Lindner K (1925) Über die Schwierigkeiten der Trachomforschung. Z Augenhlkd 57:508
95. Lippmann O (1952) Human Conjunctivitis Due to the Newcastle Disease Virus of Fowls. AJO 35:1021
96. Löhlein W (1912) Klinischer und experimenteller Beitrag zur Frage der Bedeutung der am Auge gefundenen Epitheleinschlüsse. Graefes Arch Ophth 70:392
97. Mahoney JB, Chernessky MA (1985) Effect of Swab Type and Storage Temperature on the Isolation of C.Trachomatis from Clinical Specimens. J Clin Microbiol 22/5:865-867
98. Mardh PA, Healin I, Bobeck S (1980) Colonization of Pregnant and Puerperal Women and Neonates with C.Trachomatis. Br J Ven Dis 56:96-100
99. Martin DH, Koutzki L, Eschenbach DA et al (1982) Prematurity and Perinatal Mortality in Pregnant Size Complicated by Maternal C.Trachomatis Infections. JAMA 247:1585-1588
100. Martin DH, Pollock S, Kuo CC et al (1984) C.Trachomatis Infections in Man with Reiter's Syndrome. Ann Intern Med 100:207-213
101. Martius J, Becker I, Hartmann AA (1983) Chlamydia trachomatis im Urogenitaltrakt bei Schwangeren. Geburtsh Frauenhlkd 43:366-369
102. Mayer UM, Bialasiewicz AA (1985) Resistenzbestimmungen und Antibiotikatherapie bei bakteriellen Augenerkrankungen des Kindesalters. Klin Mbl Augenhlkd 187:517-520
103. McKey SJ (1942) Ophthalmia Neonatorum: Etiology in 60 Consecutive Cases. AJO 1:52-58

104. Meyerhof M (1905) Über die akuten eitrigen Bindehautentzündungen in Ägypten. Klin Mbl Augenhlkd 63/2:216-237
105. Meyerhof M (1908) Follikelbildung im Hornhautpannus bei Trachom. Klin Mbl Augenhlkd 66/2:353-359
106. Mitsui Y, Hanabusa J, Minoda R et al (1957) Effect of Inoculating Adenovirus Type 8 in the Human Volunteers. AJO 43/2:84
107. Mitsui Y, Hanna L, Minoda R et al (1959) Experiments in Human Volunteers with Adenovirus Type 8. Br J Ophthalmol 43:540
108. Mitsui Y (1964) Relation between Trachoma and Inclusion Conjunctivitis. Rev Int Trach 41:252
109. Mordhorst CH (1977) In: Hobson D, Holmes KK (eds) Nongonococcal Urethritis and Related Infections. Am Soc Microbiol Washington. pp 126-134
110. Morris R, Metzger A, Stone R (1974) HLA B 27 a Clue to the Diagnosis and Pathogenesis of Reiter's Syndrome. New Engl Med 290:554-556
111. Neidhart FC, Halverson HO, Hausler WJ (1982) The Chlamydia Problem. ASM News 48:306
112. Neubauer H (1921) Die Kölner Epidemie von Badconjunctivitis. Med Klin 279
113. Oriel JD, Powes PA, Reeve P (1974) Chlamydial Infections of the Cervix. Br J Ven Dis 50:11
114. Ostler HB, Schachter J, Dawson CR (1969) Acute Follicular Conjunctivitis of Epizootic Origin. Arch Ophthalmol 82:587-591
115. Paderstein R (1925) Was ist Schwimmbadconjunctivitis? Klin Mbl Augenhlkd 74:63-66
116. Paraavonen J, Brunham R, Tiviat N et al (1982) Cervicitis: Etiology, Clinical and Histopathologic Findings. In: Mardh PA, Holmes KK, Oriel JD et al (eds) Chlamydial Infections. Elsevier Biomed Press Amsterdam. pp 141-145
117. Pascheff C (1909) Über die Chlamydozoen der Trachomkörperchen und andere eigenartige Körperchen / Epithelzelleneinschlüsse. Graefes Arch Ophth 73/1:175-183
118. Peuckert W, Huys J, Pringsheim W et al (1981) Chlamydienpneumonien im jungen Säuglingsalter. Mschr. Kinderhlkd 129:575
119. Piura B, Sarov I, Sarov B et al (1985) Serum IgG and IgA Specific for C.Trachomatis in Salpingitis Patients as Determined by Immuno Peroxidase Assay. Eur J Epidemiol 1/2:110-116
120. Rake G (1957) The Etiologic Role of the Virus of Herpes Simplex in Ophthalmic Disease. AJO 43/2:113-118
121. Rees E, Tait IA, Hobson D et al (1977) Neonatal Conjunctivitis Caused by N.Gonorrhoeae and C.Trachomatis. Br Ven Dis 53:173
122. Reiter H (1916) Über eine bisher unerkannte Spirochäteninfektion. Dtsch Med Wchschr 42:1535-1536
123. Ripa KT, Mardh TA (1977) Cultivation of C.Trachomatis in Cyclohexamide Treated McCoy Cells. J Clin Microbiol 6:328-331
124. Rönnerstam R, Persson K, Hansson H (1985) Prevalence of Chlamydial Eye Infection in Patients Attending an Eye Clinic or a VD Clinic and in Healthy Persons. Br J Ophthalmol 69:385-388
125. Rohrschneider W (1926) Die Schwimmbadconjunctivitis und ihr endemisches Auftreten in Berlin. Klin Mbl Augenhlkd 76:619
126. Rohrschneider W (1926) Statistisches zur Berliner Schwimmbadconjunctivitis-Endemie. Z Augenhlkd 59:126
127. Roos R (1985) Entwicklung der klinischen Infektiologie. Die USA als Schrittmacher. Dt Ärztebl B 82/9:555-557
128. Saikku P, Paavonen J (1978) Single Antigen Immunofluorescent Test for Chlamydial Antibodies. J Clin Microbiol 8/2:119-122

129. Schachter J, Rose L, Meyer KF (1967) The Venereal Nature of Inclusion Conjunctivitis. Am J Epidemiol 85:445-452
130. Schachter J, Hanna L, Dewell IC et al (1975) Are Chlamydial Infections the Most Prevalent Venereal Disease? JAMA 231/12:1252-1255
131. Schachter J, Dawson CR (1977) Comparative Efficiency of Various Diagnostic Methods for Chlamydial Infections. In: Hobson D, Holmes KK (eds) Nongonococcal Urethritis and Related Infections. Am Soc Microbiol, Washington,DC.pp. 337-341
132. Schachter J, Holt J , Goodner E et al (1979) Prospective Study of Chlamydial Infection in Neonates. Lancet II:377-379
133. Schachter J, Grossman M (1981) Chlamydial Infections. Ann Rev Med 32:45-61
134. Schachter J, Osoba AO (1983) Lymphogranuloma Venereum. Br Med Bull 39:151-154
135. Schachter J, Sweet RL, Grossman M et al (1986) Experience with the Routine Use of Erythromycine for Chlamydial Infections in Pregnancy. New Engl J Med 314:276-279
136. Schaefer D, Harrison HR, Boyce WB et al (1985) Illness in Infants born to Women with C.Trachomatis Infection. Am J Child 139:127-133
137. Schmeichler L (1909) Über Chlamydozoenbefunde bei nichtgonorrhoischer Blennorrhoe der Neugeborenen. Berl Klin Wchschr 46:2057
138. Schmeichler L (1909) Aussprachebemerkungen zu K. Lindner: Demonstration von Prowazek'schen Einschlüssen. Z Augenhlkd 22:271
139. Schmitt R (1933) Züchtungsversuche der Einschlußkörper in die Gewebskultur. Klin Mbl Augenhlkd 91:683
140. Schneller A (1892) Über die Behandlung der follikulären Bindehauterkrankungen. Graefes Arch Ophth 38/4:52-95
141. Seefelder A (1906) Beiträge zur Lehre von den fötalen Augenentzündungen. Graefes Arch Ophth 64/1:224-236
142. Seitz GR, Linnemann CC, Brookman RR (1981) Chlamydia Trachomatis Cervical Infections in Female Adolescents. J Ped 98:981-985
143. Sexually Transmitted Disease (STD) Treatment Guide Lines (1985) MMWR 34/45:77-78
144. Simon C, Hoeger P, Toeller W et al (1982) Vorkommen und Diagnostik von C.trachomatis-Infektionen bei Neugeborenen und Säuglingen. Infektionen 10/2:79-83
145. Smith DL, Bennett RM, Reagan NG (1980) Reiter's Disease in Women. Arthritis and Rheumatism 23/3:335-340
146. Stamm WE, Holmes KK (eds) (1981) Chlamydial Infections. West J Med 135:226-229
147. Stargardt K (1908) Epithelzellen vom akuten Trachom mit Prowazek-Halberstaedter'schen Körperchen. Ber Dtsch Ophth Ges 35:329
148. Stargardt K (1909) Über Epithelzellveränderungen bei Trachom und anderen Conjunctivalerkrankungen. Graefes Arch Ophth 69/3:525-542
149. Sundmacher R, Harnisch P, Darougar S et al (1981) Chlamydienerkrankungen des Auges. Klin Mbl Augenhlkd 179:149-156
150. Sweet RL, Schachter J, Landers DV (1983) Chlamydial Infections in Obstetrics and Gynecology. Clin Obstet Gyn 26:143-164
151. Tang FF, Chang HL, Huang YK et al (1957) Studies on the Etiology of Trachoma with Special Reference to Isolation of the Virus in Chick Embryo. Nt Chin Med J 43:81-86
152. Taylor HR, Agarwala N, Johnson SL (1984) Detection of Experimental C.Trachomatis Eye Infection in Conjunctival Smears and in Tissue Culture by Use of Fluorescein-Conjugated Monoclonal Antibody. J Clin Microbiol 20/3:391-395

153. Taylor-Robinson D, Thomas BJ (1980) The Role of Chlamydia Trachomatis in Genital Tract and Associated Diseases. J Clin Path 33:205-233
154. Thompson SE, Tretter RH (1982) Epidemiology and Treatment of Chlamydial Infections in Pregnant Women and Infants. Rev Inf Dis 4:747-757
155. Thorsteinsson SB (1982) Lymphogranuloma Venereum: Review of Clinical Manifestations, Epidemiology, Diagnosis, and Treatment. Scand J Inf Dis 32:111-115
156. Thygeson P (1934) The Etiology of Inclusion Blennorrhea. AJO 17:1019
157. Thygeson P (1939) Cultivation of Trachomatous Conjunctival Epithelium in Vitro. Arch Ophthalmol 21:229-234
158. Ticho A (1915) Frühjahrskatarrh in Palästina. Klin Mbl Augenhlkd 154:510
159. Viswalingham ND, Wishart M, Woodland RM (1983) Adult Chlamydial Ophthalmia (Paratrachoma). Br Med Bull Chlamydial Dis 39:193
160. Wilpula AH, Illikerttula UI, Ahlroos AK et al (1981) Chlamydial Isolation and Serology in Reiter's Syndrome. Scand J Rheumatol 10:181-185
161. Wishart PK, James C, Wishart MS et al (1984) Prevalence of Acute Conjunctivitis Caused by Chlamydia, Adenovirus and Herpes Simplex Virus in Ophthalmic Casualty Department. Br J Ophthalmol 68:653-655
162. Witmer R, Iwamoto T (1968) Electron Microscopic Observation of Herpes-Like Particles in the Iris. Arch Ophthalmol 70:331-335
163. Wölner-Hanssen P, Weström L (1983) Second Look Laparascopy after Acute Salpingitis. Obstet Gyn 61:702-704
164. Woolfitt JMG, Watt L (1977) Chlamydial Infection of the Urogenital Tract in Promiscuous and Nonpromiscuous Women. Br J Ven Dis 53:93
165. Yly-Kerttula YLI, Selander UI, Takaterho PE et al (1984) The Nature of Urogenital Involvement in Female Uroarthritis with Special Reference to Chlamydial Infection. Clin Rheumatol 3:155-162

VII. Reiter's Syndrome

Pathogenesis of Reiter's Syndrome

T.E.W. Feltkamp

Abstract. Reiter's syndrome consists of arthritis, urethritis and conjunctivitis and is a non-purulent reaction to infections with Gram-negative intestinal bacteria or Chlamydia trachomatis.
The syndrome shows a strong association with HLA-B27. Probably HLA-B27 negative Reiter's syndrome follows another pathogenic pathway, since this type contrary to the syndrome in HLA-B27 positive individuals, rarely becomes chronic and is almost never complicated by sacroiliitis and acute anterior uveitis.

It is possible that the HLA class I molecule B27 itself is involved in the pathogenesis. The pathogenetic mechanism is, however, far from clear. The molecular mimicry between the HLA-B27 molecule and proteins of Klebsiella and Yersinia is probably not of pathogenetic significance. Also the studies on HLA-B27 transgenic animals unfortunately gave still no solid indication of a pathogenetic role of this molecule. Two clinical studies on small numbers suggested that there is no preference for one of the seven subtypes of HLA-B27. If this is so, the so-called "45 pocket" of the molecule is possibly of pathogenetic importance.

Apart from HLA-B27 other genetic factors are also involved in the pathogenesis. The genes for these factors are probably not situated on the short arm of chromosome 6 or on the tip of the long arm of chromosome 14. The rest of the genome is open for further studies.

Introduction

Reiter's syndrome consisting of arthritis, urethritis and conjunctivitis is a syndrome, which may occur as a part of the so- called "reactive arthritides". The term "reactive arthritis" indicates the non-purulent arthritis, which may complicate an infection elsewhere in the body (1). Reiter's syndrome can occur secondary to infections with Gram-negative intestinal bacteria (Campylobacter, Clostridium difficile, Salmonella, Shigella, Yersinia) and Chlamydia trachomatis. These bacteria are responsible for reactive arthritides which are strongly associated with the genetic marker and cell membrane protein HLA-B27. No association with HLA-B27 is observed in the reactive arthritis due to group A, ß-hemolytic Streptococcus pyogenes, known as rheumatic fever, and the reactive arthritis as a part of Lyme disease due to Borrelia burgdorferi.

HLA-B27

The frequency of HLA-B27 in patients with Reiter's syndrome is 80% (15). In normal controls from the same population the frequency is 9%. The relative risk, being the number of positive patients times the number of negative controls, divided by the number of negative patients times the number of positive controls is 37. This indicates a very strong association. It is possible that this association is even stronger if the HLA-B27 negative patients with Reiter's syndrome are considered as having another type of Reiter's syndrome. Linssen (9), compiling figures from McCluskey and coworkers, Calin and Fries, Nicholls and Willkens and coworkers showed that the HLA-B27 positive patients are more frequently males having a more severe and chronic disease, which is more frequently complicated by balanitis, spondylitis and acute anterior uveitis than the disease of the HLA-B27 negative patients (Tab.1).

Such discrepancies between HLA-B27 positive and HLA-B27 negative patients have also been described for acute anterior uveitis, ankylosing spondylitis and for the non-Reiter's syndrome reactive arthritides. In general, it can be stated that the HLA-B27 positive patients have an onset of their disease ten years earlier than the HLA-B27 negative patients. The male to female ratio of the HLA-B27 positive patients is about 1.5:1 and of the HLA-B27 negative patients 1:1. The HLA-B27 positive patients frequently show an overlap of ankylosing spondylitis and acute anterior uveitis. They more often have peripheral arthritis and bamboo spine lesions, and they sometimes show a familial aggregation. The HLA- B27 negative patients, on the other hand, sometimes have psoriasis, inflammatory bowel disease (Crohn's disease, ulcerative colitis), erythema nodosum and a uveitis with mutton fat keratic precipitates. The common characteristics of the HLA-B27 positive patients stimulated the introduction of the term "HLA-B27 associated diseases" (Fig.1) and suggested that HLA-B27 itself might play a pathogenetic role.

The notion that HLA-B27 might be of pathogenetic importance, was further supported by the fact that the association between these diseases and HLA-B27 is observed in all racial groups, also in those where the normal HLA-B27 frequency is extremely low. On the other hand, it should be kept in mind that only about 2% of the HLA-B27 positive individuals actually develop such diseases. This points to other pathogenetic factors which are probably of exogenous nature.

Molecular Mimicry

Discussing Reiter's syndrome, our thoughts, of course, are directed to intestinal and genital bacterial infections. Exciting hypotheses have been proposed recently suggesting that such bacteria, by mimicking HLA-B27, might lead to a cross-reactivity of antibacterial antibodies to the HLA-B27 molecules on the host cells, and thus to autoimmune phenomena. It is also possible that such a mimicry could lead to a cross-tolerance in which the normal non-reactivitiy against autologous HLA antigens causes an immunological tolerance for the resembling of bacterial antigens.

Schwimmbeck and coworkers (14) have, indeed, shown that a hexamer of HLA-B27 is identical to Klebsiella pneumoniae nitrogenase. Lahesmaa and coworkers (8) have found that four of these six amino acids are identical to an outer membrane protein of Yersinia enterocolitica 0:3 and Yersinia pseudotuberculosis III. However, the indications that this leads to a cross-reactivity are poor.

It is therefore unlikely that this mimicry phenomenon is of pathogenetic significance.

Transgenic animals

The knowledge of the pathogenetic role of HLA-B27 would, of course, increase enormously if animals, in which the human genetic information of HLA-B27 was introduced, would develop phenomena of the so-called HLA-B27 associated diseases. It is, indeed, surprising that transgenic HLA-B27 positive mice show somewhat more and earlier phenomena of ankylosing enthesopathy than mice, which are only transgenic for human ß2m (7). Unfortunately, proper controls studying mice transgenic for other HLA class I types have not yet been performed. Experiments performed by other workers in this field have revealed that HLA-B27 mice are somewhat more sensitive to lethal abscesses due to Yersinia infections, but on the other hand less sensitive to "collagen induced arthritis" and less vulnerable for demyelinisation due to viral encephalomyelitis (6). Taurog and coworkers (16) have studied HLA-B27 transgenic rats. They have observed that rats carrying more than 50 copies of HLA-B27 developed inflammatory bowel disease with perianal fistulas, psoriasis-like phenomena, urinary tract infections and heart disease. Their controls carrying less copies of HLA-A2 have not shown these phenomena.

Although all of these findings are highly interesting, they are far from conclusive up to now.

Other Genetic Factors

Family studies on ankylosing spondylitis and acute anterior uveitis have revealed that, although it is evident that HLA-B27 is a predisposing genetic factor, other genetic factors must also play a pathogenetic role (Tab.2) (3,16). It is also possible that not all of the seven subtypes, which are now distinguishable (Fig.2) are involved in the pathogenetic process to the same degree. Only two small studies, both performed in the Netherlands, have suggested that ankylosing spondylitis and acute anterior uveitis are associated in the same degree to HLA-B*2702 as to HLA-B*2705 (2,4). These studies have to be extended and reproduced in other parts of the world.

If, however, the "HLA-B27 associated diseases" are indeed equally associated with all HLA-B27 subtypes this would mean that the pathogenic site of the HLA-B27 molecules is probably situated on the part of the molecule, which is equal to all distinct HLA-B27 molecules and different from all non-HLA-B27 types. Only the amino acid residues Lys70 and Asn97 are unique for all HLA-B27 subtypes. It is supposed that the so-called "45 pocket" involving the residues 24, 26, 34, 45 and 67 together with the polymorphic residues close to this pocket being 9, 32, 63, 69 and 71 is the critical part of the HLA-B27 molecules (Fig.3) (12).

In the past it has often been suggested that HLA-B27 is only a marker for the actual pathogenetic gene(s) next to the B locus on chromosome 6. There are now, however, no indications that any other HLA class I or II antigen is associated with the aforementioned diseases if compared to HLA-B27 positive normal controls. Also, haplotype studies both on ankylosing spondylitis by Lochead and coworkers (13) and on acute anterior uveitis by Derhaag and coworkers (5) have shown that it is unlikely that other genes of pathogenetic importance might be located on the short arm of chromosome 6, leaving the rest of the genome open for further studies. Only the tip of the long arm of chromosome 14 has been studied previously - but also with a negative result (10).

Conclusions

In conclusion, it can be stated that the HLA-B27 associated diseases probably have a common causal pathway in the form of a dysfunction of this MHC class I molecule. One may suppose that peptides of intracellular bacteria are presented in a particular way to cytotoxic T-cells. This is the subject of further studies.

Table 1. HLA-B27+ Reiter's Syndrome Versus HLA-B27- Reiter's Syndrome

	HLA-B27^{+} n=297	HLA-B27^{-} n=73
Chronic course	94%	9%
Low back pain	44%	22%
Fever/weight loss	62%	26%
Abnormal SI joints	31%	9%
Ankylosing Spndylitis	22%	4%
Acute anterior uveitis	49%	0%
Balanitis/vulvovaginitis	45%	10%
Mucocutaneous manifestations	50%	19%
Males	97%	50%

<Compiled from the literature by Linssen (9)>

Table 2. Prevalence of Ankylosing Spondylitis (AS) and Acute Anterior Uveitis (AAU) in the General Population and Relatives of Patients

Prevalence	of AS	of AAU
Population	0.2%	0.2%
HLA-B27+ population	1.0%	1.3%
HLA-B27+ 1st degree relatives over 45 years of age of B27+ patients	21.0%	18.0%

<Based on studies by van der Linden and coworkers (16) and Derhaag and coworkers (3)>

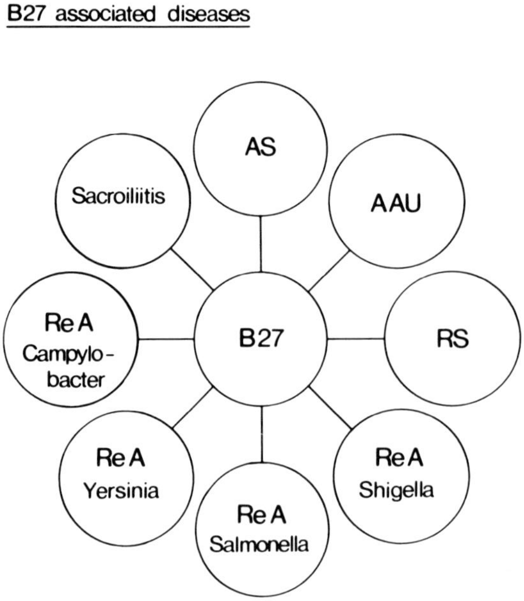

Fig.1.HLA-B27 as the pivotal point of its associated diseases (11)
AS = Ankylosing spondylitis
AAU= Acute anterior uveitis
RS = Reiter's syndrome
ReA= Reactive arthritis
(with permission from the Ann.Rheumat.Dis. (1988)47:431-439))

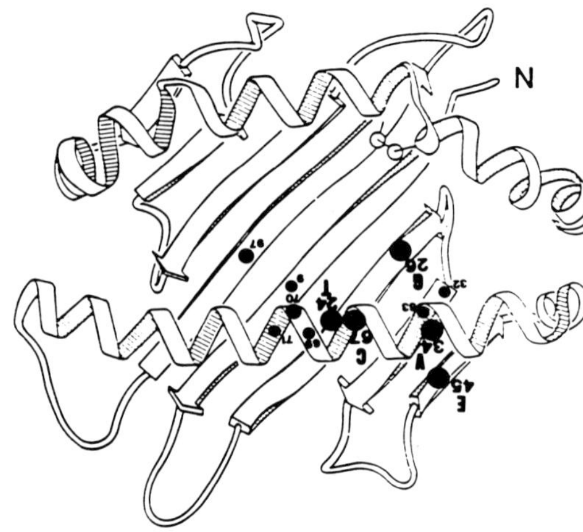

Fig. 3. This figure was made by Lopez de Castro and coworkers (12) and shows the combination of polymorphic residues unique to HLA-B27 and common to all HLA-B27 subtypes. Large dots indicate residues determining the "45 pocket". Medium dots are residues spicific to HLA-B27 molecules (lys70 an Asn97). Small dots are polymorphic residues located close to the "45-pocket". The combination of Thr24, Cys67 and Glu 45 is specific to HLA-B27 among the class I types of known structure. (With permission of the Scand. J. Rheumatol. (1990) Suppl.87:21-31

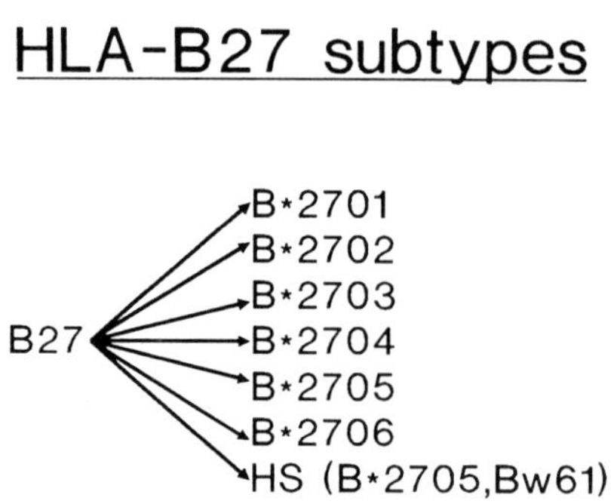

Fig. 2

References

1. Aho K, Ahvonen P, Lassus A et al (1973) HLA-Antigen 27 and Reactive Arthritis. Lancet ii:157
2. Breur-Vriesendorp BS, Neefjes JJ, Huis B et al (1986) Identification of New B27 Subtypes (B27C and B27D) Prevalent in Oriental Populations. Hum Immunol 16:163-168
3. Derhaag PJFM, Linssen A, Broekema N et al (1988) A Familial Study of the Inheritance of HLA-B27 Positive Acute Anterior Uveitis. Am J Ophthalmol 105:603-606
4. Derhaag PJFM, de Waal LP, Linssen A et al (1988) Acute Anterior Uveitis and HLA-B27 Subtypes. Invest Ophthalmol Vis Sci 29:1137-40
5. Derhaag PJFM, de Waal LP, Linssen A et al (1989) HLA-B27$^+$ Acute Anterior Uveitis and Other Antigens of the Major Histocompatibility Complex. Invest Ophthalmol Vis Sci 30:2160-2164
6. Feltkamp TEW (ed)(1990) The Pathogenetic Role of HLA-B27. Scand J Rheumatol Suppl 87
7. Ivanyi P (1990) B27-Transgenic Mice and Disease. Scand J Rheumatol Suppl 87:97
8. Lahesmaa R, Skurnik M, Granfors K et al (1990) A Tetrapeptide Shared by Yersinia Outer Membrane Protein Yop1 and LA-B27. Scand J Rheumatol Suppl 87:70-71
9. Linssen A (1990) B27$^+$ Disease Versus B27$^-$ Disease. Scand J Rheumatol Suppl 87:111-119
10. Linssen A, Rothova A, Feltkamp TEW et al (1987) Genes on Chromosome 14q and Their Role in the Pathogenesis of HLA-B27 Associated Diseases. Clin Exp Rheumatol 5/S1:89-95
11. Linssen A, Feltkamp TEW (1988) B27 Positive Diseases Versus B27 Negative Diseases, a View-point. Ann Rheumat Dis 47:431-439
12. Lopez de Castro JA, Bragado R, Lauzurica P et al (1990) Structure and Immune Recognition of HLA-B27 Antigens: Implications for Disease Association. Scand J Rheumatol Suppl 87:21-31
13. Lochead JA, Chalmers IM, Marshall WH et al (1983) HLA-B27 Haplotypes in Family Studies of Ankylosing Spondylitis. Arthr Rheumat 26:1011-1016
14. Schwimmbeck PL, Yu DTY, Oldstone MBA (1987) Autoantibodies to HLA-B27 in Sera of Patients with Ankylosing Spondylitis and Reiter's Syndrome. J Exp Med 166:173-81
15. Tiwari JL, Terasaki PI (1985) HLA and Disease Associations. Springer Berlin Heidelberg New York
16. Van der Linden SM, Valkenburg HA, De Jongh BM et al (1984) The Risk of Developing Ankylosing Spondylitis in HLA-B27 Positive Individuals. Arthr Rheumat 27:241-249

Molecular Mimicry of Bacteria and Viruses

Manfred Zierhut

Abstract. The term "molecular mimicry" is used for a phenomenon in which viruses and bacteria share epitopes with host-cell proteins. After general considerations, the molecular mimicry of HLA-B27 with Gram-negative bacteria (Shigella flexneri, Klebsiella pneumoniae and Yersinia pseudotuberculosa) are discribed. HLA-B27 is associated with a group of diseases including seronegative arthritis and Reiter's syndrome, and is closely related to anterior uveitis.

The possible role of molecular mimicry for the induction of auto-immune phenomena is discussed.

Introduction

A close resemblance of one organism to another or to some objects in its environment, as in the case of some insects to leaves or twigs of plants, is called mimicry. Mimicry is an important mechanism of these animals or plants to fool their enemies.

The term "molecular mimicry" was introduced into immunology by George Snell in 1968. He suggested that the major histocompatibility complex system and viruses encode similar antigens, which cause the host to regard an infecting virus as "self" and not to mount an immune response.

Research of the last few years has changed this concept. The present definition of molecular mimicry is: "an immune response mounted against a specific determinant of an infecting agent, which cross-reacts with a similar host antigen, leading to tissue injury and autoimmune disease". "Similar" in all the studies previously published and reviewed in this article always means sequence homology, identical primary structure. Whether or not mimicry of secondary or tertiary protein structures has any importance for the induction of autoimmunity is still unknown and is subject to controversial discussion, especially in the field of HLA B27-related diseases.

The probability that a random six amino acid sequence will be identical in two dissimilar proteins assuming that all amino acids are represented equally is estimated at $1:20^6$. Presently it is not clear how many amino acids of a protein have to be identical before the immune system cannot differentiate them any more. It seems that in the case of a foreign antigen three shared amino acids may be enough to mimic a self-antigen structure.

For the induction of cross-reactivity, the amount of shared amino acids seems to be less important than the localization of sequence homology. Cross-reactions will only be found if the sequence is located in a biologically meaningful domain. If a viral antigen has a sequence homology to an autoantigen structure, which is anchored in the basement membrane, no cross-reacting antibodies will be found.

Srinivasappa and coworkers in 1986 analysed over 600 monoclonal antibodies produced against 11 different DNA and RNA viruses for cross-reactivity with host determinants (22). They found that almost 4% of their anti-viral antibodies bound to self-antigens expressed on uninfected tissue, several antibodies reacting with antigens in more than one organ.

Even cross-reacting T-cells have been described. Bahmanyar and coworkers (2) reported that monoclonal antibodies to measles can cross-react with normal human T lymphocytes.

Investigations of molecular mimicry were made possible through the growing experience in identification of protein structures and the production of respective monoclonal antibodies. The complete amino acid sequence for HLA-B27, a major area of molecular mimicry research was published in the last years (review in 15). Today, computer libraries with the complete primary structures of various proteins are commercially available.

This review concentrates on the molecular mimicry in areas related to Ophthalmology. It includes findings for the two classic autoimmune models, experimental allergic encephalitis and experimental autoimmune uveitis and discusses the most conclusive findings reported to date for HLA-B27-associated Gram-negative bacteria.

Molecular Mimicry and Myelin Basic Protein

Experimental allergic encephalitis is a paralytic disease similar in many ways to multiple sclerosis, which can be induced in animals by immunization with myelin basic protein, a neural tissue antigen. Fujinami and Oldstone (10) have shown that some viral proteins contain sequences homologous to the encephalitogenic site of myelin basic protein. One example is the hepatitis B virus polymerase sequence 592-597, which is the same as 69-74 in the myelin basic protein molecule. Humoral and cellular immune responses have been elicited in rabbits inoculated with the viral protein. Inoculation of the viral protein had caused accumulation of inflammatory cells around blood vessels of central nervous tissue in the same way as inoculation of the myelin basic protein.

Today a few hypothesis are discussed for activation of myelin basic protein-reactive T-cells (31). One of these, the molecular mimicry theory, suggests that viral antigen is presented to peripheral T-cells. These T-cells enter the blood-brain barrier and are not able to differentiate between myelin basic protein and the viral antigen, leading to experimental allergic encephalitis. The appearance of disseminated encephalomyelitis subsequent to viral infections is well-known clinically.

Molecular Mimicry of Retinal S-Antigen

Experimental autoimmune uveitis results from inoculation of susceptible animals with retinal antigens. Retinal S-antigen is the best characterized autoantigen for the induction of experimental autoimmune uveitis. In primates, experimental autoimmune uveitis induced by retinal S-antigen resembles sympathtic ophthalmia and birdshot retinochoroidopathy. Singh and coworkers in 1989 demonstrated sequence homology among the five amino acid peptides 303-307 of retinal S-antigen and 106-110 of yeast histone H3 (20). This S-antigen sequence is part of the uveitogenic peptide M, which also can induce experimental autoimmune uveitis (6).

Inoculation of native yeast histone or a small synthetic peptide including the mimicking structure result in experimental autoimmune uveitis. Finally, experimental autoimmune uveitis has adoptively been transferred in immunologically naive rats by lymph node cells (20).

In 1990 the same group (21) found evidence that various different virus peptides (e.g. hepatitis B virus DNA polymerase) with at least three consecutive amino acids identical to a uveitogenic epitope of S-antigen can induce experimental autoimmune uveitis. The importance of these findings for human uveitis is unclear at the moment.

Molecular Mimicry and HLA-B27

The association of HLA-B27 with ankylosing spondylitis (18) and acute anterior uveitis (4) has been known since 1973. While only 6% to 8% of Caucasians are HLA-B27 positive, 85-96% of patients with ankylosing spondylitis and 43-60% of patients with acute anterior uveitis harbor this surface marker. If ankylosing spondylitis and acute anterior uveitis are present, HLA-B27 is expected to be found in 83-100%. There seems to be a difference in the clinical patterns of systemic disease between HLA-B27 positive and HLA-B27 negative patients (8). The differences in clinical manifestations of uveitis are not clear. Some authors have reported a higher recurrence rate in HLA-B27 positive patients.

Salmonella, Shigella and Yersinia-reactive arthritis also occur predominantly in HLA-B27 positive individuals (1).

Serologic examinations of patients with Reiter's disease or ankylosing spondylitis have shown higher titers of antibody against these Gram-negative gut bacteria, and also Klebsiella.

HLA-B27 positive patients with anterior uveitis also have higher antibody titers against Yersinia (27), but not Klebsiella (14). While White and coworkers (29) have found an increase in Klebsiella in the feces of patients with anterior uveitis, others were unable to confirm these findings (28,30).

Molecular Mimicry and Klebsiella

First evidence for cross-reactivity between Klebsiella and HLA-B27 had been reported by Ebringer and coworkers in 1976 (7). Geczy and coworkers in 1979 have found that antiserum from rabbits immunized against Klebsiella also reacts with lymphocytes from HLA-B27 positive ankylosing spondylitis patients, but not with healthy HLA-B27 positive or negative subjects (11). Other laboratories have not been able to reproduce these important results (13).

Comparing Klebsiella proteins with the HLA-B27 structure by database, Schwimmbeck and coworkers (19) have found a six aminoacid sequence shared by Klebsiella pneumoniae-nitrogenase and HLA-B27. These experiments have been repeated in various laboratories with different results. While some researchers had not been able to reproduce Schwimmbeck's results, Ewing and coworkers (9) have found these cross-reacting antibodies only in 20-25% of patients, and in some patient populations even this figure has appeared too high (25). Husby and coworkers (12) have found that antiserum against this cross-reacting peptide stains infiltrating inflammatory cells and vascular endothelium of inflamed synovial tissue of HLA-B27 positive patients. However, tissues of healthy HLA-B27 positive individuals had not been examined.

Molecular Mimicry and Shigella

A different approach in the search for molecular mimicry has been taken by Stieglitz and coworkers (23) in 1989. They have looked for common plasmids in Shigella strains differentiating in arthritogenic and non-arthritogenic strains. Plasmids are bacterial DNA-structures encoding proteins. The authors have identified a 2Md plasmid common to all arthritogenic strains but not found in non-arthritic strains. This plasmid encodes one protein which has a sequence homology to the alpha 1 domain of HLA-B27.

In 1990 Tsuchiya and coworkers using anti-2Md plasmid antibody, have demonstrated strong cross-reactivity of these plasmids to HLA-B27 in the serum of HLA-B27 positive patients (26). Comparing the titers of anti-Klebsiella nitrogenase antibody and anti-2Md Shigella plasmid, they have found much higher titers for the Shigella antibody.

Molecular Mimicry and Yersinia

Chen and coworkers in 1987 have screened multiple bacteria with anti-HLA B27 monoclonal antibodies (5). They have found a strong reaction of two strains of Yersinia pseudotuberculos is with these antibodies and were able to demonstrate molecular mimicry with the peptide sequence 69-83 of HLA-B27. Recently, the same group has also found a plasmid-encoded protein of Yersinia enterocolitica with sequence homology to HLA-B27 (Hamachi and coworkers, in press).

What is the Role of Molecular Mimicry in HLA-B27 related Diseases? To answer this question, we have to look more closely at the initiation of autoimmune T- and B-cell formation.

Normally, the immune system does not produce autoantibodies or autoreactive T-cells. The developing immune system recognizes self-reactive clones, which will be negatively selected mainly from the thymus. Then self-tolerance inhibits production of autoimmune cells.

This state of self-tolerance may be compromised for various reasons. Recognition of microbes is one of them: The immune response seems to depend on the amount of antigen, major histocompatibility complex genes, and supposedly on the extent of homology as well. If anti-microbial antibody formation leads to a recognition of self-antigen, a break at the T- or B-cell level may occur. If the stimulus is strong enough, the existence of autoreactive B- or T-cells can continue without the persistence of the initiating antigen (hit-and-run event). It is obvious that antibiotic treatment is unsuccessful at this time.

Currently, two theories are discussed to explain the role of bacteria in HLA-B27 related diseases:

- the cross-tolerance theory based on molecular mimicry, and
- the receptor theory.

The cross-tolerance theory suggests that antibodies directed against bacteria may cross-react with antigens on the surface of HLA-B27 positive cells producing autoantibodies. The facts that

- antibodies against mimicking peptides e.g. against Klebsiella pneumoniae nitrogenase are not very often found in the serum of these patients, and that
- proteins like the outer membrane proteins (OmpA proteins) show strong cross-reactivity to HLA-B27 without having any sequence homology (32), seem to point to a different model for HLA-B27 related diseases, e.g. the receptor model. On the other hand, instead of looking for cross-reacting autoantibodies in the serum it may seem to be more appropriate to investigate the local immune systems (e.g. synovia of the joint and anterior segment of the eye).

Since the first publication of the three-dimensional structure of the HLA-A2 molecule, the T-cell-receptor-antigen-major histocompatibility complex has received much attention (3). Analogous to HLA-A2, the HLA-B27 molecule seems to present antigen to the T-cell in an antigen pocket. The groove of this pocket is surrounded by positively charged amino acids, which can complex with lipopolysaccharides. Bacterial lipopolysaccharides have been known for many years to induce arthritis in animal models. At the moment some groups are working to find the lipopolysaccharides that may fit into the HLA-B27 groove.

In conclusion, these theories suggest that molecular mimicry of Gram-negative bacteria may initiate an autoimmune reaction at the synovial, maybe also at the uveal sites. It is also possible that the particular biochemical structure of HLA-B27 may be important for the perpetuation of the HLA-B27 related diseases.

Further work is necessary to find a clear path through this complex field of theories.

Future Aspects

At the moment, molecular mimicry research concentrates on the role of the T-cell receptor against cross-reactive peptide structures and cross-reactive T-cells in general.

Moreover, it seems that molecular mimicry is not only limited to sequence homologies (primary structure). Secondary and even tertiary structures have to be evaluated.

One of the most promising models in this field uses the HLA-B27 transgenic mouse and rat. First results of Nickerson and coworkers have suggested that these mice have a higher incidence of arthritis than the control mice (17). After infection with Yersinia enterocolitica, the incidence of arthritis had increased to almost 100%. This group has also noticed a higher frequency of paravertebral abscess formation in their transgenic mice than in the controls following intravenous injection of the bacteria (16). However, working with these animals seems to be tricky, because Taurog and coworkers using mice from a different genetic background, were unable to reproduce these results (24).

Conclusions

Molecular mimicry seems to be one of the mechanisms leading to induction of autoimmune diseases. While this mechanism, which has been found in experimental allergic encephalitis, has been suggested as one of the possible pathogenic factors in multiple sclerosis after viral infection, the significance of findings in experimental autoimmune uveitis with regard to the induction of uveitis in man is still unclear.

Molecular mimicry between Klebsiella pneumoniae nitrogenase or arthritogenic strains of Shigella or Yersinia pseudotuberculosa and the HLA-B27 antigen may explain the link of HLA-B27 associated diseases (like ankylosing spondylitis or Reiter's disease) with Gram-negative gut bacteria.

Since cross-reacting antibodies are not often detectable in the serum of diseased patients, the cross-tolerance theory seems to be less preferable than the "receptor-theory" at present. The latter suggests that the crucial role of HLA-B27 in the induction of arthritis may lie in its special biochemical structure allowing for the presentation of bacterial lipopolysaccharides to the T-cell receptor.

References

1. Aho K, Ahvonen P, Lassus A et al (1973) HLA-B27 in Reactive Arthritis. Lancet ii:157
2. Bahmanyar S, Srinivasappa J, Casall P et al (1987) Antigenic Mimicry Between Measles Virus and Human T-Lymphocytes. J Infect Dis 156:526-527
3. Bjorkman PJ, Saper MA, Samraoui B et al (1987) Structure of the Human Class I Histocompatibility Antigen: HLA-A2. Nature 329:506-512
4. Brewerton DA, Caffrey M, Hart FD et al (1973) Ankylosing Spondylitis and HLA-B27. Lancet i:904-907
5. Chen JH, Kono DH, Yong Z et al (1987) A Yersinia Pseudotuberculosis Protein which Cross-Reacts with HLA-B27. J Immunol 139:3003-3011
6. Donoso LA, Merryman CF, Shinohara T et al (1987) S-Antigen. Experimental Autoimmune Uveitis Following Immunization with a Small Synthetic Peptide. Arch Ophthalmol 105:838-840
7. Ebringer A, Cowling P, Ngawa Suh N et al (1976) Cross-Reactivity Between Klebsiella Aerogenes Species and B27 Lymphocyte Antigens as an Aetiological Factor in Ankylosing Spondylitis. INSERM (Paris) 58:27
8. Ebringer A (1990) Theoretical Models to Explain the Association of HLA-B27 with Ankylosing Spondylitis. Scand J Rheumatol Suppl S87:151-163
9. Ewing C, Ebringer R, Tribbick G et al (1990) Antibody Activity in Ankylosing Spondylitis Sera to Two Sites on HLA B27.1 at the MHC Groove Region (Within Sequence 65-85), and to a Klebsiella pneumoniae Nitrogenase Reductase Peptide (Within Sequence 181-199). J Exp Med 171:1635-1647
10. Fujinami RS, Oldstone MBA (1985) Amino Acid Homology Between the Encephalitogenic Site of Myelin Basic Protein and Virus: Mechanism for Autoimmunity. Science 230:1043-1045
11. Geczy AF, Yap J (1979) HLA-B27, Klebsiella, and Ankylosing Spondylitis. Lancet i:719-720
12. Husby G, Tsuchiya N, Schwimmbeck PL et al (1989) Cross-Reactiv Epitope with Klebsiella Pneumoniae Nitrogenase in Articular Tissue of HLA-B27^{+} Patients with Ankylosing Spondylitis. Arthr Rheumat 32:437-445
13. Ivanji P (1990) Dysfunction of HLA-B27. Scand J Rheumatol (Suppl) 87:51-69
14. Kijlstra A, Luyendijk L, van der Gaag R et al (1986) IgG and IgA Immune Response Against Klebsiella in HLA-B27-Associated Anterior Uveitis. Br J Ophthalmol 70:85-88
15. Lopez de Castro JA (1989) HLA-B27 and HLA-A2 Subtypes: Structure, Evolution and Function. Immunology Today 10:239-246
16. Nickerson CL, Luthra HS, David CS (1990) Role of Enterobacteria and HLA-B27 in Spondyloarthropathies: Studies with Transgenic Mice. Ann Rheum Dis 49:426-433
17. Nickerson P, Hogen KL, Luthra HS et al (1990) Effect of H_2 Genes on Expression of HLA-B27 and Yersinia-Induced Arthritis. Scand J Rheumatol (Suppl) S87:85-90
18. Schlosstein L, Terasaki PJ, Bluestone R et al (1973) High Association of an HLA Antigen w27 with Ankylosing Spondylitis. New Engl J Med 288:704
19. Schwimmbeck PL, Yu DTY, Oldstone MBA (1987) Autoantibodies to HLA-B27 in the Sera of HLA-B27 Patients with Ankylosing Spondylitis and Reiter's Syndrome. J Exp Med 166:173-181
20. Singh VK, Yamaki K, Donoso LA et al (1989) Yeast Histone H3-Induced Experimental Autoimmune Uveitis. J Immunol 142:1512-1517
21. Singh VK, Kalra HK, Yamaki K et al (1990) Molecular Mimicry Between a Uveitopathogenic Site of S-Antigen and Viral Peptides. J Immunol 144:1282-1287
22. Srinivasappa J, Saegusa J, Prabhaker BS et al (1986) Molecular Mimicry: Frequence of Reactivity of Monoclonal Anti-viral Anti-

bodies with Normal Tissue. J Virol 57:397-401

23. Stieglitz H, Fosmire S, Lipsky P (1989) Identification of a 2-MD Plasmid from Shigella Flexneri Associated with Reactive Arthritis. Arthr Rheumat 32:937-946
24. Taurog JD (1990) Immunology, Genetics and Animal Models of the Spondyloarthropathies. Curr Opin Rheumatol 2:586-591
25. Tsuchiya N, Husby G, Williams RC Jr (1989) Studies of Humoral and Cell-mediated Immunity to Peptides Shared by HLA-B27.1 and Klebsiella Pneumoniae Nitrogenase in Ankylosing Spondylitis. Clin Exp Immunol 76:354-360
26. Tsuchiya N, Husby G, Williams RC Jr (1990) Autoantibodies to the HLA-B27 Sequence Cross-React with the Hypothetical Peptide from the Arthritis-Associated Shigella Plasmid. J Clin Invest 86:1193-1203
27. Wakefield D, Stahlberg TH, Toivanen A et al (1990) Serologic Evidence of Yersinia Infection in Patients with Anterior Uveitis. Arch Ophthalmol 108:219-221
28. Warren RE, Brewerton DA (1980) Fecal Carriage of Klebsiella by Patients with Ankylosing Spondylitis and Rheumatoid Arthritis. Ann Rheum Dis 39:37-44
29. White L, McCoy R, Tait B et al (1984) A Search for Gram-negative Enteritic Microorganisms in Acute Anterior Uveitis: Association of Klebsiella with Recent Onset of Disease. Br J Ophthalmol 68:750-755
30. Willshaw HE (1981) Acute Anterior Uveitis and Klebsiella Aerogenes: A Causal Relationship? Br J Ophthalmol 65:796-797
31. Wucherpfennig KW, Weiner HL, Hafler DA (1991) T-Cell Recognition of Myelin Basic Protein. Immunol Today 12:277-282
32. Zhang JJ, Hamachi M, Hamachi T et al (1989) The Bacterial Outer Membrane Protein that Reacts with Anti-HLA-B27 Antibodies is the OmpA Protein. J Immunol 143: 2955-2960.

Reiter's Syndrome: Dermatological Features

Sandor Marghescu

Abstract. In Reiter's syndrome, the lesions of the skin and mucous membranes are very distinct. In most cases, the clinical diagnosis can be made without any other work-ups. Palms and soles show keratotic plaques and reddish scaling patches are seen on fingers and toes. Nail deformities with discoloration occur and, considering all of these manifestations, they are very similar to psoriatic alterations. The lesions of glans and oral mucous membranes are circinate, linear, crusted erosions that must be differentiated from candidiasis in these locations.

Histopathologically, the skin lesions are indistinguishable from pustular psoriasis.

Considering the alternatives of antipsoriatic agents, systemic Etretinate therapy is most effective to clear the lesions from the skin, mucous membranes and nails.

Clinical Features

In Reiter's syndrome, characteristic lesions can frequently in addition to the classical triad of urethritis, conjunctivitis and arthritis be observed and may involve the skin, mucous membranes and nails. The incidence of palmoplantar keratosis was found to be about 10%, mucous membrane lesions occur in 20-40% and nail changes in 20-30% of cases. The dermatological findings consist of palmoplantar keratoderma, exudative psoriasiform lesions, nail dystrophy, balanitis circinata and/or uranitis circinata (1).

The palmoplantar keratoderma (Fig.1) begins with abortive or fully developed sterile pustules as a result of the immigration of leucocytes into the epidermis and formation of subcorneal sterile abscesses. After the eruptive pustular phase, confluent keratotic lesions arise on the soles and palms. The keratotic masses contain serous fluid and have a succulent aspect.

Psoriasiform lesions (Fig.2) are frequently seen in the paraungual area. They are sharply delineated and show an arched configuration and an elevated dark red erythema with coarse scales.

Nail dystrophy (Fig.3) is associated with a yellow discoloration and destruction of the distal part of the nail plates with subungual hyperkeratosis.

Balanitis circinata (Fig.4) appears as an erosive area encircled by round or circinate small whitish linear lesions. Analogous lesions were observed on the mucous membranes of the palate called "uranitis circinata" (4). Furthermore, elevated dark red patches on the buccal or pharyngeal mucous membranes not covered by membranes have been observed (6).

Histopathology

The histopathologic changes of the skin lesions consist of orthohyperkeratosis with parakeratotic areas, subcorneal spongiform pustules, acanthosis of the epidermis, papillomatosis and polymorphous dermal infiltrates.

Differential Diagnosis

Clinically and histopathologically, the skin lesions are almost indistinguishable from true psoriasis. Morphologically Reiter's syndrome exhibits features of psoriasis vulgaris and psoriasis pustulosa.

In fact, the lesions of Reiter's syndrome are more of an exudative, inflammatory and succulent nature compared to those of psoriasis vulgaris, and sterile pustules are only apparent on palms and soles and in the early phase of the disease.

Balanitis circinata is pathognomonic for Reiter's syndrome, but similar lesions may be seen on the buccal mucous membranes of patients with psoriasis pustulosa generalisata. Aside from psoriasis, there are other diseases, which have to be differentiated from Reiter's syndrome.

It is demanding to exclude a secondary (infectious) pustulosis with pustules on palms and soles in its early phase. The absence of bacteria in the pustules and the lack of lymphangitis with persisting disease argue in favor of Reiter's syndrome.

Balanitis and uranitis circinata may be mistaken for circinate lesions of candidiasis of the mucous membranes. Mycologic cultures may be indicated.

Finally, the described lesions of the nails are clinically indistinguishable from tinea. The lack of fungal elements in the culture argue in favor of psoriasis or Reiter's syndrome.

The treatment of skin, mucocutaneous and nail lesions of Reiter's syndrome can only be symptomatic. Except for local and systemic corticosteroids other immunosuppressive drugs have been used with variable success. Etretinate alone (2) and in combination with Methotrexate and Prednisolone (3) has resulted in marked remissions. Furthermore, photochemotherapy (psoralene+UV-A) has been shown successful.

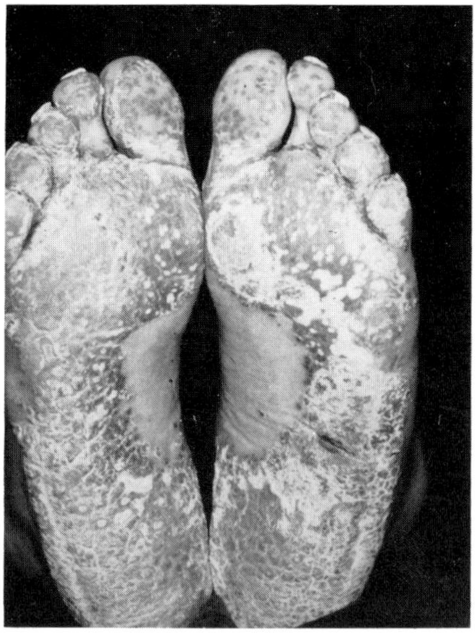

Fig.1. Reiter's syndrome: plantar keratoderma

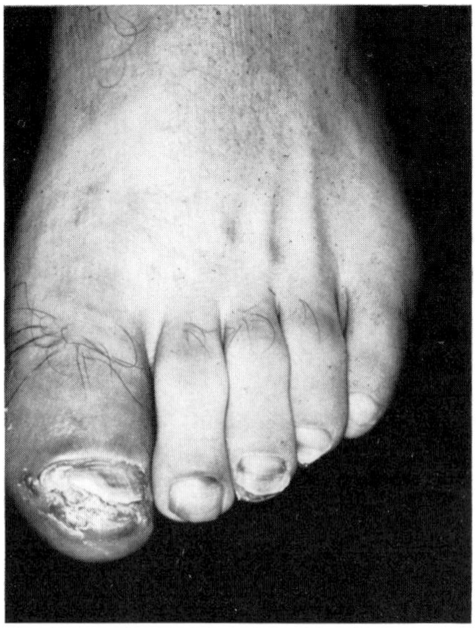

Fig.3. Reiter's syndrome: nail dystrophy

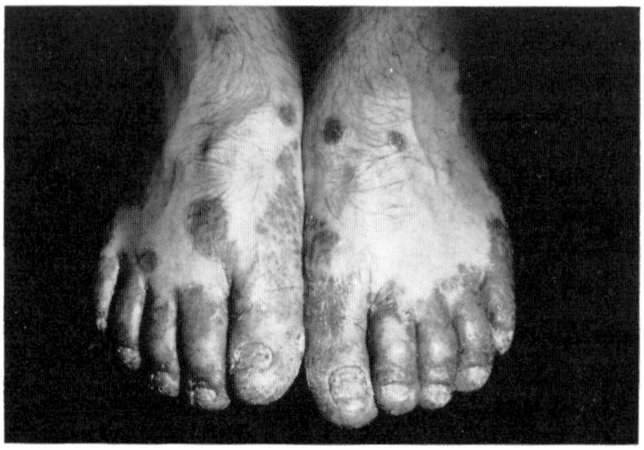

Fig.2. Reiter's syndrome: psoriasiform lesions

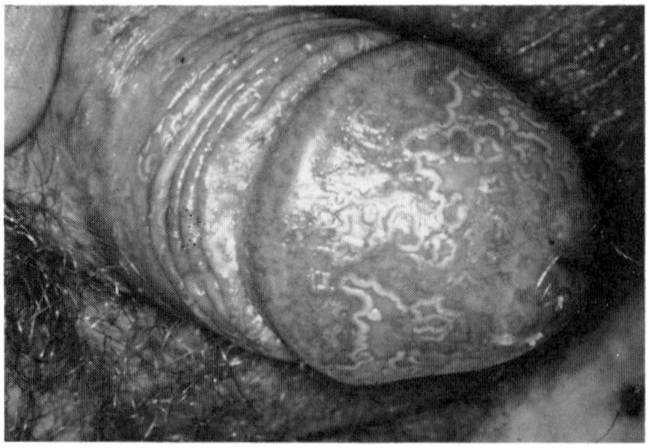

Fig.4. Reiter's syndrome: balanitis circinata

References

1. Braun-Falco O, Plewig G, Wolff HH (1984) Dermatologie und Venerologie. 3rd ed. Springer, Heidelberg
2. Lassus A, Eskelinen A, Säilä K et al (1985) Treatment of Reiter's Disease with Etretinate. In: Saurat,JH (ed.) Retinoids: New Trends in Research and Therapy. Karger, Basel
3. Luderschnmidt CH, Balda BR (1983) M.Reiter: Erfolgreiche Kombinations-Chemotherapie mit Methotrexat, Etretinat und Prednisolon. Münch Med Wchschr 125:936-940
4. Marghescu S, Kock BW, Lubach D (1985) Balranitis circinata bei M.Reiter. Therapie mit Etretinat (Tigason[R]). Hautarzt 36:291-293
5. Miehle W (1979) Reiter-Syndrom.Teil 1: Definition, Pathogenese, klinisches Bild. Fortschr Med 97:134-138
6. Montgomery MM, Poske RM, Barton EM et al (1959) The Mucocutaneous Lesions of Reiter's Syndrome. Ann Intern Med 51:99-109.
7. Tholen S, Lubach D (1987) Mundschleimhautveränderungen bei Psoriasis pustulosa generalisata. Hautarzt 38:419-421

Rheumatological Features of Infection-Related Disease (Reiter's Syndrome)

Henning Zeidler

Abstract. In recent years, an increasing number of rheumatic disorders triggered by bacterial infections (Yersinia, Campylobacter, Salmonella, Clostridium difficile, Chlamydia) and sterile joint inflammations has been described and termed "reactive arthritis". The disease most often affects young adults. Women suffer from reactive arthritis as often as men, however, classical "Reiter's Syndrome" is seen more frequently in men.
Mono- or oligoarticular joint involvement is most frequent, but an asymmetric synovitis is also not unusual. The weight-bearing joints of the lower limbs are usually affected: the knees, ankles and less frequently the hips. Other large joints, e.g. elbows or wrists may also be inflamed as well as single small joints of the feet and hands.
Not only the joints are involved, but also the periarticular structures of the enthesis. Plantar fasciitis with heel pain, various insertitides and inflammations of the tendons are commonly seen. Lumbar pain due to sacroiliitis is a frequent feature, but clear radiologic changes are particularly seen in later stages of the disease.
Systemic features are frequent and may be classified in two groups. Bacterial infections

may lead to visceral and organic manifestations at the entry sites or by ascending spread of the microbes. Further systemic manifestations are caused by the host's immune reaction and/or by dissemination of the infectious pathogens.

The severity of reactive arthritis may vary from mild arthralgias to invalidating, life-threatening systemic disease and from an acute, self-limiting to a slowly progressive chronic disease. Chronic joint and spinal diseases are seen in 30-70% of patients.

Introduction

The term reactive arthritis, which had in the past been most often used in the context of HLA-B27 associated rheumatological manifestations has recently been more frequently applied to other nonpurulent arthritides like rheumatic fever, Lyme-arthritis, Brucella reactive arthritis and most recently to some rheumatic syndromes related to human immunodeficiency virus infections (Tab.1) (1, 2, 3, 8).

This survey only refers to the HLA B27-associated reactive arthritides because Reiter's syndrome is restricted to this group of diseases.

Rheumatological Manifestations (Tab.2)

A number of epidemics have shown that only 1-4% of persons infected with the respective enteric or urogenic bacteria develop reactive arthritis. No more than 10-30% of these patients with reactive arthritis show the classic triad of Reiter's syndrome.

The disease most often affects young adults, aged 20 to 40 years, but also elderly persons of more than 60 years have been reported. In arthritis associated with enteric infections the male to female ratio approximates 1:1, whereas sexually acquired reactive arthritis and classical Reiter's syndrome are reported more frequently in men. According to our own experience and other observations, chlamydia-induced arthritis has been underdiagnosed in women because of more frequent persistent, clinically inapparent chlamydial infections in the female urogenital tract (12,14,15). The gender ratio is more even when the diagnosis is based on the detection of the causative organism and not only on clinical symptoms and even more on the classical triad of Reiter's syndrome.

Usually, reactive arthritis begins one to three weeks after the onset of gastroenteritis or urethritis with a range between one day and more than six weeks. The interval from infection to arthritis has been reported less than 30 days in 80 to 94% of patients in different studies (7). However, it must be taken into account that genitourinary symptoms may precede arthritis up to several years in chlamydial infections, particularly in females suffering from salpingitis.

Joint symptoms vary from mild arthralgia to severe, immobilising arthritis. The synovitis with the classic symptoms of pain, swelling, increased local warmth and restricted movement generally occurs as an acute phenomenon over several hours or one to two days or subacutely over several days. In very severe reactive arthritis the joints, particularly those of the toes and fingers, are frequently reddish and therefore a misdiagnosis of purulent arthritis, phlegmonia, gout, other crystal synovitis and psoriatic arthropathy may occur at first.

Reactive arthritis most often shows an oligoarticular manifestation involving two to five joints (Tab.3). However, monoarticular and polyarticular (more than 5 affected joints) forms are also encountered. An asymmetric pattern of involvement is typical with preference for the weight-bearing joints of the lower limbs. Knee and ankle joints are most commonly affected. Larger joints of the upper extremities, e.g. the elbows or wrists are also often inflamed as well as single small joints of the feet and hands. In principle, however, any joint including central ones like the sterno-clavicular and mandibular joints may be involved.

Dactylitis or "sausage-like digit" otherwise typical for psoriatic arthritis may also not infrequently be seen in reactive arthritis, which is generally restricted to one finger or toe. Occasionally the disease may closely resemble the polyarticular joint pattern of rheumatoid arthritis.

Not only the joints are involved, but also inflammatory lesions of the periarticular structures and especially of the entheses are characteristic for this group of infection-related rheumatological diseases (Tab.3). The most frequent symptom is heel pain usually representing inflammation at the tendinous insertion of the plantar fascia into the calcaneous (calcaneodynia) or more rarely resulting from the involvement of the Achilles tendon (Achillodynia). Other sites of tendon or fascial attachments may also be affected mono- or polylocularly and in rare instances may give rise to a polytopic fibromyalgia syndrome. The reasons for this characteristic site of involvement remain undetermined. The special anatomical structures with collagen fibers and cartilagenous tissues have been hypothesized as the common pathogenic denominator for these enthesopathies but local vasculature and local innervation have also been suggested as contributing factors (6,10). Finally, inflammation of periarticular structures with a synovia-like membrane may also occur leading to tenosynovitis, including synovitis of the digital tendon sheath, and bursitis most frequently affecting the bursa subachillea.

Each of these lesions may be seen in other rheumatoid factor negative rheumatic diseases like ankylosing spondylitis and psoririatic arthritis as well emphasizing the overlap between reactive arthritis and other members of the spondylarthritis group. Therefore, in view of the whole spectrum of clinical features the term reactive spondylarthritis may describe more precisely the rheumatological manifestations of reactive arthritis.

Axial involvement presenting as low-back pain is noted frequently varying between 9% in mild short-lived disease and 31-91% in patients with typical Reiter's syndrome (7). Although it may be difficult to determine the origin of low-back pain, the positive sacroiliac joint signs, especially positive Mennell's sign, and positive scintiscans most frequently indicate the presence of a sacroiliitis (7,11,14). Each part of the spine can be involved leading to cervical, dorsal or lumbal pain of the inflammatory type i.e. with morning stiffness and night pain, however, symptoms may also be atypical and of the more mechanical type. Finally, the involvement of the costo-vertebral and sterno-costal joints give rise to thoracic pain often misinterpreted as cardiac pain, pleural or lung disease.

Extra-Articular Organ Manifestations

Extraarticular systemic features are multiple and may be classified in two groups:
1. Visceral and organ manifestations at the entry site of the causative infection inclusive the ascending or local spread of the microbial organisms.
2. Systemic manifestations due to immune reactions and/or by dissemination of the infectious pathogens with both of these alternatives potentially being the underlying pathogenetic mechanism.

Classification and Diagnostic Criteria

Both the rheumatological and systemic manifestations show one organism causing many disorders. Moreover, the high variability in presentation and the overlap of clinical features make the development of diagnostic and classification criteria difficult.

Nowadays, the term "Reiter's syndrome" can only be used to describe clinical manifestations of a subgroup of patients and a designation "Reiter's disease" in the sense of a disease entity is totally out of time because of its multiple etiology. Furthermore, preliminary criteria for "Reiter's syndrome" are no longer appropriate because they do not include the bulk of patients with rheumatologic manifestations and no overt symptoms of the initiating infection (13). The only criteria available, but unfortunately not well-known and only rarely used, have been stated by Amor and the French Society of Rheumatology (1) (Tab.4). These criteria including clinical, genetic and aetiological features have been tested by us for their diagnostic significance in an early synovitis out-patient clinic. The sensitivity of 92% and the specificity of 99% seems to be appropriate for the diagnostic situation in most university tertiary referral centre (5).

More recently, we have proposed classification criteria for chlamydia induced arthritis defining possible and definite diseases (14,16) and including clinical, microbiological and serological parameters. These criteria have been useful for case definitions, but have to be further evaluated for diagnostic validity.

Course and Prognosis

Usually reactive arthritides are considered to be non-destructive joint diseases with a self-limited benign course, but most follow-up studies (6,8,9) describe recurrent arthralgias and attacks of synovitis, chronic arthritis, remittent or chronic enthesopathy, low-back pain, sacroiliitis and spondylitis leading to severe long-term morbidity in a substantial number of patients with Reiter's syndrome, Yersinia arthritis and Salmonella arthritis (Tab.5). Chronic joint and spinal diseases are seen in 30-70% of the patients (9). The typical relapsing synovitis of palindromic rheumatism occasionally has been noticed indicating the variability of the natural history of reactive arthritis.

Altogether, there is certainly a high variability in the natural history of reactive arthritis which may make it difficult to foresee and to determine the efficacy of any new therapeutic regimen in an individual patient. Nevertheless, radiological erosive changes of the peripheral joints are very rare and characteristically occur in the forefoot, with a predilection for asymmetric involvement of metatarsal-phalangeal and interphalangeal joints. Usually, X-ray examinations of the peripheral joints only reveal soft tissue swelling, periarticular osteoporosis and mild periostitis. Chronic enthesopathy may lead to erosions and spurs representing local repair phenomena preferentially at the site of the insertion of the plantar fascia, less common at the site of insertion of the Achilles tendon and occasionally at any other site of enthesopathy.

The axial involvement more frequently leads to radiographic changes. By X-ray, sacroiliitis is seen in up to 25% of acutely diseased patients and in 50-70% of patients with chronic Reiter's syndrome and persisting symptoms for two or more years(7). Sacroiliitis is often asymmetric or unilateral as opposed to idiopathic ankylosing spondylitis, in which symmetric changes in the sacroiliac joints are generally seen. A complete sacroiliac and spine ankylosis indistinguishable from ankylosing spondylitis has rarely been documented in patients with severe relapsing Reiter's syndrome (7).

A genetic factor plays an important role in the development of chronic spinal disease. In a 10-year follow-up of Yersinia reactive arthritis, radiological evidence of sacroiliitis or spondylitis was more common in the HLA B27-positive group than in the HLA B27-negative group (51% vs.16% resp.). The development of sacroiliac changes did not correlate with the number of attacks of Reiter's syndrome (9). Paravertebral ossification, the principal and characteristic spinal change other than sacroiliitis also may occur in the absence of clinical sacroiliitis or back symptoms suggesting an "unusual response to minor spinal trauma among genetically predisposed persons" (7). The nonmarginal syndesmophytes or parasyndesmophytes (= vertical osseous bridges extending across the intervertebral disc separated by a clear space from the disk and vertebral body) commonly involve the lower thoracic vertebrae and the upper lumbal vertebrae. Paravertebral ossification may be an early finding or be seen in advanced disease as a typical marker for prior Reiter's syndrome.

Conclusions

The present review emphasizes the high variability of reactive arthritis. In the clinical situation the most troubling point is due to the fact that one organism may cause many rheumatological syndromes and that the reactive arthritides of different etiology clinically resemble each other. In addition to the rheumatological features the organic manifestations overlap to a significant degree with those seen in other spondylarthropathies. Moreover, triggering infections that are abortive and asymptomatic frequently complicate the finding of an etiologically related diagnosis with regard to the underlying infective organism. The clinical course and prognosis also show a high variability, which may make it difficult to prognosticate in the individual patient.

We need more data to understand the mysteries why reactive arthritis is self-limited in some patients and chronic in others as well as why some patients suffer only from arthritis and/or spinal disease and others exhibit systemic manifestations.

Finally, there is important clinical evidence for a key role of bacterial persistence (Tab.6) in chronic inflammatory diseases demanding to elucidate the pathophysiology of chronic infections and to find new strategies for efficient antimicrobial treatment (16).

Table 1. Classification of reactive arthritis

HLA-B27 associated		Other
enteric	urogenital	
Yersinia	Chlamydia	Rheumatic fever
Salmonella	Neisseria gonorrhoeae (?)	Lyme-Borreliose
Shigella	Mycoplasma (?)	Brucellosis
Campylobacter	Ureaplasma urealyticum (?) HIV infection	
Clostridium		

Table 2. Characteristic features of reactive arthritis

- Attack rate 1%-4% of infected individuals in unselected populations
- Mono-/oligoarticular joint involvement, asymmetric, lower extremities
- Enthesopathy
- Axial involvement (sacroiliitis, spondylitis)
- Systemic manifestations (e.g. carditis, nephritis, neuritis, hepatitis)

Table 3. Joint lesions in reactive arthritis (Keat 1983)

- Affected joints	2.8 - 3.7
- Joints most often affected	knee, ankle, wrist, MTP
- Monoarthritis (%)	4 - 19
- Radiological sarcoiliitis (%)	7 - 16
- Tendinitis / dactylitis (%)	8 - 13
Fasciitis / enthesopathy (%)	22

Table 4. Criteria for reactive arthritis (Amor 1983)

- Arthritis
  -- asymmetric oligoarthritis
  -- low back pain, sacroiliitis, heel pain, dactylitis
- Enteritis
- Conjunctivitis
- Urethritis, cervicitis
- Stomatitis, balanitis
- Genetic disposition, HLA-B27
- Triggering infection

4 criteria positive = reactive arthritis

Table 5. Course and prognosis of reactive arthritis (In 30-70% of patients)

- Recurrent arthralgia and arthritis
- Chronic arthritis
- Remittent or chronic enthesopathy
- Low back pain, sacroiliitis, ankylosing spondylitis

Table 6. Evidence for bacterial persistence

- Recurrent dysenteria or urogenital symptoms
- Asymptomatic urogenital chlamydial infection and asymptomatic persistence of yersinia in intestinal mucosa
- IgA-antibodies positive in active joint disease
- Benefical effect of antibiotic treatment

References

1. Amor B (1983) Reiter's Syndrome and Reactive Arthritis. Clin Rheumatol 2:315-319
2. Aho K, Ahvonen P, Lassus A et al (1973) HLA Antigen 27 and Reactive Arthritis. Lancet II:157-161
3. Espinoza LR, Aguilar JL, Bormen et al (1989) Review. Rheumatic Manifestations Associated with the Human Immunodeficiency Virus Infection. Arthr Rheum 32:1615-1622
4. Ford D (1987) Editorial. One Syndrome - Many Infectious Agents. J Rheumatol 14:650-652
5. Hülsemann JL, Zeidler H, Krech T (1989) Diagnostische Charakteristika früher Arthritiden und Spondarthritiden. Akt Rheumatol 14:115-118
6. Inman RD (1990) Reiter's Syndrome and Reactive Arthritis. Spine 4:627-634
7. Keat A (1983) Reiter's Syndrome and Reactive Arthritis in Perspective. New Engl J Med 309:1606-1615
8. Lahesmaa-Rantala R, Toivanen A (1988) Clinical Spectrum of Reactive Arthritis. In: Toivanen A, Toivanen P (eds) Reactive arthritis. CRC Press, Boca Raton
9. Leirisalo-Rep G, Skylv G, Kousa M (1987) Follow-up Study of Reiter's Disease and Reactive Arthritis. Factors Influencing the Natural Course and the Prognosis. Clin Rheumatol 6(Suppl 2):74-82
10. Moll JMH (1983) Pathogenetic Mechanisms in B27 Associated Diseases. Br J Rheumatol 22(Suppl.2):93-103
11. Russel LAS, Davis P, Percy JS et al (1977) The Sacroiliitis of Acute Reiter's Syndrome. J Rheumatol 4:293-296
12. Taylor-Robinson D, Thomas BJ, Dixey J et al (1988) Evidence that Chlamydia trachomatis Causes Seronegative Arthritis in Women. Ann Rheum Dis 47:295-299
13. Willkens RF, Arnett FC, Bitter T (1981) Reiter's Syndrome; Evaluation of Preliminary Criteria for Definite Disease. Arthr Rheum 24:844-849
14. Wollenhaupt HJ, Schneider C, Zeidler H et al (1989) Klinische und serologische Charakterisierung der Chlamydien-induzierten Arthritis. Dtsch Med Wschr 114:1949-1954
15. Yli-Kerttula UJ, Vilpulla AH (1988) Reactive salpingitis. In: Toivanen A, Toivanen P (eds) Reactive Arthritis. CRC press, Boca Raton, pp 125 - 131
16. Zeidler H, Wollenhaupt J (1991) Chlamydia-Induced Arthritis. The Clinical Spectrum,

Serology and Prognosis. In: Lipsky PE, Taurog JD (eds) HLA-B27 Spondyloarthropathies, Elsevier, New York, pp 175 - 187

Reiter's Syndrome: Ocular Features

K. Matti Saari

Abstract. Reactive conjunctivits or reactive iritis may occur together with reactive arthritis and/or urethritis as a part of complete or incomplete Reiter's syndrome. Occasionally reactive ocular inflammation may occur without any joint or urethral involvement as an independent disease (19). However, different symptoms of Reiter's syndrome may appear alone or in different combinations simultaneously or at irregular intervals for even months or years. The association of reactive conjunctivitis or acute anterior uveitis with reactive arthritis, sacroiliitis, and HLA-B27, would still implicate it either as an independent disorder or as a aymptom of Reiter's syndrome with an HLA-B27 associated rheumatic disease.

Introduction

In 1916 Hans Reiter published his famous observations on a soldier who developed nongonococcal urethritis, conjunctivitis, and arthritis 8 days after bloody diarrhea (15). Later, the same patient suffered from iritis and chronic polyarthritis. In 1942, Bauer and Engelman published the first case of nongonococcal urethritis, conjunctivitis, and arthritis in the American literature, and they called it Reiter's disease, a syndrome of unknown etiology (4). Since that time, the combination of conjunctivitis, arthritis, and urethritis has been referred to as Reiter's syndrome.

Now the triad of Reiter's syndrome may be defined as reactive arthritis, urethritis or cervicitis, and reactive ocular inflammation. The term reactive arthritis (introduced by Aho and coworkers (1)) means an acute nonpurulent arthritis following a bacterial infection elsewhere in the body. The term reactive ocular inflammation, reactive conjunctivitis, and reactive iritis (introduced by Saari and coworkers (19)) mean acute ocular inflammations following certain bacterial infections elsewhere in the body. The causative agent can be isolated neither in reactive arthritis from the synovial fluid of the involved joint, in reactive conjunctivitis from the conjunctiva, nor in reactive iritis from the aqueous humor. Exceptionally, however, reyctive iritis may be associated with inclusion conjunctivitis caused by a chlamydial infection. Reactive ocular inflammation in Reiter's syndrome may become manifest after Yersinia, Salmonella, Shigella, Campylobacter, and Chlamydia infections in individuals with a genetically determined predisposition indicated by HLA-B27 (17,19,20,21,23).

Ophthalmological Findings in Reiter's Syndrome

Several ocular manifestations may be seen in Reiter's syndrome. They are generally transient and, except for iritis, usually mild. Reactive conjunctivitis is the most common ocular finding in Reiter's syndrome. It is usually bilateral and may precede but often follows the urethritis; it may be catarrhal or purulent.

Blepharitis and episcleritis have been occasionally reported in patients with Reiter's syndrome. They are not typical findings of this disease and might represent a coincidence. A superficial keratitis with punctate infiltrations beneath the Bowman's membrane may be seen in patients with longstanding conjunctivitis. Corneal ulceration is a rare ocular finding in Reiter's syndrome. Reactive iritis is often seen in Reiter's syndrome. Papillitis, and macular edema or retinitis without iritis are rare findings in Reiter's syndrome.

Incidence of Eye Inflammation in Reiter's syndrome

Ahvonen (3) observed eye inflammation in 12 cases (11.5%) of 104 patients with Yersinia-triggered reactive arthritis, including four cases with iritis and 8 cases with conjunctivitis. Of the 23 patients with Yersinia-triggered ocular inflammation reported by Saari and coworkers (19) reactive iritis occurred in 17 and reactive conjunctivitis in 9 patients.

Yersinia-triggered ocular inflammation is rarer in children. Lang and coworkers (12) reported a 13-year-old boy with acute anterior uveitis and arthritis associated with Yersinia infection, and Saari and coworkers (20) reported one 4-year-old girl and five 10- to 14-year-old children with reactive arthritis and ocular inflammation in association with Yersinia infection. The very rare occurence of reactive iritis and conjunctivitis before the age of 10 years suggests that after that age the reactive immunological response and the clinical characteristics of reactive ocular inflammations resemble those found in adults (20).

Reiter's syndrome after Salmonella infection occurs rarely; it occurred only in one case in an epidemic afflicting 2800 patients (12). Saari and coworkers (23) reported 8 patients with ocular inflammation in Reiter's syndrome after Salmonella enteritis including seven patients with reactive conjunctivitis, three with acute anterior uveitis, and one patient with keratitis.

Of about 150000 cases of Shigella dysentery, Reiter's syndrome developed in 334 (0.2%). All three cardinal symptoms of Reiter's syndrome occurred in 233 cases (69.8%). The joints and the eyes were affected in 56 cases (16.8%), the eyes and the urogenital system in four (1.2%), and the eyes alone in five cases (1.5%) (14).

Eye involvement was the initial symptom, alone or in any combination, in altogether 48.6% of the postdysenteric cases with Reiter's syndrome (14). Ocular inflammation occurred altogether in 298 cases (89.2%) including conjunctivitis in 239 cases, keratoconjunctivitis in 13, acute anterior uveitis in 12, keratoiritis in 10, corneal ulcer in four, and feeling speck in the eye and purulent discharge without noticeable redness in 20 cases (14). In only two cases was iritis and in one case keratoconjunctivitis the primary ocular diagnosis. In all other cases involvement of the iris and the cornea was preceded by a conjunctivitis which had either become entirely asymptonatic or at least improved considerably in the meantime. The fundus was normal in all examined cases (14).

Reiter's syndrome after Campylobacter enteritis is rare. We reported an 18-year-old woman who developed acute polyarthritis one week and bilateral, acute, mucopurulent conjunctivtis and sterile pyuria two weeks after the onset of Campylobacter jejuni enteritis (17).

The incidence of Reiter's syndrome among cases of nongonococcal urethritis varies from 0.8 to 2% (8,11). In a prdominantly male material ocular involvement occurred together with urogenital and joint involvement as a complete triad of Reiter's syndrome in 50% of all cases, conjunctivitis was observed in 48%, and acute anterior uveitis in 11% of the patients (11). In another series on urogenic arthritis ocular inflammation was observed in 33% of 73 women and in 42% of 72 men including conjunctivitis in 23% of females and in 31% of males, and acute anterior uveitis in 5% of emales and in 13% of males (26).

At the Department of Ophthalmology we examined 134 patients with reactive ocular inflammations following Yersinia, Salmonella, Shigella, Campylobacter or Chlamydia infections (17,19,20,21,23). Of them, 97 patients (72%) had reactive conjunctivitis, 42 patients (31%) had reactive iritis, and only one patient had keratitis.

Reactive Conjunctivtis

Reactive conjunctivitis occurred during the first month, usually from 4 to 17 days, after onset of the triggering infection. The patients complained of redness and a smarting or burning sensation. Conjunctivitis was mostly mild. The symptoms were often bilateral and began in both eyes at the same time. However, in some cases the other eye became affected later, generally after one or two days. Chemosis was only an occasional finding. In severe cases there were slight pain or severe smarting, lacrimation, palpebral edema, severe conjunctival injection, mucopurulent exudate, and subconjunctival hemorrhages. Follicles were seen especially in longstanding or recurrent cases of conjunctivitis.

Reactive conjunctivitis following Shigella dysentery was bilateral in the great majority (95%) of all cases (14). The patients complained of smarting, photophobia, epiphora, and redness of the eyes. There were conjunctival injection, mucopurulent discharge, slight swelling of the lids, and occasionally conjunctival chemosis (14). Both the palpebral and bulbar conjunctiva showed a deep cranberry color and a velvety surface. The mucopurulent discharge was generally thin, grayish, but there were also cases in which it was purulent, even very thick (14). Bacterial cultures of the conjunctiva were negative. Conjunctivitis resolved spontaneously in two to seven days without any permanent lesions. Only occasionally conjunctivitis lasted for two to four weeks. Longer duration of the conjunctivitis is rare. Acute anterior uveitis occurred a few days to several months after disappearance of conjunctivitis.

Severe conjunctivitis may be treated with Chloramphenicol or Hydrocortisone-Chloramphenicol eye drops or oinment but often this treatment did not provide any impovement, and the symptoms subsided spontaneously in two to seven days. If the patient has chlamydial infection with inclusion conjunctivitis, local and systemic tetracycline treatment is indicated.

After the first episode recurrent episodes of conjunctivitis may be seen. In some cases it occurred once a year, in others only a few times at intervals of several years.

Keratitis

The corneal changes are characterized by epithelial edema, superficial erosions in the periphery of the cornea, superficial punctate keratitis, and infiltrations beneath Bowman's layer. The infiltrations disappear generally during several weeks without any permanent scar or residua. Corneal ulcerations and a deep diffuse interstitial keratitis were rare findings. We observed one patient who developed transient episodes of conjunctivitis that lasted for 11 months and transient episodes of keratitis and corneal erosion for two month after Salmonella enteritis (23). The corneal lesions were characterized by epithelial edema in the inferior parts of both corneas, a large corneal erosion taking fluorescein stain, and punctate epithelial erosions staining lightly. During the treatment with Chloramphenicol eyedrops and ointment, the corneal erosions healed in five days and epithelial edema disappeared ten days later, but recurrent episodes of keratitis continued. Because of severe painful joint symptoms and lower back pain, the patient took Prednisone and Azathioprine for eight months. During this time she had some conjunctival injection, but no corneal changes were seen (23).

The patients with keratitis following Shigella dysentery showed both superficial and deep corneal infiltrates, varying from round shapes, 1 to 2 mm in diameter, to large pleomorphic figures (14). One patient showed a long and narrow bow-shaped ulcer in the cornea. The duration of keratitis after Shigella dysentery varied from one to four months (14).

Reactive Iritis

Reactive iritis occurs usually from five days to one month after the onset of the triggering infection. Occasionally it may follow conjunctivitis or recurrent attacks of acute anterior uveitis and conjunctivitis may intermittently follow each others.

The patients complained of redness, photophobia and pain, and some of them dicrease of vision and increased lacrimation. Pericorneal ciliary injection was observed in all patients; occasional patients with severe exudation into the anterior chamber and vitreous developed conjunctival chemosis. Aqueous flare and cells and fine keratic precipitates were constant findings. Keratic precipitates were never mutton-fat like. Fibrinous exudation into the aqueous humur was seen in over 50% of the patients. Marked vasodilation of the iris vessels was seen in some patients. In iris angiography the iris vessels showed fluorescein leakage. The pupil was constricted and posterior synechiae were often seen.

Cases of reactive iritis with secondary glaucoma were very rare. About 50% of the patients with reactive iritis showed cells in the vitreous. Some patients developed slight macular edema but no cystic macular edema was seen. Slight edema of the disk was an occasional finding.

Reactive iritis was mostly unilateral. The duration varied between 3 and 12 (mean 6) weeks. Topical medication with corticosteroids and cycloplegics sufficed in most cases; however, in about 40% of cases because of fulminant onset of intraocular inflammation systemic corticosteroids were used.

In over 30% of cases with reactive iritis acute anterior uveitis recurred after an interval of one month to serveral years. In some cases it occurred once a year, in others only a few times at intervals of several years. The duration of recurrences varied between 2 and 11 weeks. In most cases the inflammatory signs resolved completely during the treatment.

In a follow-up study on 100 cases of post-dysenteric Reiter's syndrome, Sairanen and coworkers (25) observed recurrent acute anterior uveitis, mostly unilateral, in seven patients. In one patient with bilateral recurrent acute anterior uveitis and secondary glaucoma, the visual acuity deteriorated to 0.7 in the right eye and 0.2 in the left. The recurrences of acute anterior uveitis did not seem to be related to the joint attacks, but to occur independently (25).

Lysozyme Content in Tears of Patients with Reiter's Syndrome

We studied the lysozyme content in tears in 32 patients with Reiter's syndrome (59 eyes) and in 240 healthy subjects (479 eyes). The mean lysozyme content in tears of the healthy subjects was 1768 μg/ml. An increasing concentration of lysozyme occurred in tear fluid from children to adults, highest values were seen in the age-groups of 21 to 40 years (2090μg/ml-2388μg/ml), and a decrease of lysozyme occurred with an increase of age from 30 to 80 years (18). Among the 32 patients with Reiter's syndrome ranging in age from 6 to 62 (mean 36) years, the mean value of lysozyme titer was 2539μg/ml (range 281μg/ml - 9500μg/ml). Although the mean lysozyme content of tears in Reiter's syndrome was slightly elevated, seven (22%) of the 32 patients with Reiter's syndrome had decreased lysozyme content in tears (mean 736μg/ml, range 281μg/ml - 1250μg/ml).

Relationship of Reactive Ocular Inflammation to Other HLA-B27 Associated Rheumatic Diseases

Determination of HLA antigens was done in 39 of 134 patients with reactive ocular inflammations (17, 19, 20, 21, 23). Of the 39 HLA typed patients, 38 (97%) revealed B27, which occurs in 14% of the Finnish control population. this finding suggests that reactive ocular inflammation may become manifest after the triggering infection in individuals with a genetically determinated predisposition indicated by HLA-B27.

A highly significant association of HLA-B27 with ankylosing spondylitis (7), reactive arthritis and Reiter's syndrome (2), acute anterior uveitis (5), circinate erosive balanitis (13), and reactive conjunctivitis (17, 19, 20, 21, 23) indicated that these diseases belong to the same HLA-B27 associated group of rheumatic diseases. The same patient may have these diseases in different combinations. For example in a study of 154 patients with acute anterior uveitis, associated rheumatic diseases were observed in 64 (41.6%) including 25% with Reiter's syndrome and 27% with ankylosing spondylitis (24).

Family studies on 35 families with multiple cases of acute anterior uveitis and different rheumatic diseases in the same family suggested that HLA-B27 itself or a pleiotropic HLA-B27 linked gene with autosomal dominant inheritance, incomplete penetrance, and variable expressivity may determine the susceptibility to reactive conjunctivitis, acute anterior uveitis, sacroiliitis, ankylosing spondylitis, reactive arthritis, and Reiter's syndrome (16,22).

The patients with reactive ocular inflammations following Yersinia, Salmonella, Shigella, and Campylobacter infections provide the best examples of an association between acute anterior uveitis or reactive conjunctivitis, HLA-B27, and an identified infective agent. Evidence for the participation of infective agents in acute anterior uveitis has in the past been circumstantial. Any organsim or antigen that can cause inflammation elsewhere in the body can cause inflammation of the eye (10). However, most of the possible etiologic causes of uveitis are ubiquitous antigens, and a large proportion of the population may have had contact with these antigens, so that separating previous antigenic exposure from active infection that causes the disease is difficult (10). In the patients with reactive iritis Yersinia (19,20), Salmonella (23), or Shigella (14,21) infection always preceded acute anterior uveitis confirming the role of infecting agents in the pathogenesis of acute anterior uveitis. Similary, reactive conjunctivitis occurred during the first month after onset of Yersinia (19,20), Salmonella (23), Shigella (14,21), or Campylobacter (17) infection. On the other hand, although reactive ocular inflammation may follow inclusion conjunctivitis and symptoms of Reiter's syndrome may be associated with Chlamydia infection (9) it may in many cases take months or even for several years before symptoms of Reiter's syndrome develop after Chlamydia infection.

References

1. Aho K, Ahvonen P, Lassus A et al (1973) HL-A27 Antigen and Reactive Arthritis. Lancet 2:157
2. Aho K, Ahvonen P, Lassus A et al (1974) HL-A27 in Reactive Arthritis. A Study of Yersinia Arthritis and Reiter's Disease. Arthritis Rheum 17:521
3. Ahvonen P (1972) Human Yersiniosis in Finland. II. Clinical Features. Ann Clin Res 4:39
4. Bauer W, Engleman EP (1942) Syndrome of Unknown Etiology Characterized by Urethritis, Conjunctivitis and Arthritis (so-called Reiter's disease). Trans Assoc Am Physicians 57:307
5. Brewerton DA, Caffrey M, Nicholls A et al (1973) Acute anterior Uveitis and HL-A27. Lancet 2:994
6. Briem H, Evengard B, Jonsson M (1978) Reiter's Syndrome Complicating Salmonella enteritidis Infection Lancet 2:112
7. Caffrey MFP, James DCO (1973) Human Lymphocyte Antigen Association in Ankylosing Spondylitis. Nature 242:121
8. Csonka GW (1958) The Course of Reiter's Syndrome. Br Med J 1:1088
9. Dawson CR, Schachter J, Ostler HB et al (1970) Inclusion conjunctivitis and Reiter's Syndrome is a Married Couple. Arch Ophthalmol 83:300
10. Kaufman HE (1968) The Testing of Microbial Allergies in Uveitis. In: Aronson SB, Gamble CN, Goodner EK, O'Connor GR (eds) Clinical Methods in Uveitis. C.V.Mosby, St.Louis p.177
11. Kousa M (1978) Clinical Observations on Reiter's Disease with Special Reference to the Venereal and Non-venereal Aetiology. Acta Derm Venereol 58(Suppl)81)
12. Lang GK, Knapp W, Völcker HE (1983) Yersinia-Uveitis. Klin Mbl Augenheilk 182:156

13. Lassus A, Tiilikainen A, Stubb S et al (1975) Circinate Erosive Balanitis and HL-A27. Acta Derm Venereol 55:199
14. Paronen I (1948) Reiter's Disease. A Study of 344 Cases Observed in Finland. Acta Med Scand Suppl 212:1
15. Reiter H (1916) Über eine bisher unbekannte Spirochaeten Infektion (Spirochaetosis arthritica). Dtsch Med Wschr 42:1535
16. Saari KM (1983) Genetic Background of Uveitis. In: Henkind,P (ed) Acta XXIV Int Congr Ophthalmol. J.B.Lippincott Co. Philadelphia pp.46-48
17. Saari KM, Kauranen O (1980) Ocular Inflammation in Reiter's Syndrome Associated with Campylobacter jejuni Enteritis. Am J Ophthalmol 90:572
18. Saari KM, Klockars M (1983) Lysozyme Content in Tears of Patients with Various Inflammatory Diseases. In: Henkind P (ed) Acta XXIV Int Congr Ophthalmol J.B.Lippincott Co.Philadelphia pp.834-837
19. Saari KM, Laitinen O, Leirisalo M et al (1980) Ocular Inflammation Associated with Yersinia Infection. Am J Ophthalmol 89:84
20. Saari KM, Mäki M, Päivönsalo T et al (1986) Acute anterior Uveitis and Conjunctivitis Following Yersinia Infection in Children. Int Ophthalmol 9:237
21. Saari KM, Miettinen P, Saari R (1981) Reaktive Augenentzündungen nach Yersinia-, Salonellen-, Shigellen, Campylobacter- und Chlamydieninfektionen. Ber Dtsch Ophthalmol Ges 78:203
22. Saari KM, Solja J, Häkli J et al (1981) Genetic Background of Acute Anterior Uveitis. Am J Ophthalmol 91:711
23. Saari KM, Vilppula A, Lassus A et al (1980) Ocular Inflammation in Reiter's Disease After Salmonella Enteritis. Am J Ophthalmol 90:63
24. Saari R, Lahti R, Saari KM et al (1982) Frequency of Rheumatic Diseases in Patients with Acute Anterior Uveitis. Scand J Rheumatol 11:121
25. Sairanen E, Paronen I, Mähönen H (1969) Reiter's Syndrome: A Follow-up Study. Acta Med Scand 185:57
26. Yli-Kerttula U (1984) Reiter's Syndrome or Uro-arthritis in Females with Special Emphasis on Chlamydial Infections. Acta Univ Tamperensis Ser A 177.1

VIII. TROPICAL INFECTIOUS DISEASES

- Trachoma

Immunology of Trachoma

Judith A. Whittum-Hudson and Hugh R. Taylor

Abstract. The pathogenesis of trachoma results in part from the immune response to Chlamydia trachomatis infection of the conjunctiva. Recent advances have increased our understanding of anti-chlamydial immunity which develops after infection, in large part because of studies in animal models. These studies have provided new information on the immunopathogenesis of chlamydia-induced disease, and have directed the efforts in many laboratories toward vaccine development. The fine antigen specificity of serologic responses has been characterized and the chlamydial major outer membrane protein (MOMP) identified as a major immunogen during chlamydial infection. Anti-chlamydial MOMP monoclonal antibodies have been shown to be neutralizing for infectious chlamydia. For these reasons several laboratories have focussed on characterization of the chlamydial MOMP and its use as a recombinant or protein vaccine. In addition, the local cell-mediated and B cell responses to ocular chlamydial infection have been investigated. Studies in the primate model of trachoma have shown that high frequencies of chlamydia-specific T and B cells accumulate in the conjunctiva during infection. These cells are found during peak inflammation, and their presence supports a chlamydia-specific component in the inflammatory response. These findings have been strengthened by the observation of large numbers of T and B cells in the conjunctiva of patients with late-stage cicatricial trachoma.

Introduction

The immunology of ocular chlamydial infections has been under intense investigation for more than twenty years. A better understanding of the immunologic responses to chlamydia is important to both understanding the pathogenesis of the disease trachoma as well as to efforts to control ocular infections by immunologic modulation via vaccination. Evidence has accumulated that an immunologic balance must be struck between deleterious and protective immune responses if the blinding sequelae of trachoma are to be prevented.

Attempts have been made experimentally and clinically for many years to define the immunologic requirements for control of ocular chlamydial infections, but immunologic control of chlamydial infections has proven elusive. Some of the recent advances in chlamydial immunology are summarized in Table 1. Experimental attempts to induce protection from ocular Chlamydia trachomatis infection have shown that protection better than that induced by recovery from a natural infection has not been achieved (30).

Early vaccination attempts were unsuccessful or even worsened disease. Guinea pigs have been a useful experimental animal for immunopathologic studies (14,17), but the comparability of results of studies with nonhuman biovars of C.psittaci to C.trachomatis is not fully known. In the guinea pig, a primary chlamydial infection induces protective immunity which persists for weeks to months, and this differs from results in man and monkeys.

The target tissue of chlamydial infection is the mucosal epithelium, and the immune responses at mucosal surfaces, particularly by T cells, are believed to be critical to successful protection from chlamydial infection. Unfortunately, the mucosal immune responses to chlamydia remain poorly understood. The potential importance of neutralizing secretory IgA (sIgA) in tears at sites of infection was demonstrated in guinea pigs and owl monkeys (4,17); hence, most strategies for stimulation of protective immunity against chlamydia have been aimed at induction of a local sIgA response.

Immunopathogenesis

The mononuclear infiltrate in the infected conjunctiva had been described (31,33), but the lymphocyte subset distribution was not known until immunohistochemical studies were performed on chlamydia-infected tissues. Normal monkey and human conjunctiva contain very few lymphocytes, and those present appear to be predominantly subepithelial $CD8^+$ suppressor-cytotoxic cells. Following ocular chlamydial infection, large numbers of T cells are found surrounding the B cell-containing follicles where $CD8^+$ cells greatly out-number $CD4^+$ T cells. B cells expressing all the major immunoglobulin classes were found exclusively within the follicles. Similar results have been obtained from the monkey model and from trachoma patients (10,21,39). In addition, the majority of the lymphocytic infiltrates express major histocompatibility complex Class II antigens (22; Zhang and coworkers, in preparation, 1992). While immunohistochemical studies provided new information regarding the immunopathogenesis of trachoma, it remained unknown how much of the conjunctival infiltrate was antigen-specific versus part of the nonspecific chronic inflammatory response induced by ocular chlamydial infection.

Functional assays with peripheral blood mononuclear cells have been used for in vitro studies of immune responses to ocular chlamydial infection in subhuman primates and man (13,40,41). $CD8^+$ suppressor T cells have been demonstrated in experimental infection models, but their role in disease pathogenesis remains unknown (40,41). While chlamydia-specific proliferative responses by peripheral blood mononuclear cells were observed in human and experimental ocular infection, studies of conjunctival and regional lymph node populations have shown that higher antigen-specific responses occur locally. Studies in the cynomolgus monkey allowed isolation of conjunctival lymphocytes during ocular infection and testing for the presence of chlamydia-specific T and B cells. Our first indication that the expected chlamydia-specific B cells were present was the detection of chlamydia-specific IgG and IgA secreted into culture supernatants (38).

Recently the ELISPOT technique has allowed enumeration of the relative frequency of chlamydia-specific B cells present in isolated conjunctival lymphocyte populations. High frequencies of IgG-secreting B cells were observed in the range of 100 chlamydia-specific cells/million total mixed lymphocytes (18,37). The frequency of chlamydia-specific T cells in the same population was shown to range from 100-1000 chlamydia-specific proliferating T cells/10^6 cells (19,37) (Table 2). The precise nature of these T cells (e.g., $CD4^+$ vs. $CD8^+$) has not yet been determined because of limited numbers of available conjunctival cells. However, similar frequencies of chlamydia-specific T and B cells were found in regional draining cervical lymph nodes of infected monkeys, and this tissue should provide sufficient cells to further investigate the functions of chlamydia-specific lymphocytes.

The possibility exists that local immune responses account primarily for the pathogenesis of disease, rather than partial protective immunity. Recently the 57kD chlamydial protein was shown to be homologous to the 60kD heat shock protein (15,16). Studies in guinea pigs (36) and the monkey model (31) showed that ocular exposure of immune animals to the 57kD protein elicited a local hypersensitivity reaction. Lymphocytes isolated from immune monkey conjunctivae during the response to the 57kD protein exhibited a high frequency of chlamydia specificity (18,37). These results further support a role for the 57kD chlamydial antigen in the immunopathogenesis of trachoma. Information regarding other potentially pathogenic responses during ocular infection is limited but is under active investigation by several laboratories.

Another chlamydial heat shock protein, a 75kD protein, has been identified (12). Monoclonal antibodies to the 75kD protein were found to neutralize infectious organisms in vitro (12,32). However, the same antibody when mixed with elementary bodies prior to ocular challenge failed to neutralize in vivo infection (Taylor, Whittum-Hudson, Maclean and Brunham, unpublished observation). The chlamydial 75kD protein does not induce an ocular hypersensitivity reaction when applied to conjunctiva of immune monkeys, and therefore probably does not contribute to the pathogenesis of trachoma (32). Furthermore, this protein did not protectively immunize monkeys against infectious ocular challenge. Women with chlamydia-induced salpingitis appear to have lower antibody responses to the 75kD protein than patients who do not develop this genital infection, suggesting that anti-75kD antibodies have a protective role in vivo (9).

The role of several cytokines in chlamydial infection has been studied recently (11,22-25). Most of these studies were performed in vitro, but tears of chlamydia-infected patients and monkeys appeared to have elevated levels of interleukin-1 (22). Recent in vitro studies showed the inhibitory effects of gamma-interferon on chlamydial infectivity (11) and the increased production of several cytokines including tumor necrosis factor-alpha by infected monocytes (24,25). The relationship of the various cytokines to the pathogenesis of trachoma remains to be further elucidated (2,3).

Protective Immunity and Vaccine Development

Antichlamydial vaccine development depends upon clearer understanding of the immunology of trachoma, as well as increased knowledge of the chlamydial organism. Molecular biologic approaches have revolutionized the field of chlamydial research in recent years. This, plus the detailed information provided by the protein biochemists, have now directed much of the effort toward identification of chlamydial antigens which are immunogenic and, therefore, potential vaccine candidates.

MOMP: The best understood chlamydial antigen is the major outer membrane protein, which is a membrane protein consisting of four variable domains (3,26). The variable domains have been the focus of subunit vaccine development, and we will be hearing more about these efforts in the future. The immunogenicity of MOMP is unarguable, because this is the major specificity of immune sera and tears from animals and patients. The relative importance of the four variable domains in protective immunity is not clear at present, although the presence of T cell epitopes in variable domains 1 and possibly 3 and 4 is believed to be important for optimal immunogenicity (1,28). Elegant studies with synthetic peptides of different amino acid lengths of the MOMP molecule have deduced the minimum recognition sequence required to elicit antibody responses in vivo (20). Studies with monoclonal antibodies suggested initially that only the variable domains 1,2 and 4 were exposed on the elementary bodies' surface (28), but recently variable domain 3 was demonstrated to be exposed (1), perhaps after conformational changes in the other variable domains. These types of studies will be invaluable to development of a successful trachoma vaccine.

In studies in our laboratories, recombinant forms of the MOMP variable domains have been tested for immunogenicity and as vaccine candidates in the monkey model. Monkeys were immunized with MOMP variable domains 2 or 4 both mucosally by the oral and ocular routes and systemically (intraperitoneally) before challenge with infectious chlamydia. A slight degree of clinical protection was induced by recombinant variable domain 2, but not by variable domain 4 (34). None of the monkeys developed significant anti-chlamydial serologic or cell-mediated responses to whole elementary bodies prior to infectious challenge, although post-challenge antibody titers were elevated and resembled those seen during a secondary immune response. A subsequent vaccination attempt with recombinant variable domain 2 plus an associated T cell epitope was performed in another study, but this candidate antigen failed to induce protection. These antigens have been shown to be immunogenic in rodents, generally after systemic immunization. The protective capacity of subunit vaccines at mucosal surfaces in primates may depend upon different factors, including the choices of adjuvant, dosage, temporal factors, etc.

The importance of the conformation of MOMP in immunogenicity has been demonstrated by several studies (6,7,29). When MOMP is extracted from elementary bodies by harsh detergents, it loses its native conformation, and this change may explain the failure of such extracts to protect from experimental ocular infection (30). Recent studies with MOMP extracted with milder detergents (sarkosyl and octylglucopyranoside) have suggested that such a nonionic detergent preserved the native confirmation of MOMP because vigorous serologic and cell-mediated responses to whole elementary bodies were induced by systemic vaccination with octylglucopyranoside (OGP) - extracted MOMP. Guinea pigs so immunized were protected from genital infection with C.psittaci (6), and sheep were significantly protected from chlamydia-induced abortions (29).

Based on the OGP-MOMP results in guinea pigs and sheep, we attempted to protect monkeys against ocular infection with OGP-MOMP extracted from a human Chlamydia trachomatis biovar. Using the extraction method of Bavoil (7), monkeys were immunized with OGP-MOMP either mucosally or systemically. Cholera toxin was mixed with OGP-MOMP for mucosal immunization; OGP-MOMP was administered intramuscularly with complete Freund's adjuvant for the initial systemic immunization, followed by antigen in incomplete Freund's adjuvant for the boosting immunization.

As shown in Fig.1, OGP-MOMP induced substantial serum and tear IgG responses to whoule chlamydial elementary bodies prior to infectious challenge on day 0. Only systemic immunization induced tear IgA prior to challenge. In addition, both immunization groups appeared to have developed anti-chlamydial cell-mediated immune responses prior to challenge, but these were short-lived. Immunoblotting revealed that serum and tear antibody was directed primarily against MOMP after immunization. Despite obvious immunization by OGP-MOMP, monkeys were not protected from clinical disease; the reason for the failure of OGP-MOMP to protect from ocular infection is not yet clear. The two most obvious possibilities are that insufficient IgA was induced at the conjunctival surface prior to challenge, or that there are different immunization requirements for protection against trachomatis and C.psittaci. The vigorous immunity to OGP-MOMP may have contributed to the observed disease rather than preventing it.

Anti-Idiotypic Antibody: The potential of anti-idiotypic antibody to serve as a vaccine against trachoma is another area beginning to be investigated with C.trachomatis. An exoglycolipid (GLXA) obtained from viable chlamydia (27) was used to raise a monoclonal antibody (AB1) against which an anti-idiotypic antibody (AB2) was raised. We tested the ability of an anti-anti-idiotypic antibody (AB3) raised against anti-idiotypic antibody AB2 to neutralize infectivity of chlamydia in the monkey eye. Infectious elementary bodies were incubated in vitro with anti-anti-idiotypic antibody AB3, pre-immune IgG or medium, after which each eye received an inoculum containing 1000 IFU. The microbiologic result of these pre-treatments on positive ocular isolates over three weeks post-challenge indicated that anti-anti-idiotypic antibody AB3 substantially reduced the infectivity of the elementary bodies challenge, while the infectivity in either control group was not reduced. These results are summarized in Table 3. Most importantly, the reduction in clinical disease scores appeared to parallel the reduced culture positivity in the recipients of elementary bodies plus anti-anti-idiotypic antibody AB3 (2; MacDonald and coworkers, manuscript in preparation). These results suggest that an anti-idiotype for ocular chlamydial infection may be a feasible vaccine, and studies are planned to test this possibility.

There are important studies on the immunology of chlamydial infections being conducted primarily with C.psittaci in smaller animals, using routes of infection other than the eye (e.g., genital tract). It is generally believed that chlamydial infections of the various mucosal tissues (gut, genital tract, lung and eye) will be shown to have similar immunologic requirements for protection. Until it is clear that C.trachomatis and C.psittaci induce similar immunological responses relevant to protective immunity, some caution must be used in extrapolating results to C.trachomatis infections in man.

Conclusions

In summary, our understanding of the immunology of trachoma is that long-lasting anti-chlamydial immunity is difficult to induce. Because anti-chlamydial immune responses can worsen disease, protective (neutralizing) immunity must precede or block progression to pathogenic responses. Clearly, the successful vaccine candidate will have to

- avoid induction of 57kD protein-mediated local hypersensitivity,
- stimulate appropriate mucosal immunity,
- be long-lasting.

The cumulative results from the chlamydia research community also suggest that the first successful vaccine may be a cocktail of chlamydial antigens including those already associated with protection from infection:

- the 75kD protein,
- the exoglycolipid,
- the cysteine-rich 60kD protein,
- protective epitopes on the MOMP.

Acknowledgment. Support for studies in our laboratories came in part from the U.S. Department of Health and Human Services, National Institutes of Health, and the Edna McConnell Clark Foundation, New York, NY.

Table 1. Recent immunologic landmarks in trachoma research

1. Chlamydia-specific anti-MOMP antibody in serum and tears (32)
2. MOMP as a major immunogenic chlamydial protein (6,10,13,40)
3. High frequencies of chlamydia-specific T and B lymphocytes in infected conjunctiva (18,19,37,38)
4. Immunogenicity of 57kD chlamydial protein (15,16,18,35)
5. Immunogenicity of MOMP variable domains (1,28)

See References 5 and 8 for additional immunologic investigations.

Table 2. High frequencies of chlamydia-specific T and B lymphocytes locally during ocular infection

Mean frequencies of antigen-specific cells			
T cells		B cells	
Conjunctiva	PBMC	Lymph node	PBMC
494 ± 409	15 ± 18	238 ± 251	19 ± 19

Mean ± S.D. of results from 4-6 monkeys at varying times after secondary challenge with infectious C serovar or 57kDa protein. See references 18 and 19 for details.

Table 3. Neutralization of infectivity by anti-anti-idiotype

	No. of Positive results (%)		
	EBs preincubated with:		
Assay	AB3	preimmune IgG	None
Culture	9/48 (19)	17/24 (70)	19/24 (79)
DFA	2/48 (4)	16/24 (67)	19/24 (79)

Cumulative results from individual eyes of monkeys challenged with C serovar EB (1000 IFU) preincubated with anti-anti-Id (AB3), preimmune IgG, or no antibody before topical ocular application.

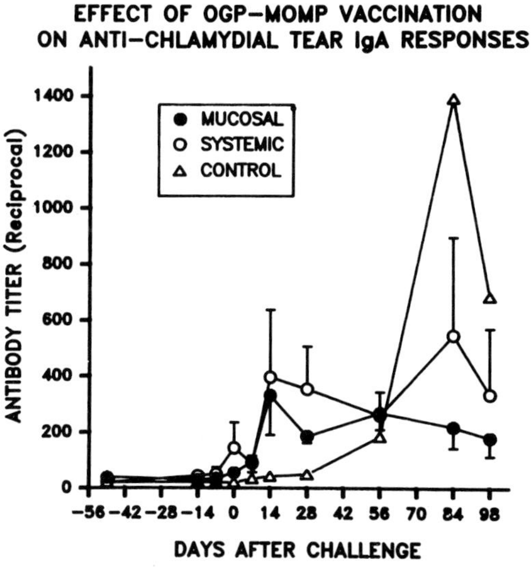

Fig.1. Serum and tear antibody responses to Chlamydia trachomatis after immunization with octylglucopyranoside-major outer membrane protein; (a) serum IgG, (b) tear IgA. Antibody titers against whole C serovar elementary bodies were determined by enzyme linked immunosorbent assays using cross-reactive anti-human heavy chain-specific second antibodies.

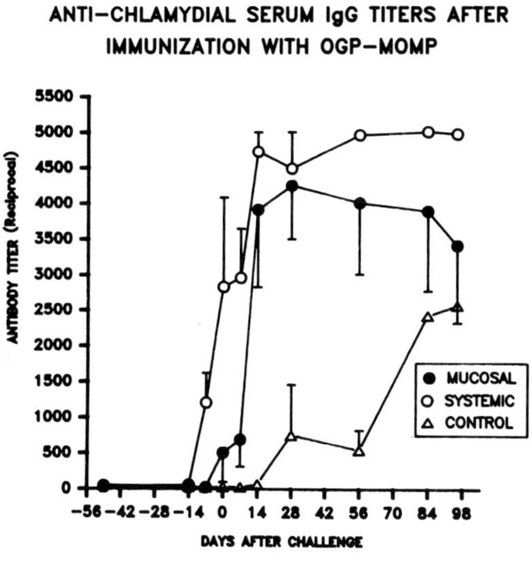

Fig.2.

References

1. Allen JE, Locksley RM, Stephens RS (1991) A Single Peptide from the Major Outer Membrane Protein of Chlamydia trachomatis Elicits T-Cell Help for the Production of Antibodies to Protective Determinants. J Immunol 147:674-679
2. An LL, Whittum-Hudson JA, Taylor HR et al (1991) An Anti-Idiotype Antibody Mimics Glycolipid Antigen of C.trachomatis. Abstr Am Soc Microbiol p.120
3. Baehr W., Zhang Y-X, Joseph T et al (1988) Mapping Antigenic Domains Expressed by Chlamydia trachomatis Major Outer Membrane Protein Genes. Proc Natl Acad Sci 85:4000-4004
4. Barenfanger J, MacDonald AB (1974) The Role of Immunoglobulin in the Neutralization of Trachoma Infectivity. J Immunol 113:1607-1617
5. Barron AL (ed) (1988) Microbiology of Chlamydia. CRC Press, Boca Raton
6. Batteiger BE, Rank RG, Soderberg LSF (1990) Immunization of Guinea Pigs with Isolated Chlamydial Outer Membrane Protein. In: Bowie WR et al (eds) Chlamydial Infections. Cambridge Univ Press, Cambridge pp.265-268
7. Bavoil P, Ohlin A, Schachter J (1984) Role of Disulfide Binding in Outer Membrane Structure and Permeability in Chlamydia trachomatis. Infect Immun 44:479-485
8. Bowie WR, Caldwell HD, Jones RP et al (eds) (1990) Chlamydial Infections. Cambridge Univ Press, Cambridge
9. Brunham RC, Peeling R, Maclean I et al(1987) Postabortal Chlamydia trachomatis Salpingitis: Correlating Risk with Antigen-Specific Serological Responses and with Neutralization. J Infect Dis 155:749-755
10. Burd EM, Tabbara KF, Nasr AM et al (1988) Conjunctival Lymphocyte Subsets in Trachoma. Int Ophthalmol 12:53-57
11. Byrne GI, Carlin JM, Merkert TP et al (1989) Long-term Effects of Gamma Interferon on Chlamydia-Infected Host Cells: Microbicidal Activity Follows Microbistasis. Infect Immun 57:1318-1320
12. Danilition SL, Maclean IW, Peeling R et al (1990) The 75kD Protein of Chlamydia trachomatis: A Member of the Heat Shock Protein 70 Family. Infect Immun 58:189-196
13. Mabey DCW, Holland MJ, Bailey RL et al (1990) In vitro Studies of Cell-Mediated Immunity to Chlamydial Antigens in Trachoma. In: Bowie WR et al (eds) Chlamydial Infections. Cambridge Univ Press, Cambridge pp.283-286
14. Monnickendam MA, Darougar S, Treharne JD et al (1981) Development of Chronic Conjunctiviti with Scarring and Pannus, Resembling Trachoma. B.J Ophthalmol 64:284-290
15. Morrison RP, Belland RJ, Lyng K et al (1989) Chlamydial Disease Pathogenesis: The 57kD Chlamydial Hypersensitivity Antigen is a Stress Response Protein. J Exp Med 170:1271-1283
16. Morrison RP, Lyng K, Caldwell HD (1989) Chlamydial Disease Pathogenesis: Ocular Hypersensitivity Elicited by a Genus-Specific 57kD Protein. J Exp Med 169:663-675
17. Murray ES, Charbonnet LT, MacDonald AB (1973) The Role of Circulatory and Secretory Antibodies in Resistance to Reinfection with Guinea Pig Inclusion Conjunctivitis. J Immunol 110:1518-1525
18. Pal S, Taylor HR, Huneke RB et al (1992) Frequency of Antigen-Specific B Cells During Experimentel Ocular Chlamydia trachomatis Infection. Infect Immun 60: 5294 - 5291
19. Pal S, Zhang P, Huneke RB et al (1991) Chlamydia-Specific Lymphocytes in Conjunctiva During Ocular Infection: Limiting Dilution Analysis. Region Immunol 3:171-176

20. Pickett MA, Ward ME, Clarke IN (1988) High Level Expression and Epitope Localisation of the Major Outer Membrane Protein of Chlamydia trachomatis Serovar L1. Mol Microbiol 2:681-685
21. Reacher MH, Taylor HR (1990) Trachoma. Curr Opinion Infect Dis 3:549-554
22. Reacher MH, Pe'er J, Rapoza PA et al (1991) Tcells and Trachoma: Their Role in Cicatricial Disease. Ophthalmology 98: 334-341
23. Rothermel CD, Schachter J, Lavrich P et al (1989) Chlamydia trachomatis-Induced Production of Interleukin 1 by Human Monocytes. Infect Immun 57:2705-2711
24. Shemer-Avni Y, Holtmann H, Wallach D et al (1990) Cytokine-Cell Interactions Resulting in Chlamydia trachomatis Inhibition - Mechanisms Involved. In: Bowie WR et al. (eds) Chlamydial Infections. Cambridge Univ Press, Cambridge pp.173-176
25. Shemer-Avni Y, Wallach D, Sarov I (1989) Reversion of the Antichlamydial Effect of Tumor Necrosis Factor by Tryptophan and Antibodies to Beta Interferon. Infect Immun 57:3484-3490
26. Stephens RS, Wagar EA, Schoolnik GK (1988) High Resolution Mapping of Serovar-Specific and Common Antigenic Determinants of the Major Outer Membrane Protein of Chlamydia trachomatis. J Exp Med 167:817-831
27. Stuart ES, MacDonald AB (1989) Some Characteristics of a Secreted Chlamydial Antigen Recognized by IgG from C.trachomatis Patient Sera. Immunology 68:469-473
28. Su H, Caldwell HD (1991) In vitro Neutralization of Chlamydia trachomatis by Monovalent Fab Antibody Specific to the Major Outer Membrane Protein. Infect Immun 59:2843-2845
29. Tan TW, Herring AJ, Anderson IE et al (1990) Protection of Sheep Against Chlamydia psittaci Infection with a Subcellular Vaccine Containing the Major Outer Membrane Protein. Infect Immun 58:3101-3108
30. Taylor HR (1990) Development of Immunity to Ocular Chlamydial Infection. Am J Trop Med Hyg 42:358-364
31. Taylor HR, Johnson SL, Schachter J et al (1987) Pathogenesis of Trachoma: The Stimulus for Inflammation. J Immunol 138:3023-3027
32. Taylor HR, Maclean IW, Brunham RC et al (1990) Chlamydial Heat Shock Proteins and Trachoma. Infect Immun 58:3061-3063
33. Taylor HR, Prendergast RA, Dawson CR et al (1981) An Animal Model for Cicatrizing Trachoma. Invest Ophthalmol Vis Sci 21:422-433
34. Taylor HR, Stephens RS, Whittum-Hudson JA, et al (1989) Initial Evaluation of Trachoma Subunit Vaccines. Invest Ophthalmol Vis Sci 30(Suppl):381
35. Wagar EA, Schachter J, Bavoil P et al (1990) Differential Human Serologic Response to two 60'000 Molecular Weight Chlamydia trachomatis Antigens. J Infect Dis 162:922-927
36. Watkins NG, Hadlow WJ, Moos AB et al (1986) Ocular Delayed Hypersensitivity: A Pathogenic Mechanism of Chlamydial Conjunctivitis in Guinea Pigs. Proc Natl Acad Sci 83:7480-7484
37. Whittum-Hudson JA, Taylor HR (1989) Anti-Chlamydial Specificity of Conjunctival Lymphocytes During Experimental Ocular Infection. Infect Immun 57:2977-2983
38. Whittum-Hudson JA, Taylor HR, Farazdaghi M et al (1986) Immunohistochemical Study of the Local Inflammatory Response to Chlamydial Ocular Infection. Invest Ophthalmol Vis Sci 27:64-69
39. Whittum-Hudson JA, Pal S, Zhang P et al (1990) in vitro Functional Studies of Conjunctival Lymphocytes After Ocular Chlamydia trachomatis Infection. In:

MacDonald TT et al (eds) Adv Mucosal Immunol. Kluwer Academic Publishers, Dordrecht pp.526-529

40. Young E, Taylor HR (1984) Immune Mechanisms in Chlamydial Eye Infections: Cellular Immune Responses in Chronic and Acute Disease. J Infect Dis 150:745-751
41. Young E, Taylor HR (1986) Immune Mechanisms in Chlamydial Eye Infection: Development of TSuppressor Cells. Invest Ophthalmol Vis Sci 27:616-619

Blinding Trachoma

Chandler R. Dawson

Abstract. Trachoma is still a major cause of blindness in many rural areas of developing countries: 6 to 9 million are blind from the disease and an estimated 80 million children have potentially blinding inflammatory trachoma. Conjunctival infection early in life with Chlamydia trachomatis produces a chronic follicular and papillary conjunctivitis that progresses to conjunctival scarring and corneal pannus formation. Children whose scarring is severe have a high risk of developing trichiasis/entropion in adult life and subsequently blindness from corneal scarring. Prevention of trachomatous blindness is based on improving hygienic behavior and topical antibiotic treatment of all children in endemic communities. Oral antibiotic treatment is highly effective in children with severe inflammatory disease. Systematic case finding of persons with trichiasis/entropion and corrective surgery has an immediate effect on preventing blindness. Recent studies in Egypt and elsewhere have shown that face washing of young children protects them from severe inflammatory trachoma.
Improvements in trachoma control now being tested include daily face washing of young children and new antibiotics. Vaccine development is being investigated vigorously, but there are major problems on choices of epitopes, sensitizing versus protective antigens, and definition of an appropriate response to candidate vaccines.

Introduction

Endemic trachoma is still a major cause of blindness in rural communities of the developing world (3). Trachoma affects approximately 500 million people, most of them living in poorer rural sections of developing countries, especially in arid areas. There are an estimated six million to nine million blind from trachoma, and a much larger number has suffered partial loss of vision. A simplified clinical description now allows nonspecialist health personnel to identify and treat trachoma in communities with blinding trachoma (17).

Trachoma is a chronic inflammation of the conjunctiva and cornea that regularly leads to conjunctival scarring and corneal vascularization. C.trachomatis is the specific etiologic agent of trachoma, but other pathogenic microorganisms often contribute to the disease process (8). In its communicable, inflammatory phase trachoma is characterized by the presence of lymphoid germinal centers (lymphoid follicles) surrounded by diffuse infiltration and hyperemia (papillary hypertrophy) in the conjunctiva, and by the growth of a superficial vascular membrane or pannus over the cornea.

Trachomatous inflammation can undergo spontaneous resolution without serious sequelae or progress to severe conjunctival scarring which causes inturned eyelashes. The misdirected lashes constantly abrade the cornea, eventually producing corneal ulceration and permanent opacity. The final visual acuity may range from normal vision to total blindness.

Etiology: C.trachomatis eye infections occur in two distinct epidemiological settings. The first pattern is the potentially blinding disease of developing countries that is spread by eye-to-eye transmission of infection, and is defined as endemic trachoma. It is caused by C.trachomatis, almost always serotypes A, B, Ba or C (20).

The second pattern is infection of the eye by sexually transmitted C.trachomatis (usually serotypes D, E, F, G, H, I, J, or K) which produces an eye disease that is often indistinguishable from the early inflammatory phases of endemic trachoma. This follicular conjunctivitis with sexually transmitted C.trachomatis strains is usually called inclusion conjunctivitis, but the term "paratrachoma" is used to describe the whole spectrum of eye disease including corneal involvement. Sexually transmitted C.trachomatis also infects newborns during delivery and causes conjunctivitis, pneumonia and gastrointestinal infection. Sporadic eye infections with sexually transmitted C.trachomatis strains rarely produce permanent visual loss, but the respiratory tract infections in infants and genital tract infections in adults are important health problems.

Some communities with trachoma of blinding severity also have seasonal epidemics of bacterial conjunctivitis which are closely associated with large numbers of eye-seeking flies (2,10). In other regions with trachoma there is a high rate of purulent conjunctivitis throughout the year. Furthermore, during these seasonal epidemics, bacterial corneal ulceration is common, and it constitutes an acute pathway to corneal blindness.

Clinical Features

Clinical Course: In communities with endemic trachoma, the disease has an insidious onset early in childhood and often presents as a mucopurulent conjunctivitis. Trachoma is characterized by conjunctival follicles which are collections of lymphocytes or lymphoid germinal centers in subepithelial conjunctiva. In children under two years, however, the conjunctiva may be heavily infiltrated and hyperemic, so that follicles even if present are hidden by the inflamed tissue. While clinical trachoma involves the entire conjunctiva, diagnosis is based on the disease process in the conjunctiva of the upper tarsal plate. The follicles may be quite prominent and larger ones are often soft and rupture easily on pressure, resulting in small hemorrhages.

Conjunctival scarring occurs as a result of chronic inflammation and has been attributed to necrosis of mature follicles. Scarring may appear during the second year of life. Moderate and severe scarring may occur as early as 10 years and some children first develop trichiasis/entropion in adolescence (1,2). Inturned eye-lashes become more common as those with conjunctival scarring become older. This is due to progressive contraction of the scarred tissue over time.

During inflammatory trachoma, epithelial and subepithelial infiltrates occur regularly at the corneal limbus, and these appear to initiate superficial corneal vascularization which is more extensive superiorly. Follicles can form at the limbus, eroding the sclera overhang and, when these resolve, they leave small depressions (Herbert's pits) which are unique to trachoma.

The presence of severe conjunctival inflammation (papillary hypertrophy) is highly predictive of later conjunctival scarring. Severe conjunctival scarring in childhood is often followed by the occurrence of trichiasis/entropion in adolescence or early adult life. These inturned eyelashes in adolescents and young adults are an important risk factor for corneal scarring in later adult life (5,6).

Descriptive clinical systems: Several systems have been used to describe the clinical features of trachoma:

- the MacCallan classification (1905) divided the natural history of the disease in four stages with the concept of active (presumably infectious), cicatricial stages and a healed stage (3,11);
- the Fourth World Health Organization Scientific Group on Trachoma Research (1966) described 22 signs with a detailed system of categorical scores for each sign (17,21);
- later World Health Organization publications (1975, 1981) described a shorter system of seven signs which emphasized the intensity of inflammatory disease and included the MacCallan stages (3,4,8); and
- a simplified system (1987) of five signs has been proposed for use by primary health care workers (17,20).

These descriptive systems (particularly the MacCallan classification and the most recent World Health Organization system) have been widely used by health authorities to guide public health policy, to evaluate treatment programs and for epidemiologic and therapeutic research studies.

Pathogenesis and Microbiology

Chlamydial tests: Laboratory tests are not essential to trachoma control programs. However, they may be used for a number of reasons:

- to support the clinical diagnosis in individual cases;
- to measure the prevalence of agent in a community where trachoma is endemic; and
- to monitor individuals or communities for the effect of therapy.

C.trachomatis infections are diagnosed by identifying the agent in clinical specimens or by a rising antibody titer. Methods to identify the agent are listed in Table 1.

The microscopic examination of Giemsa stained smears was the mainstay of laboratory diagnosis from the first decade of this century and is still a useful tool for field studies but is relatively insensitive (22). The first isolation of C.trachomatis was reported in 1956 from China by inoculation of the yolk sacs of fertile hen's eggs (16). Current isolation techniques utilize specially treated cell cultures for isolation and are very sensitive (14,15). Fluorescein labeled monoclonal antibody preparations are now easily available for fluorescent microscopy (9,13). Commercially available antigen detection tests utilize enzyme immunoassay and other techniques. Some are to large numbers of approphiate for specimens (e.g.Chlamydiazyme, Abbott Laboratories) and others can be used as single tests (e.g. Chlamydia SureCell kit, Kodak). All these newer tests have a high sensitivity and a high specificity but may be too costly for routine use in developing countries. A comparison of the sensitivity and specificity of these same tests is presented in Table 2.

Because most persons with trachoma have IgG antibody, indicating infection at some time in the past, serology has little application in detection of active chlamydial infection in individuals. Serologic tests are useful, however, for epidemiologic studies (18).

Chlamydial infection: Trachoma agent cannot be identified in all cases of clinically active trachoma. Studies with Giemsa stained conjunctival smears showed that chlamydial inclusions occurred most frequently in severe intensity cases (50% to 60% positive); less often in moderate intensity cases (10% to 20%), infrequently in mild cases (less than 5%), and very rarely in clinically inactive cases (22). The newer antigen detection and isolation tests have confirmed this general pattern, but even the most sensitive techniques detect chlamydial agent in only 50% of clinically "active" cases, suggesting that the disease process can continue in the absence of replicating chlamydial agent (15). In chronic trachoma chlamydial antigens and nucleic acids can be detected in the absence of infectious agents. The inflammatory response to these sensitizing antigens may contribute substantially to the duration and severity of chronic conjunctival inflammation.

In Egypt chlamydial agent has been recovered from the nasopharynx and rectum, and 15% of young children presenting to a rural health clinic had chlamydial infection in the eye, throat or rectum (12). Although local antibiotic treatment has only a limited effect on improving clinical trachoma, it interferes significantly with detection of agents in most laboratory tests.

Bacteriology: Bacterial studies should be an integral part of the laboratory evaluation of individuals or communities with trachoma. The important ocular bacterial pathogens include Haemophilus sp., S.pneumoniae, Neisseria sp., Moraxella sp. and S.aureus; other pathogens such as Gram negative rods and ß-hemolysine streptococci occur less frequently. Bacterial pathogens occur in higher frequency in cases with significantly greater inflammatory response (e.g. severe intensity trachoma) (8), but may also be present in the external eye of children without overt conjunctivitis (19).

Epidemiology

Trachoma has a worldwide distribution, and blinding trachoma is still a major public health problem in parts of Africa and Asia, and in limited areas of Latin America, Australia and the Pacific Islands. Non-blinding trachoma is present in a much larger area of these same regions that include most of the drier subtropical and tropical countries.

Trachoma was once prevalent and severe in many countries of Europe, North America and East Asia, but it has disappeared with rising living standards that accompanied industrialization and economic development.

In the heavily affected communities, most children are infected by the age of one or two years and, starting at age five, the prevalence of active disease declines steadily, but some adults continue to have signs of active disease (1,2). Children constitute a larger portion of the population in hyperendemic trachoma areas, so they are the chief reservoir of trachomatous infection in the community (1,2,10,12).

Blinding lesions (trichiasis/entropion and corneal scarring) are the outcome of earlier severe or moderate intensity inflammatory disease (5,6). These blinding complications are generally observed in adults but may occur in childhood due to very severe inflammatory disease. Blindness rates rise dramatically among those over 50 years due to accumulated corneal scarring and to early cataract formation (1).

Because so many more people in developing countries are surviving to adult life, the numbers of those 50 years and older is projected to increase substantially. Those who will be older than 50 in 30 years (the year 2020) are now adults and have already developed the damaging effects of childhood trachoma. The estimated blindness in Egypt can be projected for the year 2020 (Tab.3) when the blindness rate will be 3.1% and there will be 1.4 million blind compared to the estimated 338.000 blind in 1980 (1).

Transmission

Trachoma is associated with poverty. Economic development appears to eliminate or reduce the severity of the disease (2). Transmission of the disease is by direct or indirect contact with infected material (hands, clothing, towels, etc.) and by eye-seeking flies. Among the environmental and behavioral features of greatest importance are the presence of young children in the household, lack of face washing of young children and absence or non-use of latrines.

In many trachoma endemic areas, the open exposure of human and animal feces and garbage contributes to an increase in the fly population. The flies which cluster on children's eyes to feed on ocular discharges can transfer these discharges to the eyes of other children in the same family within 15 to 30 minutes (10).

Treatment and Prevention

Organization of trachoma control programs: The primary goal of public health progams for the control of trachoma is the prevention of blindness. Programs to control trachoma should be based on improving health related behavior and providing chemotherapy and necessary surgical intervention to correct lid deformities.

Both antibiotic treatment and economic development may result in a rapid reduction in the intensity and prevalence of inflammatory disease. Where there are already substantial numbers of people with severe conjunctival scarring, however, new cases of trichiasis/entropion will continue to appear for many years after active inflammatory trachoma has disappeared from the community.

Antibiotic Treatment: The objectives of chemotherapy are:

1. Reduction in the intensity of trachoma in individuals and
2. Reduction in transmission

Sulfonamides, tetracyclines, Erythromycin and other macrolides, and Rifampicin are effective in treating active trachoma. At present, topical Tetracyclines (eye ointments or suspensions) are the recommended preparations for large scale (community-wide) treatment of trachoma (3). Where communities have rates of 20% active trachoma in children, the World Health Organization recommends treatment of all children with topical Tetracycline on an intermittent schedule: Twice daily applications for five consecutive days each month for six months.

Systemic antibiotic treatment can be justified for selected cases because it may be more effective in severe intensity cases and because there is an extraocular reservoir of C.trachomatis. This "selective" therapy involves screening of the affected population for disease and assumes that children treated with oral drugs can be monitored for side effects. Studies in Tunisia indicate that for older children (over 6 to 8 years), oral Doxycycline given as a supplement to the topical Tetracycline by the same intermittent schedule is significantly better than the ointment alone in reducing trachoma intensity (7). For younger children oral Erythromycin has been the only available drug but it must be given in four divided daily doses.

The new macrolide, Azithromycin, may offer the possibility of single dose treatment for children two years and older. Oral Sulfonamides are cheaper but have unacceptably high rates of untoward reactions.

Surgery for Lid Deformities. The surgical correction of trichiasis and/or entropion (lid deformities) has an immediate impact on preventing blindness. These simple procedures can be carried out in affected communities by mobile teams. Where ophthalmologists are not available, general physicians or auxiliary personnel can be trained to do these lid operations.

Trachoma Vaccines: Although naturally occurring trachoma confers no immunity to recurrent disease, immunization as a method of prevention and treatment of the established disease has been explored by several groups. In no instance, however, has a vaccine been shown to be of value and none are in use in trachoma control programs. New advances in immunology and molecular biology, however, may yield practical vaccines for use in preventing blindness from endemic trachoma.

Behavioral Changes: Face washing of young children and latrine use by adults in the family are two forms of behavior that protect children from developing severe inflammatory trachoma. Simple health eduction methods to promote these behaviors are an essential part of trachoma control programs.

Table 1. Laboratory procedures available to detect Chlamydia trachomatis in clinical specimens

	Technology Requirements	Personnel Training	Cost
Giemsa stained smears	Low	Moderate	Low
Isolation	High	High	Expensive
Direct immunofluorescent staining (DFA)	Moderate	Moderate	Moderate to expensive
Antigen detection	Moderate	Moderate to low	Expensive to low

Table 2. Performance of diagnostic tests for C.trachomatis in conjunctival smears of Egyptian children with active trachoma (15)

Test	Sensitivity (%)	Specificity (%)
Isolation	76%	100%
Giemsa	29% *	100%
EIA (Chlamydiazyme)	73%	93%
DNA probe	84%	96%
Direct fluorescent antibody (Microtrak)-methanol fixation	78%	100%

* Significantly less sensitive than the other tests, P<0.001
Note: True positives are culture or Giemsa positive or two of the non-culture test positive; prevalence of true positives = 49.5% (45 of 91).

Table 3. Blindness projected: rural Egyptian population (1)

Year	Projected population at risk (rural)	Projected population at risk (50+years)	Blindness rate	Proportion blind 50+ of total rural blind	Projected total blind	Crude blindness rate
1980	20.98 m	2.10 m	15%	93%	338,387	1.6%
2000	32.21 m	4.51 m	15%	95%	712,021	2.2%
2020	44.66 m	8.93 m	15%	96%	1395,625	3.1%

References

1. Courtright P, Sheppard J, Schachter J (1989) Trachoma and Blindness in the Nile Delta: Current Patterns and Projections for the Future in the Rural Egyptian Population. Br J Ophthalmol 73:536-540
2. Dawson CR, Daghfous T, Messadi M et al (1976) Severe Endemic Trachoma in Tunisia. Br J Ophthalmol 60:245-252
3. Dawson CR, Jones BR, Tarizzo M (1981) Guide to Trachoma Control. WHO Geneva
4. Dawson CR, Jones BR, Darougar S (1975) Blinding and Non-blinding Trachoma: Assessment of Intensity of Upper Tarsal Inflammatory Disease and Disabling Lesions. Bull WHO 52:279-282
5. Dawson CR, Juster R, Marx R et al (1989) Limbal Disease in Trachoma and Other Ocular Chlamydial Infections: Risk Factors for Corneal Vascularisation. Eye 3:204-209
6. Dawson CR, Marx R, Daghfous T et al (1990) What Clinical Signs are Critical in Evaluating the Impact of Intervention in Trachoma ? In: Bowie WR et al (eds) Chlamydial Infections. Proc. Seventh Int.Symp. on Human Chlamydia Infections. Cambridge University Press, Cambridge
7. Dawson CR, Schachter J (1985) Strategies for Treatment and Control of Blinding Trachoma: Cost-effectiveness of Topical or Systemic Antibiotics. Rev Inf Dis 7:768-773

8. Dawson CR, Whitcher JP, Lyon C et al (1977) Response to Treatment in Ocular Chlamydial Infections. (Trachoma and Inclusion Conjunctivitis). Analogies with Non-Gonococcal Urethritis.In: Hobson D, Holmes KK (eds) Non-Gonococcal Urethritis and Other Infections. Am Soc for Microbiol Washington,DC. pp.135-139
9. Hanna L, Jawetz E, Briones O et al (1973) Antibodies to TRIC Agents in Matched Human Tears and Sera. J Immunol 110:1464-1469
10. Jones BR (1975) The Prevention of Blindness from Trachoma. Trans Ophthal Soc UK 95:16-33
11. MacCallan DF (1936) Trachoma. London, Butterworth, pp.8-26
12. Malaty R, Zaki S, Said ME et al (1981) Extraocular Infections in Children in Areas with Endemic Trachoma. J Infect Dis 143:853
13. Nowinski RC, Tam MR, Goldstein LC et al (1983) Monoclonal Antibodies for Diagnosis of Infectious Diseases in Humans. Science 219:637-644
14. Schachter J, Dawson CR (1978) Human Chlamydial Infections. PSG Publishing Co, Littleton, Mass,pp.273
15. Schachter J, Moncada J, Dawson CR et al (1988) Nonculture Methods for Diagnosing Chlamydial Infection in Patients with Trachoma: A Clue to the Pathogenesis of the Disease? J Inf Dis 158:1347-1352
16. Tang FF, Chang HL, Huang YT et al (1957) Studies on the Etiology of Trachoma with Special References to Isolation of the Virus in Chick Embryo. Chinese Med J 75:429-446
17. Thylefors B, Dawson CR, Jones BR et al (1987) A Simple System for the Assessment of Trachoma and its Complications. Bull WHO 65:477-483
18. Treharne JD, Dwyer RSC, Darougar S et al (1978) Antichlamydial Antibody in Tears and Sera, and Serotypes of Chlamydia Trachomatis Isolated from School Children in Southern Tunisia. Br J Ophthalmol 62:509-515)
19. Vastine DW, Dawson CR, Daghfous T et al (1974) Severe Endemic Trachoma in Tunisia. I. The Effect of Topical Chemotherapy on Conjunctivitis and Ocular Bacteria. Br J Ophthalmol 58:833-842
20. Wang SP, Grayston JP, Kuo CC et al (1977) Serodiagnosis of Chlamydia Trachomatis Infection with the Microimmunofluorescence Test. In: Hobson D, Holmes KK (eds) Non-Gonococcal Urethritis and Other Infections. Am Soc for Microbiol. Washington,DC. pp.237-248
21. World Health Organization (1966) Fourth WHO Scientific Group on Trachoma Research. WHO Technical Report Series No.130
22. Yoneda C, Dawson CR, Daghfous R et al (1975) Cytology as a Guide to the Presence of Chlamydial Inclusions in Giemsa Stained Conjunctival Smears in Severe Endemic Trachoma. Br J Ophthalmol 59:116-124

- Onchocerciasis

Onchocerciasis: Parasitology and Epidemiology

H.M. Seitz

Abstract. Onchocerca volvulus is a filariid worm being transmitted by the bite of simuliid flies. Third stage larvae are transferred, which develop into adult worms over months. The females produce microfilariae. These primitive larvae migrate into the skin, but they can also penetrate into the cornea and intraocularly. Protracted inflammatory reactions over many years may lead to severe damage, finally even to blindness. Control of Onchocerca transmission has been widely achieved through insecticidal measures, but now the treatment of infected people as the reservoir of the parasites is increasingly important.

Onchocerciasis or river blindness is caused by Onchocerca volvulus, a nematode belonging to the filariae. Man is the final host harbouring two phases of the parasite: the adult worms (macrofilariae) and the microfilariae. Adult females reach 50cm and more, males only 5cm. The females are coiled up and embedded in connective tissue, usually under the skin. They are viviparous and give birth to the microfilariae (approximately 350μm

Microfilariae migrating in the skin of the face can enter the cornea and the interior of the eye causing a number of lesions, which will be described in another contribution to the conference. Microfilariae can be seen in the anterior chamber of infected eyes if higher magnifications are used for observation.

The diagnosis of an Onchocerca infection is usually made by the demonstration of microfilariae in skin snips. Small biopsies (approximately 1mg) are removed from the skin and placed into saline of tissue culture fluid. If microfilariae are present, they leave the biopsy and can be seen moving around in the fluid. Serological diagnosis is not possible on a routine basis, because we have no tests for species-specific antibodies. A positive antibody titer may indicate the presence of an infection by another filaria.

long). The microfilariae migrate in the subepidermal layer of the skin causing little irritation as long as they are alive. In contrast, dying and dead microfilariae lead to inflammatory reactions in the skin and to severe itching. Later on they can cause atrophy of the skin.

The microfilariae do not develop further in man. The natural life span of the microfilariae is appoximately two years. Only those microfilariae picked up by blood-sucking flies of the genus Simulium can develop further. Within about 12 days they become third-stage larvae, which can infect human beings again during a bloodmeal, which the infected simuliid fly is taking. The time required for development for the infection to fertile worms and the appearance of microfilariae (prepatent period) is rather long, three months at minimum, usually much longer.

Onchocerca volvulus is mainly a parasite of Africa occurring in many countries of West Africa and Central Africa. Other foci are found in tropical South America and in the southern part of the Arabic peninsula.

For breeding the vector Simulium requires fast flowing rivers, which offer high levels of oxygen and nutrients to the fast growing larvae.

In West Africa the World Health Organization has carried out a very successful Onchocerciasis Control Programme, which was able to interrupt nearly completely the transmission of O.volvulus.

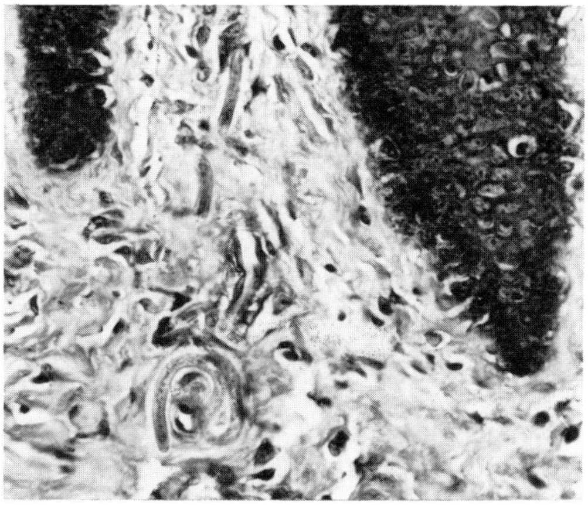

Fig.1. Onchocerca volvulus: Nodule removed from the human subcutis, histological section. The rounded structures embedded in connective tissue are cross-sections of one, maybe several, adult females, which are coiled up. In many of the cross-sections the two branches of the uterus are visible.

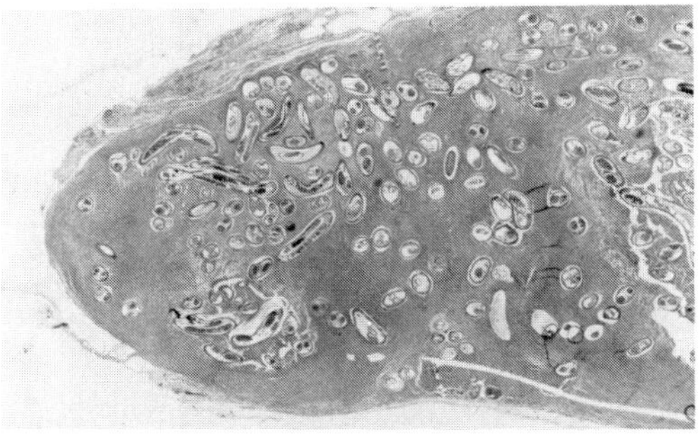

Fig.2. Human skin with several microfilariae of Onchocerca volvulus in the subepidermal tissue.

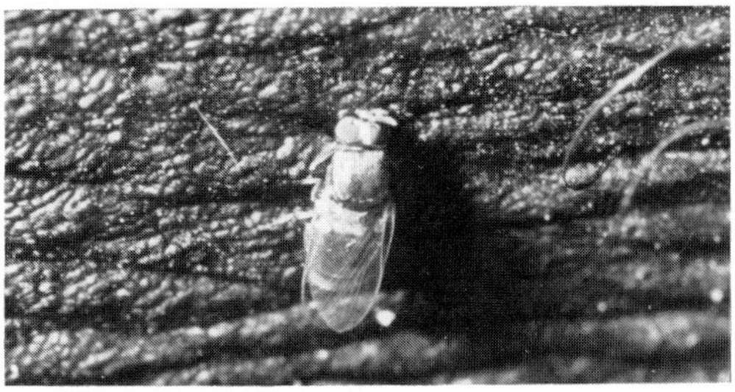

Fig.3. A simuliid fly, the vector of onchocerciasis, taking a bloodmeal on human skin.

Onchocerciasis: Clinical Features

Hugh R. Taylor

Abstract. Onchocerciasis is a devasting blinding disease caused by the parasite Onchocerca volvulus that infects about 80 million people, causing blindness and visual impairment in 1-2 million people. In hyperendemic areas, more than half of the population will become blind from Onchocerciasis before they die. Blindness is the most important effect of the disease and results, in part, from direct invasion of the eye by microfilariae.

The recent development of Ivermectin has revolutionized our ability to treat this disease. An annual oral dose of only 150mg/kg bodyweight almost completely suppressed the disease manifestations. It has been demonstrated to be safe when distributed on a mass scale and when a sufficiently large portion of the community receives treatment a decrease in transmission can be demonstrated. Programs for the community-based mass distribution of Ivermectin are now being conducted and promise to control this major blinding scourge.

Introduction

There are approximately 85 million people who live in endemic areas and 18 million people who are currently infected with Onchocerciasis (20,27). Onchocerciasis causes blindness or visual loss in up to 1-2 million of these infected people. In hyperendemic areas, more than 40% of the inhabitants above the age of 40 are blind. This high rate of blindness has a devastating socio-economic impact. More than half of the inhabitants in hyperendemic areas will become blind before they die (12). The life expectancy of those who are blind is one-third that of their sighted peers. Onchocerciasis occurs predominantly in West Africa, but endemic areas stretch across the African continent. There are also some small, isolated foci in Central and South America.

Onchocerciasis - the Disease

Onchocerciasis is caused by the filarial parasite Onchocerca volvulus. Man is the only natural host. Infective larvae are transmitted by the bite of the black flies of the Simulium species. The larvae develop into adult male or female worms that reproduce sexually. The female releases millions of microfilariae that migrate throughout the body, particularly to the skin and the eye. Microfilariae are approximately 300 microns long and die after 1-2 years if not taken up by a black fly. Adult worms may live for 10 to 15 years. Much of the pathology of Onchocerciasis is thought to be either directly or indirectly due to the death of microfilariae.

Onchocerciasis is commonly referred to as "river blindness". This is because it is found in areas adjacent to rivers and streams where black flies breed.

Skin disease related to inflammation around dead microfilaria is very common. Pruritus may occur early and be severe and debilitating. A severe reactive onchodermatitis is often seen. Significant destruction and atrophy of the skin structures may occur in advanced disease which is associated with focal changes in pigmentation.

The clinical hallmark of Onchocerciasis is the presence of subcutaneous nodules. These nodules contain adult worms coiled together like a ball of string and encapsulated by host scar tissue. Typically, they are found around the hips and waist, but may occur on the head and elsewhere.

Microfilariae can be observed in the anterior chamber of the eye. This is one of the earlier signs of ocular involvement; usually there is little reaction to the presence of the microfilariae, but at times these may be with severe anterior uveitis leading to synechia formation, secondary glaucoma and cataract.

Microfilariae also invade the cornea. Dead microfilariae form the center of small focal inflammatory infiltrates or punctate opacities. These opacities clear over several months without residual damage. Sclerosing keratitis develops as a gradual opacification of the cornea. It is more common in savannah areas where it is the major cause of blindness.

Chorioretinal changes are frequent. These may range from subtle changes in the retinal pigment epithelium and intraretinal deposits, including microfilariae, to severe destruction of the entire retina and outer choroid (21). In many areas, especially in forest areas of West Africa, chorioretinal changes are the main cause of blindness. The chorioretinal changes may in large part result from immunologically mediated changes (3,15,25). Optic atrophy is also frequently seen.

Onchocerciasis is usually diagnosed by obtaining a small punch biopsy of skin weighing 1-2mg (21). The skin snip is placed in either saline or tissue-culture medium. The emerging microfilariae are counted. Microfilarial counts may be as high as 500-600 mf/mg skin in heavily affected individuals. The finding of microfilariae in the eye also gives definitive diagnosis, as does the histopathological examination of a typical nodule.

Vector Control

The Onchocerciasis Control Program has operated in the worst affected areas of West Africa for nearly 20 years (27). It is an ambitious, large, long-term control program established by the World Health Organization, the World Bank, and other United Nations agencies. In many areas, the Onchocerciasis Control Program has eliminated the black fly vectors and stopped the transmission of Onchocerciasis by spraying the breeding sites of the black fly with a selective larvicide (2). Despite many logistic difficulties, the Onchocerciasis Control Program has been outstandingly effective and has essentially eliminated the transmission of infection in its initial area of over 700000 square kilometers involving seven countries and recently its area has been doubled. The Onchocerciasis Control Program has provided a protective umbrella for about one-quarter of those with Onchocerciasis. However, logistic and economic reasons preclude similar programs in other endemic areas.

Chemotherapy - the Revolution

Two drugs, Diethylcarbamazine and Suramin, had been available for many years to treat Onchocerciasis (21). However, both cause severe side effects and were usually reserved only for those patients with the most severe infections and the highest risk of developing blindness.

A new drug, Ivermectin, has been developed over the last few years. It has revolutionized the treatment of Onchocerciasis and it is now feasible to conduct large-scale community-based treatment of Onchocerciasis (19). Ivermectin is a semi-synthetic macrocyclic lactone that is effective against a wide range of parasites. Its pharmacological effect is as a GABA agonist.

Ivermectin has been carefully assessed through a series of clinical trials, starting with small open studies of lightly infected patients (1). Double-masked, controlled clinical trials then compared it with Diethylcarbamazine and a placebo (see (19) for a review). Subsequently, larger hospital-based studies then examined the effect of dosage and dose interval.

Ivermectin kills microfilariae and causes a rapid drop in skin-snip counts and the number of microfilariae in the eye. The reduction in skin-snip counts is prolonged so that two years after a single oral dose of Ivermectin skin microfilarial counts are only 25% of pretreatment levels. Ivermectin does not directly affect the viability of adult female worms, although it does kill some male worms (7). Ivermectin also kills the microfilariae in the uterus and it takes 6 to 9 months before embryogenesis is reinitiated (14).

The great limitation to Diethylcarbamazine treatment was the marked clinical reaction that it caused, the Mazotti reaction. This was related to the killing of microfilariae (20). Ivermectin does not induce this severe reaction and its use has remarkably few side-effects. A mild reaction may occur in approximately 15% of patients and a moderate to severe reaction in approximately 1% (6,10). This is contrasted with Diethylcarbamazine where approximately 90% of the patients will have a reaction and more than 25% will have a moderately severe reaction. Adverse reactions tend to occur more commonly in more heavily infected individuals. Adverse reactions are much less common with the retreatment. Mild reactions occur commonly in expatriates.

Unlike Diethylcarbamazine, Ivermectin does not aggravate existing ocular disease. Intraocular microfilariae disappear and there is a reduction in the presence of uveitis, limbitis, and punctate keratitis (5,18,19). The improvement in the anterior segment changes persists for up to two years following a single oral dose and becomes more marked with repeated treatment. Ivermectin treatment is not associated with the development of optic neuritis or retinal pigment epithelial abnormalities as occur with Diethylcarbamazine. Some chorioretinal changes may continue to evolve after Ivermectin treatment (5,16). The long-term impact of treatment on chorioretinal disease has yet to be established.

Treatment with Ivermectin leads to a significant improvement in skin disease and the skin symptoms related to Onchocerciasis (11, 26). Many people also pass intestinal parasites and this added bonus of treatment also contributes to its wide acceptance. Some studies have reported treatment compliance of 97% even on the third round of annual treatment (10).

A single oral dose of 150μg/kg is the optimal dosage of Ivermectin. It is recommended that the use of this dose be repeated on an annual basis (Tab.1), although some have suggested that treatment every six months for the first two years at least may lead to a more rapid lowering of skin microfilariae (20).

The reduction in skin microfilarial counts seen following individual treatment is associated with a significant decrease in the ability of that individual to contribute to transmission (4). Community-based distribution studies show that transmission rates of flies can be reduced by over 75% (13,23). To date, only one study has examined the effect of Ivermectin treatment on the acquisition of new infection (22). It showed a 45% reduction in the incidence of infection in children after the initial distribution round. Ivermectin was found not to be an effective prophylaxis against acquiring infection (17).

When Ivermectin was registered for human use in 1987, Merck Sharp & Dohme, the manufacturer announced that it would provide Mectizan, the trade name for ivermectin, at no cost to treat all patients with Onchocerciasis (24). An independent committee, the Mectizan Expert Committee, has been created in conjunction with Merck and the World Health Organization to supervise the distribution of the drug to nationally-approved treatment programs (8). Up to June 1991, over 3 1/2 million treatments have been provided and the number has roughly doubled each year (9). Mass treatment programs have been set up in each of the five Latin American countries where Onchocerciasis is endemic and in 23 of the 27 African endemic countries. In Nigeria, for example, where approximately one third of those with Onchocerciasis live, a National Onchocerciasis Control Program has been established and distribution programs are under way in 11 of the 19 endemic states. Support for distribution programs such as these has come from many sources including international agencies, bilateral agreements, national governments, non-governmental organizations and church missions. There has even been a foundation established specifically to encourage and support the distribution of Ivermectin - the River Blindness Foundation.

Despite the major advance that Ivermectin represents, continuing efforts are needed to eventually develop an effective macro-filaricidal compound to kill the adult worms. As Ivermectin does not kill the adult worm, it needs to be given on a repeated basis for at least ten years. An effective macrofilaricidal compound would only need to be given once.

Onchocerciasis, which only a decade ago was an untreatable blinding scourge, is now a disease that can be dealt with. It is not inconceivable that, given adequate resources, Onchocerciasis could be eradicated as a blinding disease by the end of this century.

Table 1. Community-based distribution of Ivermectin

Indication:	- Lives in endemic area	
Exclusion criteria:	- Pregnancy	
	- Breast feeding infant less than 7 days old	
	- Child weighing less than 15 kg	
	- Serious intercurrent illness	
Dosage :	- 15-25 kg =	0.5 tablet
	- 26-44 kg =	1 tablet
	- 45-64 kg =	1.5 tablets
	- 60 + kg =	2 tablets

References

1. Aziz MA, Diop IM, Diallo S et al (1982) Efficacy and Tolerance of Ivermectin in Human Onchocerciasis. Lancet 2:171-173
2. Bland J (1985) A Decade of Oncho Control. World Health 1985 October 1-27
3. Braun G, McKechnie NM, Connor V et al (1991) Immunological Crossreactivity Between a cloned antigen of Onchocerca

Volvulus and a Component of the Retinal Pigment Epithelium. J Exp Med 174:169-177

4. Cupp EW, Bernardo MJ, Kiszewski AE et al (1986) The Effects of Ivermectin on Transmission of Onchocerca Volvulus. Science 231:740-742
5. Dadzie KY, Remme J, De Sole G (1991) Changes in Ocular Onchocerciasis After Two Rounds of Community-Based Ivermectin Treatment in a Holo-Endemic Onchocerciasis Focus. Trans R Soc Trop Med Hyg 85:267-272
6. De Sole G, Dadzie KY, Giese J et al (1990) Lack of Adverse Reaction in Ivermectin Treatment of Onchocerciasis. Lancet 335:1106-1107
7. Duke BOL, Zea-Florea G, Castro J et al (1990) Effects of Multiple Monthly Doses of Ivermectin on Adult Onchocerca Volvulus. Am J Trop Med Hyg 43(6):657-664
8. Dull HR (1990) Mectizan Donation and the Mectizan Expert Committee. Acta Leidensia 59:399-403
9. Mectizan Program Notes, Number 3, July 1991.A publication of the Mectizan Expert Committee, Atlanta, Georgia/USA
10. Pacque MC, Dukuly Z, Greene BM et al (1991) Community-Based Treatment of Onchocerciasis with Ivermectin: Safety, Efficacy and Acceptability of Yearly Treatment. J Infect Dis 163:381-385
11. Pacque M, Elmets C, Dukuly ZD et al (1991) Improvement in Severe Onchocercal Skin Disease After a Single Dose of Ivermectin. Am J Med 90 (5):590-594
12. Prost A (1986) The Burden of Blindness in Adult Males in the Savanna Villages of West Africa Exposed to Onchocerciasis. Trans R Soc Trop Med Hyg 80:525-527
13. Remme J, Baker RHA, De Sole G et al (1989) A Community Trial of Ivermectin in the Onchocerciasis Focus of Asubende, Ghana.I. Effect on the Microfilarial Reservoir and the Transmission of Onchocerca Volvulus. Trop Med Parasitol 40:367-374
14. Schulz-Key H, Greene BM, Awadzi K et al (1986) Efficacy of Ivermectin on the Reproductivity of Female Onchocerca Volvulus. Trop Med Parasitol 37:89
15. Semba RD, Donnelly JJ, Rockey JH et al (1988) Experimental Ocular Onchocerciasis in Cynomolgus Monkeys. II. Chorioretinitis Elicited by Intravitreal Onchocerca Lienalis Microfilariae. Invest Ophthalmol Vis Sci 29:1642-1651
16. Semba RD, Murphy RP, Newland HS et al (1990) Longitudinal Study of Lesions of the Posterior Segment in Onchocerciasis. Ophthalmology 97:1334-1341
17. Taylor HR, Trpis M, Cupp EW et al (1988) Ivermectin Prophylaxis Against Experimental Onchocerca Volvulus Infection in Chimpanzees. Am J Trop Med Hyg 39:89-90
18. Taylor HR, Semba RD, Newland HS et al (1989) Ivermectin Treatment for Patients with Severe Ocular Onchocerciasis. Am J Trop Med Hyg 40:494-500
19. Taylor HR, Greene BM (1989) The Status of Ivermectin in the Treatment of Human Onchocerciasis. Am J Trop Med Hyg 41:460-466
20. Taylor HR (1990) Onchocerciasis. Int Ophthalmol 14:189-194
21. Taylor HR (1991) Onchocerciasis. In: Duane TD (ed) Chapter 62. Clin Ophthalmology, Vol 5. Hagerstown, Harper & Row.
22. Taylor HR, Pacque M, Munoz B et al (1990) Impact of Mass Treatment of Onchocerciasis with Ivermectin on the Transmission of Infection. Science 250:116-118
23. Trpis M, Childs JE, Fryauff DJ et al (1990) Effect of Mass Treatment of a Human Population with Ivermectin on Transmission of Onchocerca Volvulus by Simulium Yahense in Liberia, West Africa. Am J Trop Med Hyg 42:148-156

24. Vagelos PR (1991) Are Prescription Drug Prices High? Science 252:1080-1084
25. Van der Lelij A, Rothova A, De Vries JP et al (1991) Analysis of Aqueous Humor in Ocular Onchocerciasis. Curr Eye Res 10 (2):169-176
26. Whitworth JAG, Morgan D, Maude GH et al (1991) A Community Trial of Ivermectin for Onchocerciasis in Sierra Leone: Clinical and Parasitological Responses to the Initial Dose. Trans R Soc Trop Med Hyg 85:92-96
27. World Health Organization (1987) WHO Expert Committee on Onchocerciasis. Third Report. WHO Technical Report Series 752:1-167

- Leprosy

Ocular Leprosy - An Important Cause of Avoidable Blindness

Timothy ffytche

Abstract. Ocular leprosy is now recognized as an important cause of avoidable world blindness, although many ophthalmologists remain ignorant of its manifestations. The detection and management of ocular complications in all stages of the disease still pose clinical and therapeutic challenges to leprologists despite the successful institution of multidrug therapy in many centers.

Current knowledge on the pathogenesis of ocular involvement in leprosy will be discussed and areas of ignorance requiring further clinical research will be highlighted.

Introduction

Ocular leprosy has for long been one of the neglected areas of ophthalmology and the reasons for this are not difficult to understand. Very few ophthalmologists in the developed world have experiences with the disease, since leprosy patients do not normally form a part of their routine clinical practice. Those who have travelled to countries where the condition is endemic may not have spent more than a few weeks dealing with leprosy, and therefore they are not in a position to observe the evolution of eye complications which may have a development span of decades rather than years. The leprologists and field workers who manage leprosy on a day-to-day basis are often poorly trained in methods of ophthalmic diagnosis and therapy, and their attention is more likely to be directed towards the obvious involvement by the disease of the hands and feet, particularly with its effect on mobility and self-care.

Yet ocular complications are of fundamental importance, not only because visual impairment reduces the ability of the individual to remain independent, but also because the onset of visual deterioration may bring about a noticeable change in the patient's attitude to the disease. Ocular involvement, when it does occur, may be a significant event in the course of the disease, and when severe visual impairment or blindness follow, especially if they are added to existing deformities, the physical and psychological effects on the patient may be extreme. "Blindness in the individual who has normal skin sensitivity is enough of a handicap, but in one who has lost that faculty it is disastrous. Few have the resources, material, mental or spiritual to live with it" (1).

It is now considered that as much as 75% of world blindness can either be prevented or cured,and it is universally agreed that prevention is far more cost-effective than cure. This is especially true for ocular leprosy which is the classic preventable disease, and in many cases blindness is avoidable, not by elaborate and sophisticated medical and surgical techniques, but by simple measures, requiring little more than adequate supervision, education of the patient and common sense. In evaluating the challenge that it poses to leprologists and ophthalmologists today we should consider the clinical pathology of leprosy as it affects the eye and its ocular manifestations.

Ocular Involvement

It has always been a medical mystery that the two organisms that cause tuberculosis and leprosy, although almost identical morphologically, should behave so differently both in the laboratory and in the clinical situation. This is particularly evident in their effect on the eye, and the question must be asked as to what are the special properties of the organism causing leprosy that render the eye so susceptible to damage.

Mycobacterium leprae is a slow-growing, non-toxic intracellular organism with a special affinity for Schwann cells. Its establishment and growth in a tissue depends on the temperature, the nerve size, together with the host's immunity. The organism flourishes best in the cooler part of the body - skin, nose and eyes, and it is known that there is a temperature gradient across the eye making the anterior chamber structures approximately 4°C cooler than the posterior pole (11). Indeed the anterior part of the eye, with its high concentration of small unmyelinated nerves in the cornea, iris and ciliary body is an ideal situation for the bacillus. The fact that the organism does not produce a toxin means that endophthalmitis is not a feature of the disease despite the known presence of large quantities of mycobacteria in the anterior segment of the globe in certain types of leprosy.

The eyes can be involved in many ways, but in general, patients with paucibacillary disease are at risk from disturbances of corneal sensation and lid function, whereas those with multibacillary disease have additional problems from organisms invading the anterior segment, immune reactions and damage to the adnexae. Every affected eye, particularly one with chronic disease is at risk from secondary infection also. The manifestations of ocular disease are therefore legion, although their affect on vision is variable. The transmission of infection and the susceptibility of individuals to the disease depend on many elements. which are still not fully understood (7); but the development of ocular involvement is influenced by a number of factors which include the race of the patient, the type of leprosy, its duration, status and treatment, and, most important of all, the preventive measures that have been taken to avoid ocular damage.

It is rare for the eyes to be involved in the first few years of the disease, and this provides hope, since multidrug therapy, which was introduced by the WHO in 1982 (13) and is now standard treatment in most endemic areas, may help to eliminate the infection before eye complications develop. This should be the approach that carries the most encouragement for the future, but difficulties in case finding, patient compliance, drug resistance, and lack of governmental support in many countries, are still slowing progress.

Statistics on blindness rates and the prevalence of eye complications are difficult to obtain because, although there are numerous reports in the literature of studies made in various leprosy centres, there is a lack of conformity in methods of eye examination and evaluation. An attempt has been made to standardise data collection by means of a multicentred study of ocular involvement in the disease, which has been sponsored by LEPRA and has been carried out on cross-sections of the leprosy population examined by simple standardised techniques. More than 3.000 patients from over 30 centres in the world have been entered into the study which has been designed to give information on the incidence of eye complications over a five year period (4). Initial analysis of prevalence rates showed that 5.5% of patients examined had vision less than 3/60 (20/400) and were therefore blind by WHO standards, and 7% had vision less than 6/60 (20/200) - blind by US standards. The same study showed that 21.3% of patients had potentially sight-threatening lesions, defined as high-risk conditions likely to lead to visual loss unless preventive measures were instituted (5).

Most visual impairment or blindness resulted from four main causes which may occur on their own or in combination:

- lagophthalmos leading to exposure keratopathy,
- corneal hypaesthesia predisposing to corneal ulceration,
- acute or chronic iridocyclitis, and
- secondary cataract.

Many of these can be prevented or treated sucessfully and yet they are still responsible for the high prevalence rates of visual disability in leprosy patients in many parts of the world. Details of the management of these ocular complications and their prevention will be discussed elsewhere in this book.

Lid Involvement

The lids and adnexae may be damaged in a variety of ways, many of which pose no threat to vision. These include madarosis, blepharochalasis, lid nodules and impairment of lacrimal drainage, although the latter may provide a reservoir for secondary infection. The main problems are related to impairment of lid closure associated with lagophthalmos. The lower lid is affected through paralysis of the zygomatic branch of the facial nerve, giving rise to failure of adequate protection of the cornea. It occurs in all forms of leprosy, often as an acute event during a Type 1 reaction (Fig.1) in patients with paucibacillary and borderline disease especially where there is a reaction in a facial patch located in this region (8). Alternatively in multibacillary disease there may be a slowly advancing process associated with changes in the elastic tissue of the lower lid (Fig.2). The eye is constantly at risk, and unless measures are taken to protect it, particularly if there is an accompanying diminution of corneal sensation, exposure keratopathy is the likely outcome.

Monitoring of lid function by observing spontaneous blinking and assessing lid closure are fundamental aspects of health care in leprosy, to be taught to field workers and patients alike, and simple methods of protecting the eye can effectively reduce the frequency of corneal problems.

Significant lid involvement, defined as absent lid closure or when corrective lid surgery had been carried out, was observed in 11.5% of patients in the LEPRA multicenter survey.

Corneal Involvement

An important cause of blindness in the developing world is corneal opacity and this is particularly the case in leprosy where the cornea may be affected in all forms of the disease through impairment of corneal sensation. The corneal nerves, by virtue of their superficial position and their small size, are very susceptible to damage, and when hypaesthesia accompanies impaired lid closure the eye is at high risk for the eventual development of a severe form of exposure keratopathy. This may commence in the lower part of the cornea where exposure is greatest because of failure of adequate lid closure during sleep (Fig.3) and may spread to involve the whole cornea.

Multibacillary leprosy may be associated with a specific form of superficial stromal keratitis but this rarely causes visual loss, except in advanced cases. Other lesions such as thickened corneal nerves and pannus may be observed without affecting vision, and occasionally lepromas arising from the limbal region may encroach on the cornea.

Impaired corneal sensation predisposes to corneal damage as well by disturbing the normal epithelial metabolism, and the complications of corneal ulceration account for an important proportion of blindness in leprosy (Fig.4).

Treatment again consists of simple, commonsense methods to protect the cornea at an early stage of the condition, and therefore detection of eyes that are at risk becomes an important aspect of management. This remains the combined responsibility of the leprosy worker and the patient, since in the later stages the surgical problems presented by an opaque vascularised cornea may be insurmountable even with the most sophisticated surgical techniques.

Significant corneal involvement, defined as absent corneal sensation or corneal scarring reducing vision to below 6/36 was observed in 11.2% of patients in the LEPRA survey.

Iris Involvement

Invasion of the iris and ciliary body by Mycobacterium leprae occurs exclusively in the multibacillary form of the disease and has been called "the cause par excellence of blindness in leprosy" (12). Acute iridocyclitis is often a feature of Type 2 reactions and has all the signs of iritis due to any other cause except that pain and discomfort may not be so prominent. Rapid visual loss from the inflammation or secondary glaucoma needs to be prevented by urgent conventional therapy, and field workers and leprologists need to be instructed in the early diagnosis and management of the condition.

Chronic iridocyclitis remains the enigma of the disease and is perhaps the condition that still requires most research. In multibacillary leprosy the organisms are presumed to lodge in the ciliary body and iris during the initial bacteraemia and they remain undetected until they are well-established. The chronic disease is often asymptomatic involving a gradual diminution of ciliary body activity, a progressive loss of dilator pupillae function with a consequent increasing miosis. Indeed the minute non-functioning pupil in multibacillary disease is a potent cause of visual impairment and night blindness and in the advanced stage is not amenable to any form of medical treatment (Fig.5).

The transient appearance of iris pearls, iris atrophy, seclusio pupillae and eventual phthisis bulbi may all feature in long-standing disease, but objective signs in the early stages may be few, even with slitlamp examination, and attempts have been made to detect iris and ciliary body involvement by other clinical tests. These include the measurement of various types of pupil reactions such as pupil cycle times, light/dark reactions and pharmacological responses (10). Other studies have analysed the effect of the disease on ciliary body function, manifested by a progressive lowering of intraocular pressure and alteration in postural responses (9). Most authors now recognise that chronic iridocyclitis in multibacillary disease has a neuroparalytic element, with primary involvement of the autonomic nerves, particularly the sympathetic fibres in the iris and ciliary body. This may raise the possibility of pharmacological therapy for what can currently only be overcome by surgical intervention or photocoagulation.

Significant iris involvement, defined as either a non-reacting pupil less than 2mm in diameter, or an irregular or eccentric pupil with detectable synechiae, was observed in 8.1% of patients in the LEPRA survey.

Cataract

Cataract remains a major problem in leprosy and the question of a"leprosy cataract" has yet to be solved. Most leprosy patients live in areas of the world where cataract is common, and certainly in PB disease its presence is likely to be coincidental. In multibacillary disease cataract may be secondary to iridocyclitis, or be a complication of steroid therapy, it may also be the result of low intraocular pressure or simply be age-related.

Whatever its cause, cataract is responsible for a disproportionate amount of blindness, and can only be treated by surgery, which can be carried out effectively provided that certain operative precautions are taken. Sadly the stigma of the disease that still exists in many countries often excludes the leprosy patient with cataract from receiving the surgical services that are available to other members of the community.

Significant cataract, defined as either aphakia or visible lens opacities or an absent red reflex reducing vision to below 6/36 with no other obvious cause of visual impairment, was observed in 16.9% of patients in the LEPRA survey.

Epidemiology

Epidemiological studies in leprosy have always proved to be difficult to obtain, and estimates of important aspects in the disease such as blindness and the prevalence of sight-threatening lesions may fall wide of the mark (3).

In addition to the factors already mentioned that may determine the frequency and severity of ocular involvement, there are other less quantifiable influences such as the climate, environment, occupation and social status. This epidemiological nightmare is further aggravated by the difficulties in estimating the actual numbers of patients with the disease. Many affected individuals do not come forward for treatment and therefore do not appear on registers until late in the course of the disease. This is often due to ignorance and fear, and reflects the social stigma that still exists throughout the world. The figures are further distorted by the WHO policy of deregistering patients once they have completed multidrug therapy and have satisfied the criteria for cure - a policy that has obvious pitfalls from an ophthalmic point of view. The LEPRA survey, for example, showed that 24.3% of patients completing multidrug therapy, who might well be released from control and therefore ophthalmic supervision, had on-going eye problems that were potentially sight-threatening (6). It is not therefore difficult to see why hard epidemiological data on the prevalence of ocular complications of leprosy are scarce, and why knowledge of their incidence is almost non-existent.

Certain assumptions have therefore to be made, and if the global leprosy population is taken to be between 10 and 12 million (14), than the numbers of blind leprosy patients may reach half a million or more, making the disease rank as one of the major causes of world blindness, likely to increase proportionally as others such as trachoma, xerophthalmia and onchocerciasis become contained by modern therapy and public health measures.

Conclusions

There is no doubt that the problems of ocular leprosy will continue into the next century, and the role of the ophthalmologist must be extended beyond the traditional provision of ophthalmic care at a tertiary level. Eye doctors need to be aware that ocular complications often arise from inattention or neglect of simple problems early in the disease, which may go unnoticed by the patient because of the reduced appreciation of pain. Education of the leprologist and patient in these matters is just as important as therapy, and it is essential that young ophthalmologists acquaint themselves with the various aspects of the disease that concern the eyes. It is for this reason that this symposium is such a landmark for ophthalmology and leprosy alike.

Hansen wrote over a hundred years ago that "There is no disease which so frequently gives rise to disoders of the eye, as leprosy does" (2). A century of scientific and medical advances has hardly modified this statement at all, and the disease still remains an important cause of avoidable blindness and one of the great challenges to preventive medicine.

Acknowledgement

None of this work would have been possible without the continued support of LEPRA.

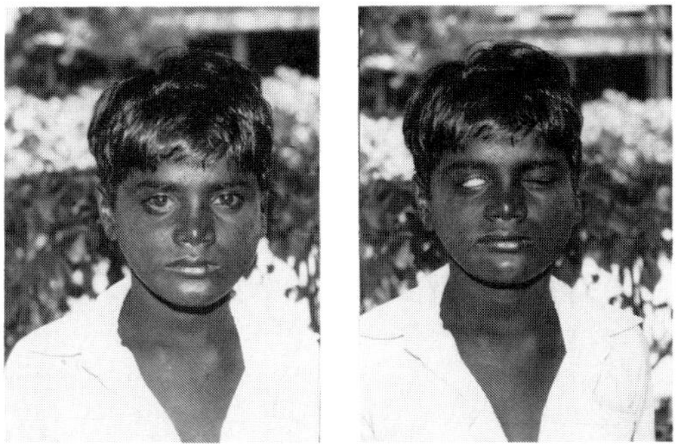

Fig.1. Acute unilateral lagophthalmos in a young boy with Type 1 reaction.

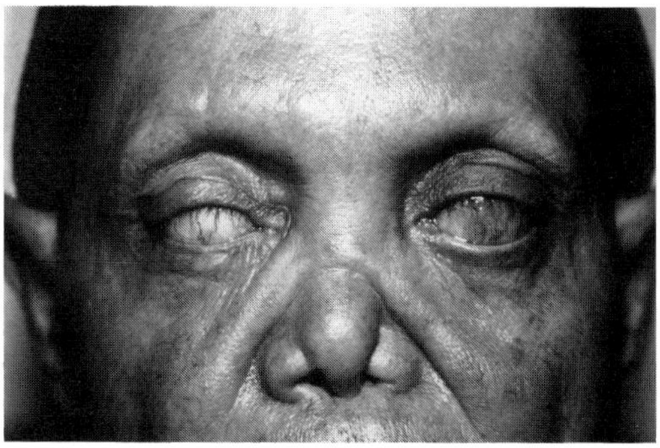

Fig.2. Chronic lagophthalmos in multibacillary disease with defective lid closure.

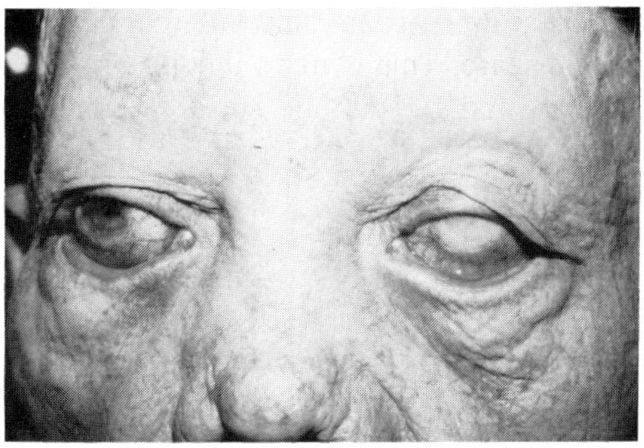

Fig.3. Exposure keratopathy affecting the inferior cornea in the right eye and causing total corneal opacification in the left eye.

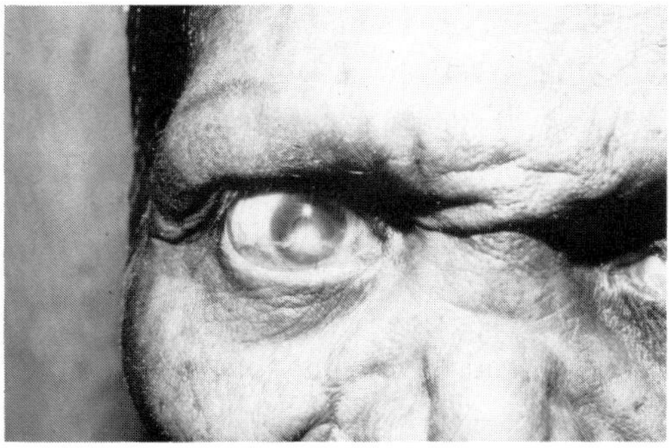

Fig.4. Corneal opacity due to healed corneal ulcer.

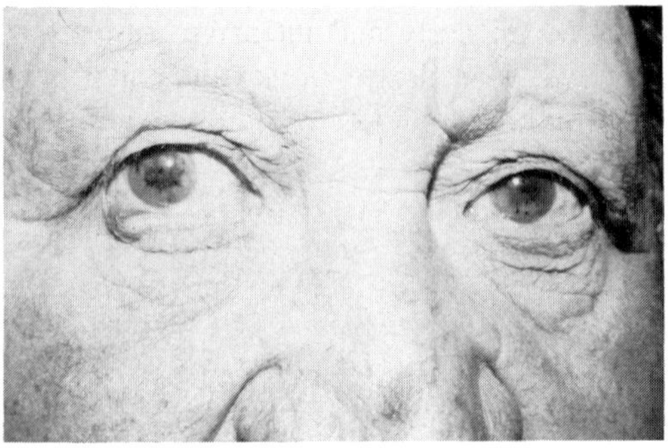

Fig.5. Chronic iridocyclitis in both eyes of patient with multibacillary leprosy. The miotic pin-point pupils are completely resistant to all forms of mydriatic therapy.

References

1. Brand MB (1980) The Care of the Eye. The Star. Carville, Louisiana
2. Bull OB, Hansen GA (1873) The Leprous Diseases of the Eye. Publ Albert Cammermeyer Christiana
3. Courtright P (1988) Defining the Magnitude of Ocular Complications from Leprosy: Problems of Methodology. Int J Lepr 56:566-573
4. ffytche TJ (1983) A Computer Form to Aid in the Collection of Data on the Ocular Complications of Leprosy. Lepr Rev 54:271-281
5. ffytche TJ (to be published) The Prevalence of Sight-Threatening Lesions in Ocular Leprosy. Proceedings of the XXVIth International Congress of Ophthalmology Singapore 1990
6. ffytche TJ (1991) Residual Sight-Threatening Lesions in Patients Completing Multidrug Therapy and Sulphone Monotherapy. Lep Rev 62:35-43
7. Fine PEM (1982) Leprosy: The Epidemiology of a Slow Bacterium. Epid Rev 4:161-188
8. Hogeweg M, Kiran KU, Suneetha S (1991) The Significance of Facial Patches and Type 1 Reaction for the Development of Facial Nerve Damage in Leprosy. Lep Rev 67:143-149
9. Hussein N, Courtright PD, Ostler HB et al (1989) Low Intraocular Pressure and Postural Changes in Intraocular Pressure in Hansen's Disease. Am J Ophthalmol 1:80-84
10. Lewallen S, Courtright PD, Ho-Sung Lee (1989) Ocular Autonomic Dysfunction and Intraocular Pressure in Leprosy. Br J Ophthalmol 73:946-949
11. Schwartz B (1965) Environmental Temperature and Ocular Temperature Gradient. Arch Ophthalmol 74:237-243
12. Weekeroon L (1969) Ocular Leprosy in Ceylon. Br J Ophthalmol 53:457-465
13. World Health Organisation Study Group (1982) Chemotherapy of Leprosy for Control Programmes. WHO Technical Report Series No.675, Geneva.
14. World Health Organisation Expert Committee on Leprosy (1988) WHO Technical Report Series No.768, Geneva.

The Medical and Surgical Treatment of Eye Complications in Leprosy

Margreet Hogeweg, Felix Brandt

Abstract. The need for early medical and surgical treatment in leprosy discussed with an emphasis on the resulting problems, both functional and cosmetic.

Introduction

Leprosy still belongs to the main blinding diseases in most developing countries. Most of the eye complications, however, can be prevented or adequately treated and therefore most of the blindness and visual impairment in leprosy is in fact avoidable and unnecessary (5).

However, it should be realized that patients may also suffer from other blinding eye diseases not directly related to leprosy, such as trachoma or corneal ulcers due to trauma, and leprosy staff should be prepared for these conditions as well, because the resulting blindness is in the same way distressing and incapacitating to the patient.

Eye complications in leprosy should be seen in relationship with the development of complications of the disease in general:

- Complications due to massive invasion of M.leprae and secondary atrophy of skin, nerves and certain organs. These complications occur only in multibacillary patients, classified as Borderline Lepromatous and Lepromatous Leprosy.
- Complications due to immune processes. Type I reactions (rever sal reaction) occur in Borderline disease, in patients classified as Borderline Tuberculoid, Borderline Borderline and Borderline Lepromatous. Type II reactions (erythema nodosum leprosum) occur only in multibacillary patients.

Treatment should therefore in principle be focussed on early and intensive antileprosy treatment in order to prevent massive proliferation of bacilli and secondly on enforced treatment of the immune reactions (8).

There are four major potentially blinding eye complications:

1. lagophthalmos with exposure keratitis,
2. corneal anesthesia,
3. iris and scleral lesions, and
4. cataract.

Treatment and possible constraints in each of these will be discussed.

Lagophthalmos

Type I reaction in the face (Fig.1), located around the eye or overlying the area of the zygomatic branch of the facial nerve will result in damage to this nerve and therefore in weakness of the orbicularis muscle and consequently in lagophthalmos (Fig.2, 3). Type I reactions occur suddenly and early in borderline disease, either before the diagnosis of leprosy is made or early, generally within the first year of anti-leprosy treatment. Therefore patients are most at risk of developing lagophthalmos either before diagnosis or early during treatment (9,13).

Type I reaction in the face or lagophthalmos of less than six months duration is treated with systemic corticosteroids, as is routine in Type I reaction with nerve damage elsewhere in the body. This may result in full recovery of the nerve function. The sooner the corticosteroid treatment is started, the more successful it will be. The initial dose is 40-60mg of frednisolone (depending on body weight) in a single morning dose slowly decreasing over a period of 4-6 months. However, relapses may occur and should be treated in the same way. The corticosteroid treatment should preferably be given on an out-patient basis to make it more acceptable to patients (11). Nerve damage that has existed for longer than six months is irreversible.

In lagophthalmos of more than six months duration and a lid gap of <5mm in mild closure (as in sleep) treatment should be conservative with protection (e.g. sunglasses) and "Think Blink" (regular conscious blinking). Lid surgery is generally unnecessary and the eye may survive for long periods of time without further complications.

However, in lagophthalmos of more than six months duration and with a lid gap of >5mm on mild closure, the eye is at risk for exposure keratitis and lid surgery is therefore indicated (Fig.4).

Tarsorraphy

Tarsorraphy (preferably Goldstein modification) (7) is the most commonly used procedure. Its main advantages are its simplicity, and the fact that only simple instruments present in any general theater are required. Disadvantages are the cosmetic results, especially in unilateral surgery, and the continuing watering of the eye. The often coexisting ectropium is not corrected by simple tarsorraphy.

However, the main and distressing complication of tarsorraphia as experienced by the patient is the loss of temporal field of vision by this procedure. This should be explained carefully to the patient beforehand.

Tarsal Strip/Fascial Sling Procedure

Tarsal strip/fascial sling procedure (1,4) gives better cosmetic and functional results and correct coexisting ectropion as well. However, they require more surgical skills, finer instruments to handle the tiny strips and good suture material for fixation of the strips to the orbital rim. They are to be considered as the procedures of choice.

Temporalis Muscle Transfer

Temporalis muscle transfer (14) is an ingenious operation, which makes "blinking" possible by chewing. However, it is major surgery, usually performed by the rare plastic surgeon working in leprosy, and it requires considerable physiotherapy afterwards. The functional final result, "spontaneous" blinking, is usually poor, although the mechanical and cosmetic results are good (Fig.5,6).

Corneal anesthesia

Although the condition is generally called "anesthesia" it usually is a relative hypesthesia, in the majority of patients less than in herpes (10). It may occur in three ways:

- as a result of Type I reaction in combination with lagophthal mos. However, to what extent corneal hypesthesia is primarily the result of the Type I reaction or secondary to the lagophthalmos is not yet determined.
- as a result of recurrent scleritis in Type II reaction, with damage to the ciliary nerves (12). This is rare but may result in deep anesthesia, not only of the cornea but also of the iris.
- due to invasion of the ciliary nerves by M.leprae and secondary atrophy of these nerves. This develops gradually in long-standing multibacillary disease. Corneal hyp/anesthesia therefore can be expected in borderline patients with lagophthalmos and in multibacillary patients.

There is no treatment for corneal hypesthesia apart from protection by (sun)glasses against foreign bodies, awareness of the danger of the "red eye" by proper health education and daily self-inspection for redness of the eyes in a mirror. The major constraint is the lack of pain as a warning sign.

Iris and Scleral Complications

Acute iritisis a well-known albeit fairly rare complication in leprosy. It is indistinguishable from acute iritis in general and it should be treated in the same way by topical corticosteroids and atropine. Although acute iritis is considered to be a type II reaction of the eye, there are usually no signs of a systemic type II reaction at the same time. On the contrary, most systemic Type II reactions occur without eye involvement. Acute iritis occurs in multibacillary patients, usually after a few years of anti-leprosy treatment or in long-standing untreated or irregularly treated disease. Once it has occurred it may recur at any time without general disease activity and even long after release from treatment. A major constraint for proper treatment of acute iritis is confusion by field staff with other conditions that give rise to a "red eye", in particular acute (bacterial/viral) conjunctivitis, which is very common in all developing countries, corneal abrasion/ulcer, herpes or possible acute glaucoma. Secondly, atropine and topical corticosteroids are often not available to field staff.

Acute Uveoscleritis

Acute uveoscleritis (Fig.7) is a rare but more severe, frequently bilateral and often almost intractable condition, that may occur in patients with severe recurrent systemic type II reactions. It particularly occurs in long-standing untreated or irregularly treated often dapsone-resistant disease and has therefore been more common in the era before dapsone or Multiple Drug Therapy existed. Acute uveoscleritis may end in bilaterally blind staphylomatous eyes in only a couple of months.

Treatment is by systemic type II reaction therapy with corticosteroids, Clofazimine (Lamprene) and thalidomide and intensive topical treatment with corticosteroids, atropine and acetazolamide as necessary.

Long-term use of clofazimine, in order to suppress further Type II reactions will give rise to dark pigmentation of the skin and a reddish/brown color of the conjunctiva. These side-effects may lead to discontinuation of the treatment by the patient.

Chronic Iritis

Chronic iritis (Fig.7) is regularly found in patients with long-term multibacillary disease and is a major cause of blindness among these patients (3). It is almost asymptomatic and there is hardly any redness or pain, in spite of low-grade flare and cells in the anterior chamber of the eye, with posterior synechiae formation. There are no signs of systemic type II reaction. It may be the result of an untreated acute iritis that smoulders on, or an idiopathic chronic iritis, or the result of a neuroparalytic iritis, due to a slow breakdown of iris tissue, secondary to invasion by M.leprae (6). The condition is often not recognized.

Treatment is by long-term atropine and corticosteroids. However, this often has hardly any effect on disease activity and may be difficult to pursue under field circumstances.

Iris Atrophy

Iris atrophy occurs in long-standing multibacillary disease. Atrophy of the iris dilator muscle may lead to a pinhole pupil that does not dilate on mydriatics (Fig.8). This may cause blindness, especially in combination with lens or corneal opacities. Later, multiple holes in the iris (policoria) may appear. Atrophy of the sphincter muscle may cause a moth-eaten pupil. The process is slowly progressive, but posterior synechiae are not formed. Intraocular pressure may be low, due to low production of aqueous as a result of atrophy of the ciliary body. This condition can probably be prevented by early and bactericidal anti-leprosy treatment as in Multiple Drug Therapy to prevent invasion and proliferation of M.leprae in the autonomous nerves of the iris and ciliary body. In case of bilateral blindness (visual acuity <3/60 in the better eye) a surgical sector iridectomy with or without lens extraction may be considered, provided mydriatics have been tried and proved not to result in sufficient sustained vision improvement. However, the iris tissue is friable and it is not easy to get a good grasp of the tissue. Surgery on a soft eye may result in postoperative phthisis.

Cataract

Cataract may well be the most important cause of bilateral blindness in leprosy (2) and the backlog in cataract blindness may even be greater among leprosy patients than in the general population, due to the stigma of the disease. Simple senile cataract may occur in all types of leprosy. Secondary cataract may occur as a side-effect of systemic corticosteroid treatment for reactions or as the result of acute/chronic iritis, iris atrophy and low intraocular pressure. Secondary cataracts are mainly found in multibacillary patients. Cataracts can be operated on in patients who are on regular treatment or have been released from therapy, provided there have been no reactions during the previous six months. There should be no active iritis and lagophthalmos and an ectropium should be corrected beforehand. Intraocular pressure must be preferably >8mm Hg to avoid possible postoperative phthisis. It should be realized that infections and ulcers elsewhere in the body will increase the risk of postoperative endophthalmitis.

In secondary cataracts the pupils will often not dilate, due to iris atrophy and posterior synechiae. Postoperatively the anterior chamber of the eye may not reform, due to insufficient aqueous production. Altogether surgery is more difficult and more prone to postoperative complications. Indications for surgery should therefore be strict.

For a minority of patients with a completely collapsed nose it may be difficult to wear aphakic glasses. However, due to the manyfold intraocular pathology and the increased risk of endophthalmitis intraocular lenses are generally contraindicated and should only be used with extreme caution and only under optimal surgical conditions.

Comment

Patients with long-standing multibacillary disease may have multiple eye complications due to leprosy, such as lagophthalmos with ectropium and corneal hypaesthesia complicated by chronic conjunctivitis and exposure keratitis. At the same time there may be chronic low-grade iritis and signs of iris atrophy with a pinhole pupil, scleral thinning and a secondary cataract. Such patients form a challenge to the ophthalmologist and need specialized ophthalmic care to prevent further deterioration and possible restauration of their eyesight.

Besides all the care for prevention of blindness in leprosy by providing medical treatment in time or in performing surgery, there always are social and cosmetic problems for the patient himself. In this context, transplantation of headhair for madarosis, the application of an artificial eye in phthisis bulbi or after an enucleation or the reconstruction of a collapsed nose with an skin-flap should never be neglected and should be provided, if possible, since a leprous patient feels very much like a non-leper human being.

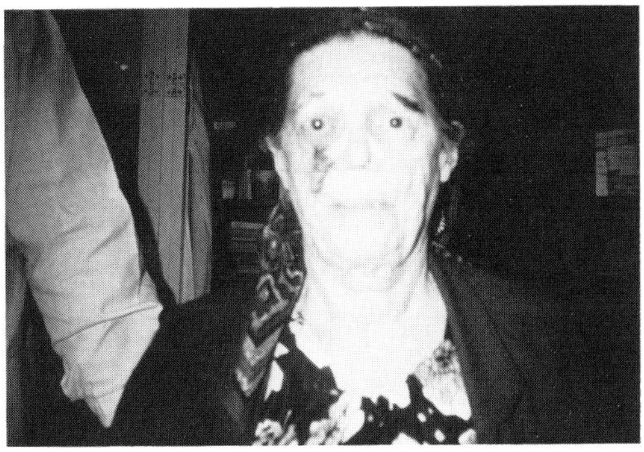

Fig.1. Acute type I reaction in face.

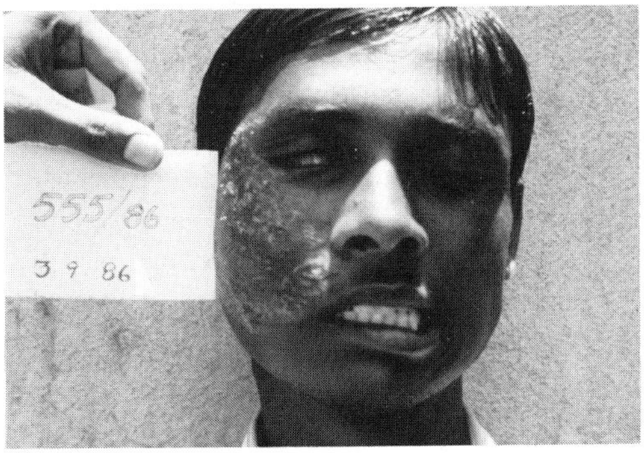

Fig.2. Type I reaction in patch with early lagophthalmos.

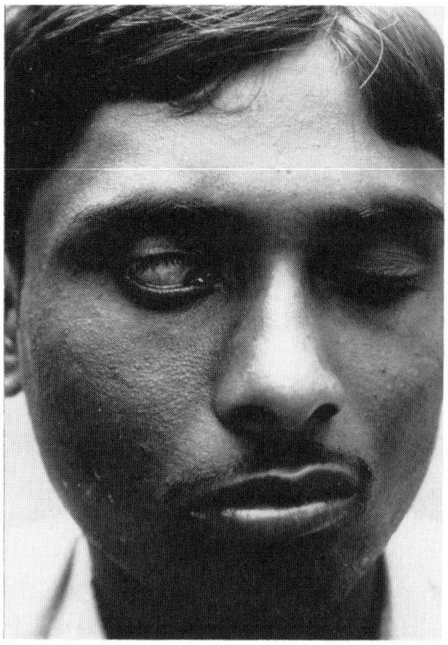

Fig.3. Resolved type I reaction, with irreversible lagophthalmos (same boy as Fig.2).

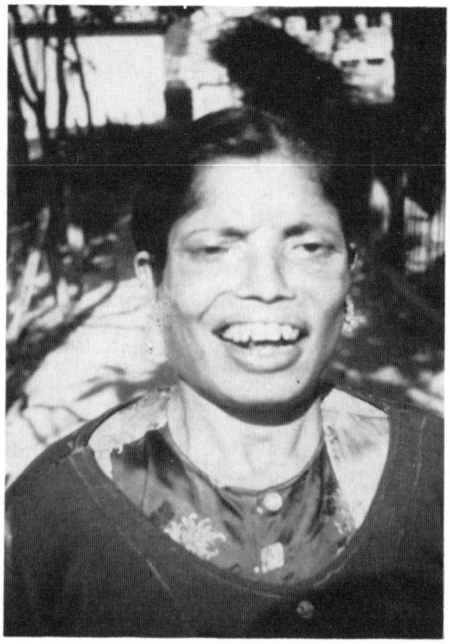

Fig.5. Temporalis muscle transfer (TMT): open eyes in an lafing face.

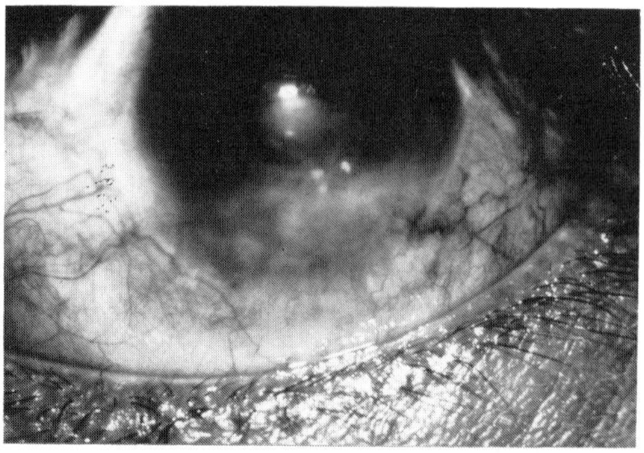

Fig.4. Exposure keratitis in lagophthalmos with lid gap of > 5mm.

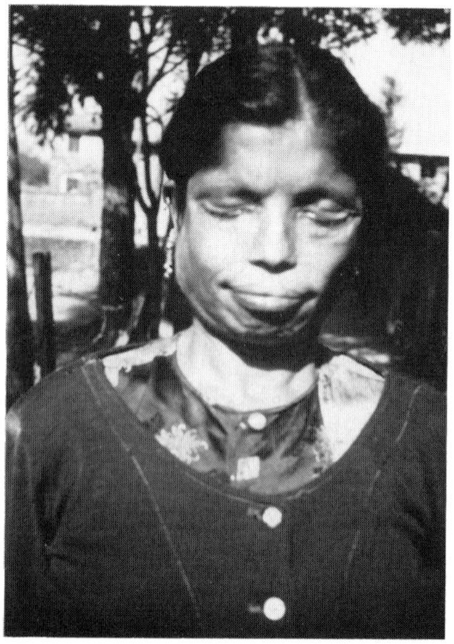

Fig.6. Temporalis muscle transfer (TMT): "blinking" eyes by chewing.

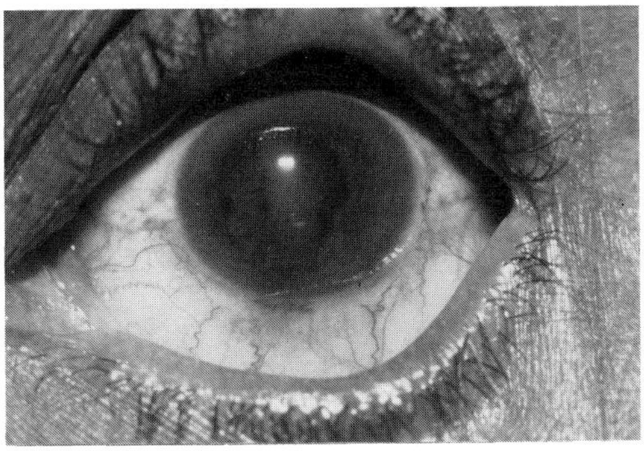

Fig.7. Chronic iritis with minimal redness and posterior synechiae (after dilatation).

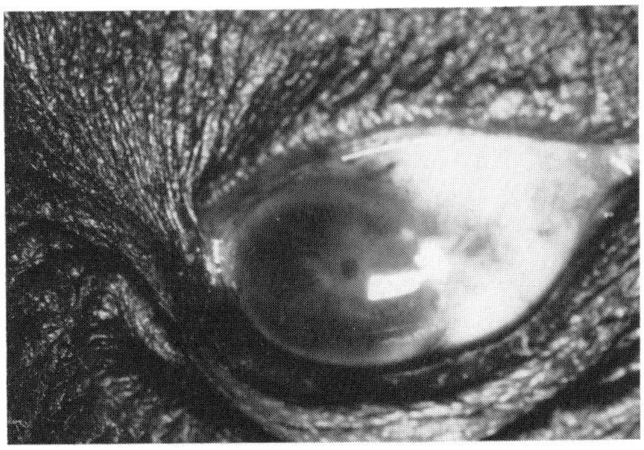

Fig.8. Pinpoint pupil with irisatrophy (after maximal dilatation).

References

1. Anderson RL, Gordy DD (1979) The Tarsal Strip Procedure. Arch Ophthalmol 97:2192-2196
2. Brandt F, Kampik A (1983) Blindness from Cataract Formation in Leprosy. Dev Ophthal 7:1-12
3. Choyce DP (1969) Diagnosis and Management of Ocular Leprosy. Br J Ophthalmol 53:217-223
4. Collin,JRO (ed) (1989) A Manual of Systematic Eyelid Surgery. Edinburgh 2nd ed. pp.131-132
5. Courtright P, Johnson GJ (1988) Prevention of Blindness in Leprosy. International Center for Eye Health, London
6. ffytche TJ (1981) Role of Iris Changes as a Cause of Blindness in Lepromatous Leprosy. Br J Ophthalmol 65:231-239
7. Fox SA (ed) (1976) Ophthalmic Plastic Surgery. Grune & Stratton, New York p.217
8. Hastings RC (1985) Medicine in the Tropics. Churchill Livingston
9. Hogeweg M, Kiran KU, Suneetha S (1991) The Significance of Facial Patches and Type I Reaction for the Development of Facial Nerve Damage in Leprosy. Leprosy Rev 62:143-149
10. Karacorlu MA, Cakiner T, Saylan T (1991) Corneal Sensitivity and Correlations Between Decreased Sensitivity and Anterior Segment Pathology in Ocular Leprosy. Br J Ophthalmol 75:117-119
11. Kiran KU, Hogeweg M, Suneetha S (1991) Treatment of Recent Facial Nerve Damage with Lagophthalmos, Using a Semistandardized Steroid Regimen. Lepr Rev 62:150-154
12. Lyne AJ (1977) Corneal Sensitivity in Scleritis and Episcleritis. Br J Ophthalmol 61:650-654
13. Naafs B, Wheate HW (1978) The Time Interval Between the Start of Anti-Leprosy Treatment and the Development of Reac

tions in Borderline Patients. Lepr Rev 49:153-157
14. Sen DK (1970) Temporalis Transplantation for Paralytic Lagophthalmos. Br J Ophthalmol 54:680-682

- Neonatal Infections

Neonatal Ophthalmia in Tropical Countries

Volker Klauß, L. Fransen

Abstract. The epidemiology of ophthalmia neonatorum (ON) in Europe and in developing countries has changed markedly over the last decades.
Chlamydia trachomatis has become more frequent than Neisseria gonorrhoeae. The etiology cannot be determined clinically. An eye smear with Gram stain represents the most valid method to prove intracellular Gram negative diplococci. Wherever possible, microbiological cultures should provide further differentiation.
Gonococcal conjunctivitis is treated with systemic antibiotics. Penicillin is the antibiotic of choice in areas with a low percentage of beta-lactamase producing strains of gonococci. Chlamydial ophthalmia neonatorum is treated with systemic Erythromycin. Treatment includes the parents of infected infants.
Credé's prophylaxis with silvernitrate has become a controversial issue because of concern about the occurrence of chemical conjunctivitis and its ineffectiveness against infections with Chlamydia trachomatis. Recent data, however, show that silvernitrate and tetracyclines are highly effective in the prevention of gonococcal ophthalmia caused by multiresistant strains but are both not very useful to prevent chlamydia conjunctivitis.
Growing populations, urbanisation and increasing promiscuity cause a rising incidence of ON in developing countries. Strategies for prevention, prophylaxis and early detection have been developed but have not been implemented in most parts of the developing world.

Introduction

Ophthalmia neonatorum (ON) represented a major health problem in Europe and was an important cause of blindness until the turn of last century. Magnus' data of 1882 demonstrate that ophthalmia neonatorum cause unilateral blindness in 6 % and bilateral blindness in 3 % of 90 children who were affected. This was before introduction of Credé's prophylaxis (6,19).

Data published by Credé show that from the introduction of silvernitrate eye drop prophylaxis in 1880 the number of cases of Ophthalmia neonatorum dropped significantly from 30 to 35 per year to 1 case in the second half of 1880 (6). The introduction of Credé's prophylaxis led to a marked improvement of the situation in Europe. Ophthalmia neonatorum became less prevalent and blindness from ophthalmia neonatorum became an exception. This is demonstrated in figures from various blind schools where before 1900 up to 50 % of the children had been blinded by ophthalmia neonatorum (15,24).

Epidemiology

Looking at today's situation figures from various countries regarding the prevalence and incidence rates of ophthalmia neonatorum incate a large difference between various countries: the situation is worst in Africa with an incidence rate of up to 24 % (2,12,20), low rates are reported from USA, Asia and Europe with a minimum of 0.04 % per 1,000 live births for gonococcal ophthalmia neonatorum and 4 per 1,000 for chlamydial ophthalmia neonatorum (3, 12, 16).

Data from Kenya show that N. gonorrhoea can be isolated in 40 % of mothers of children with ophthalmia neonatorum, 9 % of those mothers were positive for syphilis (10, 11, 12, 17, 18). Also in Kenya 1,000 mothers and children were examined for presence of Chlamydia trachomatis and Neisseria gonorrhoea, 28.5 % of mothers showed infection with Chlamydia trachomatis and 9.5 % infection with Neisseria gonorrhoae. Neonates without clinical signs had infection with chlamydia in 8.1 and with N.gonorrhoea in 5.7 % whereas in children with clinical signs of conjunctivitis chlamydia could be demonstrated in 28.7 % and gonorrhoae in 20.2 %. In industrialized countries chlamydial infections occur more frequently than infection with gonococci. The infection rate among exposed children is high, having been found to be between 25 and 50 % in studies in Africa. It is higher for N.gonorrhoea than for Chlamydia trachomatis (10, 11, 17, 18).

The epidemiologic data clarify that ophthalmia neonatorum still represents a serious health problem worldwide, but mainly in Africa with a risk of blindness. This risk may be underestimated because a number of the affected children will die during early childhood. Incidence, etiology and relative prevalence of ophthalmia neonatorum, depend on the application of silvernitrate or any other prophylaxis at birth and on the prevalence of sexually transmitted disease organisms in pregnant women.

Etiology

The etiology of ophthalmia neonatorum can be infectious or chemical in origin. The two agents of major public health importance are N.gonorrhoea and C.trachomatis. The risk of blindness depends on medical care available, which is still a problem in rural areas of developing countries and in urban slums. In Kenya 16 % of infants with gonococcal ophthalmia neonatorum showed corneal lesions (11,12). Because of penicillin resistance of N.gonorrhoea in many parts of the world treatment can be difficult or not available. Delay of treatment may be the cause of corneal lesions or generalized disease.

C.trachomatis was the most frequent identifiable cause of ophthalmia neonatorum in a prospective study in a Nairobi maternity hospital (18) in contrast to the study of infants seen at the sexually transmitted disease clinic, wherein gonorrhoea was the major cause (11). This difference may be explained by the more severe clinical symptoms in gonococcal ophthalmia which lead mothers to seek medical help. Other infectious agents like Haemophilus spp, Streptococcus pneumoniae, Staphylococcus, Escherichia coli, Enterococcus and Herpes simplex virus could be cultured in cases of ophthalmia neonatorum. Chemical conjunctivitis may be seen after use of silvernitrate in higher concentrations. In up to 40 % of infants with ophthalmia neonatorum no infectious agents can be cultured, this fact needs further investigation.

Clinical picture

Definition

Conjunctivitis of the newborn is defined as any conjunctivitis with discharge occuring during the first 28 days of life. Other terms used for this disease include ophthalmia neonatorum, blenorrhoea neonatorum and neonatal conjunctivitis.

Looking at large numbers of infants the clinical picture varies according to the causative agent which this is not necessarily true in the individual case. Thus clinical features do not allow to make a specific diagnosis. As a general rule gonococcal ophthalmia neonatorum occurs earlier after birth and produces a more purulent discharge in larger quantities than chlamydial ophthalmia neonatorum. In gonococcal ophthalmia neonatorum corneal involvement is more frequent, ulcerations and perforations however are exceptional. The clinic diagnosis is not only made by assessment of lid swelling and redness but the cornea must be inspected. As a general rule gonococcal ophthalmia neonatorum appears 3 to 7, chlamydial ophthalmia neonatorum 9 to 12 days after delivery but in case of early rupture of membranes the latter may be seen few days after delivery. Figures from Kenya indicate that newborns are taken for treatment late. The difference in age at presentation regarding different causative agents of ophthalmia neonatorum is minimal.

In chlamydial ophthalmia neonatorum pseudomembranes of the conjunctiva have been observed, follicles are not seen during the first weeks of life. The clinical picture of ophthalmia neonatorum due to other microbial agents is usually milder (pict. 1).

Chemical conjunctivitis develops during the first hours following instillation of silvernitrate drops. The signs are reddening and swelling of the lids, discharge and in exceptional cases stenosis of the lacrimal duct. Rarely silvernitrate staining of the cornea has been reported.

Laboratory Diagnosis

Treatment of ophthalmia neonatorum should not be started before a gramstain has been performed. The gramstain is most important for a quick differential diagnosis as in presence of intracellular gram negativ diplococci. Gonococcal ophthalmia neonatorum can be assumed. In the absence of intracellular gram negativ diplococci Chlamydia trachomatis is the most likely causative agent. If available additionally cultures for N.gonorrhoea and C trachomatis are useful, chlamydia can also be proven through Giemsa stain or monoclonal antibody test. The possibility of a concurrent infection with gonococci and chlamydia must be taken into consideration.

Management

Gonococcal Ophthalmia Neonatorum

Because of the seriousness of the disease and its possible complications and because a Gram stain of a conjunctival smear is highly predictive, cheap and easily feasable to make a presumptive diagnosis of gonococcal ophthalmia neonatorum, this test can be used to direct the choice of treatment immediately at the moment the child presents. The recommended treatment regimens for gonococcal ophthalmia neonatorum include multiple doses of intravenous penicillin with or without topical antimicrobial therapy and hospital admission of the infant (5). However, those regimens are only valid in areas where gonococci are not resistant to penicillin. Up to 52 % of gonococcal strains isolated from infants with ophthalmia neonatorum have been reported to be penicillinase-producing strains (11). In addition, intrinsic resistance to penicillin, not mediated by penicillinase is also increasing. A cheap, single dose treatment given to the infant as an outpatient would be better adapted to the third world countries and several such regimens have been demonstrated recently to be highly effective for treatment of ophthalmia neonatorum in areas with a high prevalence of penicillin resistant gonococci.

For areas with a penicillinase producing N.gonorrhoeae prevalence of more than 1 %, the World Health Organization recommended recently that ophthalmia neonatorum should be treated with cefotaxime 100 mg/kg or kanamycin 25 mg/kg as a single intramuscular dose with tetracycline 1 % or erythromycin 0.5 % eye ointment for 10 days (14). Spectinomycin might be equally efficient. A single dose of 75 mg kanamycin combined with topical gentamicin ointment during 7 days also has been shown to be very efficient but not always available (9). Ceftriaxone, a third generation cephalosporin with a long half life has been successfully used in gonococcal ophthalmia neonatorum without combination with topical antimicrobial therapy and it has the advantage also to eradicate oropharyngeal carriage of gonococci (13).

Chlamydial Ophthalmia Neonatorum

All above proposed regimens do not adequately treat concomitant chlamydial infections. Therefore a mixed infection treated with those regimens can result in post gonococcal conjunctivitis due to C.trachomatis.

Infants with ophthalmia neonatorum with negative laboratory tests for gonococci and with presumed or definite chlamydial ophthalmia neonatorum, can be treated with erythromycin estolate (50 mg/kg per day) for a minimum of 14 days or another derivative of erythromycin with adapted dosage. Systemic treatment is necessary. Topical antimicrobial therapy is not necessary and washing of the eyes with saline is adequate. The mother and her partner(s) should be investigated and adequately treated.

Other Microbial Causes of Ophthalmia neonatorum

Only at the highest level, laboratories are well equipped to also detect beta-lactamase producing strains of N. gonorrhoeae and to diagnose chlamydial infection. Only in this last situation a differential diagnosis can be made between chlamydial and nonchlamydial ophthalmia neonatorum. Most nonchlamydial nongonococcal conjunctivitis of the newborn can be treated with topical tetracycline hydrochloride or erythromycin eye ointment, 4 times a day for 14 days.

Prevention of Ophthalmia Neonatorum

It is an important public health measure to prevent sexually transmitted disease and their consequences in pregnant women and the neonate.

Different types of intervention strategies can be selected and the choice will depend on the relative prevalence of the causative sexually transmitted disease agents in that population or geographical area and on economic, laboratory and diagnostic facilities.

The intervention can be applied in early or late pregnancy, during labour or after delivery, in the mother or in the neonate. Different preventive regimens can be chosen: all pregnant women or all infants at the time of delivery or only high risk groups. We will here only discuss the major strategies to prevent or control ophthalmia neonatorum and its complications.

Eye Prophylaxis in the Neonate

This method was introduced by Crédé in Leipzig in the last century (6). The original procedure had two parts: first, mechanical cleaning of the newborns' eyelids as soon as the head was born and before the eyes opened, and second, instillation of an antiseptic into the conjunctival sacs as soon as possible. Crédé recommended a 2 % aqueous silver nitrate solution, but the concentration was later changed to 1 % because this was less irritating. Other silver preparations such as argyrol (5 %) have been used instead for the same reason.

This preventive measure was very effective, and within a few years the incidence of gonococcal ophthalmia (and blindness caused by it) fell from 10 % to 0.3 % of births (6,7). Later on ocular prophylaxis with silver nitrate was critisized because it causes chemical conjunctivitis or because it is not effective against extra-ocular infection by gonococci. Eye prophylaxis was abandoned in several places (21) or was changed to prophylaxis with 0.5 % erythromycin or 1 % tetracycline ointment (USA). This last method was presumed to be more effective to prevent chlamydial ophthalmia (23). Recently, it has been shown that 1 % tetracycline ointment and 1 % silver nitrate drops were equally effective prophylactic agents against gonococcal ophthalmia neonatorum, caused by multiresistant gonococci including penicillinase producing N. gonorrhoeae and strains with relatively high MIC's for tetracycline (22). In the same study both silver nitrate and tetracycline prophylaxis was not effective to prevent the incidence of chlamydial conjunctivitis (17). Alexander and Harrison reported also that tetracycline ointment does prevent chlamydial ophthalmia but that some failures occur (14). The recent data from Kenya show that both silver nitrate drops and tetracycline ointment are highly effective in the prevention of gonococcal ophthalmia caused by multiresistant strains and additionally prevent a considerable amount of chlamydial conjunctivitis (17). However, the need for prevention of chlamydial ophthalmia is less clear cut. Arguments are that chlamydial pneumonitis develops in 20 % of infected infants and may be a cause for long term pulmonary problems (4), that untreated C. trachomatis ophthalmia neonatorum might progress to scarring, corneal vascularisation and pannus formation (1,8), that the diagnosis is difficult and treatment long and costly. To prevent ophthalmia by both organisms a single application of tetracycline 1 % ointment could be used as the first choice in countries such as Kenya where the prevalence of maternal gonococcal and chlamydial infection is high and medical care facilities underdeveloped. Tetracycline ointment is widely available, cheap and has less side effects than the silver nitrate solution. However silver nitrate can still be recommended if used in monodosis and if well kept and protected from exposure to light.

In countries where the incidence of gonococcal disease in pregnant women is low and where the main sexually transmitted agent causing neonatal conjunctivitis is C. trachomatis, it could be better to replace ocular prophylaxis with silver nitrate by the following strategies if possible.

Detection and Treatment of Sexually Transmitted Disease in Pregnant Women

Another strategy to prevent infection or colonization of the neonate and also to prevent disease complications in the mother would be to detect and treat infection in the pregnant women.

This approach can only be used where medical care is well organized, i.e. where pregnant women at risk can easily be screened for sexually transmitted disease and adequately treated if infection is found. This strategy is not always possible even in industrialized countries; routine diagnosis of chlamydial infection in pregnant women is not easily and readily available and is expensive. The high risk groups for sexually transmitted disease among pregnant women are not easily motivated to be screened and they are often rapidly reinfected (22). However, in areas where this policy is feasable, treatment of infected pregnant women should be considered. This would not only eliminate neonatal infection, but also infection in the mother who is at increased risk for pre- and postpartum complications or involuntary secondary infertility.

Treatment of Ophthalmia Neonatorum in the Neonate (index case)

This strategy consists of using the infants with neonatal conjunctivits as index cases of probable sexually transmitted disease in parents, and to treat the infant, the mother and her partner(s) subsequently. This coice requires a setting where medical care is readily available, where the prevalence of gonococcal infection in pregnant women is low and where investigation and treatment for chlamydial infection is easy. This approach has the advantage not to mask disease in the mother and her partner and also to prevent disease complications and extraocular manifestations of gonococcal and chlamydial colonization (21,22,23). It has been advocated for Belgium (24) and other European countries (21,23).

Conclusions and Recommendations

Ophthalmia neonatorum is still a major public health problem in the developing world. Sexually transmitted disease agents are highly prevalent causes of ophthalmia neonatorum in those countries and the high incidence of gonococcal ophthalmia neonatorum and resistant gonococcal strains are alarming because of the threat of permanent damage of the eye as a result of corneal involvement. C. trachomatis however is also very common as a cause of ophthalmia neonatorum in those countries and parents of infants with ophthalmia neonatorum are at a high risk for sexually transmitted diseases and also need to be investigated and treated if necessary. Although each etiological agent produces a slightly different pattern of disease, there is a considerable overlap and therefore the identification of the infecting organism cannot be based on clinical signs alone.

However, to make a full differential diagnosis, all laboratoy facilities are not always available and therefore case management will depend on the level of resources. In peripheral laboratories, equipment, time and expertise are limited and the diagnosis of gonococcal conjunctivitis is restricted to Gram stained conjunctival smears which have good predictive values in areas where gonococcal prevalence is high.

At a higher level of health care facilities culture possibilities for gonococcal disease can be available and they can confirm the diagnosis made on a Gram stain and redirect treatment 2 days later if necessary.

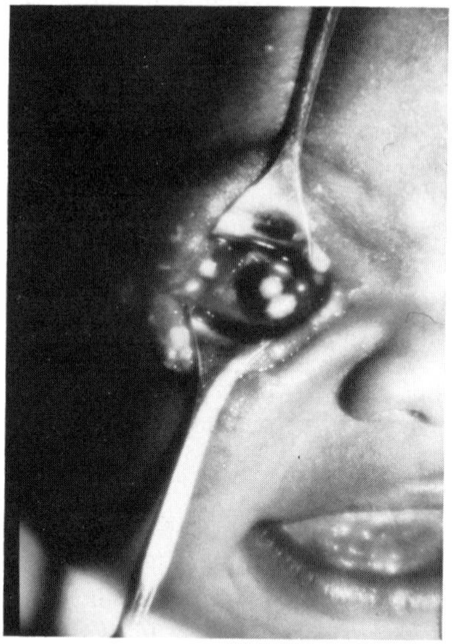

Fig.1. It is mandatory to inspect the cornea.

References

1. Allan CG, Cohen S, Kass MB et al (1979) Asymptomatic Gonorrhea in Prenatal Patients. Am J Obstet Gynecol 108:595-599
2. Armstrong JH, Zacarias F, Rein MF (1976) Ophthamia Neonatorum: A Chart Review. Pediatrics 57:884-892
3. Bijkerk H (1980) Methode van Credé, ja of nee? Ned Tijdsch Geneesk 124:716-720
4. Brasfield DM, Stagno S, Whitley RJ et al (1987) Infant Pneumonitis Associated With Cytomegalovirus, Chlamydia, Pneumocystis and Ureaplasma: Follow Up. Pediatrics 79

5. Centers for Disease Control.(1982) Sexually Transmitted Diseases: Treatment Guidelines. Rev.Inf.Dis. 4:730-746
6. Credé,CSF (1884) Die Verhütung der Augenentzündung der Neugeborenen. Berlin, Archive der Gynaecologie 17:367-370;21:179-395
7. Forbes GB, Forbes GM 1971) Silvernitrate and the Eye of the Newborn: Credé's Contribution to Preventive Medicine. Am J Dis Child 121:1
8. Forster RK, Dawson CR, Schachter J (1970) Late Follow Up of Patients With Neonatal Inclusion Conjunctivitis. Am J Ophthalmol.69:467-472
9. Fransen L, Nsanze H, D'Costa L et al (1984) Single-dose Kanamycin Therapy of Gonococcal Ophthalmia Neonatorum. Lancet ii:1234-1237
10. Fransen L, Nsanze H, D'Cosat L et al (1985) Parents of Infants With Ophthalmia Neonatorum: A High Risk Group for Sexually Transmitted Diseases. Sex Transm Dis 12:150-155
11. Fransen L, Nsanze H, Klauss V et al (1986) Ophthalmia Neonatorum in Nairobi, Kenya: The Roles of Neisseria gonorrhoeae and Chlamydia trachomatis. J Infect Dis 153:862-869
12. Fransen L, van den Bergeh Ph, Mertens A et al (1987) Incidence and bacterial aetiology of neonatal conjunctivitis. Eur J Pediatr 146:152-155
13. Haase DA, Nash RA, Nsanze H et al (1986) Single Dose Cefriaxone Therapy of Gonococcal Ophthalmia Neonatorum. Sex Transm Dis 13:53-55
14. Harrison HR, Alexander ER, Weinstein L et al (1982) Epidemiologic Correlations of Genital Infections and Outcome of Pregnancy. In: Märdh PA et al (eds) Chlamydial Infections. Elsevier Biomedical, Amsterdam pp.159-162
15. Jäger W (1968) Wandel in den Ursachen der Blindheit in den letzten 100 Jahren. Sonderdruck aus dem Jahresbericht für das Jubiläumsschuljahr 1967-1968 der Staatlichen Blindenschule Ilvesheim
16. Johnson D, McKenna H (1975) Bacteria in Ophthalmia Neonatorum Pathology 7:199-201
17. Laga M, Nsanze H, Plummer FA et al (1986) Comparison of Tetracycline and Silver Nitrate for Prophylaxis of Chlamydial and Gonococcal Ophthalmia Neonatorum. In: Oriel D, et al (eds) Chlamydial Infections. Cambridige University Press, Cambridge, p.301-304
18. Laga M, Plummer F, Nsanze H et al (1986) Epidemiology of Ophthalmia Neonatorum in Kenya. Lancet 2:1145-1148
19. Magnus H (1883) Die Blindheit - Ihre Entstehung und Verhütung. Breslau p.300
20. Meheus A, Piot (1986) Provision of Services for Sexually Transmitted Diseases in Developing Countries. In: Oriel JD, Harris JRW (eds) Recent Advances in Sexually Transmitted Diseases. Churchill Livingstone, London pp.261-271
21. Rees E, Tait IA, Hobson D et al (1977) Neonatal Conjunctivitis Caused by Neisseria gonorrhoeae and Chlamydia trachomatis. Br J Vener Dis 53:173-179
22. Schachter J, Lim L, Gooding CA et al (1975) Pneumonitis Following Inclusion Blenorrhea. J Pediatr 87:779
23. Schachter J, Grossman M, Holt J et al (1979) Prospective Study of Chlamydial Infection in Neonates. Lancet 2:377
24. Schmidt U (1986) Wandel der Ursachen für Blindheit im Kindesalter. Eine Untersuchung der ophthalmologischen Diagnosen in der Bayerischen Landesschule für Blinde bezogen auf die Geburtsjahre 1885-1976. Dissertation an der Ludwig-Maximilians-Universität, München.
25. World Health Organizatio (1986) Conjunctivitis of the Newborn. Prevention and Treatment of the Primary Health Care Level. Geneva

CONTRIBUTORS

Adam, D, Prof. & Chairman, Abtlg.für Antimikrobielle Therapie und Infektionsimmunologie Dr. v. Haunersches Kinderpital, Lindwurmstr.4, 80337 München, Germany

Alfonso, E., Bascom Palmer Eye Institute, University of Miami School of Medicine, P.O.Box 016880, Miami, FL 33101, USA

Aoki, K., 6 Kita 2-1, Hondori, Shiroishiku, Sapporo 003, Japan

Atherton, S.S., Univ.of Texas Health Sci Ctr., Dept.of Cell / Structure Biology, 7703 Floyd Curl Dr, San Antonio, TX 78284, USA

Bauernfeind, A., Prof. & Chairman, Max von Pettenkofer Institut Hyg. Med. Mikrobiol., Pettenkoferstr.9a, 80336 München, Germany

Behrens-Baumann, W., Prof.& Chairman, Klinik und Poliklinik für Augenheilkunde, Medizinische Aka-demie Magdeburg, Leipziger Str. 44, 39120 Magdeburg, Germany

Belfort, R., Prof .& Chairman, Dpt. of Ophthalmology, Escoly Paulista Medicina, CP-4086-01051 Sao Paolo SP, Brazil

Bialasiewicz, A.A., Augenklinik mit Poliklinik UKE, Martinistr.52, 20251 Hamburg, Germany

Botzenhart, K., Prof. & Chairman, Institut für Hygiene der Univ.Tübingen, Wilhelmstr.31, 72074 Tübingen, Germany

Castagna, I., Istituto di Oftalmologia, Universita di Messina, Via Consolare Valeria-Gazzi, 98125 Messina, Italy

Dawson, C.R., Prof. & Chairman, Francis I. Proctor Foundation for Research in Ophthalmology, UCSF, San Francisco, CA 94143-0411, USA

Draeger, J., Prof. & Chairman, Augenklinik mit Poliklinik UKE, Martinistr. 52, 20251 Hamburg, Germany

Emmerich, K.H., Prof. & Chairman, Augenklinik der Städt. Kliniken, Heidelberger Landstr.379, 64297 Darmstadt, Germany

Fabricius, E.-M., Seestr.99, 13353 Berlin

Feltkamp, T.E.W., Prof. & Chairman, Ophthalmic Research Inst., P.O.Box 12141, 1100 AC Amsterdam, Netherlands

ffytche, T.J., Prof.& Chairman, Dpt.of Ophthalmology, St.Thomas's Hospital, Lambeth Road, London SE1 7EH, Great Britain

Ficker, L., Moorfields Eye Hospital and Institute of Ophthalmology, City Road, London EC1 2CV, Great Britain

Franklin, R.M., LSU Eye Center, 2020 Gravier Street,Suite B, New Orleans,LA 70112, USA

Gass, J.D.M., Prof., Bascom Palmer Eye Institute, 900 NW 17th Street, Miami, FL 33101, USA

Gerling, J., Univ.-Augenklinik, Killianstr.5, 79106 Freiburg, Germany

Grabner, G., Prof. & Chairman, Augenabteilung, LKA Salzburg, Müllner Hauptstr.46, 5020 Salzburg, Austria

Green, W.R., Prof. & Chairman, Eye Pathology Laboratories, The Wilmer Institute,Johns Hopkins Hospital, 600 N.Wolfe Street, Baltimore, MD 21287-9248, USA

Griffiths, M.F.P., Moorfields Eye Hospital and Institute of Ophthalmology, City Road, London EC1V 2PD, Great Britain

Guex-Crosier, Y., Dpt. of Ophthalmology, Hopital Jules Gonin, Univ. of Lausanne, 15 Avenue de France, 1004 Lausanne, Switzerland

Herbort, C.P., Dpt. of Ophthalmology, Hopital Jules Gonin, Univ. of Lausanne, 15 Avenue de France, 1004 Lausanne, Switzerland

Hofmann, A.E.A., Max von Pettenkofer Institut, Pettenkoferstr.9a, 80336 München,Germany

Hogeweg, M., Dpt.of Ophthalmology, Erasmus University, Nieuwe Plantage 11, 2611 XH Delft, Netherlands

Holland, G.N., Jules Stein Eye Institute, UCLA, 100 Stein Plaza, Los Angeles CA, 90024-7003, USA

Huber-Spitzy, V., II. Univ.-Augenklinik, Alserstr.4, 1090 Wien, Austria

Jahn, G.J., Prof. & Chairman, Abtlg. für Medizinische Mikrobiologie und Epidemiologie der Viruskrankheiten, Silcherstr.7, 72076 Tübingen, Germany

Kampik, A., Prof. & Chairman, Univ.-Augenklinik, Josef Schneider Str.11, 97080 Würzburg, Germany

Kaufman, H.E., Prof. & Chairman, LSAU Eye Center, Louisiana State University Med. Center, School of Medicine, 2020 Gravier Street/Suite B, New Orleans, LA 70112-2234, USA

Kelly, L., A-157 Dpt.of Ophthalmology,Stanford Medical Center, Stanford, CA 94305-5308, USA

Kijlstra, A., Prof., Ophthalmic Research Inst., P.O.Box 12141, 1100 AC Amsterdam, Netherlands

Kirkness, C.M., Prof. & Chairman, Tennent Inst. of Ophthalmology,38 Church Street,Glasgow G11 6NT, Scotland

Klauß, V., Prof., Univ.-Augenklinik, Mathildenstr.8, 80336 München, Germany

Knorr, H.J., Univ.-Augenklinik Erlangen - Nürnberg, Schwabachanlage 6, 91054 Erlangen, Germany

Lemmen, S., Institut für Klinikhygiene, Univ. Freiburg, Hugstetter Str.55, 79106 Freiburg, Germany

Luger, A., Prof. & Chairman, Ludwig-Boltzmann Institut für Dermato-Venerologische Serodiagnostik, Wolkersbergenstr.1, 1130 Wien, Austria

Marghescu, S., Prof. & Chairman, Hautklinik Linden der Medizinischen Hochschule und der Landeshauptstadt Hannover, Ricklinger Str.5, 30449 Hannover, Germany

McCulley, J.P., Prof. & Chairman, Dpt. of Ophthalmology, University of Texas Southwestern Med. Center at Dallas, 5323 Harry Hines Blvd., Dallas, TX 75235-9057, USA

McGill, J., Prof. & Chairman, Southampton Eye Hospital, Wilton Avenue, Southampton,Hampshire,Great Britain

Miehlke, M.E.A., Inst. für Med. Mikrobiologie und Infektionsimmunologie der FU, Hindenburgdamm 27, 12203 Berlin, Germany

Pepose, J.S., Prof., Dpt. of Ophthalmology and Vis. Sciences, Washington Univ. School of Medicine, 660 S. Euclid Avenue, St. Louis, MO 63110, USA

Pflugfelder, S.C., Bascom Palmer Eye Institute, 900 NW 17th Street, Miami, FL 33136, USA

Phillipp, W., Univ.-Klinik für Augenheilkunde, Anichstr.35, 6020 Innsbruck, Austria

Roth, H.W., Institut für Wissenschaftliche Kontaktoptik, Im Grund 73, 89079 Ulm, Germany

Rüchel, R., Prof., Institut für Med. Mikrobiologie und Institut für Hygiene der Univ. Göttingen, Kreuzbergring 57, 37075 Göttingen, Germany

Saari, M., Prof. & Chairman, Dpt. of Ophthalmology, Univ. Central Hospital, Künamyllynkatu 4-8, 20520 Turku, Finland

Salvanet-Bouccara, A., Service d' Ophthalmologie, Hopital de Villeneuve - St.-Georges, 40 Allée de la Source, 94195 Villeneuve-St.Georges CEDEX, France

Schadewaldt, H., Prof. & Chairman, Institut für Geschichte der Medizin der Universität, Moorenstr. 5, 40225 Düsseldorf, Germany

Schein, O.D., Eye Research Institute, Harvard Med. School, 20 Staniford Street, Boston, MA 02114, USA

Schönherr, U., Univ.-Augenklinik Erlangen-Nürnberg, Schwabachanlage 6, 91054 Erlangen, Germany

Seitz, H.M., Prof. & Chairman, Institut für Med. Parasitologie der Universität, Sigmund Freud Str.25, 53127 Bonn, Germany

Silverstein, A.M., Prof., Institute of the History of Medicine, The Johns Hopkins Medical School, East Monument Street, Baltimore, MD 21204, USA

Streilein, W., Prof. & Chairman, Dpt. of Microbiology and Immunology, Univ. of Miami School of Medicine, 1600 NW 10th Avenue, Miami, FL 33136, USA

Strobel, J., Prof. & Chairman, Univ.-Augenklinik, Bachstr.18, 07743 Jena Germany

Sundmacher, R., Prof. & Chairman, Univ.-Augenklinik, Moorenstr.5, 40225 Düsseldorf, Germany

Tabbara, K.F., Prof. & Chairman, Dpt. of Ophthalmology, King Saud Univ. & King Khaled Eye Specialist Hospital, P.O.Box 7191, 11462 Riyadh, Saudi Arabia

Taylor, H.R., Prof. & Chairman, Dpt. of Ophthalmology, University of Melbourne, 32 Gisborne Street, East Melbourne, Victoria 3002, Australia

Tervo, T., Dpt. of Ophthalmology, Helsinki University Central Hospital, Haartmanink 4c, 00290 Helsinki, Finland

Tetz, M.R., Univ.-Augenklinik, Im Neuenheimer Feld 400, 69129 Heidelberg, Germany

Thiel, H.J., Prof. & Chairman, Univ.-Augenklinik, Schleichstr.12, 72076 Tübingen, Germany

Tittarelli, R., Prof. & Chairman, Clinica Oculistica Università di Ancona, Ospedale Reg. di Torrette, 60020 Ancona, Italy

Tost, M.F.W., Prof. & Chairman, Univ.-Augenklinik, Leninallee 8, 06097 Halle,Germany

Underdown, B., Prof. & Dean, Dpt. of Pathology, Faculty of Health Sciences, 1200 Main Street West, Hamilton, ON L8N 3Z5, Canada

von Graevenitz, A., Prof. & Chairman, Institut für Med. Mikrobiologie der Univ. Zürich, Gloriastr. 30, 8028 Zürich, Switzerland

van Setten, G.-B., Karolinska Institute St Eriks Eye Clinic, Fleminggatan 22, 11282 Stockholm, Sweden

Vojvodic-Ruzir, C.M., Centro Oftalmologico de Alta Complejidad,

Sanchez de Bustamente 1086 (1173), Buenos Aires, Argentina

Wegener, A., Univ.-Augenklinik, Abtlg. für Exp. Ophthalmologie, Sigmund Freud Str.25, 53127 Bonn, Germany

Whittum-Hudson, J., The Wilmer Institute, The Johns Hopkins Hospital, 600 N. Wolfe Street, Baltimore, MD 21287-9142, USA

Wilhelmus, K.R., Prof., Cullen Eye Institute, Baylor Coll.of Medicine, 6501 Fannin-NC200, Houston, TX 77030, USA

Wright, P., Moorfields Eye Hospital and Institute of Ophthalmology, City Road, London EC1 2CV, Great Britain

Zeidler, H., Prof. & Chairman, Med. Hochschule Hannover, Abtlg.Rheumatologie, Konstanty Gutschow Str.8, 30625 Hannover, Germany

Zierhut, M., Univ.-Augenklinik Tübingen, Schleichstr.12, 72076 Tübingen, Germany